Radiotherapy for Head
and Neck Cancers
INDICATIONS AND TECHNIQUES
FIFTH EDITION

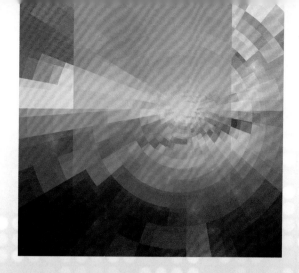

Radiotherapy for Head and Neck Cancers

INDICATIONS AND TECHNIQUES

FIFTH EDITION

ADAM S. GARDEN, MD

Professor of Radiation Oncology
Head and Neck Radiation Oncology
Department of Radiation Oncology
The University of Texas M.D. Anderson Cancer Center
Houston, Texas

BETH M. BEADLE, MD, PHD

Associate Professor of Radiation Oncology
Head and Neck Radiation Oncology
Department of Radiation Oncology
Stanford University
Stanford, California

G. BRANDON GUNN, MD

Associate Professor of Radiation Oncology
Head and Neck Radiation Oncology
Department of Radiation Oncology
The University of Texas M.D. Anderson Cancer Center
Houston, Texas

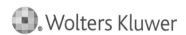 Wolters Kluwer

Philadelphia • Baltimore • New York • London
Buenos Aires • Hong Kong • Sydney • Tokyo

Acquisitions Editor: Ryan Shaw
Product Development Editor: Kristina Oberle
Editorial Coordinator: Lindsay Ries
Marketing Manager: Rachel Mante Leung
Production Project Manager: Kim Cox
Design Coordinator: Holly McLaughlin
Manufacturing Coordinator: Beth Welsh
Prepress Vendor: SPi Global

5th edition

Library of Congress Cataloging-in-Publication Data
Names: Garden, Adam S., author. | Beadle, Beth M., author. | Gunn, G. Brandon, author. | Preceded by (work): Ang, K. K. (K. Kian). Radiotherapy for head and neck cancers.
Title: Radiotherapy for head and neck cancers : indications and techniques / Adam S. Garden, Beth M. Beadle, G. Brandon Gunn.
Description: Fifth edition. | Philadelphia : Wolters Kluwer Health, [2018] | Preceded by Radiotherapy for head and neck cancers / K. Kian Ang, Adam S. Garden. 4th ed. c2012. | Includes bibliographical references and index.
Identifiers: LCCN 2017009535 | ISBN 9781496345899
Subjects: | MESH: Head and Neck Neoplasms—radiotherapy
Classification: LCC RC280.H4 | NLM WE 707 | DDC 616.99/4910642—dc23 LC record available at https://lccn.loc. gov/2017009535

Dedication

The current edition is dedicated to the memory of K. Kian Ang. Kian was a cherished mentor, colleague, and friend.

Over his career, he led multiple seminal phase III trials in head and neck cancer, with a focus on radiation. He helped define the role of altered radiation fractionation, as well as the role of cetuximab, the first biologic agent approved as a radiation enhancer for the treatment of head and neck cancer. He spearheaded international efforts in clinical research of radiation and head and neck cancer through his role as leader of the RTOG head and neck section in the 1990s and 2000s. He further enhanced the role of radiation as a former president of the American Society for Radiation Oncology (ASTRO).

Kian was the principal author of this text. He cowrote the original edition over 25 years ago and was the principal author of subsequent editions, such that the text was often referred to as "The Ang Manual." It was a great honor and privilege to cowrite the previous three editions with him. He was always insistent that each edition combine common and still-used techniques with the latest advances in the field, through clinical applications of both biology and physics. Prior to his passing, we had several conversations regarding this work and its direction. I hope he would be proud of this current edition that continues the legacy of a teaching manual of head and neck radiotherapy aimed at a wide audience of both those new to the specialty and those experienced and interested in the latest advances.

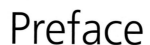

Preface

It is difficult to believe that the first edition of this textbook was conceived over 25 years ago. My two mentors, Lester Peters and Kian Ang along with our fellow at the time, Johannes Kaanders, wrote this original work based on a desire to create a handbook useful for a day-to-day reference. Based on encouragement from our residents and many visitors, the three authors took a compilation of teaching materials, and in particular case studies, and created the first edition.

Lester and Johannes moved on to continue successful careers as leaders in the head and neck radiotherapy field in Australia and Europe, and Kian asked me to join him to write the second edition. There was an 8-year gap between the first and second edition; during that time in the late 1990s and early 2000s, many advances had been made, including the more routine integration of systemic therapy with radiation for treating head and neck cancer and technologic advances in radiation planning and delivery with the development of intensity modulated radiotherapy (IMRT). However, concurrent chemoradiation and IMRT were just starting to be brought into the clinic, and this 2nd edition included just a few examples, ultimately serving as a "sneak preview" of things to come. Additionally, the results of radiation fractionation trials had been completed, and the 2nd edition incorporated these schedules when applicable into our dose/fractionation regimens.

The 3rd edition saw two changes. The most significant change, just 10 years ago, was the incorporation of color images into the text. The second change was due to the recognition that IMRT was practice changing and likely to become the standard of care for the mode of radiation for head and neck cancers. As such we expanded the case examples, showing more case studies of IMRT for most of the site-specific chapters and began to formalize our presentation. IMRT not only was a newer way to plan and deliver radiation, but also represented a change in how to think about head and neck cancer with regard to treating with radiation. This principal change was a shift from field design based on anatomic landmarks (principally on two-dimensional images), to designing treatment based on identifying and delineating target volumes. The most common sites investigated for a role of IMRT at that time were the oropharynx, nasopharynx, and paranasal sinuses; the text introduced target definitions (GTV, CTV, and PTV) for tumors originating from those sites.

The 4th edition, published in 2012, mainly reflected the change in practice from conventional therapy to IMRT. For the clinician, target definition involves identification of the gross target (GTV) and clinical target volumes. Many patients come to radiation after other therapies (surgery or chemotherapy), and as such the original GTV is altered, so we also included the concept of a virtual GTV (vGTV). Further, we formalized CTV definitions to high-dose, intermediate-dose, and low-dose targets (CTV$_{HD}$, CTV$_{ID}$, CTV$_{ED}$). Each site-specific section was expanded to include guidelines for target definitions. This edition also evolved with the times and included online access. Additionally, we added a chapter on reirradiation, as conformal therapies are now allowing us to retreat patients with recurrent cancers or second primary cancers that develop in irradiated tissues. The hard copy version was expanded 50%, but our goal was still to keep it more as a manual rather than an encyclopedic tome.

The current edition attempts to continue to both be a day-to-day reference and also incorporate the advances in the field. To the best of our ability, we have attempted to update the suggested readings and background tables. Based on feedback, we have added a "bridge" chapter between general concepts and site-specific chapters. As target delineation is the main activity for clinicians to design their patients' radiation treatments, we include guidelines for normal tissues as well. We expanded the case examples and also included cases of patients treated with proton therapy, as this half-decade has seen an introduction of proton therapy being used for head and neck cancer. Similar to IMRT a decade ago, we are starting to see in the literature retrospective clinical series reflecting the use of protons and anticipate prospective and multiinstitutional trials to be the next step in exploring and developing this technology.

We are excited to share new advances in the field, but we also recognize that many are still not able to use the latest technologic advances to treat patients. As such, while we have removed some examples of 2D therapy, we have kept those principles of field design in the current edition. We hope this 5th edition both reflects our current practices and provides general guidelines for clinicians to help treat their patients who will be irradiated for head and neck cancer.

Preface to the First Edition

Primary cancers of the head and neck region are relatively rare. The estimated yearly number of new cases, excluding skin cancers located in the head and neck area, is about 42,000, which represents 4% to 5% of the total number of cancers diagnosed per annum in the United States. Although the vast majority of head and neck cancers arise from epithelial elements, their natural history differs considerably according to the disease location. This is related to regional anatomical peculiarities that dictate patterns of contiguous and lymphatic spread. The extent of the lesion and the presence of numerous critical normal tissues in the head and neck area, injury to which could result in serious functional impairment, are obstacles to local-regional disease eradication. Therefore, failure to achieve local-regional control is the leading cause of cancer-related death in patients with head and neck neoplasms.

Radiotherapy plays a very important role in the management of patients with head and neck cancers. In early-stage lesions, radiotherapy is frequently preferred because it is as effective as surgery in controlling the disease and is generally better in preserving cosmetic and organ functions. In advanced tumors, radiation treatment is complementary to surgery in obtaining maximal local-regional control. Sound knowledge of the behavior of various head and neck cancers is essential for selecting proper indications for radiotherapy for different subsets of patients. Thorough command of the regional anatomy, technical bases of radiotherapy, and awareness of available data on radiation effects on critical normal tissues are necessary for optimizing the treatment outcome. The choice of radiation target volume and dose is based on the best trade-off between control probability and likelihood of severe treatment-induced complication.

The natural history of head and neck cancers, general treatment strategies, and therapy results obtained at different institutions are summarized in a number of textbooks and chapters. However, so far there is no handbook on the technical detail of radiotherapy for head and neck cancers. This manual serves as a practical reference to head and neck radiotherapy. We chose to present the basic concepts and specific indications and techniques for various common types of head and neck cancers, i.e., carcinoma and melanoma, as practiced at The University of Texas M.D. Anderson Cancer Center rather than compiling all available techniques in an encyclopedic fashion. The treatment policies described in this manual evolved during the past one-half century through gradual refinements based on results of systematic analysis of causes of failure and complications in cohorts of patients treated in a disciplined and consistent way. This philosophy introduced by the late Dr. Gilbert H. Fletcher has continued to the present day.

Contents

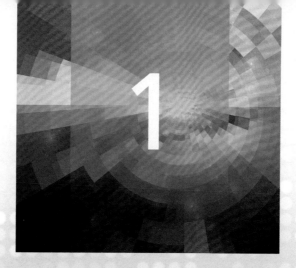

General Principles of Head and Neck Radiotherapy

Head and neck cancers have been the subject of intensive laboratory research and clinical investigations. Advances in molecular biology techniques have facilitated research addressing molecular epidemiology, genetic predisposition, genetic tumor progression models, and personalization of treatment. Because of the ease of clinical assessment and a relatively low incidence of systemic spread, head and neck cancers are good models for testing the efficacy of new therapy concepts that are aimed primarily at improving locoregional disease control. Most of the clinical radiobiology research on altered fractionation and combinations of radiation with chemotherapy or novel agents, for example, has been conducted on patients with locally advanced head and neck squamous cell carcinoma (HNSCC).

Long-term investment in cancer research has come to fruition for certain cancers. After increasing for decades, the mortality rate of most cancers in the United States has decreased since 1975.[1] More recent data, for example, showed that while the incidence of all cancer has been stable in men and has increased by 0.3% annually in women between 1993 and 2002, the overall death rate has declined by an annual rate of 1.1% during this period.[2] This improvement has been attributed, at least in part, to advances in cancer treatment and better dissemination of guideline-based treatment into the community.

Many advances have been achieved in the understanding of the biology, natural history, and treatment of HNSCC. A detailed depiction of recent progress is beyond the scope of this handbook—this brief introductory summary highlights a few recent findings contributing to the better understanding of the biology of the disease and to expanding treatment options for head and neck cancers.

Overview of Recent Advances

BIOLOGY OF HEAD AND NECK SQUAMOUS CELL CARCINOMA

Key Points

- HNSCCs are classically associated with tobacco and alcohol exposure. However, the incidence of HPV-related oropharyngeal carcinomas has been increasing steadily in the industrialized world since the 1970s.

- Advances in molecular studies, accompanied by research into HPV-associated cancer, have led to a recognition that HNSCCs represent a group of biologically heterogeneous carcinomas. For the present time, the most prominent subdivision of these cancers is into two subgroups: those that are viral associated (HPV or Epstein-Barr virus [EBV]) and those that are not.

- Clonal genetic changes occur early in malignant cellular transformation and in the histopathologic continuum of tumor progression.

- Newer molecular assay techniques, such as comparative genomic hybridization and next-generation sequencing technology, have greatly increased the ability to interrogate genetic changes and thereby improve the understanding of genetic predilection (host susceptibility) and cancer biology.

- Whole genome sequencing has confirmed *TP53* is the most commonly mutated gene in HPV-negative HNSCC; *NOTCH1* is the second most commonly mutated gene.

- The understanding of tumorigenesis of nasopharyngeal carcinoma (NPC) continues to grow. Adding to the recognition of an endemic group with genetic predilection (including deletions on 3p and 9p) harboring latent EBV infection are findings of numerous oncogenes and tumor suppressor genes that lead to initiation of tumorigenesis, and EBV then contributes to transformation.

- HPV has an active role in carcinogenesis, particularly of oropharyngeal cancers, mainly through the actions of E6 and E7 oncoproteins. HPV-positive tumors have fewer mutations than HPV-negative tumors.

Lifestyle-Related Risk Factors

Tobacco and alcohol exposure have long been recognized as the dominant risk factors for HNSCC. Other risk factors include low fruit and vegetable consumption and betel quid chewing. In an overview, Petti[3] estimated that, worldwide, 25% of HNSCCs are attributable to tobacco use, 7% to 19% to alcohol consumption, 10% to 15% to dietary deficiency, and, in regions of prevalence, >50% to betel quid chewing. Carcinogenicity is dose dependent and magnified by exposures to multiple carcinogens.

Although tobacco and alcohol consumption is estimated to account for a significant proportion of oral and pharyngeal carcinomas in the United States,[4] neoplasms develop in only a small fraction of exposed individuals. This intriguing information raised the notion of the contribution of genetic susceptibility or predisposition and other cofactors (for examples of cofactors, see "Viral Etiology" section) to carcinogenesis. The potential pathways are thought to include genetic polymorphisms influencing environmental carcinogen absorption and detoxification and individual sensitivity to carcinogen-induced genotypic alterations, among others. These ideas can now be tested more comprehensively because of recent progress in molecular biology concepts and assay methodology. For example, the ability to identify smokers at high risk for developing cancer will have important practical clinical implications in selecting individuals for more aggressive screening programs or for enrollment into intensive chemoprevention trials.

VIRAL ETIOLOGY

Epstein-Barr Virus

Although the association between EBV and NPC has been recognized for almost four decades, elucidating the association between EBV and oncogenesis has been challenging. The advances in molecular technology have allowed for greater insight into the relationship between EBV and NPC. The EBV genome was characterized (reviewed by Liebowitz)[5] to consist of a linear, 172-kb, double-stranded DNA having five unique sequences separated by four internal repeats and two terminal repeats. The DNA circularizes by homologous recombination at random locations within terminal repeats in the nucleus of infected cells. The length of the terminal repeat is specific for each infected cell, and this is the basis for clonality assays, which may be useful in determining the putative primary tumor in patients presenting with nodal metastasis from an unknown source. The genome encodes several families of proteins, such as early antigens, Epstein-Barr nuclear antigens (EBNAs), and latency membrane proteins (LMPs). Many of these proteins control viral behavior and affect cell proliferation regulatory mechanisms; these are thought to play a role in transformation and carcinogenesis and to influence tumor response to therapy. EBNA-1 regulates viral genome replication during cell division and was found to induce growth and dedifferentiation of an NPC cell line not infected by EBV.[6] LMP1 and LMP2A drive clonal expansion and transformation.

More work has been done on the molecular genetics of NPC. Similar to other tumors, NPCs appear to follow a multistep tumorigenesis model. Among the questions regarding NPC and EBV are whether the presence of EBV is ubiquitous and why is EBV associated with NPC in Southern China and with Burkitt lymphoma in equatorial Africa but not clearly related to other neoplasms elsewhere in the world. One observation is that many NPCs have been found to have dele-

tions of the short arm, or some regions of the short arm, of chromosomes 3 and 9, suggesting the possibility of the existence of tumor suppressor genes (TSGs) in these regions.[7,8] Next-generation sequencing technologies have shown that a frequent deletion region is one covering the *CDKN2A* gene of 9p21.[9]

While these chromosomal changes are consistent in NPC, irrespective of the patient's origin, studies of normal nasopharyngeal epithelium show a preponderance of these findings among the people of Southern China, lending evidence to an underlying genetic susceptibility for NPC. This has led to a hypothesis that these genetic changes lead to premalignant changes due to p16 inactivation or cyclin D1 overexpression that promotes maintenance of latent EBV infection.[10]

Once a stable EBV infection has been established, latent gene proteins will drive rapid clonal expansion and transformation. During this phase, multiple events will occur, including alteration of host immune response, microenvironmental changes, as well as altered genetics and epigenetics. These and additional events will occur through progression and metastasis.

Additional new findings using whole-exome and targeted deep sequencing in over 100 NPC cases include observing a relatively low mutational rate, though one with wide diversity. In particular, high rates of derangements in chromatin modification, ERBB–PI3K signaling, and autophagy machinery were observed. ERBB–PI3K mutations were linked to more advanced-staged cases with poorer survival.[9]

Human Papillomavirus

The causal relation between HPVs and some human neoplasms has long been appreciated. First described for carcinoma of the uterine cervix, it has also been associated more recently with anal, penile, and oropharyngeal cancers. HPV DNA is categorized into low- and high-risk groups. Low-risk HPV includes HPV-6 and HPV-11, which are associated with benign lesions. The most common of the high-risk types associated with malignancies are HPV-16 and HPV-18.[11] Cell culture studies clearly demonstrated that the high-risk HPVs can transform and immortalize epithelial cells from the cervix, foreskin, and oral cavity.[12–14] Expression of the *E6* and *E7* open reading frames of HPV-16 or HPV-18 genome is sufficient for immortalization.[15,16]

The evidence implicating HPVs in carcinogenesis of tonsillar carcinomas is quite strong because these tumors not only contain HPV DNA in most of the cells but also express readily detectable levels of HPV RNA.[17] In a series of 253 patients, Gillison et al.[18] detected HPV in 25% of tumors, with HPV-16 present in 90% of the positive neoplasms. The presence of HPV was most common in oropharyngeal carcinoma occurring in individuals with no history of smoking or alcohol consumption whose tumors were of a basaloid subtype without TP53 mutation. Laboratory data showing the persistence of transcriptionally active, integrated HPV-16 DNA in an oral carcinoma cell line with features indistinguishable from those of the primary tumor[19] provide strong evidence that HPV has an active role in carcinogenesis.

HPV infection is extremely common, and in the vast majority of cases, the infection is cleared and malignancy does not occur. Epidemiologic studies have identified social risk factors associated with HPV-associated oropharyngeal cancer,[20] but further understanding of risk factors associated with and causing viral persistence leading to oncogenesis remains under study. The question of how high-risk HPV induces cell transformation has been studied mostly in cervical cancer, and the findings have been summarized in several review articles.[21–23] Briefly, two viral oncoproteins, E6 and E7, are crucial in the transformation process. E6 binds to and inactivates the tumor suppressor protein p53, affecting many cellular functions including impairment of DNA repair after damage by other agents and suppression of the ability of cells to die by apoptosis. E7 degrades pRb, thereby releasing transcription factors such as E2F, which in turn induces the expression of other cellular proteins including p16. The increase in p16 expression has led to p16 immunohistochemical staining to be used as a surrogate test for HPV association. E6 and E7 can also directly bind to several other host proteins, such as Bak and p21[Cip1], thereby contributing to amplification of genetic instability. The expression of E6 and E7 alone does not seem to be sufficient for transforming cells, but the additional genetic alterations necessary for neoplastic conversion remain uncertain. Recent profiling of head and neck cancers performed by the Cancer Genome Atlas network[24] has demonstrated that the genomics of HPV-positive cancers are very different from HPV-negative cancers. HPV-positive cancers have fewer mutations and in particular rarely have mutations of TP53. HPV-associated cancers are dominated by mutations in *PIK3CA*, amplification of the cell cycle gene E2F1, and loss of TRAF3, a gene associated with antiviral activity.

Numerous studies conducted over the last decade support a global trend in an increase in oropharyngeal cancer. Chaturvedi et al.[25] used data from the *Cancer Incidence in Five Continents* (CI5) Volumes VI to IX (1983 to 2002) and observed that the incidence of oropharyngeal cancer increased significantly, particularly in economically developed countries. The magnitude of increase among men was significantly higher in younger men. The Surveillance, Epidemiology, and End Results (SEER) program has a separate Residual Tissue Repository (RTR). Using oropharyngeal cancer samples from the RTR, Chaturvedi et al. divided the samples obtained over two decades into four calendar groups and analyzed the samples for the presence of HPV. The authors showed that HPV prevalence increased over the four calendar periods, with a fourfold increase from 1984 to 1989 to 2000 to 2004. Based on this data, the group predicted that by 2030, HPV-associated head and neck cancer will continue to increase and account for nearly half of all head and neck cancers.

An increasingly large body of data shows that the prognosis for patients with HPV-related oropharyngeal carcinomas (OPSCCs) is consistently better than for those with HPV-unrelated OPSCCs after treatment with surgery,[26] radiotherapy,[27,28] induction chemotherapy followed by chemoradiation,[29] and concurrent radiation plus cisplatin.[30] The principle hypothesis for this improvement in response to chemotherapy and radiation and overall improved prognosis is based on genomic studies describing fewer mutations in and less cellular dysregulation of HPV-associated cancers. The high survival rates seen in patients with HPV-associated oropharyngeal cancer have led to investigations of treatment deintensification. The RTOG recently completed a study (RTOG 1016) testing if cetuximab is less toxic as a concurrent radiation agent than cisplatin for HPV-associated oropharyngeal cancer. The NRG is now conducting a trial testing lower doses and elimination of systemic therapy for the most favorable patients (those with smaller tumor burden and minimal tobacco exposure). However, until such trials yield conclusive results, head and neck oncologists should not change the current treatment policies for patients with HPV-positive OPSCCs.

Genetic Alterations in Non–Viral-Associated Head and Neck Cancers

For head and neck carcinomas, Califano et al.[31] described a preliminary tumor progression model using allelic loss or imbalance as a molecular marker for oncogene amplification or TSG inactivation. They identified *p16* (9p21), *p53* (17p), and *Rb* (13q) as candidate TSGs and cyclin D1 (11q13) as a candidate protooncogene. About one third of histopathologically benign squamous hyperplasias already consist of a clonal population of cells with shared genetic anomalies characterizing head and neck cancer. Identification of such early events facilitates discovery of genetic alterations associated with further transformation and aggressive clinical behavior.

The introduction of newer molecular assay techniques has greatly increased the ability to detect genetic changes and thereby improve the understanding of cancer biology in general. An overview by Ha et al.[32] summarizes recent findings on genetic alterations in HNSCC grouped by assay techniques, such as comparative genomic hybridization, *in situ* hybridization, single nucleotide polymorphism, and microarray technology, and provides excellent illustrations of the complexity of HNSCC and how that complexity will require much more research to reveal the full picture. This complexity has been further explored with whole-exome sequencing. Two separate studies[33,34] confirmed mutations in many known genes, including the most common mutation of TP53, but additionally found mutations in other genes known to regulate squamous differentiation including NOTCH1, which was the second most frequently mutated gene after TP53. The Cancer Genome Atlas Network[24] reported their preliminary analysis of 279 samples of HNSCC. The majority were HPV negative, obtained from the oral cavity or larynx, from a patient population predominantly consisting of heavy smoking males. The analysis again confirmed near universal loss-of-function TP53 mutations but also identified 10 other mutations occurring frequently enough to warrant further study. CDKN2A inactivation was common as was high genomic instability reflected by a mean of 141 copy number alterations. With further validation, this knowledge will contribute a great deal to the development of screening strategies focusing on the earlier steps of genetic alterations required to generate an invasive tumor phenotype and to the conception of early pharmacologic or genetic therapy approaches.

BIOMARKERS

Key Points

- Three strong prognostic biomarkers have emerged for HNSCC. The absence of circulating EBV DNA titer, the presence of HPV in cancer cells, and low tumor EGFR expression are associated with better outcome after current standard therapies for patients with nasopharyngeal cancer, oropharyngeal carcinoma, and HNSCC not associated with EBV or HPV, respectively.

- Patients with NPC and persistent circulating EBV DNA after completion of radiotherapy with concurrent cisplatin have a high distant relapse rate and are thus suitable candidates for intensification of systemic therapy.

- With current standard therapies, patients with HPV-associated OPSCCs have much better locoregional control and overall survival rates than those with HPV-unrelated OPSCCs.

- HPV-associated OPSCC is now considered a distinct cancer entity, and protocols focusing on reducing long-term morbidity are being designed for such patients.

- The search for biomarkers that can predict the likelihood that a certain cancer subset will respond to a given therapy (predictive marker) has not yielded promising leads.

- High-EGFR–expressing HNSCCs are more proficient in repairing radiation-induced DNA injury and hence recur more frequently after radiotherapy, but whether inhibitors of EGFR can preferentially enhance the radiation response of these tumors has not been resolved.

- Because the cost of cancer treatment has been increasing steeply with only modest improvements in efficacy, the identification, standardization, and validation of predictive biomarkers are crucial for rational selection of specific therapies for a given subset of patients to improve outcome, reduce overall toxicity, and contain cost.

Although mortality rates from cancer have gradually declined in the United States over the past 10 years,[35] the cost of cancer therapy has increased drastically during that time (American Cancer Society report on *Cancer Facts & Figures 2009*). This increase in cost results from progressive intensification of therapies, such as the addition of chemotherapy to radiation or to surgery plus radiation, the emergence of expensive novel agents, and the lack of validated markers to guide rational patient selection for available therapies. Consequently, expensive and complex combined therapy regimens have often been prescribed to large groups of patients that benefit only a small subset of those patients and often at the cost of increased acute and long-term morbidity. Therefore, identification and validation of biomarkers to guide the rational selection of specific therapy for a given subset of patients have become critical for improving the outcome, reducing the toxicity burden, and containing the costs of cancer treatment.

Progress in searching for useful markers for early detection of tumor, estimation of tumor burden, prediction of response to therapy, and monitoring disease progression has been slow. A prototypical marker is prostate-specific antigen, which proved to be quite useful for prostatic cancer screening, prognostic grouping, and monitoring of response to therapy. Unfortunately, equivalent markers have yet to be identified for most other solid tumors. However, recent studies in head and neck carcinomas have generated some optimism, as discussed in the sections that follow.

Prognostic and Predictive Biomarkers

The distinction between prognostic and predictive biomarkers has not been widely appreciated. Therefore, until recently, these terms have been used rather loosely and interchangeably. Figure 1.1 illustrates the concept and definition for different classes of markers. The rates and extent of separation among the curves will vary with the disease type and stage and the efficacy of therapy, but the general principles and the relative ranking are applicable. In Figure 1.1A, marker X represents an aggressive tumor feature, the presence of which is associated with poorer survival rate after both treatment (Rx) regimens 1 and 2, though Rx 2 is more effective than Rx 1. Marker Y (Fig. 1.1B), on the other hand, exemplifies a predictive marker for response to Rx 2. Hence, its presence is associated with better survival after Rx 2 (solid brown curve). Figure 1.1C illustrates that some markers could have both prognostic and predictive values. The absence of marker Z is associated with better prognosis (solid and dotted black curves vs. dotted purple curve). However, since this marker also predicts response to Rx 2, its presence is associated with a better outcome after Rx 2 (solid purple curve) relative to Z+ after Rx 1 (dotted purple curve) and Z– after Rx 2 (solid black curve).

Figure 1.1 shows that carefully designed clinical trials incorporating patient stratification according to biomarkers and randomizing patients to received distinct

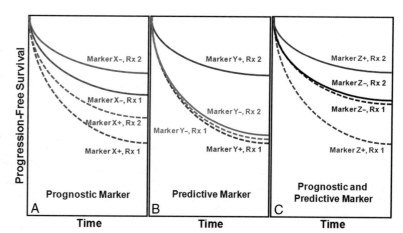

Figure 1.1 Schematic illustration of prognostic and predictive biomarkers. X and Y **(A,B)** represent pure prognostic and predictive markers, respectively, whereas Z **(C)** stands for a marker that predicts favorable response to treatment (Rx) 2 in addition to prognosis (see text for details).

therapy modalities are needed to yield a conclusive answer as to whether a marker is prognostic, predictive, both, or neither.

Three potent prognostic biomarkers for HNSCC have emerged in recent years. Two of these biomarkers are related to virus-associated head and neck carcinomas: circulating EBV titer for NPC and the presence of the HPV genome or its surrogate marker, p16, for OPSCC. The third biomarker, epidermal growth factor receptor (EGFR), seems to be more applicable for other HNSCCs.

Circulating EBV DNA Titers in Nasopharyngeal Carcinoma

The association between EBV and NPC was summarized in a previous section. Lo et al.[36] have developed a real-time quantitative polymerase chain reaction assay for measuring circulating levels of tumor-derived EBV DNA in the serum or plasma of patients with NPC. They found in a longitudinal follow-up of 17 patients that elevations in serum EBV DNA titer could be detected as early as 6 months before clinical manifestation of recurrence, whereas the titer stayed low or undetectable in patients who remained in remission. A subsequent study of patients treated with radiation, with or without chemotherapy, at the same center[37] showed that having a pretreatment EBV DNA titer exceeding 4,000 copies per mL was associated with a 2.5-fold higher risk of NPC recurrence. More interestingly, having a high posttreatment EBV DNA titer was found to be an even stronger marker for poor overall outcome, that is, an 11.9-fold increase in recurrence rate. Conversely, having a posttreatment titer of <500 copies per mL was associated with favorable overall survival and relapse-free survival rates (Fig. 1.2) and also correlated with low relapse rate. Similar results were reported by Lin et al.[38] in a series of patients treated with weekly neoadjuvant chemotherapy (cisplatin alternating with fluorouracil for a total of 10 doses) followed by radiotherapy.

The combination of intensity-modulated radiotherapy (IMRT), as discussed in the section "High-Precision Radiotherapy" below, with concurrent cisplatin has yielded locoregional control rates of around 90% even among patients presenting with locally advanced NPC. Consequently,

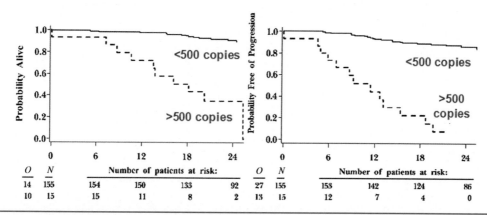

Figure 1.2 Overall survival **(left)** and progression-free survival **(right)** curves of patients treated with radiation with or without chemotherapy as a function of posttreatment EBV DNA titers analyzed using a cutoff value of 500 copies per mL. O, numbers observed; N, numbers at risk. (Modified from Chan ATC, Lo YMD, Zee B, et al. Plasma Epstein-Barr virus DNA and residual disease after radiotherapy for undifferentiated nasopharyngeal carcinoma. *J Natl Cancer Inst* 2002;94:1614–1619.)

distant metastasis has become the main pattern of relapse for this neoplasm. One question that is of interest is the role of adjuvant chemotherapy. An international collaboration has designed a study incorporating posttreatment titers to better address this question. The design is to enroll patients, have them treated with concurrent chemo-IMRT, and assess their titers post treatment. Those with negative titer levels will be observed, while those with elevated titers will receive chemotherapy even in the absence of radiographic evidence of disease.

Human Papillomavirus and p16 in Oropharyngeal Carcinomas

A thorough correlative study was undertaken to quantify the magnitude of impact of tumor HPV status on tumor outcome in patients enrolled in a large phase III trial of the Radiation Therapy Oncology Group (RTOG 0129) treated with a combination of radiation with concurrent cisplatin.[30] Patients with locally advanced HNSCC were assigned to receive either accelerated fractionation with a concomitant boost (72 Gy in 42 fractions over 6 weeks) or standard fractionation (70 Gy in 35 fractions over 7 weeks) regimens. Chemotherapy consisted of intravenous cisplatin at a dose of 100 mg/m^2 on days 1 and 22 in the accelerated fractionation group or on days 1, 22, and 43 in the standard fractionation group.

Of the 743 patients enrolled, 60% had OPSCC. Pretreatment biopsy specimens from the patients with OPSCC were evaluated for HPV-16 DNA by using *in situ* hybridization, and HPV-16–negative tumors were further assayed for 12 additional oncogenic HPV types (types 18, 31, 33, 35, 39, 45, 51, 52, 56, 58, 59, and 68). Tumor expression of the cyclin-dependent kinase inhibitor p16, induced as a consequence of pRb inactivation by viral oncoprotein E7,[39] was evaluated by immunohistochemical staining with a mouse monoclonal antibody. Strong agreement between tumor HPV status as determined by *in situ* hybridization and p16 expression was

observed, but some discrepancies were noted as well. Overall, 64% of OPSCCs were found to be positive for HPV DNA and 68% were positive for p16. Figure 1.3 shows the differences in overall survival according to HPV or p16 status. A strength of the p16 assay is that it is not HPV-type specific and is therefore an excellent surrogate for tumor HPV status. Analysis of patterns of failure among these groups showed that the locoregional failure rate at 3 years was significantly lower for patients with HPV-positive OPSCC (13.6% vs. 35.1%; $P < 0.001$), but rates for distant metastasis were not (8.7% vs. 14.6%; $P = 0.23$). Also, the cumulative incidence of second primary tumors (SPTs) was significantly lower for patients with HPV-positive OPSCC (3-year rates 5.9% vs. 14.6%; $P = 0.02$), largely because of lower rates of smoking-related cancers in that group.

These observations of improvement in outcomes have been reported in other secondary analyses of randomized head and neck trials, including the subsequent RTOG 522 trial,[40] which randomized patients to either concurrent cisplatin cetuximab and radiation or cisplatin and radiation. The 3-year overall survival rates were 85.6% versus 60.1% for patients with p16-positive tumors and p16-negative tumors, respectively ($P < 0.001$). Similar to RTOG 0129, the locoregional failure rate was lower for patients with p16-positive tumors (17.3% vs. 32.5%, respectively; $P < 0.001$), but the rate of distant recurrence was also lower for patients with p16 positive OPSCC (6.5% vs. 17.0%, respectively; $P = 0.005$).

Tobacco smoking was also found to be independently associated with overall survival and progression-free survival, both in patients with OPSCC and in the entire study population. A secondary analysis of patients in RTOG 0129 as well as RTOG 9003 (a four-arm randomized trial evaluating differing schedules of altered fractionation) revealed that the risk of death increased significantly by 1% per each pack-year increase in tobacco use, and magnitudes of effect were similar for patients with HPV-positive OPSCCs (hazard ratio [HR] 1.01, 95% confidence interval [CI] 1.00 to 1.02) and HPV-negative OPSCCs (HR 1.01, 95% CI 1.00 to 1.03).[41]

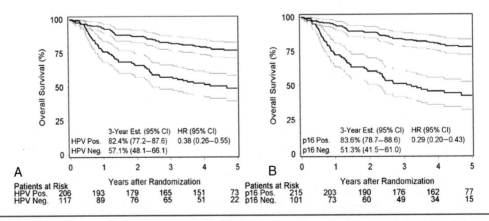

Figure 1.3 Kaplan-Meier estimates with 95% confidence intervals for overall survival for patients with oropharyngeal squamous cell cancer stratified by HPV status **(A)** and by p16 status **(B)**. Patients with HPV-positive tumors had significantly better overall survival compared to patients with HPV-negative tumors (two-sided log-rank test $P < 0.001$) with an absolute benefit in overall survival of 25% (95% CI 11 to 40) at 3 years. The difference was slightly larger when stratified by p16 status. (Modified from Ang KK, Harris J, Wheeler R, et al. Human papillomavirus (HPV) and survival of patients with oropharynx cancer. *N Engl J Med* 2010;363:24–35.)

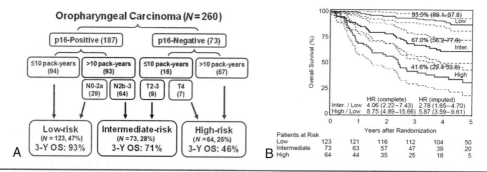

Figure 1.4 A: Survival tree developed with recursive partitioning analysis using S-Tree software to identify which prognostic factors found to be significant in a proportional hazards model (age, T classification, N classification, race, smoking, HPV status, anemia, performance status, treatment assignment, sex) had the most influence on overall survival and to segregate patients into groups at low, intermediate, or high risk of death. **B:** Kaplan-Meier estimates, with 95% CIs, for overall survival among patients with oropharyngeal cancer stratified by RPA risk group. (Modified from Ang KK, Harris J, Wheeler R, et al. Human papillomavirus (HPV) and survival of patients with oropharynx cancer. *N Engl J Med* 2010;363:24–35.)

Recursive partitioning analysis performed on the data from RTOG 0129[30] indicated that tumor HPV status was the major determinant of overall survival, followed by tobacco smoking (≤10 vs. >10 pack-years) and then nodal category (N0-2a vs. N2b-3) for patients with HPV-positive OPSCCs and primary tumor category (T2-3 vs. T4) for patients with HPV-negative OPSCCs (Fig. 1.4A). Recursive partitioning led to the classification of patients with OPSCC into three risk groups: low risk (reference group, with a 3-year overall survival rate of 93%), intermediate risk (HR 3.54, 95% CI 1.91 to 6.57; 3-year overall survival rate of 70.8%), and high risk (HR 7.16, 95% CI 3.97 to 12.93; 3-year overall survival rate of 46.2%) of death (Fig. 1.4B).

Additional work has been done to identify which patients with HPV-associated tumors have the best prognoses for targeting for treatment deintensification trials. O'Sullivan et al.[42] evaluated 382 patients with HPV-positive OPSCC. Within this population, they identified a "low-risk" group with T1-3, N0-2c disease, whose 3-year locoregional control and distant control were 93% and 91%, respectively. However, the group expressed concern that the high distant control achieved in patients with N2c disease was with the most intensified therapies, leading to their recommendation to exclude these patients (for now) as deintensification candidates. The current NRG phase II trial is testing 60 Gy in 5 weeks and 60 Gy in 6 weeks with cisplatin. The trial is open to patients with stage III and IVA disease, T1-3, N0-2b, and <10 years of smoking. To further be consistent with the improved prognosis of HPV-positive OPSCC, the AJCC has created a separate staging for this entity, including a major change in clinical nodal staging that is more akin to that used for nasopharyngeal cancers. This new staging will drastically downstage many patients, as the majority of patients formerly staged as IV will now be stage I.[43]

Tumor Expression of Epidermal Growth Factor Receptor

EGFR is composed of four extracellular domains (I to IV), including the ligand-binding regions (domains I and III), a hydrophobic transmembrane domain, a juxtamembrane domain, an intracellular protein tyrosine kinase domain containing the ATP-binding pockets, and a regulatory carboxyl terminal domain. It is monomeric in the absence of ligands. Binding of a ligand to the extracellular domains I and III alters the spatial configuration of these domains, creating an extended and stabilized conformation that promotes homodimerization and heterodimerization[44] and activates signal transduction.

The EGFR-signaling pathway has evoked considerable attention as a potential biomarker for radiation response. EGFR is overexpressed in many neoplasms, for example, in 80% to 100% of HNSCCs, and perturbation of EGFR signaling is regarded as a major cause of malignant transformation.[45] An extensive correlative biomarker analysis using tumor biopsy specimens from patients with locally advanced HNSCC enrolled in a phase III trial of conventionally fractionated radiation (70 Gy in 2-Gy fractions, five times a week) showed no correlation between EGFR expression and T or N classification, American Joint Committee on Cancer (AJCC) disease stage grouping, and recursive partitioning analysis classes[46] (r: −0.07 to +0.17).

EGFR overexpression, defined in terms of some level above the median mean optical density or a staining index measured using an image analysis–based immunohistochemical assay, was found to be a strong and independent marker for higher locoregional relapse rate (68% vs. 50% at 5 years; P = 0.0031) and inferior overall survival rate (20% vs. 40%; P = 0.006).[46] These findings led to a belief that pretreatment level of tumor EGFR expression would predict response to EGFR antagonists leading to personalized therapy. Unfortunately, correlative studies testing these agents in the metastatic setting[47,48] and more recently in the concurrent chemoradiation setting[40] have not been able to demonstrate that EGFR expression can predict response.

Over the past 10 to 20 years, over 100 articles have been published in the medical literature. A recent meta-analysis[49] limited to 37 papers that provided sufficient data for analysis revealed significant heterogeneity in the studies (with regard to tumor subsites and methodology of EGFR assessment). The ultimate results revealed that high EGFR expression was associated with worse overall survival (pooled HR 1.69, 95%

CI 1.43 to 2.00), but a weaker association for disease-free survival (pooled HR 1.28, 95% CI 1.04 to 1.58). As RTOG 0522 was designed to test the additive efficacy of an EGFR inhibitor (cetuximab), EGFR staining was performed. EGFR staining performed on 235 tumor samples revealed no significant differences in survival end points nor pattern of relapse.[40]

Collectively, the available data at this time indicate that EGFR is a predictor of the response of HNSCC to radiation. Unfortunately, the inconsistency in the results of these trials, the inability to demonstrate any correlation with targeted therapy, and results of genomics analyses suggesting other druggable targets other than EGFR have tampered the enthusiasm for using high EGFR expression as a utile biomarker.

Treatment of Advanced Cancers

Refinement in surgical resection and reconstructive techniques and advances in radiotherapy planning and delivery technology yield excellent outcomes for most patients with early head and neck cancers. Unfortunately, therapy consisting of surgical resection and preoperative or postoperative radiotherapy still achieves only fair results in terms of disease control, preservation of organ function, or both in patients with locally advanced cancer. Consequently, the search continues for better treatment approaches. The largest gains to date with regard to tumor control have been with the combining of chemotherapy with radiation. This approach though often leads to increased toxicity. The use of high-precision radiotherapy has helped head and neck patients achieve improved functional outcomes, with better posttreatment quality of life.

COMBINING RADIATION WITH CHEMOTHERAPY

Key Points

- The combination of radiation with chemotherapy for the treatment of HNSCC has been extensively investigated in phase III trials since the early 1970s.

- A thorough meta-analysis of 16,485 patients in 87 trials revealed that adding concurrent chemotherapy to radiation increased the absolute 5-year survival rate to a greater extent than did combining non–taxane-containing induction chemotherapy with radiation (6.5% vs. 2.4%).

- No significant difference in the magnitude of benefit was detected between concomitant chemotherapy trials addressing frontline and adjuvant therapy and conventional and altered fractionation and using single-agent and multiagent regimens.

- In the single-agent group, the effect of chemotherapy was significantly higher for platinum-based compounds than with other agents; cisplatin, at a dose of 100 mg/m^2 three times throughout the course of radiotherapy, has been a common standard regimen used in combination with radiotherapy.

- The effect of chemotherapy on survival decreased with increasing patient age. Plausible explanations include that older patients more often die from causes other than cancer, which makes it more difficult to detect the benefit in these patients, or that chemotherapy increases the number of deaths from causes other than cancer in older patients.

- Analyses of long-term follow-up data indicated that adding platinum-based concurrent chemotherapy to radiation increases the incidence of late morbidity, such as swallowing dysfunction and soft tissue fibrosis or necrosis.

- A recent phase III trial showed no difference in overall survival, other tumor outcome end points, or toxicity profile between an accelerated regimen plus two cycles of cisplatin and conventional fractionation with three cycles of cisplatin, suggesting that both regimens can serve as a platform to which new agents can be added.

- Postoperative adjuvant radiation with concurrent cisplatin is recommended only for patients with histologically proven extracapsular extension, positive surgical margins, or both. Postoperative radiotherapy alone (without chemotherapy) remains the standard of care for patients with intermediate-risk features such as perineural invasion, close margins, and positive nodes without extracapsular extension.

Meta-analyses of Concurrent Versus Induction Chemotherapy Regimens

Combining radiation with chemotherapy has been extensively investigated in patients with HNSCC. However, most of the regimens that have been studied have evolved empirically by administering drugs found to have some activity against tumors of interest in a dose and time sequence known to be tolerated in the setting of single-modality therapy. Meta-analyses of available data of randomized trials in head and neck cancer undertaken years ago showed that in spite of a high initial response rate, multiagent chemotherapy given before radiation treatment (i.e., neoadjuvant therapy) had only a small impact on locoregional control and survival rates.[50,51] Concurrent radiation and chemotherapy, on the other hand, has yielded survival rates up to 10% higher than those of radiation alone.[52] Unfortunately, the complication rates of combined regimens are also higher than those of radiotherapy alone.[52]

The Meta-Analysis of Chemotherapy on Head and Neck Cancer (MACH-NC) Collaborative Group undertook a very extensive meta-analysis[52] and updated the analysis nearly a decade later. The updated meta-analysis included 87 trials with 16,485 patients comparing various locoregional treatments with or without chemotherapy.[53] Updated follow-up was obtained for most of the trials, and the overall median follow-up time was 5.6 years. Given the substantial impact that this thorough analysis will continue to have on treatment policy, pertinent results are summarized below.

Overall Effect of Concomitant Chemotherapy

The HR of death was 0.81 (95% CI 0.78 to 0.86; $P < 0.0001$) in favor of concomitant chemotherapy with an absolute benefit of 6.5% at 5 years. The magnitude of the benefit was identical for trials conducted during two periods (1965 to 1993 and 1994 to 2000), and no significant heterogeneity ($P = 0.27$) was found in the most recent trials. Cancer-related and non–cancer-related deaths could be distinguished from one another in the recent trials because the cause of death was missing in <4% of the patients without recurrence. The benefit of chemotherapy was due to reduction of deaths related to HNSCC (HR 0.78, 95% CI 0.73 to 0.84; $P < 0.0001$) with no effect on noncancer deaths (HR 0.96, 95% CI 0.82 to 1.12; $P = 0.62$). Results were similar for event-free survival, with an HR of 0.79 (95% CI 0.76 to 0.83; $P < 0.0001$) and an absolute benefit of 6.2% at 5 years (29.3% vs. 23.1%).

Subset analyses revealed no significant difference in benefit between the group of trials testing postoperative radiotherapy (HR 0.79, 95% CI 0.68 to 0.91) and curative radiotherapy given in either conventional fractionation (HR 0.83, 95% CI 0.78 to 0.88) or altered fractionation (HR 0.73, 95% CI 0.65 to 0.82). No significant difference was seen between single-agent chemotherapy (HR 0.84) and multiagent chemotherapy (HR 0.78). In the single-agent chemotherapy group, the effect of chemotherapy was significantly higher ($P = 0.006$) for platinum-based compounds than for other agents.

Consistent with the previous findings, the effect of chemotherapy on survival decreased with increasing patient age (test for trend; $P = 0.003$). Recent trials with more complete data showed that the cause of death, as expected, varied markedly according to age. The proportion of deaths not related to HNSCC increased progressively with age from 15% in patients younger than 50 years to 39% in those over 70 years of age.

Overall Effect of Induction Chemotherapy

The HR of death was 0.96 (95% CI 0.90 to 1.02; $P = 0.18$) with an absolute difference of 2.4% at 5 years. The effect did not vary ($P = 0.23$) according to the type of chemotherapy: the HRs were 0.90 (0.82 to 0.99) for cisplatin–fluorouracil, 1.01 (95% CI 0.91 to 1.12) for other multiagent regimens, and 0.99 (95% CI 0.84 to 1.18) for single agents (no trial was done with cisplatin alone). Results for event-free survival were similar, with an HR of 0.99 (95% CI 0.93 to 1.05; $P = 0.67$)

and an absolute benefit of 1.3% at 5 years (27.6% vs. 26.3%). The HRs of death were not significantly different ($P = 0.68$) between trials using radiotherapy alone, surgery plus postoperative radiotherapy, or other locoregional treatment.

Effects of Concomitant and Induction Chemotherapy on Locoregional Relapses and Distant Metastasis

Locoregional relapse data were available for 50 concomitant and 30 induction trials. The benefit of concomitant chemotherapy was significant (HR 0.74, 95% CI 0.70 to 0.79; $P < 0.0001$), whereas induction chemotherapy had no effect (HR 1.03, 95% CI 0.95 to 1.13; $P = 0.43$). The two HRs were significantly different ($P < 0.0001$) in favor of the concomitant group.

Distant metastasis data were available for 44 concomitant and 26 induction trials. Both concomitant and induction chemotherapy were found to have significant effects, with HRs of 0.88 (95% CI 0.77 to 1.00; $P = 0.04$) for concomitant therapy and 0.73 (95% CI 0.61 to 0.88; $P = 0.001$) for induction therapy. Although the HR of induction chemotherapy was smaller than that of the concomitant regimens, the comparison of the two HRs did not yield a significant difference ($P = 0.12$).

Summary of Meta-analysis

The authors of the meta-analysis concluded that adding data from the 24 more recent trials with minimal heterogeneity did not change the magnitude of the observed survival benefit resulting from the addition of chemotherapy that had been reported previously, which stayed at around 4% at 5 years. This benefit was firm for concomitant chemotherapy (HR 0.81) but was not demonstrable for induction regimens. Important observations were that concomitant chemotherapy markedly improved locoregional control, which was not observed for induction chemotherapy. On the other hand, induction chemotherapy had a more pronounced effect on distant metastases compared with concomitant regimens, suggesting the need to use relatively high doses of chemotherapy to influence the manifestation of distant metastases.

Cisplatin alone, cisplatin or carboplatin plus fluorouracil, or other multiagent regimens including either cisplatin or fluorouracil yielded the same magnitude of benefit. In contrast, drugs given alone (except for cisplatin) had inferior results and, therefore, should not be recommended in routine practice. Single-agent cisplatin seems to be a common standard regimen in combination with radiotherapy. Most of the randomized trials used high-dose cisplatin regimens, that is, 100 mg/m² given three times throughout the course of radiotherapy (cumulative dose of 300 mg/m²). Interestingly, the only negative "cisplatin-alone" trial in this meta-analysis used a cumulative dose of 140 mg/m² (20 mg/m² × 7), suggesting that the cumulative dose of cisplatin could be important.

The benefit of concomitant chemotherapy seems to be similar regardless of whether the radiotherapy was given in conventional or altered fractionation, but the magnitude of the benefit was less in older patients. One explanation is that older patients more often die from causes other than cancer, which makes it more difficult to detect the benefit in these patients (dilution effect). Alternatively, chemotherapy could increase the number of deaths from causes other than cancer in older patients.

Long-Term Toxicity of Concurrent Chemoradiotherapy

The meta-analysis presented above focused on tumor control end points. Data on compliance and toxicity were not available for analysis. Notably, the recording and reporting of late morbidity associated with concurrent chemoradiotherapy have not been sufficiently consistent or systematic.[54]

In the long-term evaluation of RTOG 9111,[55] the authors report 10-year cumulative rates of grade 3 to 5 late toxicities ranging from 30.6% to 38% for patients in the three treatment arms with no significant differences in cumulative incidence between the treatment groups (i.e., between those that received or did not receive concurrent cisplatin). There were fatal events in all three groups.

More mature data have also been released from RTOG 129,[56] the study that randomized over 700 patients receiving cisplatin concomitant with radiation to either 6 or 7 weeks or therapy. This study still used conventional modes of radiation planning and delivery. The incidence of grade 3 to 5 late toxicity was approximately 37% and essentially similar in the two arms. At 2 years, 5.9% of the surviving patients treated with standard fractionation had a feeding tube, compared to 13.2% of those treated with accelerated radiation ($P = 0.08$). The subsequent RTOG 522 trial[40] randomized 940 patients. All patients were treated with accelerated radiation and cisplatin (with or without cetuximab), and approximately 86% were treated with IMRT. The rate of feeding tube dependency at 2 years was similar to that in RTOG 129 (13.5% and 11.9% in the two arms). Setton and colleagues performed a retrospective multi-institutional analysis of gastrostomy tube dependence in patients with oropharyngeal cancer treated with IMRT. In over 1,000 patients with stage III and IV disease treated with concurrent chemotherapy and radiation, the 1- and 2-year gastrostomy rates were 8.6% and 3.7%.[57]

Adjuvant Therapy for Locally Advanced HNSCC

Although data from several trials addressing adjuvant chemoradiation were included in the meta-analyses, the results of two larger-scale trials done by the RTOG[58] and the EORTC[59] are briefly summarized here because they contributed to refining the standard of care. Both studies randomly assigned patients with high-risk surgical pathologic features to surgery followed by conventionally fractionated postoperative radiotherapy alone or combined with cisplatin (100 mg/m^2 every 3 weeks for three cycles). The RTOG allowed a dose range of 60 to 66 Gy, and 18% of patients were treated to 66 Gy,[60] while the EORTC had a fixed dose of 66 Gy for all patients. While the treatment schema was relatively similar,

there were differences in the two groups with regard to the definition of "high-risk" pathologic features. In the initial report of the RTOG trial,[58] radiochemotherapy significantly reduced the risk of locoregional recurrence compared with radiation alone (HR 0.61; $P = 0.01$) but did not improve overall survival. However, in a subsequent report of long-term follow-up, the significant difference in locoregional control was no longer evident ($P = 0.10$).[61] In contrast, the EORTC trial[59] showed significant improvement in progression-free survival (HR 0.75; $P = 0.04$) and overall survival (HR 0.70; $P = 0.02$) in addition to locoregional control. Long-term follow-up has not been reported yet. Notably, both trials found that the addition of cisplatin had no significant effect on the incidence of distant metastases. Both studies (including the initial RTOG report) also found that cisplatin considerably increased the rate of grade 3 or higher adverse events (from 34% to 77% [$P < 0.001$] in the RTOG trial and from 21% to 41% [$P = 0.001$] in the EORTC trial). However, with long-term follow-up, the additional toxicity due to chemotherapy was harder to define. The increased toxicity appeared to be greatest in the first year of follow-up, but the data did not suggest a continued disproportionate increase in toxicity in the patients treated with chemotherapy in the later years of follow-up.

To determine which patients are most likely to benefit from intensive postoperative radiochemotherapy, a pooled analysis of data from both trials was performed.[60] This analysis revealed that in both trials, only patients with extracapsular extension and positive surgical margins benefited from radiochemotherapy. This combined analysis thus contributed to refining the criteria for the high-risk category and the treatment algorithm. While the overall results presented in the long-term RTOG analysis were negative, an unplanned subgroup analysis of those patients with microscopically involved margins and/or extracapsular extension did reveal improved locoregional control, disease-free survival, and overall survival for those patients receiving chemotherapy with radiation (P-value ranging from 0.02 to 0.07 for the three end points). Adjuvant radiation with concurrent cisplatin is now recommended only for patients with histologically proven extracapsular extension, positive surgical margins, or both. For those with intermediate-risk features (e.g., positive nodes without extracapsular extension, perineural invasion, close margins), the current standard of care is postoperative radiotherapy without chemotherapy. Efforts are underway to test the combination of radiotherapy, with or without chemotherapy depending on the risk features, with molecular therapeutics for this subset of patients.

Taxane-Based Chemotherapy

The success of taxanes in the treatment of other solid tumors has generated interest the integration of taxanes into chemotherapy and chemoradiation regimens used in HNSCC. The greatest efforts have been put into incorporation of taxanes into adjuvant regimens.

Results of three randomized trials addressing the efficacy of neoadjuvant docetaxel, cisplatin, and fluorouracil regimen (TPF) relative to cisplatin and fluorouracil (PF) for patients with locally advanced HNSCC were reported, all favoring the regimens that incorporated a taxane.[62-64] Table 1.1 summarizes the published results of these trials.

Encouraged by the results suggesting that the addition of a taxane to the classic PF regimen improved outcomes (with regard to disease control), and a subgroup analysis of the data collected by the MACH analysis focusing on induction therapy with PF demonstrating a survival advantage, several investigators tested a hypothesis that the optimal induction regimen of TPF combined with the optimal local therapy, that is, concurrent chemoradiation, should improve survival compared to chemoradiation.

The DeCIDE trial[65] evaluated two cycles of docetaxel 75 mg/m^2 and cisplatin 75 mg/m^2 on day 1, combined with fluorouracil 750 mg/m^2 on days 1 to 5. A total of 285 patients (of a planned 400 patients) with N2 or N3 HNSCC were randomized to receive either this induction regimen or no induction. All patients were then planned for chemoradiation with gross disease treated to 75 Gy with 1.5-Gy fraction delivered twice daily every other week. The concurrent drugs used were docetaxel, fluorouracil, and hydroxyurea. There was no difference in the primary end point, overall survival, with the HR = 0.91 (95% CI = 0.59 to 1.41).

The PARADIGM trial was nearly similar in design.[66] The eligibility was a diagnosis of stage III to IVB HNSCC. The induction regimen was relatively similar to the DeCide regimen with minor differences (docetaxel 75 mg/m^2 and cisplatin 100 mg/m^2 on day 1, combined with fluorouracil 1,000 mg/m^2 on days 1 to 4). The radiation planned was 70 Gy in 7 weeks. Patients received concurrent carboplatin (weekly AUC 1.5) if they either did not randomize to induction therapy or responded favorably. Patients who had a poor response were planned for concurrent weekly docetaxel with radiation. A total of 145 patients (of a planned 330 patients) were enrolled. The 3-year survival in the induction therapy group was 73% compared to 78% for the chemoradiotherapy group.

Despite concerns regarding poor accrual, these two trials demonstrated little if any gain in survival and additional toxicity when using taxane-based induction regimens to treat patients with HNSCC. However, if induction regimens are to be used, taxane-based regimens are considered standard, and there remain several areas of ongoing investigation.

The role of adjuvant and neoadjuvant therapy still remains unclear in NPC. A recent meta-analysis[67] evaluated 19 randomized trials, and conclusions were similar to those seen in the MACH analyses; concomitant chemoradiation improves overall survival. The interaction between induction therapy alone and radiation did not appear to confer benefit. However, similar to the general HNSCC studies, it is believed that the role of taxanes incorporated into an adjuvant regimen needs further exploration and studies are ongoing.

While data is lacking in demonstrating survival improvements with taxane-based induction therapy, the question of induction therapy's role in laryngeal preservation remains unanswered. In their initial report,[68] the authors of RTOG 91-11, a study randomizing patients with advanced cancers to radiation alone, induction chemotherapy followed by radiation (or surgery), or concomitant chemoradiation, concluded that concomitant chemoradiation was most efficacious in meeting the end point of optimal laryngectomy-free survival. In their recent update[55] reporting long-term results, the authors noted that locoregional control and larynx preservation were best in patients on the concomitant radiation

TABLE 1.1 Efficacy of Neoadjuvant Docetaxel, Cisplatin, and Fluorouracil (TPF) Versus Cisplatin and Fluorouracil (PF) Followed by Radiation Alone or Combined with Weekly Carboplatin for the Treatment of Locally Advanced Head and Neck Squamous Cell Cancer

End points	EORTC 24971 (n = 358)			TAX 324 (n = 501)		
	TPF	PF	P-Value	TPF	PF	P-Value
Response rate (%)	68	54	0.006	72	64	0.07
Median progression-free survival (mo)	11.0	8.2	0.007	36	13	
3-Yr survival rate (%)	37	26	—	62	48	0.002
Median overall survival (mo)	18.6	14.2	0.005	71	30	0.006
Hazard ratio	0.73 (0.56–0.94)		0.02	0.70 (0.54–0.90)		0.006

Median follow-up times were 32.5 mo in the EORTC trial[62] and 42 mo in the TAX 324 study[63].

arm; induction therapy (with PF) followed by radiation had a similar efficacy with concomitant therapy for the composite end point of laryngectomy-free survival, and further, fewer noncancer deaths were observed with long-term follow-up in patients treated with induction therapy compared to concomitant therapy.

In one of the three PF versus TPF trials described above,[64] GORTEC 2000-01 was a trial designed to test whether using TPF induction therapy leads to better larynx preservation compared to PF. While not demonstrating improvement in survival, long-term follow-up demonstrated 10-year larynx preservation rates of 70% and 47% in patients treated with TPF compared to PF ($P = 0.01$).[69] The authors concluded that if an induction approach is taken for larynx preservation, TPF is the regimen of choice (followed by radiation), but the clear role of TPF, and the role of concomitant chemoradiation alone, or following TPF for laryngeal preservation remains unclear.

Taxane therapy has not been well tested as a concurrent agent to be used with radiation. Several phase I and II trials have suggested that it is efficacious as either a single agent or combined with other drugs, but phase III trials have not been done. Building on the postoperative chemoradiation trial described above (RTOG 9501), the RTOG randomized operated patients with high-risk findings to 60 Gy in 6 weeks with either weekly cisplatin (30 mg/m²) combined with weekly cetuximab and weekly docetaxel (15 mg/m²) with cetuximab.[70] The results of the docetaxel arm were favorable, with a 2-year survival rate of 79%. This has led to a current randomized phase III trial for high-risk postoperative patients that is further exploring the role of both taxane and cetuximab.

ALTERED FRACTIONATION

Key Points

- Results of meta-analysis of large randomized trials assessing the effects of biologically sound fractionation schedules show that, on the whole, altered fractionation yielded a significant survival benefit (3.4% increase in 5-year survival rate) relative to conventional fractionation, with highly significant reductions in cancer-related death and in local tumor failure without increases in late treatment morbidity.

- Hyperfractionation and accelerated fractionation by concomitant boost or six weekly fractions have been adopted in many centers for the treatment of some patients with intermediate-stage HNSCC or those with locally advanced HNSCC who are not suitable for or decline chemotherapy.

Radiobiologic concepts derived from close to three decades of integrated laboratory and clinical investigations led to the conception of two classes of altered fractionation schedules for the treatment of head and neck cancers. These altered fractionation regimens are referred to as *hyperfractionation* and *accelerated fractionation* schedules. Hyperfractionation exploits the difference in fractionation sensitivity between tumors and normal tissues manifesting late morbidity. Commonly used regimens are 80.5 to 81.6 Gy given in 1.15 to 1.2 Gy per fractions, twice a day with a 6-hour interval, over 7 weeks. In contrast, accelerated fractionation schedules attempt to reduce tumor proliferation as a major cause of radiotherapy failure. Although there are many permutations in accelerating radiation treatment, the existing schedules can be conceptually grouped into two categories: those with and without reduction of the conventional total dose (66 to 70 Gy). Two accelerated fractionation regimens that have been tested in large clinical trials are a concomitant boost regimen (designed by investigators at MD Anderson)[71] that delivers 54 Gy in 30 fractions over 6 weeks plus an 18-Gy boost dose given in 1.5-Gy fractions as second daily fractions during the last 2.5 weeks, and a regimen involving delivery of six 2-Gy fractions per week used by Danish investigators.[72] These radiobiologically sound fractionation regimens have been extensively tested in patients with intermediate and advanced head and neck carcinomas.

Bourhis et al.[73] reported a meta-analysis regarding fractionation regimens that included updating of individual data for 6,515 patients enrolled in 15 phase III trials. The main primary tumor sites were the oropharynx (3,079 patients, 44%) and larynx (2,377 patients, 34%), and most patients (5,221, 74%) had stage III to IV disease. The length of follow-up ranged from 4 to 10 years, with a median of 6 years. The treatment regimens tested were divided into three categories: hyperfractionated and accelerated fractionation with or without dose reduction. Table 1.2 summarizes the benefit of altered fractionation versus conventional fractionation on different outcome end points. On the whole, altered fractionation yielded a significant survival benefit relative to conventional fractionation ($P = 0.003$), with highly significant reductions in cancer-related death ($P = 0.0002$) and in local tumor failure ($P < 0.0001$). Moreover, the benefit was significantly higher in younger than in older patients ($P = 0.007$ for test for trend). An update to this meta-analysis is currently in preparation.

Overall, the magnitude of the survival benefit was significantly higher in the hyperfractionation group than in the two accelerated fractionation groups ($P = 0.02$). However, the authors emphasized that the populations included in the three groups were dissimilar, as the accelerated fractionation without dose reduction group enrolled more patients with early-stage or laryngeal cancer. Relapses in the latter group could be effectively salvaged, as shown in the RTOG larynx preservation trial[68,74] and thus have little impact on the survival end point. Indeed, in the only phase III trial in which hyperfractionation and accelerated fractionation with concomitant boost were tested simultaneously against conventional fractionation, both regimens were found to yield a similar magnitude of effect.[71]

TABLE 1.2 Absolute Improvements at 5 Years, with Hazard Ratios and 95% CI, of Hyperfractionated Versus Accelerated Fractionation Schedules for Locally Advanced Head and Neck Squamous Cell Cancer

End point	Overall Benefit	P-Value	Hyperfractionation	Accelerated Fractionation without Dose Reduction	Accelerated Fractionation with Reduced Dose
Improvements at 5 yr					
Overall survival	+3.4%[a]	0.003	+8.2%	+2.0%	+1.7%
Locoregional control	+6.4%	<0.0001	+9.4%	+7.3%	+2.3%
Hazard ratios					
Total death	0.92 (0.86–0.97)	0.003	0.78 (0.69–0.89)	0.97 (0.89–1.05)	0.94 (0.84–1.05)
Cancer death	0.88 (0.83–0.94)	0.0002	0.78 (0.68–0.90)	0.91 (0.83–1.00)	0.93 (0.83–1.05)
Local relapse	0.77 (0.71–0.83)	<0.0001	0.75 (0.63–0.89)	0.74 (0.67–0.83)	0.83 (0.71–0.96)
Regional relapse	0.87 (0.79–0.97)	0.01	0.83 (0.66–1.03)	0.90 (0.77–1.04)	0.87 (0.72–1.06)
Locoregional relapse	0.82 (0.77–0.88)	<0.0001	0.76 (0.66–0.89)	0.79 (0.72–0.87)	0.90 (0.80–1.02)
Metastatic relapse	0.97 (0.82–1.15)	0.75	1.09 (0.76–1.58)	0.93 (0.74–1.19)	0.95 (0.68–1.32)

[a]An 8% reduction in the risk of dying.
Modified from Bourhis J, Overgaard J, Audry H, et al. Hyperfractionated or accelerated radiotherapy in head and neck cancer: a meta-analysis. *Lancet* 2006;368:843–854.

Evidence generated from numerous randomized trials indicates that altered fractionation is a reasonable option for the treatment of some patients with intermediate-stage (i.e., T2N0-1 or exophytic T3N0-1) HNSCC or those with locally advanced HNSCC who are not suitable for or decline chemotherapy. However, the use of altered fractionation regimens has declined in recent years owing to advances in the development of high-precision radiation treatment technology, particularly IMRT, which combines the principles of both hyperfractionation with accelerated fractionation as discussed below.

Role of Altered Fractionation in Concurrent Chemoradiotherapy

As presented above, both altered fractionation regimens and concurrent chemoradiotherapy can improve locoregional control, survival, or both over conventionally fractionated radiotherapy alone. Of two trials designed to address this comparison, results of one trial (RTOG 0129) have been reported to date.[56] In that large phase III trial, 743 patients were stratified according to tumor site (larynx vs. other), nodal classification (N0 vs. N1-N2b vs. N2c-N3), and Zubrod performance status (0 vs. 1) and assigned to receive high-dose cisplatin concurrent with either accelerated fractionation by concomitant boost or standard fractionation. The accelerated schedule delivered 72 Gy in 42 fractions over 6 weeks, which included twice-a-day irradiation for 12 treatment days (as previously reported),[71] whereas the standard schedule consisted of 70 Gy in 35 fractions (2 Gy per

fraction) over 7 weeks. Chemotherapy consisted of intravenous cisplatin at a dose of 100 mg/m^2 on days 1 and 22 in the accelerated group or on days 1, 22, and 43 in the standard fractionation group.

No significant differences were observed between the accelerated and standard fractionation groups with regard to overall survival the two groups (8-year overall survival rate 48% for accelerated vs. 48% for standard fractionation; $P = 0.18$). Additionally, no differences were detected in any disease control end points. There also was no difference between the two arms in incidence of acute or late toxicity. Thus, altered fractionation (at least with a mild accelerated regimen) appeared to be neither beneficial nor detrimental. As most patients receive systemic therapy with radiation, the role of altered fractionation has diminished.

HIGH-PRECISION RADIOTHERAPY

Key Points

- IMRT can incorporate principles of both hyperfractionation and accelerated fractionation by generating a gradient of lower dose per fraction to normal tissues and by administering twice-a-day fractions during some treatment days. This feature, coupled with the ability to reducing the total dose to critical normal tissues, makes IMRT more popular than altered fractionation for the treatment of HNSCC.

- Data from both single-institution and multicenter trials on the use of IMRT for the treatment of nasopharyngeal and oropharyngeal carcinomas demonstrate high locoregional control and reduction of xerostomia.

- Further developments needed to fully benefit from IMRT include quantification of and adapting to intrafraction and interfraction variation and topographic and biologic tumor imaging to improve target definition, among others.

- The observation that most recurrences are situated within the high-dose region indicates that radiation dose escalation alone will improve outcome in only a subset of patients.

Advances in computerized radiotherapy planning and delivery technology open the possibility of conforming irradiation to irregular tumor target volumes, an approach commonly referred to as *conformal radiotherapy* (CRT).[75] Consequently, it is feasible to reduce the radiation dose to the crucial normal tissues surrounding the tumor without compromising dose delivery to the intended target volume, resulting in a reduction in morbidity. Reduced toxicity would, in turn, permit escalation of the radiation dose or combining radiotherapy with intensive chemotherapy, each of which has the potential for improving HNSCC control. The clinical application of precision radiotherapy, however, requires basic expertise in anatomy, imaging, and patterns of tumor spread.

Precision radiotherapy can be accomplished by the use of an array of x-ray beams individually shaped to conform to the projection of the target, which is referred to as *three-dimensional conformal radiotherapy* (3-D CRT). In addition, technology is also available to modify the intensity of the beams across the irradiation field as an added degree of freedom to enhance the capability of conforming dose distributions in three dimensions. This radiotherapy technique is called *intensity-modulated radiotherapy* (IMRT). Proton beams potentially offer an even higher magnitude of normal tissue sparing, and the role of protons, particularly *intensity-modulated proton therapy* (IMPT), is an area of active investigation.

With IMRT, all target volumes are irradiated during every radiation session, but lower doses are delivered to the subclinical disease volume at each fraction. For example, when 70 Gy is delivered in 35 fractions (at 2 Gy per fraction) to the gross disease, the low-risk subclinical target volumes receive doses ranging from 56 to 59.5 Gy, also in 35 fractions (corresponding to 1.70 to 1.75 Gy per fraction). Normal tissues outside these volumes receive even lower total doses given in lower-dose

fractions. Hence, IMRT incorporates some degree of normal tissue sparing by lowering the dose per fraction.

The role of 3-D CRT and, particularly, IMRT in reducing morbidity and, perhaps, in improving disease control has undergone fairly extensive evaluation over the past decade. The first toxicity that investigators have attempted to minimize with IMRT was xerostomia. Eisbruch et al.[76] revealed that IMRT is effective in sparing parotid glands from receiving high radiation doses, thereby diminishing radiation-induced permanent xerostomia in some patients. Further work has tried to define dose–volume effects for parotid sparing.[77]

The encouraging single-institution experiences demonstrating parotid gland sparing and reduction in severity of xerostomia led to several randomized prospective trials designed to further validate that IMRT is an efficacious radiation technique for xerostomia reduction without compromising disease control. Investigators in Hong Kong completed two phase III trials. The study reported by Kam et al.[78] showed that patients given IMRT had a lower incidence of observer-rated severe xerostomia than did patients given 2-D radiotherapy, results that paralleled higher fractional-stimulated rates of parotid flow and whole saliva flow rates. However, there was only a trend toward improvement in patient-reported outcome after IMRT relative to 2-D radiotherapy. In the second study, Pow et al.[79] showed that patients given IMRT had fewer xerostomia-related symptoms than did patients given conventional radiotherapy at 12 months after radiotherapy and that symptoms that were experienced improved consistently over time. Global health scores showed continuous improvement in quality of life after both treatments ($P < 0.001$), but after 12 months, the subscale scores for role-physical, bodily pain, and physical function were significantly higher in the IMRT group, indicating overall better condition in that group.

In the United Kingdom, investigators conducted the PARSPORT trial.[80] This trial, conducted at six centers, randomized patients with oropharyngeal and hypopharyngeal cancer to either parotid-sparing IMRT or conventional radiotherapy (3-D conformal therapy with parallel-opposed fields). Ninety-four patients were randomized. The trial demonstrated a significant reduction in grade 2 or worse xerostomia (29% vs. 83% for patients treated with IMRT and conventional therapy, respectively) at 24 months. Additionally, patients treated with IMRT had significant improvements in dry mouth–specific and global quality of life scores measured at 1 and 2 years post therapy.

Reduction in xerostomia is not confined to general gland sparing. Recent work from the University of Groningen has demonstrated that dose to the region of the salivary gland containing the stem/progenitor cells predicted the function of the gland 1 year post therapy.[81] The feasibility of precision radiotherapy to target this section with in the larger parotid gland needs further testing. In addition to the parotids, sparing of the submandibular glands has garnered recent interest. Part of this move has been data suggesting that level

1B nodes may be at low risk of involvement in pharyngeal cancers,[82] and by not targeting these nodes, submandibular gland avoidance is achievable. Retrospective studies[83] have reported on the feasibility of submandibular gland sparing, as well as describing further improvements in xerostomia reduction than that seen with parotid sparing alone.

Conformal techniques have not only focused on xerostomia reduction, but also on reducing other toxicities. Chronic dysphagia can be a significant problem for many survivors of HNSCC. Similar to xerostomia, the specific causes of dysphagia are varied and complex, and further methods of defining dysphagia are numerous, including differing subjective scoring systems and differing objective end points. However, studies[84,85] have suggested that mean doses to swallowing organs correlate with long-term swallowing dysfunction, and conformal therapies, particularly IMRT designed to spare these organs, can reduce the incidence of dysphagia. The potential for proton therapy, specifically IMPT, to further reduce the incidence of dysphagia is of current interest. The Rococo cooperative group has done dosimetric analyses to demonstrate that IMPT can lower doses to swallowing organs even lower than that achieved with IMRT.[86] Clinical trials to further test IMPT are ongoing.

NPC and paranasal sinus cancers often require treatment near or to the skull base (and adjacent brain) and/or visual structures. Conformal techniques are clearly advantageous in these situations. Evaluating the evolution of NPC treatment, Lee et al.[87] noted a neurological toxicity rate of 1.8% in patients treated with IMRT, compared to 7.4% and 3.5% in patients treated with 2-D or 3-D techniques. Similarly, in a retrospective study Al-Mamgani et al.[88] described their experience treating paranasal sinus cancer and noted both a significant reduction in overall late toxicity with IMRT compared to 3-D conformal therapy as well as an improvement in visual preservation with IMRT.

While the principal efforts of conformal therapy, with state-of-the-art conformal therapy being IMRT, are designed to reduce toxicity, it is hoped that IMRT can improve disease control. While imaging improvements over time, and incorporation of chemotherapy have contributed to improved disease control, there are suggestions that IMRT may also be a contributory factor to improved outcomes. Data from studies on NPC and paranasal sinus cancer have suggested improvement in local control.[87,88] Using SEER-Medicare data, Beadle and colleagues demonstrated that in over 3,000 patients with head and neck cancer, those treated with IMRT had a better cause-specific survival rate (84%) than those treated with non-IMRT techniques (66%).[89]

It has been hypothesized that high-precision radiation may allow for dose escalation in the tumor while avoiding normal tissues. Although the results of IMRT and particle therapy are encouraging, the observation that most recurrences originated from the high-dose region indicates that radiation dose escalation alone will improve outcome in only a subset of patients. However, as the technology improves to allow for more precise delivery, with imaging improvements to deliver this precise treatment with greater accuracy, it is anticipated that further improvements in the therapeutic ratio will be realized.

COMBINING RADIATION WITH AGENTS TARGETING SIGNALING PATHWAYS (TARGETED AGENTS)

Key Points

- A phase III trial demonstrated that adding the EGFR inhibitor cetuximab to radiation significantly improves locoregional control and survival rates; this has now been compared to concurrent treatment with cisplatin, and results are forthcoming on relative benefits and toxicity profiles.

- While cetuximab concurrent with radiation has been proven in a phase III setting to be superior to radiation alone, testing of other drugs that inhibit EGFR has been less successful.

- Future studies will likely investigate immunotherapy, check-point inhibitors and other targeted agents both independently and combined with radiation.

The results of correlative biomarker analyses and preclinical work on modulating tumor radiation response by targeting EGFR, as summarized above, provided the impetus for launching and completing a multinational phase III study (IMCL-9815) testing the efficacy of the combination of the EGFR inhibitor cetuximab with radiation relative to radiation alone for patients with locally advanced HNSCC.[90] A total of 424 patients from 73 centers in the United States and 14 other countries were randomly assigned to receive high-dose radiotherapy alone (predominantly in accelerated fractionation by concomitant boost) or the same radiotherapy regimens plus eight doses of cetuximab (starting 1 week before and continuing during the course of radiotherapy). As summarized in Table 1.3, this proof-of-principle, highly referenced trial demonstrated that the addition of cetuximab resulted in significant improvement in locoregional control rate and survival without increasing radiation-induced side effects, such as mucositis and dysphagia. Notably, the antibody did induce an acneiform rash, common to EGFR antagonists, and a few patients could not receive this treatment because of infusion reactions.

An update of the results of this cetuximab trial[91] yielded a median overall survival time of 49.0 months (95% CI 32.8 to 69.5) for patients treated with cetuximab and radiotherapy versus 29.3 months (95% CI 20.6 to 41.4) in the radiotherapy alone group (HR 0.73, 95% CI 0.56 to 0.95; $P = 0.018$). The 5-year overall survival rate was 45.6% in the cetuximab plus

TABLE 1.3 Efficacy of Radiotherapy with Cetuximab Versus Radiotherapy Alone for the Treatment of Locally Advanced HNSCC

End points	Radiotherapy Alone	Radiotherapy + Cetuximab	Hazard Ratios (5% CI)	P-Values
Locoregional control				
Median duration (mo)	14.9	24.4	0.68 (0.52–0.89)	0.005
Rate at 2 yr	41%	50%		
Progression-free survival				
Median duration (mo)	12.4	17.1	0.70 (0.54–0.90)	0.006
Rate at 2 yr	37%	46%		
Overall survival				
Median duration (mo)	29.3	49.0	0.74 (0.57–0.97)	0.03
Rate at 3 yr	45%	55%		
Distant metastasis[a]				
Rate at 1 yr	10%	8%		NS
Rate at 2 yr	17%	16%		

[a]Cumulative incidence.
Modified from Bonner JA, Harari PM, Giralt J, et al. Radiotherapy plus cetuximab for squamous-cell carcinoma of the head and neck. *N Engl J Med* 2006;354:567–578.

radiotherapy group and 36.4% in the radiotherapy alone group. An additional finding was that overall survival was significantly better among patients who experienced an acneiform rash of at least grade 2 severity compared with patients with grade 0 or grade 1 rash (HR 0.49, 95% CI 0.34 to 0.72; $P = 0.002$).

Two questions followed from the development of this novel agent. The first is whether cetuximab could add synergistically to further improve results of concurrent chemoradiation. A randomized trial, RTOG 0522, was performed in which patients were randomized between chemoradiation with cisplatin with and without cetuximab; there was no additional benefit to patients who were treated with concurrent cetuximab.[41] Of 891 analyzed patients enrolled on this trial, patients receiving cetuximab had more frequent treatment breaks and more acute toxicity, including an approximate 10% increase in the rate of grade 3 to 4 mucositis. Further, there were no difference in 3-year overall survival, locoregional failure, or distant metastasis. Additionally, tumor EGFR expression did not distinguish outcome.

The second question is whether cetuximab can substitute for cisplatin when using curative-intent chemoradiotherapy for advanced head and neck cancer. Many trials have tried to answer whether cetuximab is as efficacious as cisplatin when combined with radiation. The TREMPLIN trial, a randomized phase II study compared concurrent cisplatin–radiation with cetuximab–radiation following induction chemotherapy for patients with stage III to IV laryngeal and hypopharyngeal cancers.[92] The study concluded that there was no evidence that

one treatment was better. Nien and colleagues evaluated retrospectively 339 patients with HPV-associated oropharyngeal cancer treated with chemoradiation. They also observed similar efficacy between platin agents and cetuximab with regard to overall survival and disease control. A retrospective secondary analysis of IMCL 9815 to test the efficacy of cetuximab in HPV-positive and HPV-negative patients recently demonstrated that cetuximab added to radiation resulted in improved 3-year locoregional control for both the p16-positive and p16-negative subgroups (HR 0.31 [95% CI 0.11 to 0.88] and HR 0.78 [95% CI 0.49 to 1.25], respectively).[93] The answer to the efficacy of cetuximab compared with platin may ultimately be answered by the recently completed RTOG 1016 trial, a phase III trial comparing the two drugs as concurrent agents.

Despite the success of cetuximab, the role of other drugs targeting EGFR inhibition has been less compelling. A phase II multi-institutional trial of panitumumab that compared this biologic agent with radiation to chemoradiation showed a worse progression-free survival rate in the patients treated with panitumumab, as well as greater toxicity with the biologic agent.[94] However, the greatest effort has been to combine these agents with chemoradiation. A variety of agents, including gefitinib, erlotinib, panitumumab, and lapatinib, were tested as an additional agent to cisplatin-based chemoradiation, and all used radiation doses of 70 Gy in 35 fractions (Table 1.4). Unfortunately, none of the trials demonstrated improved outcomes with the addition of the EGFR inhibi-

TABLE 1.4 Studies of Combination EGFR-Targeted Agents with Chemoradiotherapy

Drug	Phase	Patient Number	Median Follow-Up	Primary End Point
Gefitinib (1)	II	226	ND	PFS (OR = 0.9, *P* = 0.61) 2-yr LDCR
Erlotinib (2)	II	204	26 mo	PFS (HR = 0.9, *P* = 0.71)
Panitumumab (3)	II	153	106–110 wk	LRC (HR = 1.33, *P* = 0.31)
Lapatinib (4)	III	688	35.3 mo	DFS (HR = 1.1, *P* = 0.45)

OR, odds ratio; LDCR, local disease control rate; ND, not described; PFS, progression-free survival; HR, hazards ratio; LRC, locoregional control; DFS, disease-free survival.

Table adapted from (1) Gregoire V, Hamoir M, Chen C, et al. Gefitinib plus cisplatin and radiotherapy in previously untreated head and neck squamous cell carcinoma: a phase II, randomized, double-blind, placebo-controlled study. *Radiother Oncol* 2011;100:62–69; (2) Martins RG, Parvathaneni U, Bauman JE, et al. Cisplatin and radiotherapy with or without erlotinib in locally advanced squamous cell carcinoma of the head and neck: a randomized phase II trial. *J Clin Oncol* 2013;31:1415–1421; (3) Mesía R, Henke M, Fortin A, et al. Chemoradiotherapy with or without panitumumab in patients with unresected, locally advanced squamous-cell carcinoma of the head and neck (CONCERT-1): a randomised, controlled, open-label phase 2 trial. *Lancet Oncol* 2015;16:208–220; (4) Harrington K, Temam S, Mehanna H, et al. Postoperative adjuvant lapatinib and concurrent chemoradiotherapy followed by maintenance lapatinib monotherapy in high-risk patients with resected squamous cell carcinoma of the head and neck: a phase III, randomized, double-blind, placebo-controlled study. *J Clin Oncol* 2015;33:4202–4209.

tor, and some of the trials also demonstrated additional toxicity exhibited by patients treated with the biologic agent, dampening the enthusiasm for further investigations of EGFR inhibitors combined with cisplatin-based radiation in locally advanced head and neck cancer. However, in the postoperative setting, and described above, RTOG 0234[70] did note in a phase II trial that the combination of docetaxel and cetuximab resulted in improved outcomes compared to historic controls (RTOG 9501[58]) and based on these encouraging results have initiated a phase II to III trial that is testing the efficacy of taxane-based therapy compared to cisplatin as well as whether adding a biologic agent to a taxane will improve disease control and survival rates.

PREVENTION OF HEAD AND NECK CANCERS

Key Points

- The primary method to prevent HNSCC has been the avoidance of carcinogen exposure. In countries with a decreased incidence of smoking, the incidence of HNSCC (not linked to viruses) has declined. Prevention of HPV-associated cancers can be achieved with immunization.

- Patients exposed to carcinogens experience field cancerization resulting from interactions between prolonged exposure and individuals' genetic profiles; this renders an individual who survives an upper aerodigestive cancer susceptible to developing a second primary tumor (SPT) in the same anatomic region.

- A large multi-institutional randomized trial launched based on the encouraging results of smaller studies did not show a benefit for isotretinoin (*cis*-retinoic acid) in reducing the rate of SPTs.

- Identification of key genetic changes resulting in the development of malignant clones and markers of multistep carcinogenesis will aid in identifying patients at highest risk so that they can be enrolled in future chemoprevention trials. One such effort was testing an oral EGFR inhibitor for patients with premalignant lesions that demonstrated loss of heterozygosity (LOH). While the drug could not demonstrate efficacy in cancer prevention, it did demonstrate that patients with lesions with LOH were at great risk for malignancy.

- A vital component in HNSCC and SPT prevention is the development of novel agents with low toxicity profiles that target key molecular pathways that are disrupted early in the carcinogenesis.

The principle mechanism of head and neck cancer prevention is avoidance of carcinogens. While sounding simplistic, data on the incidence of cancer through SEER database analysis and worldwide databases suggest that efforts to decrease tobacco exposure have led to decreases in the incidence of HNSCC linked to smoking. Unfortunately, the data also strongly suggests an increase in HPV-associated oropharyngeal cancer. It is unlikely that exposure to HPV per se can be targeted, but there are effective vaccines to combat the most prevalent high-risk HPV viruses associated with carcinogenesis. Initially developed for women at risk for uterine cervical cancer, the dramatic increases noted in oropharyngeal cancer has led the Centers for Disease Control (CDC) to expand their recommendations for vaccination for boys as well. The current recommendation is for vaccination with 9vHPV (Gardasil 9, Merck and Co., Inc.). This latest vaccine immunizes against nine high-risk HPV strains. The recommendation is for vaccination for all children age 11 or 12 years old, though also recommending vaccination for females age 13 to 26 and males age 13 to 21 who have not been vaccinated.[96]

While tobacco avoidance can minimize the risk of HNSCC, and cessation is strongly recommended, people with a history of past smoking, and those with a history of non-HPV HNSCC are still at risk. The concepts of field cancerization[96] and multistep carcinogenesis form the basis for research on better understanding the reasons these people have increased risk and are potential subjects for cancer chemoprevention.

Results of relatively large series revealed that patiets cured of their first head and neck cancer had a projected lifetime risk of developing SPTs of more than 20%. The estimated annual SPT development rate ranged from 4% to 6% for at least 8 years after the diagnosis of the first cancer.[97,98] In fact, SPTs are the leading cause of death among patients with early-stage head and neck cancers.[99] This patient population has served as a model for addressing the efficacy of *adjuvant chemoprevention* regimens. Unfortunately, a large multi-institutional randomized trial showed that isotretinoin did not significantly reduce the rate of SPTs (HR 1.06, 95% CI 0.83 to 1.35) or increase survival (HR 1.03, 95% CI 0.81 to 1.32) compared with placebo for patients with early-stage HNSCC.[100] However, this trial did show that current smokers had a higher rate of SPTs than did those who had never smoked (HR 1.64, 95% CI 1.08 to 2.50) or had formerly smoked (HR 1.32, 95% CI 1.01 to 1.71). Major sites of SPTs included the lung (31%), oral cavity (17%), larynx (8%), and pharynx (5%).

The observation of overexpression of EGFR in HNSCC led to interest in using orally available EGFR tyrosine kinase inhibitors for chemoprevention. The EPOC trial[101] tested erlotinib in a phase III placebo-controlled trial. This trial was unique in that the patients selected for trial were defined as being at risk due to identification of oral premalignant lesions (OPLs). Further, the OPLs were tested for loss of heterozygosity (LOH), and patients with OPLs that were LOH positive were eligible for randomization. The number of enrolled patients was 379, of whom 254 were LOH positive and 150 randomized to placebo or erlotinib. The study concluded with several interesting findings. Patients treated with erlotinib did not have an improvement in cancer-free survival (CFS), with 3-year rates of CFS 74% versus 70% for patients treated with placebo versus erlotinib, respectively ($P = 0.45$). However, the study did reveal that an erlotinib-induced rash was associated with improved CFS and LOH was associated with a poorer 3-year CFS (74% vs. 87% for LOH-positive vs. LOH-negative patients) ($P = 0.01$).

While the EPOC trial did not meet its primary end point, it did set an example for future trials. The principle effort is the development of novel agents with low toxicity profiles that target key molecular pathways that are disrupted early in the pathogenesis of carcinogenesis. The continued rapid growth in our understanding of the molecular genesis of HNSCC through a variety of omics-based research will hopefully lead to success in this endeavor.

SUMMARY

It has been exciting and gratifying to participate in laboratory research and clinical trials on head and neck cancer during the past three decades. Advances in technology have improved the precision with which radiation can be conformed to irregular target volumes and thereby reduce normal tissue toxicity. Progress in molecular biology techniques has opened new research avenues yielding new concepts or knowledge, such as the multistep tumor progression model, genetic susceptibility to environmental carcinogen-induced tumorigenesis, and processes of virus-induced changes in cellular behavior, factors, and mechanisms governing cellular and tissue radiation response. Some of the new wisdom has already found applications in developing novel therapy strategies that have completed or are undergoing preclinical and clinical testing. All in all, the basic and translational research efforts have finally paid off in that the head and neck cancer mortality rate in the United States has declined since the inception of record-keeping. For example, the annual death rate for men due to oral cavity and pharyngeal cancers in the United States decreased by an average of 1.9% and 3% between 1975 to 1993 and 1993 to 2001, respectively.[1]

It is very likely that the pace of discovery will increase in the coming years. For example, it is reasonable to envisage that, before long, sensitive methods for detecting occult tumor foci for screening and staging purposes will be developed and new approaches in characterizing the molecular profiles and signatures of individual cancers will accurately depict their virulence, predict their response to therapy, and guide the selection of treatment. Optimism in developing rational novel therapeutic strategies aimed at specific molecular targets to prevent malignant transformation or to reverse malignant phenotype is also increasing. Hopefully, the new insights and technologies gained from further research will have an additional sizable impact in reducing the mortality caused by head and neck cancers.

The fast pace of new discoveries and the large number of research directions make determining what constitutes standard therapy for a variety of patient subsets increasingly complex. In situations where several treatment options can yield approximately the same locoregional tumor control rate, other determinants to be taken into account in selecting the treatment of choice include cosmetic and functional outcome, acute and long-term morbidity (quality of life), resource utilization (cost), physician expertise, and patient convenience.

REFERENCES

1. Jemal A, Clegg LX, Ward E, et al. Annual report to the nation on the status of cancer, 1975–2001, with a special feature regarding survival. *Cancer* 2004;101:3–27.
2. Edwards BK, Brown ML, Wingo PA, et al. Annual report to the Nation on the Status of Cancer, 1975–2002, featuring population-based trends in cancer treatment. *J Natl Cancer Inst* 2005;97:1407–1427.
3. Petti S. Lifestyle risk factors for oral cancer. *Oral Oncol* 2009;45:340–350.
4. Blot WJ, McLaughlin JK, Winn DM, et al. Smoking and drinking in relation to oral and pharyngeal cancer. *Cancer Res* 1988;48:3282–3287.
5. Liebowitz D. Nasopharyngeal carcinoma: the Epstein-Barr virus association. *Semin Oncol* 1994;21:376–381.
6. Sheu LF, Chen A, Meng CL, et al. Enhanced malignant progression of nasopharyngeal carcinoma cells mediated by the expression of Epstein-Barr nuclear antigen 1 in vivo. *J Pathol* 1996;180:243–248.
7. Choi PHK, Suen MWM, Path MRC, et al. Nasopharyngeal carcinoma: genetic changes, Epstein-Barr virus infection, or both. *Cancer* 1993;72:2873–2878.
8. Huang DP, Lo KW, van Hasselt CA, et al. A region of homozygous deletion on chromosome 9p21–22 in primary nasopharyngeal carcinoma. *Cancer Res* 1994;54:4003–4006.
9. Lin DC, Meng X, Hazawa M, et al. The genomic landscape of nasopharyngeal carcinoma. *Nat Genet* 2014;46:866–871.
10. Lo K-W, Chung GT, To K-F. Deciphering the molecular genetic basis of NPC through molecular, cytogenetic and epigenetic approaches. *Semin Cancer Biol* 2012;22:79–86.
11. zur Hausen H, Schneider A. The role of papillomaviruses in human anogenital cancer. In: Salzman NP, Howley PM, eds. *The papovaviridae*. New York, NY: Plenum Publishing, 1987.
12. Kaur P, McDougall JK. Characterization of primary human keratinocytes transformed by human papillomavirus type 18. *J Virol* 1988;62:1917–1924.
13. Park NH, Min BM, Li SL, et al. Immortalization of normal human oral keratinocytes with type 16 human papillomavirus. *Carcinogenesis* 1991;12:1627–1631.
14. Woodworth CD, Bowden PE, Doniger J, et al. Characterization of normal human exocervical epithelial cells immortalized in vitro by papillomavirus types 16 and 18 DNA. *Cancer Res* 1988;48:4620–4628.
15. Barbosa MS, Schlegel R. The E6 and E7 genes of HPV-18 are sufficient for inducing two-stage in vitro transformation of human keratinocytes. *Oncogene* 1989;4:1529–1532.
16. Munger K, Phelps WC, Bubb V, et al. The E6 and E7 genes of the human papillomavirus type 16 together are necessary and sufficient for transformation of primary human keratinocytes. *J Virol* 1989;63:4417–4421.
17. Snijders PJ, Cromme FV, van den Brule AJ, et al. Prevalence and expression of human papillomavirus in tonsillar carcinomas, indicating a possible viral etiology. *Int J Cancer* 1992;51:845–850.
18. Gillison ML, Koch WM, Capone RB, et al. Evidence for a causal association between human papillomavirus and a subset of head and neck cancers. *J Natl Cancer Inst* 2000;92:709–720.
19. Steenbergen R, Hermsen M, Walboomers J, et al. Integrated human papillomavirus type 16 and loss of heterozygosity at 11q22 and 18q21 in an oral carcinoma and its derivative cell line. *Cancer Res* 1995;55:5465–5471.
20. Gillison ML, D'Souza G, Westra W, et al. Distinct risk factor profiles for human papillomavirus type 16-positive and human papillomavirus type 16-negative head and neck cancers. *J Natl Cancer Inst* 2008;100:407–420.
21. zur Hausen H. Papillomaviruses and cancer: from basic studies to clinical application. *Nat Rev Cancer* 2002;2:342–350.
22. Chung CH, Gillison ML. Human papillomavirus in head and neck cancer: its role in pathogenesis and clinical implications. *Clin Cancer Res* 2009;15:6758–6762.
23. Psyrri A, Gouveris P, Vermorken JB. Human papillomavirus-related head and neck tumors: clinical and research implication. *Curr Opin Oncol* 2009;21:201–205.
24. The Cancer Genome Atlas Network. Comprehensive genomic characterization of head and neck squamous cell carcinomas. *Nature* 2015;517:576–582.
25. Chaturvedi AK, Anderson WF, Lortet-Tieulent J, et al. Worldwide trends in incidence rates for oral cavity and oropharyngeal cancers. *J Clin Oncol* 2013;31:4550–4559.
26. Licitra L, Perrone F, Bossi P, et al. High-risk human papillomavirus affects prognosis in patients with surgically treated oropharyngeal squamous cell carcinoma. *J Clin Oncol* 2006;24:5630–5636.
27. Lindquist D, Romanitan M, Hammarstedt L, et al. Human papillomavirus is a favourable prognostic factor in tonsillar cancer and its oncogenic role is supported by the expression of E6 and E7. *Mol Oncol* 2007;1:350–355.
28. Lassen P, Eriksen JG, Hamilton-Dutoit S, et al. Effect of HPV-associated p16INK4A expression on response to

radiotherapy and survival in squamous cell carcinoma of the head and neck. *J Clin Oncol* 2009;27:1992–1998.

29. Fakhry C, Westra WH, Li S, et al. Improved survival of patients with human papillomavirus-positive head and neck squamous cell carcinoma in a prospective clinical trial. *J Natl Cancer Inst* 2008;100:261–269.

30. Ang KK, Harris J, Wheeler R, et al. Human papillomavirus (HPV) and survival of patients with oropharynx cancer. *N Engl J Med* 2010;363:24–35.

31. Califano J, van der Riet P, Westra W, et al. Genetic progression model for head and neck cancer: implications for field cancerization. *Cancer Res* 1996;56:2488–2492.

32. Ha PK, Chang SS, Glazer CA, et al. Molecular techniques and genetic alterations in head and neck cancer. *Oral Oncol* 2009;45:335–339.

33. Agarwal N, Frederick MJ, Pickering CR, et al. Exome sequencing of head and neck squamous cell carcinoma reveals inactivating mutations in *NOTCH1*. *Science* 2011;333:1154–1157.

34. Stransky N, Egloff AM, Tward AD, et al. The mutational landscape of head and neck squamous cell carcinoma. *Science* 2011;333:1157–1160.

35. American Cancer Society. *Cancer Facts & Figures 2009.* Atlanta, GA: American Cancer Society, 2009.

36. Lo YM, Chan LYS, Chan ATC, et al. Quantitative and temporal correlation between circulating cell-free Epstein-Barr virus DNA and tumor recurrence in nasopharyngeal carcinoma. *Cancer Res* 1999;59:5452–5455.

37. Chan ATC, Lo YMD, Zee B, et al. Plasma Epstein-Barr virus DNA and residual disease after radiotherapy for undifferentiated nasopharyngeal carcinoma. *J Natl Cancer Inst* 2002;94:1614–1619.

38. Lin J-C, Wang W-Y, Chen KY, et al. Quantification of plasma Epstein-Barr virus DNA in patients with advanced nasopharyngeal carcinoma. *N Engl J Med* 2004;350:2461–2470.

39. Nakao Y, Yang X, Yokoyama M, et al. Induction of p16 during immortalization by HPV 16 and 18 and not during malignant transformation. *Br J Cancer* 1997;75:1410–1416.

40. Ang KK, Zhang Q, Rosenthal DI, et al. Randomized phase III trial of concurrent accelerated radiation plus cisplatin with or without cetuximab for stage III to IV head and neck carcinoma: RTOG 0522. *J Clin Oncol* 2014;32:2940–2950.

41. Gillison ML, Zhang Q, Jordan R, et al. Tobacco smoking and increased risk of death and progression for patients with p16-positive and p16 negative oropharyngeal cancer. *J Clin Oncol* 2012;30:2102–2111.

42. O'Sullivan B, Huang SH, Siu, LL, et al. Deintensification candidate subgroups in human papillomavirus-related oropharyngeal cancer according to minimal risk of distant metastasis. *J Clin Oncol* 2013;31:543–550.

43. Lydiatt WM, Patel SG, O'Sullivan B, et al. Head and neck cancers- major changes in the American Joint Committee on cancer eighth edition cancer staging manual. *CA Cancer J Clin* 2017;67:122–137.

44. Burgess AW, Cho HS, Eigenbrot C, et al. An open-and-shut case? Recent insights into the activation of EGF/ErbB receptors. *Mol Cell* 2003;12:541–552.

45. Grandis J, Tweardy D. Elevated levels of transforming growth factor alpha and epidermal growth factor receptor messenger RNA are early markers of carcinogenesis in head and neck cancer. *Cancer Res* 1993;53:3579–3584.

46. Ang KK, Berkey BA, Tu X, et al. Impact of epidermal growth factor receptor expression on survival and pattern of relapse in patients with advanced head and neck carcinoma. *Cancer Res* 2002;62:7350–7356.

47. Soulieres D, Senzer NN, Vokes EE, et al. Multicenter Phase II Study of erlotinib, an oral epidermal growth factor receptor tyrosine kinase inhibitor, in patients with recurrent or metastatic squamous cell cancer of the head and neck. *J Clin Oncol* 2004;22:77–85.

48. Burtness B, Goldwasser MA, Flood W, et al. Phase III randomized trial of cisplatin plus placebo compared with cisplatin plus cetuximab in metastatic/recurrent head and neck cancer: an Eastern Cooperative Oncology Group Study. *J Clin Oncol* 2005;23:8646–8654.

49. Keren S, Shoude Z, Lu Z, et al. Role of EGFR as prognostic factor for survival in head and neck cancer: a meta-analysis. *Tumour Biol* 2014;35:2285–2295.

50. Munro AJ. An overview of randomised controlled trials of adjuvant chemotherapy in head and neck cancer. *Br J Cancer* 1995;71:83–91.

51. El-Sayed S, Nelson N. Adjuvant and adjunctive chemotherapy in the management of squamous cell carcinoma of the head and neck region. A meta-analysis of prospective and randomised trials. *J Clin Oncol* 1996;14:838–847.

52. Pignon JP, Bourhis J, Domenge C, et al. Chemotherapy added to locoregional treatment for head and neck squamous-cell carcinoma: three meta-analyses of updated individual data. *Lancet* 2000;355:949–955.

53. Pignon J-P, Maître Al, Maillard E, et al. Meta-analysis of chemotherapy in head and neck cancer (MACH-NC): an update on 93 randomised trials and 17,346 patients. *Radiother Oncol* 2009;92:4–14.

54. Trotti A, Bentzen SM. The need for adverse effects reporting standards in oncology clinical trials. *J Clin Oncol* 2004;22:19–22.

55. Forastiere AA, Zhang Q, Weber RS, et al. Long-term results of RTOG 99-11: a comparison of three nonsurgical treatment strategies to preserve the larynx in patients with locally advanced larynx cancer. *J Clin Oncol* 2013;31:845–852.

56. Nguyen-Tan PF, Zhang Q, Ang KK, et al. Randomized phase III trial to test accelerated versus standard fractionation in combination with concurrent cisplatin for head and neck carcinomas in the Radiation Therapy Oncology Group 0129 trial: long-term report of efficacy and toxicity. *J Clin Oncol* 2014;32:3858–3866.

57. Setton J, Lee NY, Riaz N, et al. A multi-institution pooled analysis of gastrostomy tube dependence in patients with oropharyngeal cancer treated with definitive intensity-modulated radiotherapy. *Cancer* 2015;121:294–301.

58. Cooper JS, Pajak TF, Forastiere AA, et al. Postoperative concurrent radiotherapy and chemotherapy for high-risk squamous-cell carcinoma of the head and neck. *N Engl J Med* 2004;350:1937–1944.

59. Bernier J, Domenge C, Ozsahin M, et al. Postoperative irradiation with or without concomitant chemotherapy for locally advanced head and neck cancer. *N Engl J Med* 2004;350:1945–1952.

60. Bernier J, Cooper JS, Pajak TF, et al. Defining risk levels in locally advanced head and neck cancers: a comparative analysis of concurrent postoperative radiation plus chemotherapy trials of the EORTC (#22931) and RTOG (#9501). *Head Neck* 2005;27:843–850.

61. Cooper JS, Zhang Q, Pajak TF, et al. Long-term follow-up of the RTOG 9501/intergroup phase III trial: postoperative concurrent radiation therapy and chemotherapy in high-risk squamous cell carcinoma of the head and neck. *Int J Radiat Oncol Biol Phys* 2012;84: 1198–1205.

62. Vermorken JB, Remenar E, van Herpen C, et al. Cisplatin, fluorouracil, and docetaxel in unresectable head and neck cancer. *N Engl J Med* 2007;357:1695–1704.

63. Posner MR, Hershock DM, Blajman CR, et al. Cisplatin and fluorouracil alone or with docetaxel in head and neck cancer. *N Engl J Med* 2007;357:1705–1715.

64. Pointreau Y, Garaud P, Chapet S, et al. Randomized trial of induction chemotherapy with cisplatin and 5-fluorouracil with or without docetaxel for larynx preservation. *J Natl Cancer Inst* 2009;101:498–506.

65. Cohen EE, Karrison TG, Kocherginsky M, et al. Phase III randomized trial of induction chemotherapy in patients with N2 or N3 locally advanced head and neck cancer. *J Clin Oncol* 2014;32:2735–2743.

66. Haddad R, O'Neill A, Rabinowits G, et al. Induction chemotherapy followed by concurrent chemoradiotherapy (sequential chemoradiotherapy) versus concurrent chemoradiotherapy alone in locally advanced head and neck cancer (PARADIGM): a randomized phase 3 trial. *Lancet Oncol* 2013;14:257–264.

67. Blanchard P, Lee A, Marguet S, et al. Chemotherapy and radiotherapy in nasopharyngeal carcinoma: an update of the MAC-NPC meta-analysis. *Lancet Oncol* 2015;16:645–655.

68. Forastiere AA, Goepfert H, Maor M, et al. Concurrent chemotherapy and radiotherapy for organ preservation in advanced laryngeal cancer. *N Engl J Med* 2003;349:2091–2098.

69. Janoray G, Pointreau Y, Garaud P, et al. Long-term results of a multicenter randomized phase III trial of induction chemotherapy with cisplatin, 5-fluorouracil, +/– docetaxel for larynx preservation. *J Natl Cancer Inst* 2015;108.

70. Harari PM, Harris J, Kies MS, et al. Postoperative chemoradiotherapy and cetuximab for high-risk squamous cell carcinoma of the head and neck: Radiation Therapy Oncology Group ROTG-0234. *J Clin Oncol* 2014;32:2486–2495.

71. Fu KK, Pajak TF, Trotti A, et al. A radiation therapy oncology group (RTOG) phase III randomized study to compare hyperfractionation and two variants of accelerated fractionation to standard fractionation radiotherapy for head and neck squamous cell carcinomas: first report of RTOG 9003. *Int J Radiat Oncol Biol Phys* 2000;48:7–16.

72. Overgaard J, Hansen HS, Specht L, et al. Five compared with six fractions per week of conventional radiotherapy of squamous-cell carcinoma of head and neck: DAHANCA 6 and 7 randomized controlled trial. *Lancet* 2003;362:933–940.

73. Bourhis J, Overgaard J, Audry H, et al. Hyperfractionated or accelerated radiotherapy in head and neck cancer: a meta-analysis. *Lancet* 2006;368:843–854.

74. Weber RS, Berkey BA, Forastiere A, et al. Outcome of salvage total laryngectomy following organ preservation therapy: the Radiation Therapy Oncology Group trial 91–11. *Arch Otolaryngol Head Neck Surg* 2003;129:44–49.

75. Verhey LJ. Comparison of three-dimensional conformal radiation therapy and intensity-modulated radiation therapy systems. *Semin Radiat Oncol* 1999;9:78–98.

76. Eisbruch A, Ten Haken RK, Kim HM, et al. Dose, volume, and function relationships in parotid salivary glands following conformal and intensity-modulated irradiation of head and neck cancer. *Int J Radiat Oncol Biol Phys* 1999;45:577–587.

77. Dijkema T, Raaijmakers CP, Ten Haken RK, et al. Parotid gland function after radiotherapy: the combined Michigan and Utrecht experience. *Int J Radiat Oncol Biol Phys* 2010;78:449–453.

78. Kam MKM, Leung S-F, Zee B, et al. Prospective randomized study of intensity-modulated radiotherapy on salivary gland function in early-stage nasopharyngeal carcinoma patients. *J Clin Oncol* 2007;25:4873–4879.

79. Pow EHN, Kwong DLW, McMillan AS, et al. Xerostomia and quality of life after intensity-modulated radiotherapy vs. conventional radiotherapy for early-stage nasopharyngeal carcinoma: initial report on a randomized controlled clinical trial. *Int J Radiat Oncol Biol Phys* 2006;66:981–991.

80. Nutting CM, Morden JP, Harrington KJ, et al. Parotid-sparing intensity modulated versus conventional radiotherapy in head and neck cancer (PARSPORT): a phase 3 multicentre randomized controlled trial. *Lancet Oncol* 2011;12:127–136.

81. van Luijk P, Pringle S, Deasy JO, et al. Sparing the region of the salivary gland containing stem cells preserves saliva production after radiotherapy for head and neck cancer. *Sci Transl Med* 2015;7:305.

82. Sanguinetti G, Califano J, Stafford E, et al. Defining the risk of involvement for each neck nodal level in patients with early T-stage node-positive oropharyngeal carcinoma. *Int J Radiat Oncol Biol Phys* 2009;74:1356–1364.

83. Gensheimer MF, Liao JJ, Garden AS, et al. Submandibular gland-sparing radiation therapy for locally advanced oropharyngeal squamous cell carcinoma: patterns of failure and xerostomia outcomes. *Radiat Oncol* 2014;9:255.

84. Feng FY, Kim HM, Lyden TH, et al. Intensity-modulated chemoradiotherapy aiming to reduce dysphagia in patients with oropharyngeal cancer: clinical and functional results. *J Clin Oncol* 2010;28:2732–2738.

85. Paleri V, Roe JW, Strojan P, et al. Strategies to reduce long-term postchemoradiation dysphagia in patients with head and neck cancer: an evidence-based review. *Head Neck* 2014;36:431–443.

86. van der Laan HP, van de Water TA, van Herpt HE, et al. The potential of intensity-modulated proton radiotherapy to reduce swallowing dysfunction in the treatment of head and neck cancer: a planning comparative study. *Acta Oncol* 2013;52:561–569.

87. Lee AW, Ng WT, Chan LL, et al. Evolution of treatment for nasopharyngeal cancer—success and setback in the intensity-modulated radiotherapy era. *Radiother Oncol* 2014;110:377–384.

88. Al-Mamgani A, Monserez D, Roook PV, et al. Highly-conformal intensity-modulated radiotherapy reduced toxicity without jeopardizing outcome in patients with paranasal sinus cancer treated by surgery and radiotherapy or (chemo)radiation. *Oral Oncol* 2012;48:905–911.

89. Beadle BM, Liao KP, Elting LS, et al. Improved survival using intensity-modulated radiation therapy in head and neck cancers: a SEER-Medicare analysis. *Cancer* 2014;120:702–710.

90. Bonner JA, Harari PM, Giralt J, et al. Radiotherapy plus cetuximab for squamous-cell carcinoma of the head and neck. *N Engl J Med* 2006;354:567–578.

91. Bonner JA, Harari PM, Giralt J, et al. Radiotherapy plus cetuximab for locoregionally advanced head and neck cancer: 5-year survival data from a phase 3 randomised trial, and relation between cetuximab-induced rash and survival. *Lancet Oncol* 2010;11:21–28.

92. Lefebvre JL, Pointreau Y, Roland F, et al. Induction chemotherapy followed by either chemoradiotherapy or bioradiotherapy for larynx preservation: the TREMPLIN randomized phase II study. *J Clin Oncol* 2013;31:853–859.

93. Rosenthal DI, Harari PM, Giralt J, et al. Association of human papillomavirus and p16 status with outcomes in the IMCL-815 phase III registration trial for patient with locoregionally advanced oropharyngeal squamous cell carcinoma of the head and neck treated with radiotherapy with or without cetuximab. *J Clin Oncol* 2016;34:1300–1308. doi:10.1200/JCO.2015.62.5970.

94. Giralt J, Trigo J, Nuyyts S, et al. Panitumumab plus radiotherapy versus chemoradiotherapy in patients with unresected, locally advanced squamous-cell carcinoma of the head and neck (CONCERT-2): a randomized, controlled, open-label phase 2 trial. *Lancet Oncol* 2015;16:221–232.

95. Slaughter DP, Southwick HW, Smejkal W. "Field cancerization" in oral stratified squamous epithelium: clinical implications of multicentric origin. *Cancer* 1953;6:963–968.

96. Meites E, Kempe A, Markowitz LE. Use of a 2-dose schedule for Human Papillomavirus vaccination — Updated recommendations of the Advisory Committee on Immunization Practices. *MMWR Morb Mortal Wkly Rep* 2016;65:1405–1408. DOI: http://dx.doi.org/10.15585/mmwr.mm6549a5

97. Cooper JS, Pajak TF, Rubin P, et al. Second malignancies in patients who have head and neck cancer: incidence, effect on survival and implications based on the RTOG experience. *Int J Radiat Oncol Biol Phys* 1989;17:449–456.

98. Vokes EE, Weichselbaum RR, Lippman SM, et al. Head and neck cancer. *N Engl J Med* 1993;328:184–193.

99. Lippman SM, Hong WK. Second malignant tumors in head and neck squamous cell carcinoma: the overshadowing threat for patients with early stage disease. *Int J Radiat Oncol Biol Phys* 1989;17:691–694.

100. Khuri FR, Lee JJ, Lippman SM, et al. Randomized phase III trial of low-dose isotretinoin for prevention of second primary tumors in stage I and II head and neck cancer patients. *J Natl Cancer Inst* 2006;98:441–450.

101. William Jr WN, Papadimitralopoulou V, Lee JJ, et al. Erlotinib and the risk of oral cancer: the erlotinib prevention of oral cancer (EPOC) randomized clinical trial. *JAMA Oncol* 2016;2:209–216. doi:10.1001/jamaoncol.2015.4364

2

Modes of Therapy

PRIMARY RADIOTHERAPY

Key Points

- External beam radiotherapy, generally using 6-MV x-rays, has an important role in frontline therapy for patients with carcinoma of the oropharynx, larynx, or hypopharynx; its aim is to eradicate tumors while preserving organ structure and function.

- Intensity-modulated radiation therapy (IMRT) has been widely adopted because of its ability to better target tumors and reduce late morbidity by diminishing the radiation dose to salivary glands and other critical organs.

- Proton therapy may provide more conformality in the treatment of head and neck cancers and is an area of active investigation.

- Chemotherapy is often given to improve control of locally advanced carcinomas. The greatest benefit is when chemotherapy is given concurrently with radiation. Recent studies suggest that the benefits of sequential chemotherapy and chemoradiation are minimal.

- Surgery remains the preferred therapy for cancers of the oral cavity, paranasal sinuses, salivary glands, and thyroid and also for less common head and neck neoplasms.

- Postoperative radiation, alone or combined with concurrent chemotherapy when indicated, is an established adjuvant treatment for patients with adverse surgical pathologic features, such as multiple positive lymph nodes, extranodal disease extension, positive surgical margins, and perineural invasion, among others.

External Beam Irradiation (Teletherapy)

Primary frontline radiotherapy is generally preferred for the treatment of patients with carcinoma of the oropharynx, larynx, or hypopharynx. Such therapy is most often delivered through external beam irradiation with 6-MV x-rays. Selected cases may benefit from incorporating higher-energy photon beams for deeper-seated targets. The increasing capabilities to modulate photon beams to provide ideal dose distributions have diminished the use of electron beams. However, electrons of 6 to 20 MeV still have occasional benefits for the treatment of superficial tumors and as boost treatments, particularly for nodal disease. The choice of the beam type and energy is based on the location and geometric parameters of the target volumes. Occasionally, orthovoltage x-rays can be useful, for example, for the treatment of skin cancers or for intraoral cone therapy for accessible, well-circumscribed tumors of the oral cavity or anterior oropharynx. Proton therapy may provide an improvement in desired dose distributions and is a modality that is being actively investigated.

The initial target volume for external beam therapy includes both the gross tumor, as determined by clinical examinations and diagnostic imaging, and the potential routes of subclinical (microscopic) disease spread. Historically, a shrinking field technique was widely used in which the target volume is reduced after a dose sufficient to sterilize subclinical disease is reached and then an additional boost dose is delivered to the demonstrable gross tumor. The boost dose may be given after or concomitantly with the initial large-field target volume irradiations. In the latter scenario, the boost irradiations are administered as second daily fractions.[1] The concept of treating a larger volume and then reducing the "fields" of radiation is still used with IMRT occasionally but has largely been replaced with simultaneous integrated boosts (SIBs). As intensity-modulated treatment allows delivery of differing doses to differing targets within one treatment, the SIB concept is to deliver the maximal dose to the gross target volume(s) with margin, while lower doses are delivered "simultaneously" to subclinical sites of disease.

The common practice in the United States until the late 1990s was to administer primary radiotherapy in 2-Gy fractions, once a day, 5 days a week, to total doses ranging from 66 to 70 Gy depending on the tumor stage and site. As summarized in Chapter 1, intensive clinical investigations conducted during the past three decades revealed the superiority of altered fractionation when radiation is delivered as a single modality.[2,3] When chemotherapy is delivered concurrently, the advantages of altered fractionation are moot. Thus, most treatment regimens remain once daily, 5 days a week. Subtle acceleration with concurrent chemotherapy and IMRT is occasionally done to deliver 70 Gy in 33 fractions. This fractionation was principally designed due to concerns of lowering the fractional subclinical dose, but particularly with concurrent chemotherapy and the shape of the dose–response curve being relatively linear and flat, these concerns may be overstated. The observation that oropharyngeal cancer associated with human papillomavirus (HPV) appears to have increased radiosensitivity has led to investigations of both lower dose per fraction and lower total doses, but to date, there is no sufficient evidence to modify dose nor dose per fraction for this disease.

Intensity-Modulated Radiation Therapy

As presented in Chapter 1, advances in computing and engineering technologies have greatly improved the flexibility and precision of aiming radiation beams at irregular volumes. Such precision radiotherapy can be achieved with intensity-modulated photon beams in IMRT. With IMRT, all target volumes are irradiated during every radiation session, but with a properly shaped dose gradient, a higher dose per fraction (e.g., 2 Gy) is delivered to the clinical target volume (CTV), which encompasses the gross tumor (primary lesion and involved nodes) with 1- to 1.5-cm margins (CTV_{HD}), a lower elective dose (e.g., 1.6 Gy per fraction) to subclinical disease target volumes (CTV_{ED}), and, when desired, an intermediate dose (e.g., 1.8 Gy per fraction) to intermediary volumes (CTV_{ID}) surrounding the CTV_{HD}. It should be noted, however, that in addition to delivering radiation in smaller fractions, the overall radiotherapy time for treating

subclinical disease is prolonged from the conventional 5 weeks (50 Gy in 25 fractions) up to 6 to 7 weeks (30 to 35 fractions). Therefore, it is prudent to adjust the dose to the electively irradiated regions to correct for these changes. Consequently, when IMRT is given in 6 weeks to deliver a total dose of 66 Gy in 30 fractions to CTV_{HD} such as in the treatment of T1 to T2 oropharyngeal carcinoma, we currently prescribe 54 Gy (1.8 Gy per fraction) to the elective volume. When a total dose of 70 Gy is given in 35 fractions (2.0 Gy per fraction) to CTV_{HD} for treatment of larger tumors, we prescribe 56 Gy (1.6 Gy per fraction) to CTV_{ED} and 63 Gy to CTV_{ID}. In the latter scenario, IMRT can be given in conventional fractionation over 7 weeks by delivering five daily fractions per week or in accelerated fractionation over 6 weeks by administering six fractions per week (usually by prescribing two fractions a day, with a 6-hour interfraction interval, 1 day a week, for 5 weeks), a schedule modeled after the regimen used by Danish investigators.[4]

Brachytherapy

Brachytherapy is usually combined with external beam therapy. The rationale for this combination is that areas at risk of harboring subclinical disease are irradiated with external beams to a dose sufficient to sterilize microscopic deposits and that the gross lesion is boosted with a brachytherapy system to higher doses. This approach results in exposing a smaller volume of normal tissues to high radiation doses. Therefore, if applied appropriately by an experienced team, high tumor control rates can be obtained with generally low treatment morbidity.

Brachytherapy is used in the form of interstitial implants (e.g., for primary cancer of the base of tongue or tonsillar fossa extending into the base of tongue), molds (e.g., for lesions of the hard palate), or intracavitary applicators (e.g., for recurrent nasopharyngeal cancer).

In selected situations, brachytherapy is used alone. Examples of such applications include treatment of superficial lip cancers, small nasal vestibule neoplasms, and alveolar ridge carcinomas. Brachytherapy alone is also used occasionally for reirradiation to minimize the volumes of tissue exposed to cumulative very high doses.

High-precision external beam radiation techniques such as IMRT can better conform the high-dose region to the tumor with narrow margins. Therefore, IMRT has gradually been substituted for brachytherapy in the treatment of head and neck cancer.

Proton Therapy

The advent of commercially available proton delivery systems has created an increase in interest in proton therapy. Protons are one of several particles that are available for radiotherapeutic purposes. To date, the principal theoretical advantage of protons is based on its physical properties to deliver an improved dose distribution. The biologic advantages remain speculative.

For all practical purposes, proton therapy can be considered a type of conformal therapy; therapy aimed at delivering optimal doses to tumor targets while avoiding dose to normal tissues. However, rather than using numerous beam paths typically all aimed at targets while spreading out dose to non-target tissue as with photons, protons accomplish their conformality based on the beam properties inherent and unique to proton therapy. These properties include a modest entrance dose, a fairly uniform dose within the target, and then a rapid falloff of dose at the distal end of the range of the beam. This description may sound similar to electron beam characteristics, but protons have a much sharper fall off of dose at the distal range, can be more penetrating, and thus are able to treat deeper targets.

A Bragg curve is a graph of the linear energy transfer (LET) of a charged particle through a range of a given material. As described above, protons have a fairly uniform energy transfer on entrance through a material and dependent on the energy of the proton beam will have a very high but narrow deposition of its energy and then dissipate to close to zero energy very rapidly. This narrow high-energy transfer followed by rapid falloff is called the Bragg peak and is the basis for the therapeutic advantage of protons. Since tumor targets are broader than the narrow Bragg peak, it is necessary to widen it, creating a spread out Bragg peak (SOBP) that will allow for the high dose to be deposited in a wider target while still maintaining the rapid falloff of dose at the distal end of the range.

There are two methods to deliver protons with current technology. Passive scattering is accomplished by broadening the incoming narrow proton beam. A combination of an individually designed collimator and tissue compensator shapes the beam in the radial dimensions and creates conformality at the distal aspect of the target. The second method, active scanning, uses a series of "pencil beams" that are steered and deflected with the use of magnets. These beams are successively layered by varying the energy of the protons to create desired dose distributions. Active scanning has several advantages over passive scattering. There is less neutron contamination with active scanning, as there is less interaction with devices between the beam and patient. Additionally, individual devices do not have to be fabricated for each patient. This not only saves in general costs but also allows for easier adaption of plans should there be a change in the patient or tumor that could alter the precise and accurate delivery of dose. An additional advantage to active scanning is the ability to perform intensity-modulated proton therapy (IMPT). Akin to its photon counterpart (IMRT), IMPT allows for additional conformality to try to create the optimal plan that achieves the desired goals of therapy. IMPT plans can be designed with either single-field optimization (SFO) **(Case Study 2.1)** or multiple-field optimization (MFO) **(Case Study 2.2)**. These terms can be confusing since both plans use multiple fields. The principle difference is that with SFO, each field is optimized individually, and then the doses from each beam are summated. In IMPT planned with MFO, all the fields are optimized simultaneously. This allows for

improved conformality. However, currently, this complexity in computer-generated beam design can lead to increased sensitivity to patient setup and anatomic changes and the need for more frequent verification.

At the present, the biologic advantages of protons are moot. The radiobiologic equivalence used is 1.1, a generally accepted figure, though animal studies have suggested this number falls in a range between 1.05 and 1.25. Compared to other particle therapy, that is, neutrons or heavy particles, this is still a relatively low RBE. However, questions remain regarding not only the general RBE but also whether there is a varying RBE within each proton beam. Specifically, some are questioning whether the RBE increases at the distal end of the Bragg peak, and if so, can this be taken advantage of. For the present, protons are advocated for the potential of greater conformality and also avoidance of the low-dose bath seen with IMRT that is considered "safe" but is unnecessary and may have underappreciated consequences.

Concurrent Radiation and Chemotherapy

As presented in Chapter 1, data from several clinical trials have demonstrated that concurrent radiation–chemotherapy regimens improve the local–regional control of locally advanced head and neck cancers, and some regimens also improve survival rates over those of radiation alone. Sufficient studies have been conducted such that concurrent chemotherapy and radiation is considered standard of care for locally advanced head and neck cancer. There is general agreement that patients with T3 or T4 disease (treated without surgery) benefit from this combined approach. Since, by definition, any patient with lymphadenopathy is considered to have locally advanced disease, most guidelines recommend concurrent chemoradiation for those patients as well, though a patient with low-volume primary and nodal disease may be adequately treated with radiation alone. The indications for concurrent chemotherapy and radiation in the postoperative setting are for patients identified as "high risk" for recurrence. The data from randomized trials have identified patients with nodal extracapsular extension or positive margins as "high risk."[5]

Outside of the protocol study setting, for patients treated definitively with radiation, the combination of conventional fractionation (70 Gy in 35 fractions over 7 weeks) with three cycles of cisplatin (100 mg/m^2) given during weeks 1, 4, and 7 is often recommended (even for patients with HPV-associated oropharyngeal carcinoma) because this regimen has the longest and most solid track record. Results of phase III trials have shown that as primary therapy, this regimen improves local–regional control and survival as compared with radiation alone for patients with locally advanced nasopharyngeal carcinoma[6,7] and other head and neck carcinomas.[8] It also increases the likelihood of laryngeal preservation.[9] The combination of conventionally fractionated radiotherapy with cisplatin given as postoperative adjunctive therapy also improves local–regional control, disease-free survival,[10,11] and survival[11] in patients with high-risk surgical pathologic features.[5]

CASE STUDY 2.1

A 50-year-old gentleman on chronic immunosuppressants due to a renal transplant presented to our center with a multiply recurrent cutaneous squamous carcinoma of the right upper lip.

He underwent wide local excision and reconstruction of the surgical defect with an Abbe flap. Surgical margins were negative. Pathology revealed poor differentiation and extensive perineural invasion.

He was then treated with postoperative proton therapy using passive scattering technique to the tumor bed (60 Gy[RBE]), operative bed (57 Gy[RBE]), and nerve tracts at risk (54 Gy[RBE]) all in 30 fractions. Dose distributions at the level of the tumor bed are shown (Fig. 2.1A) and highlight the rapid falloff deep to the targets. The brass aperture (Fig. 2.1B) used to shape one of the five fields and the associated acrylic compensator (Fig. 2.1C) are shown.

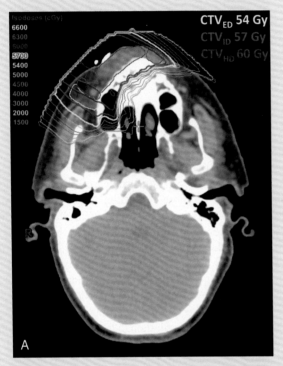

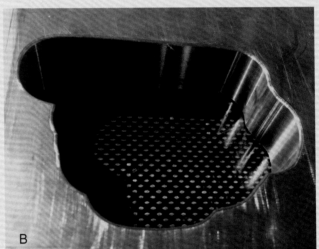

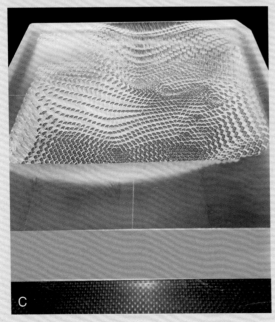

Case Figure 2.1 A–C

CASE STUDY 2.2

A 33-year-old female noticed anisocoria with associated headache and nasal congestion, which prompted evaluation with an otolaryngologist. A nasopharyngeal mass was evident with clival destruction and sphenoid sinus involvement. Biopsy revealed adenoid cystic carcinoma. There were no regional or distant metastases, and the tumor was judged to be unresectable.

She was treated with definitive concurrent chemoradiation using active scanning proton therapy, IMPT-MFO technique. Following CT simulation, she underwent volumetric MRI in the treatment position, which was fused with the treatment planning CT in order to accurately delineate targets and avoidance structures at the base of skull. She was treated to 70 Gy(RBE) in 33 fractions to the GTV with narrow margin. Aspects of the GTV adjacent to the brainstem, temporal lobes, and optic structures were targeted to 66 Gy(RBE), but were optimized to respect critical structure tolerance. Surrounding soft tissue regions at risk were treated to 56 Gy(RBE). The three CTVs are shown (Fig. 2.2A) on a representative axial slice of the fused MRI.

Two anterior oblique and a single vertex field were used. IMPT dose distributions are displayed on the MRI in both the axial (Fig. 2.2B) and sagittal planes (Fig. 2.2C) and highlight the sparing of brain and oral cavity. A mouth-opening tongue-depressing oral stent and bite block were used for simulation and treatment. She initially received weekly cisplatin (40 mg/m²), but was transitioned to carboplatin toward the end of treatment due to ototoxicity.

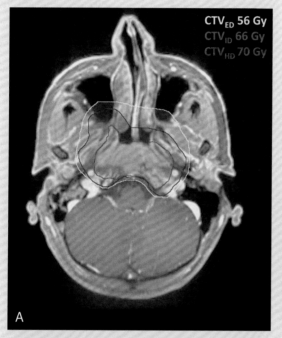

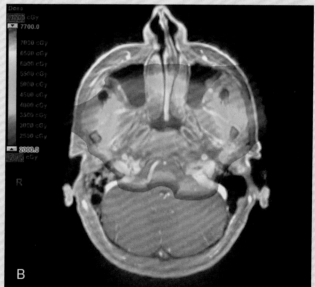

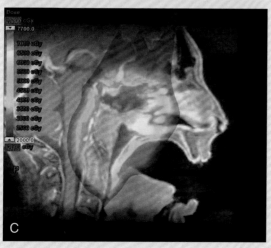

Case Figure 2.2 A–C

The large meta-analysis on the role of chemotherapy in head and neck cancer concluded that concurrent chemoradiation provides a survival advantage over radiation alone.[12] Secondary analyses of this pool of data suggested that single-agent chemotherapy was most efficacious, and platins were the most efficacious single agents. A review of the platin-based trials in the meta-analysis reveals that the majority were with cisplatin. While carboplatin is very similar to cisplatin, and often substituted for cisplatin, there is no strong evidence to advocate carboplatin as routine.

Additionally, the majority of data on cisplatin, as described above, is by administering cisplatin in high doses, every 3 weeks. There is great interest in administering cisplatin as a weekly drug in doses of 30 to 40 mg/m^2. It is believed that the cumulative dose of a weekly regimen would be equivalent to the q3 week high-dose regimens and may provide more radiosensitization by allowing more frequent interaction with radiation. Further, a weekly regimen of cisplatin is used concurrent with radiation to treat uterine cervical carcinoma. While there is no strong evidence to support superiority or even equivalency of a weekly regimen compared with the q3 week high-dose regimen, these regimens are becoming more popular and are even being incorporated into clinical trials in lieu of the standard high-dose schedules. Our retrospective experience suggests no major detriment with using concurrent weekly cisplatin compared to cisplatin delivered q3 weeks; however, the weekly regimen also did not appear to be significantly less toxic.[13]

Concurrent Radiation and Cetuximab

Data from a single randomized trial showed that adding eight weekly doses of cetuximab to radiation improves local–regional control and survival rates without increasing radiation-induced side effects such as mucositis and dysphagia when compared to radiation alone.[14] Consequently, this biologically oriented combined regimen has become one of several currently approved standard frontline therapies for locally advanced carcinoma of the oropharynx, larynx, or hypopharynx. As the toxicity profile of concurrent cetuximab–radiation was demonstrated to be similar to radiation alone, while nearly all trials demonstrate increased toxicity when cisplatin is added to radiation, the RTOG recently completed a large phase III trial comparing cetuximab–radiation to cisplatin–radiation for patients with HPV-associated oropharyngeal cancer. It is hoped that cetuximab–radiation will be noninferior with regard to survival outcomes and demonstrate less toxicity.

Radiotherapy after Chemotherapy

Neoadjuvant chemotherapy can produce complete tumor responses in up to 20% of patients and partial tumor response in up to 60% of patients. Despite these occasional impressive responses, there is a paucity of data suggesting neoadjuvant chemotherapy improves ultimate outcomes. As described in Chapter 1, two recent phase III trials showed that taxane-based neoadjuvant chemotherapy given before concurrent chemoradiation did not yield superior overall survival rates compared with concurrent chemoradiation.[15,16]

The long-term results of RTOG 91-11[9] left questions of the benefit of neoadjuvant chemotherapy compared with concurrent chemoradiation when laryngeal preservation is a component of the treatment goals. The two chemotherapy regimens tested in this trial resulted in equivalent outcomes for the primary end-point, laryngectomy-free survival. Patients treated with concomitant cisplatin–radiation had improved larynx preservation rates compared to patients treated with induction therapy, but there was a suggestion that the reverse was true for overall survival. Patients treated with concomitant therapy had a higher rate of death not attributed to larynx cancer.

Induction therapy remains controversial and continues to be studied in patients with nasopharyngeal cancer. The relatively high rates of distant disease in patients with nasopharyngeal cancer have made it a disease where effective systemic therapy should be beneficial. However, since original trial design incorporated not only concurrent therapy but also adjuvant therapy, the benefit of each individual change remains unclear. Extrapolating from other head and neck disease sites combined with the results of a recent meta-analysis,[17] it is generally agreed that the concomitant component of therapy provides significant benefit, while the gains from adjuvant therapy remain moot. As neoadjuvant therapy is preferred in most situations over postradiation adjuvant chemotherapy, several trials have incorporated induction therapy. However, randomized trials are still ongoing to resolve the question of benefit of chemotherapy sequenced with concomitant chemoradiation. Recently, preliminary results of NPC-0501 were reported.[18] This complex trial attempted to answer several questions including changing from concurrent-adjuvant to induction-concurrent chemoradiotherapy. The conclusions did not show a significant benefit to this change. The study not only highlighted whether there is a benefit to any sequential program but also demonstrated that adjuvant or induction therapy may be dependent on the specifics of the drugs used and so should not be thought of only in abstract conceptual terms.

For patients receiving induction chemotherapy, our policy is to irradiate the entire anatomical region containing the original tumor volume with adequate margins to doses equivalent to those from primary radiotherapy alone. A small dose reduction is sometimes made when the tumor is adjacent to critical organs, such as locally advanced nasopharyngeal carcinoma adjacent to optic structures or with intracranial extension, or when acute reactions are excessive.

Adjuvant Postoperative Radiotherapy

Surgery is the preferred treatment for cancer of the oral cavity, paranasal sinuses, salivary glands, and thyroid.

Advanced carcinomas of the oropharynx, larynx, or hypopharynx (e.g., those invading the mandible or neck soft tissues) are often also treated with a combination of surgery and radiation. The general indications for postoperative radiotherapy include close or positive surgical margins, perineural spread, lymphovascular invasion, contiguous tumor extension into bone or neck soft tissue, multiple positive nodes, and extracapsular extension of nodal disease. Radiation with 6-MV x-rays often includes consideration of using a 3-mm scar bolus to deliver sufficient dose to the subcutaneous tissues.

As a general principle, the entire operative bed is included in the postoperative target volume. The donor site(s) for skin grafts or myocutaneous flaps is not considered part of the operative bed in this context. With conventional techniques, several field reductions may be necessary to deliver desired doses to the undissected nodal basins, surgical bed, and regions at high risk of recurrence, such as sites of extensive extracapsular extension or positive margins. IMRT is also being increasingly used for postoperative treatment because of its ability to better distribute radiation dose according to high-risk features while sparing salivary glands and other critical normal tissues. The target volume that is to receive higher doses and the total doses prescribed are based on surgical pathologic findings.

In the presence of perineural invasion of major or named nerves, our general policy is to treat the course of involved major nerves at least to the skull base. However, if only minor unnamed nerves are histologically involved, slightly larger portals (e.g., with margins of an additional 2 or 3 cm) are generally selected with more limited tracking of the nerves at risk.

The general rule is to start radiotherapy as soon as the surgical wound has healed, usually 3 to 4 weeks after surgery. With good communication between surgical, radiation, and dental oncologists, treatment simulations generally can take place 3 to 4 weeks after surgery, and radiotherapy can start within a week for most patients. This approach requires that dental assessment occur before surgery to determine the need for extractions when postoperative radiotherapy is contemplated. When postoperative radiotherapy is recommended, dental care can be provided at the time of cancer surgery to avoid the need for a second anesthesia for full-mouth tooth extraction and unnecessary delay in initiating radiotherapy.

Our series revealed that completion of combined therapy within 11 weeks yielded better local–regional control and better survival rates than completion of treatment in 11 to 13 weeks, and finishing combined therapy in more than 13 weeks resulted in a much worse outcome.[19] When delayed wound healing postpones postoperative radiation beyond 5 to 6 weeks after surgery, we prescribe accelerated fractionation to reduce the overall treatment time by 1 week to avoid the potential deleterious effects of prolonged cumulative treatment time. Using this strategy, a dose of 60 Gy is given in 5 weeks, which may induce more severe mucositis but does not increase the rate of late complications.

Our general dose guidelines for postoperative radiation are to deliver 60 Gy to the tumor bed, 56 to 57 Gy to the operative bed, and 50 to 54 Gy to subclinical sites at risk that have not been surgically violated. Treatment is planned to be delivered in 30 fractions. The range of doses above is dependent on technique; for conventional techniques with shrinking fields, where all sites get 2 Gy per fraction, the lower doses are selected. If IMRT is used, and all targets are treated simultaneously, due to the slightly lower fractional dose, the doses at the higher end of the range are used.

The benefit of doses above 60 Gy to high-risk areas remains controversial. A randomized study demonstrated that dose escalation above 63 Gy (at 1.8 Gy per fraction) did not improve the therapeutic ratio.[20] This study was of radiation alone postoperatively. The two seminal trials of postoperative chemoradiation had dose ranges of 60 to 66 Gy (2 Gy per fraction).[5] They were not designed nor able to resolve the radiation dose question. Thus, while the benefit of higher doses remains questionable, the ability of IMRT to limit this high-dose area if appropriately identified seems to allow a reasonable compromise in many situations. More dose can be given to the highest risk region, while the potential for increased toxicity can be minimized if the volume identified is small.

Preoperative Radiotherapy

Preoperative radiotherapy is rarely used in our practice because of the surgeons' preference to operate in an unirradiated field where frozen section control of surgical margins can be obtained. In certain circumstances, however, planned preoperative radiotherapy may be given.

These include situations in which the cancer is marginally resectable or has a very rapid growth history. Patients with small radiocurable primary tumors and large adenopathy may be treated with definitive radiation to the primary tumor and preoperative radiation to the neck with a planned neck dissection to follow radiation. This strategy is particularly appealing for patients with bulky disease in the level IV nodal region, to eliminate the need to administer a total dose of 70 Gy to the brachial plexus. Neck dissection is performed approximately 6 weeks after radiotherapy.

For most preoperative treatments, the dose is limited to that required for sterilization of subclinical disease, that is, 50 Gy in 25 fractions over 5 weeks. For very advanced tumors, a dose of 60 Gy in 30 fractions over 6 weeks may be administered. Surgery may also be performed, however, after full-dose primary radiotherapy if residual disease persists at 6 or more weeks after completion of treatment. This situation occurs mostly in the presence of a large nodal mass. The timing for surgery is generally about 6 weeks after completion of radiation.

REFERENCES

1. Ang KK, Peters LJ, Weber RS, et al. Concomitant boost radiotherapy schedules in the treatment of carcinoma of the oropharynx and nasopharynx. *Int J Radiat Oncol Biol Phys* 1990;19:1339–1345.
2. Bourhis J, Overgaard J, Audry H, et al. Hyperfractionated or accelerated radiotherapy in head and neck cancer: a meta-analysis. *Lancet* 2006;368:843–854.
3. Fu KK, Pajak TF, Trotti A, et al. A Radiation Therapy Oncology Group (RTOG) phase III randomized study to compare hyperfractionation and two variants of accelerated fractionation to standard fractionation radiotherapy for head and neck squamous cell carcinomas: first report of RTOG 9003. *Int J Radiat Oncol Biol Phys* 2000;48:7–16.
4. Overgaard J, Hansen HS, Specht L, et al. Five compared with six fractions per week of conventional radiotherapy of squamous-cell carcinoma of head and neck: DAHANCA 6 and 7 randomised controlled trial. *Lancet* 2003;362:933–940.
5. Bernier J, Cooper JS, Pajak TF, et al. Defining risk levels in locally advanced head and neck cancers: a comparative analysis of concurrent postoperative radiation plus chemotherapy trials of the EORTC (#22931) and RTOG (# 9501). *Head Neck* 2005;27:843–850.
6. Al-Sarraf M, LeBlance M, Shanker PG, et al. Chemoradiotherapy versus radiotherapy in patients with advanced nasopharyngeal cancer: phase III randomized intergroup study 0099. *J Clin Oncol* 1998;16: 1310–1317.
7. Wee J, Tan EH, Tai BC, et al. Randomized trial of radiotherapy versus concurrent chemoradiotherapy followed by adjuvant chemotherapy in patients with American Joint Committee on Cancer/International Union against cancer stage III and IV nasopharyngeal cancer of the endemic variety. *J Clin Oncol* 2005;23:6730–6738.
8. Adelstein DJ, Li Y, Adams GL, et al. An Intergroup Phase III Comparison of standard radiation therapy and two schedules of concurrent chemoradiotherapy in patients with unresectable squamous cell head and neck cancer. *J Clin Oncol* 2003;21:92–98.
9. Forastiere AA, Zhang Q, Weber RS, et al. Long-term results of RTOG 91-11: a comparison of three non-surgical treatment strategies to preserve the larynx in patients with locally advanced larynx cancer. *J Clin Oncol* 2013;31:845–852.
10. Cooper JS, Pajak TF, Forastiere AA, et al. Postoperative concurrent radiotherapy and chemotherapy for high-risk squamous-cell carcinoma of the head and neck. *N Engl J Med* 2004;350:1937–1944.
11. Bernier J, Domenge C, Ozsahin M, et al. Postoperative irradiation with or without concomitant chemotherapy for locally advanced head and neck cancer. *N Engl J Med* 2004;350:1945–1952.
12. Pignon JP, le Maitre A, Maillard E, et al.; MACH-NC Collaborative Group. Meta-analysis of chemotherapy in head and neck cancer (MACH-NC): an update on 93 randomised trials and 17,346 patients. *Radiother Oncol* 2009;92:4–14.
13. Nien HH, Sturgis EM, Kies MS, et al.; Comparison of systemic therapies used concurrently with radiation for the treatment of human papillomavirus-associated oropharyngeal cancer. *Head Neck* 2016;38 Suppl1:E1554–1562.
14. Bonner JA, Harari PM, Giralt J, et al. Radiotherapy plus cetuximab for locoregionally advanced head and neck cancer: 5-year survival data from a phase 3 randomised trial, and relation between cetuximab-induced rash and survival. *Lancet Oncol* 2010;11:21–28.
15. Haddad R, O'Neill A, Rabinowits G, et al. Induction chemotherapy followed by concurrent chemoradiotherapy (sequential chemoradiotherapy) versus concurrent chemoradiotherapy alone in locally advancer head and neck cancer (PARADIGM): a randomized phase 3 trial. *Lancet Oncol* 2013;14:257–264.
16. Cohen EE, Karrison TG, Kocherginsky M, et al. Phase III randomized trial of induction chemotherapy in patients with N2 or N3 locally advanced head and neck cancer. *J Clin Oncol* 2014;32:2735–2743.
17. Blanchard P, Lee A, Marquet S, et al.; MAC-NPC Collaborative Group. Chemotherapy and radiotherapy in nasopharyngeal carcinoma: an update of the MAC-NPC meta-analysis. *Lancet Oncol* 2015;16:645–655.
18. Lee AW, Ngan RK, Tung SY, et al. Preliminary results of trial NPC-0501 evaluating the therapeutic gain by changing from concurrent-adjuvant to induction-concurrent chemoradiotherapy, changing from fluorouracil to capecitabine, and changing from conventional to accelerated radiotherapy fractionation in patients with locoregionally advanced nasopharyngeal carcinoma. *Cancer* 2015;121:1328–1338.
19. Ang KK, Trotti A, Brown BW, et al. Randomized trial addressing risk features and time factors of surgery plus radiotherapy in advanced head and neck cancer. *Int J Radiat Oncol Biol Phys* 2001;51:571–578.
20. Peters LJ, Goepfert H, Ang KK, et al. Evaluation of the dose for postoperative radiation therapy of head and neck cancer: first report of a prospective randomized trial. *Int J Radiat Oncol Biol Phys* 1993;26:3–11.

Practical Aspects of External Beam Therapy

- Patient positioning and immobilization are critical components for planning external beam radiotherapy.

- Supine position is best for the vast majority of patients.

- Positional or shielding stents are useful for decreasing radiation dose to normal tissues in certain cases.

- CT-based plan with heterogeneity correction is the current standard method.

- Target definition and delineation (and normal tissue delineation) have become the key components for treatment plan development regardless of the technology used to plan and deliver the treatment. Once appropriately defined, current techniques including 3-D conformal, IMRT (including volumetric modulated arc therapy [VMAT]), or proton therapy can potentially improve target coverage while reducing radiation exposure of normal tissues including salivary glands and neurologic tissues.

- The complexity of therapy including the desire to shape radiation to tumor targets and away from normal tissues has required increased verification processes. Image-guided radiation therapy (IGRT) is the process of acquiring 2-D (often KV images) or 3-D images (cone beam CT or CT on rails) for setup verification.

- Research and consensus guidelines continue to help define the nodal regions at risk. However, for many patients, bilateral neck irradiation remains the standard. Ipsilateral radiation may be appropriate for patients with well-lateralized primary tumors such as cancers of the buccal mucosa and parotid.

- While the introduction of IMRT provides better conformation of radiation to the target volumes, many head and neck cancers require treatment to relatively superficial tissues. Bolus remains an important device to improve superficial dosing. Other devices such as individualized missing tissue compensators are used less frequently, though wedges still remain important for 2-D and 3-D treatments, such as therapy for early glottic cancer.

PATIENT POSITIONING

The supine position is most frequently used to deliver radiation with the conventional technique or intensity-modulated radiation therapy (IMRT, volumetric modulated arc therapy [VMAT], or intensity-modulated proton therapy [IMPT]). An isocentric technique is applied for matching opposed lateral fields or IMRT upper neck portals to an anterior or anterior–posterior (AP-PA) lower neck portal(s). Nonmatching techniques (i.e., techniques in which the entire volume is treated with each field, such as "whole-field" IMRT, VMAT, or IMPT) still rely on an isocenter for field localization and facilitate portal verification.

The "open neck" position, in which the head is rotated on the trunk, resulting in flattening of the contours of the neck, is used for irradiating lateralized tumors and the ipsilateral neck. This position is suitable for irradiations with adjoining appositional electron fields or with a wedge-pair photon portal matched to an appositional electron field for the lower neck.

The seated position is used very rarely, primarily for those who have difficulty managing their secretions or those who have difficulty breathing in the supine position. Treatment is accomplished using a specially designed chair mounted to the treatment couch. This chair enables the same immobilization and allows the same treatment accessories to be used as in the supine position. The chair is used only if other options are not feasible because complex treatment planning and dosimetry are difficult and because computed tomography (CT) scanners cannot accommodate patients in this position. Research in developing devices to allow for the seated position is ongoing.

PATIENT IMMOBILIZATION

Virtually all patients nowadays are immobilized with thermoplastic masks that are individually made in the desired treatment position. A variety of commercial neck pads and head holders are available for the purpose of immobilization in different positions. When making a mask, care should be taken to stretch the thermoplastic sufficiently thin to avoid unwanted bolus effect. For treatments limited to the neck region, the mask can be constructed so as to avoid the portals altogether. Figures 3.1 and 3.2 outline briefly the general procedure of constructing immobilization devices.

Introduction of IMRT to reduce radiation morbidity or to escalate radiation dose to improve tumor control demands more precise and reproducible immobilization technology. Several methods have been introduced, which can be grouped into invasive and noninvasive techniques. Invasive techniques use head immobilization frames similar to those

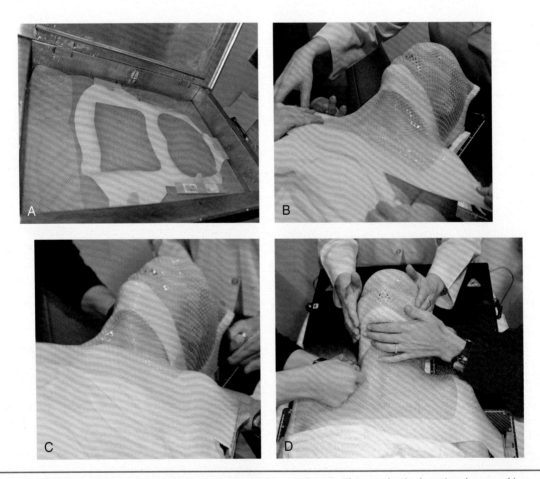

Figure 3.1 Procedure for making a thermoplastic mask in a supine position. **A:** Thermoplastic sheet is submerged in a warm water bath (72°C) until it becomes flexible. **B,C:** The thermoplastic sheet is placed over the head and shoulders of the patient, aligned in the desired position, and the frames are then fixed to a head holder by clamps. Care is taken to stretch the thermoplastic sheet sufficiently thin to avoid unwanted bolus effect. **D:** Gentle pressure is applied to make the thermoplastic sheet conform to the contours of the head and shoulder while cooling off and becoming more rigid.

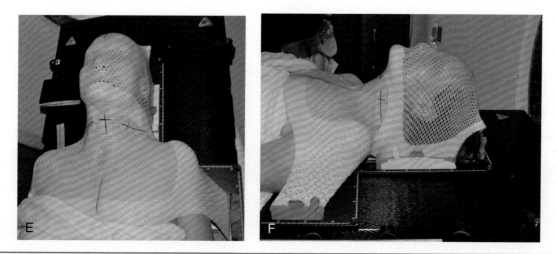

Figure 3.1 (*Continued*) **E,F:** Isocenter or reference point is marked, and thin-slice CT images are obtained for delineation of target volumes or portals and dosimetric planning.

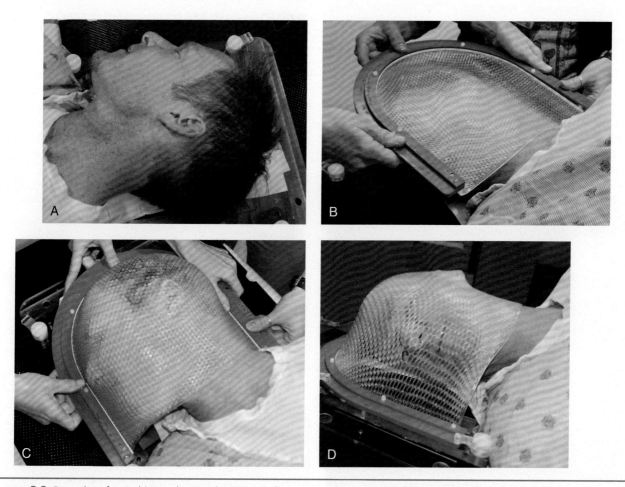

Figure 3.2 Procedure for making a thermoplastic mask for treatment in an open neck position. **A:** The patient is positioned with the head rotated on the trunk to flatten the contours of the neck. **B–D:** The thermoplastic sheet is stretched over the head of the patient, and the frame is then fixed to a head holder.

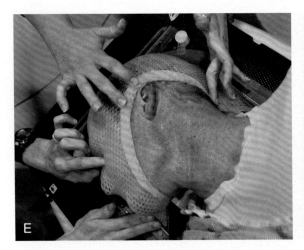
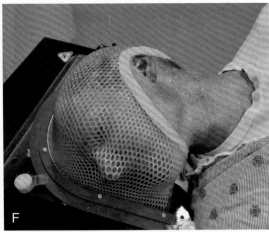

Figure 3.2 (*Continued*) **E,F:** Gentle pressure is applied to make the thermoplastic sheet conform to the contour of the patient, and the sheet is rolled up cranially to expose the area of irradiation to minimize perturbation of electron beams. Simulation can take place while the mask is cooling down and becoming more rigid.

used for stereotactic radiosurgery. The frame is affixed to the patient's skull by several screws, usually placed by a neurosurgeon.

Numerous noninvasive immobilization techniques have been described. They are based on thermoplastic mask immobilization or customized polyurethane cradles. Some systems add individualized cradles for support of the occiput (see Figure 3.3 and **Case Study 18.6**). We currently use a longer headboard for attachment of a mask that extends from the vertex of the scalp to the upper chest, giving additional support to the upper neck and shoulder (Fig. 3.1). Additionally, a "bite block" (Fig. 3.3) or customized stent (see below) will have an anterior extension that allows for "locking" the block or stent into the mask to reduce day-to-day variations in neck flexion/extension.

RADIOPAQUE MARKERS AND STENTS

Although CT scan–based simulation and dosimetry are widely used, radiopaque markers can still be useful for delineating the scars, skin and external soft tissue grafts, and, in select cases, the primary lesion. It is important to realize that it is often difficult to visualize superficial tumors in the diagnostic or planning CT scan. This simple procedure helps in designing treatment portals to minimize the risk of a geographic miss and to avoid unnecessary inclusion of normal tissues.

Wires and seeds placed on the skin, on the thermoplastic mask, or inserted into the tissue are helpful in marking the boundaries of the primary tumor, nodal biopsy sites, or surgical scar.

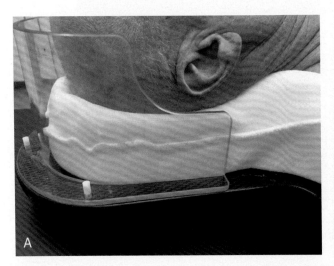
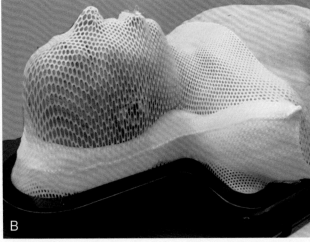

Figure 3.3 A patient immobilized with the Klarity AccuCushion. **A:** Prior to the fabrication of the mask, the patient is set in the cushion for customized support of the occiput, neck, and shoulders. **B:** The thermoplastic mask is fabricated to immobilize the patient laying in the AccuCushion. Additional immobilization is provided with a bite block that is locked into the mask.

Several types of custom-made stents are useful in reducing the volume of normal tissues irradiated.

Stents can be custom-made, such as those used to depress or shield the tongue or to protrude the lip. In general, these devices can be categorized into two basic types: shielding stents and positional stents. A shielding device serves to reduce the radiation dose administered to normal tissues by incorporating shielding material, whereas a positional device serves to displace normal tissues out of the treatment fields (Figs. 3.4–3.7).

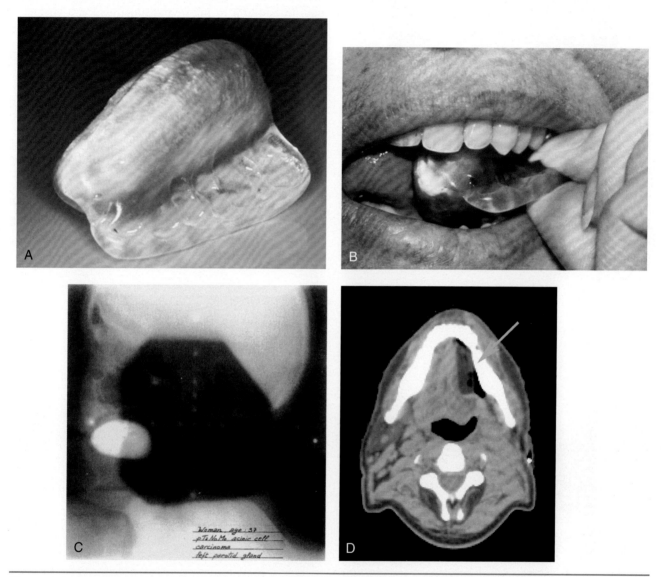

Figure 3.4 A 37-year-old woman presented with a 1.5-cm mass at the left angle of the mandible. The head and neck examination was otherwise unremarkable, and the facial nerve function was intact. Material for cytologic study was obtained by fine needle aspiration and was interpreted as pleomorphic adenoma. At surgery, the tumor was found to be mainly located in the deep lobe of the parotid gland. It was well encapsulated and was dissected out along with the surrounding normal parotid tissue. The facial nerve was preserved. Pathologic examination revealed an acinic cell carcinoma measuring 2.4 cm in maximum diameter. All gross tumor was resected, but tumor cells extended to the surgical margin. Therefore, postoperative radiotherapy was recommended. The left parotid bed was treated with an ipsilateral appositional field using a combination of 20-MeV electrons and 18-MV photons, weighted 4:1, respectively. A dose of 56 Gy was delivered in 2-Gy fractions, specified at the 90% isodose line. To reduce the dose to the underlying brain during the electron treatments, 2 cm of beveled bolus was placed over the superior part of the field. After a dose of 44 Gy, the field was reduced off the spinal cord, and treatment to the postauricular and posterior cervical area was completed with 12-MeV electrons. A custom-made intraoral stent containing cerrobend (Lipowitz's metal, Cerro Metal Product, Bellefonte, PA, or Belmont Metal Inc., Brooklyn, NY) with a flange containing occlusal registration (**A**) was used to shield the tongue and contralateral oral mucosa from the electron beam treatments. The stent was held in place by the teeth fitting in the flange on the lateral side (**B**), which positioned the main stent between the alveolar processes and the tongue and, thereby, shielding as shown on the portal image (**C**) and displacing the tongue toward the contralateral side as shown on planning CT scan (*green arrow*) (**D**). Because 80% of the dose was delivered by electrons, there was still a significant protection of the tongue and contralateral oral mucosa so that mucositis could be prevented.

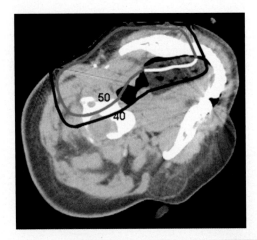

Figure 3.5 Axial computed tomographic (CT) scan images of patient with parotid carcinoma treated with an appositional 16-MeV electron field. A dose of 50 Gy was prescribed to the 90% line. To avoid artifact, a wax pattern of the stent was used for obtaining CT scan images. The stent captures the 50-Gy line at the edge of where the lateral tongue would normally be positioned. Without the stent, the 40-Gy line would have penetrated to the midline of the oral tongue.

An ancillary function of positional stents is to facilitate the use of internal bolus to fill surgical cavities, for example, to fill the cavity after maxillectomy or orbital exenteration (Fig. 3.8). Fortunately, progress in reconstructive techniques allows the surgeon to fill such tissue defects, even the palate, using a myocutaneous vascular flap. In addition to improving functional and cosmetic outcome, such a flap eliminates the need to use internal bolus.

SIMULATION

Simulation is a crucial procedure in planning the technical aspects of radiotherapy. The general treatment strategy (target volumes, organ at risk, field arrangement, treatment unit, etc.) should be determined before the onset of simulation. During simulation, attention is paid to mark relevant structures, to set up and immobilize patients in the desired position, and to obtain CT scan images for portal design. The following sequence is usually applied.

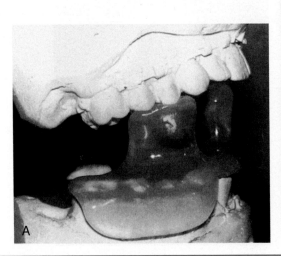

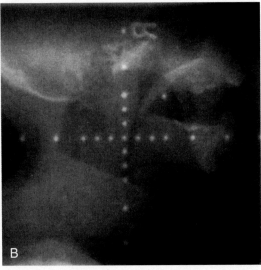

Figure 3.6 A 49-year-old woman presented with a 3-month history of enlarging neck masses. On examination, she was found to have a 3-cm exophytic lesion on the left side of the tongue base, extending laterally to the glossopharyngeal sulcus. Mobility of the tongue was normal. There were three palpable nodes in the neck (a 3.5 × 3 cm right upper jugular node, a 2.5 × 2 cm left jugulodigastric node, and a 2 × 2 cm left midjugular node). Biopsy of the primary lesion revealed squamous cell carcinoma. The patient received radiotherapy followed by neck dissection. The primary tumor and upper neck nodes were treated with lateral parallel–opposed portals with 6-MV photons to a dose of 45 Gy in 25 fractions, delivered to the isocenter. Reduction of the spinal cord was made, and therapy was continued to a tumor dose of 54 Gy in 30 fractions. The posterior cervical strips were supplemented with electron beams. The mid and lower jugular nodes were treated through an anterior appositional field and were supplemented with a smaller posterior field to a tumor dose of 54 Gy in 30 fractions. During the last 2.5 weeks of this basic treatment, the primary tumor and palpable nodes were boosted to a total tumor dose of 72 Gy. The boost was delivered in 1.5 Gy per fraction, given as second daily treatments using the concomitant boost technique. The stent for this patient consisted of a horizontal tongue positioner with protrusions fitting the occlusal surfaces of the mandibular and maxillary teeth, which served to separate the upper and lower jaws. The horizontal portion depressed the tongue so that it could be treated with adequate margins without encompassing the hard palate, upper gums, and most of the buccal mucosa. **A:** Stent mounted on maxillary and mandibular casts. **B:** Portal film showing the position of the tongue held down by the depressor and the mouth kept open by the stent so that the palate, gum, and most of the buccal mucosa were excluded from the field. (From Kaanders JHAM, et al. Devices valuable in head and neck radiotherapy. *Int J Radiat Oncol Biol Phys* 1992;23:639–645.)

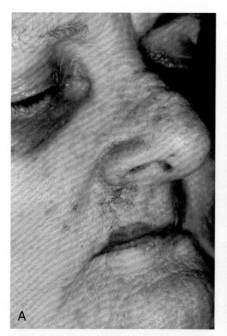
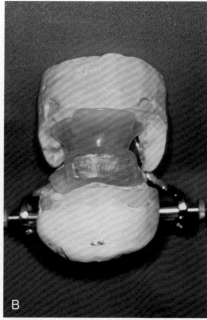
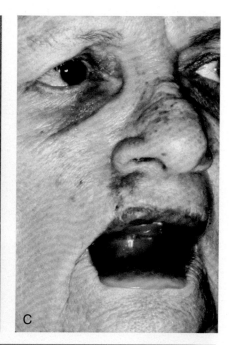

Figure 3.7 A 76-year-old woman presented with a lesion on the right side of the upper lip. On examination, there was a slightly raised, erythematous lesion extending from the vermilion of the upper lip to the nasal ala with upward retraction of the lip (**A**). The lesion was 2.2 cm in largest dimension and involved almost the entire thickness of the lip. The inner mucosal lining was, however, intact. There were no palpable lymph nodes in the neck. A biopsy of this lesion showed basal cell carcinoma of which the patient received radiation therapy through an appositional 9-MeV electron field, which encompassed the tumor and a 1-cm margin of normal tissue. A lead cutout was used for skin collimation, and a bolus of 1 cm thickness was placed over the skin to ensure an adequate dose at the surface of the tumor. Also, a bolus was placed in the right nostril to enhance the dose homogeneity. A dose of 50 Gy was given in 25 fractions, specified at the 90% isodose line, which was followed by an implant with radium needles. A stent was placed over the upper and lower alveolar processes to open the mouth and separate the lips, thereby excluding the lower lip from the radiation field (**B,C**). It also displaced the tongue posteriorly so that it was out of the range of the electron beam. To shield the gum, the part of the stent that was between the upper lip and the alveolar ridge was filled with cerrobend. Acrylic coating prevents overdosage to the mucosa of the upper lip by backscatter. At the completion of electron beam treatment, confluent mucositis occurred at the upper lip mucosa, whereas no appreciable reaction was observed on the mucosa of the gum. **A:** A woman with a slightly raised lesion extending from the vermilion of the upper lip to the nasal ala with upward retraction of the lip. **B:** The stent used mounted on an articulator. The upper part of the stent that separated the upper lip from the alveolar process contained cerrobend to shield the latter. **C:** The stent in treatment position. The lower flange held the lower lip away from the radiation field. (From Kaanders JHAM, et al. Devices valuable in head and neck radiotherapy. *Int J Radiat Oncol Biol Phys* 1992;23:639–645.)

Marking Anatomic Structures and Patient Positioning

When indicated, wires are used to mark the boundaries of the nodes or surgical scars and to delineate relevant structures (e.g., orbital canthi, lacrimal gland, external auditory canals, and oral commissures). For accessible tumors, seeds can be implanted to indicate the borders. The next step, before making an immobilization mask, is to set up the patient in a suitable position and to verify the appropriate orientation of the patient's anatomy (e.g., no axial rotation and the desired degree of neck extension) and, when applicable, stent position (e.g., tongue depressor) by acquiring a scout image using CT simulator (or with fluoroscopy). Subsequently, the thermoplastic mask is made, and the patient's position is preserved. Care must be taken to ensure that the marking wires are not displaced when the mask is put in position, or a geographic miss may result when the portals are planned. The final step is to choose the optimal site for isocenter.

Determining Isocenter

The choice of the isocenter depends on the technique used for portal junction. For monoisocentric (or half-beam) junction technique using asymmetric collimator jaw setting, the isocenter is placed on the desired junction location. When techniques are to be used to cover the primary tumor and all cervical nodal regions ("whole-field" IMRT, VMAT, IMPT), the isocenter is placed near the center of the target volumes. Although the flexibility and automation available in modern equipment reduce these concerns, it is still beneficial to get the setup correct at the outset, because adjustments after simulation are a source of potential errors.

For parallel-opposed fields, the isocenter is generally placed at the midplane of the central axis. Appositional fields are generally treated using the source-to-surface distance technique. The isocenter for wedge-pair or three-field techniques is determined on the basis of the shape and size of the target volume.

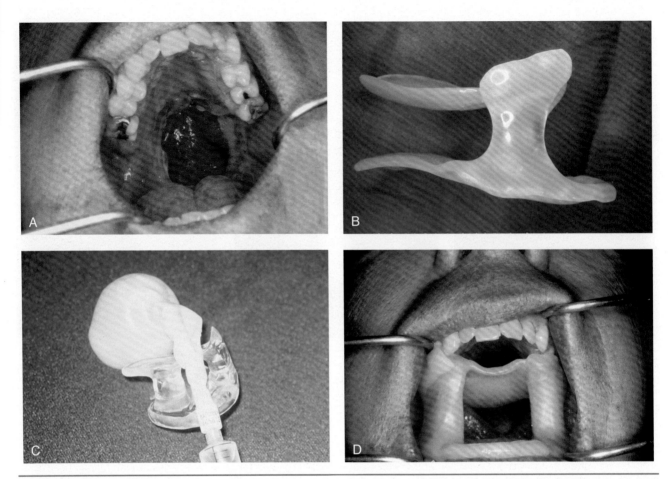

Figure 3.8 A 41-year-old man sought medical attention because of a 2-year history of a slowly enlarging soft palate mass. On physical examination, he was found to have a 4-cm submucosal soft tissue mass involving the left side of the soft and hard palate extending to the left maxillary tuberosity. The neck had no palpable nodes. The patient subsequently underwent a wide resection of the tumor with partial palatectomy and partial maxillectomy. Pathologic examination showed an adenoid cystic carcinoma measuring 3 cm in largest diameter. The surgical margins were close and, therefore, he received postoperative radiotherapy. He was treated in the supine position with right and left lateral parallel–opposed 6-MV photon fields, which encompassed the surgical bed and upper neck. A dose of 60 Gy in 2-Gy fractions was delivered to the isocenter. A field reduction was made after 44 Gy. A modification of the stent as described in Figure 3.7 was used. It served to open the mouth and depress most of the oral tongue out of the radiation field. The surgical procedure left a relatively large air cavity, which could compromise the dose homogeneity in the target volume (**A**). For this reason, a balloon filled with water (tissue equivalent for radiation absorption) was placed in the surgical defect. To support the balloon, a cradle was added on top of the tongue-depressing part (**B,C**). A space was provided between the upper incisors and the blade to insert the balloon (**D,E**). The position of the balloon can be verified by filling it with contrast material during simulation (**F**). **A:** Surgical defect after left partial palatectomy and partial maxillectomy in a patient with an adenoid cystic carcinoma. **B:** A balloon-supporting stent: the lower blade serves to depress the tongue and the cradle supports a water-filled balloon. **C:** Side view of the position of the balloon. **D:** Stent in position: a space was created to facilitate filling of balloon.

Computed Tomography Simulation

CT scan simulation allows for defining the target volumes on digitally reconstructed images. Following appropriate immobilization, cross-sectional images are acquired for delineation of clinical target volumes (CTVs) and normal tissue avoidance structures, commonly referred to as *organs at risk (OARs)*, for dosimetric planning. At the time of the scan, either the actual isocenter or reference points are marked on the mask and/or patient. As presented above, it is beneficial to select the desired isocenter at the outset whenever possible, because adjustments after simulation are sources of potential errors.

TREATMENT PLANNING

The majority of patients with head and neck cancer are now treated with conformal techniques, which can effectively restrict the dose to the tumor while reducing radiation exposure to normal tissues and thereby diminishing the morbidity of radiotherapy (e.g., xerostomia, fibrosis, and neuropathy). Expertise in the anatomy of the head and neck region, clinical examination, interpretation of diagnostic tumor imaging, and knowledge of pattern of tumor spread are crucial for delineation of specific CTVs

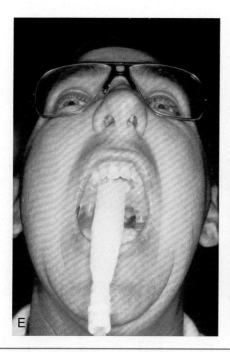
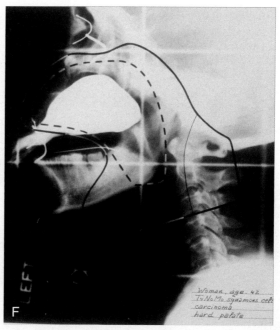

Figure 3.8 (*Continued*) **E:** Stent and balloon in position. **F:** Simulation film: the tongue blade was marked by a radiopaque wire, and the balloon was filled with contrast material to indicate the position of the device relative to the normal tissues; the lateral orbital canthi and oral commissures were also marked; the *solid and dotted black lines* represent the large and boost fields, respectively. (From Kaanders JHAM, et al. Devices valuable in head and neck radiotherapy. *Int J Radiat Oncol Biol Phys* 1992;23:639–645.)

to receiving irradiation to minimize the likelihood of geographic miss, leading to marginal relapse. Close teamwork between the radiation oncologist, physicists, dosimetrists, and radiation therapists is essential for proper planning and delivery of IMRT.

Intensity-Modulated Radiation Therapy

IMRT (as well as VMAT [a variation of IMRT] and IMPT) is planned using *inverse* treatment planning systems. With these systems, treatment portals are created using a complex mathematical optimization process, based on user-defined target dose prescription and normal tissue dose limits. Inverse planning actually requires that radiation oncologists explicitly define the desired doses to various CTVs and the acceptable dose limits to normal structures (OARs). Thus, the procedure starts with delineation of clinically and radiologically demonstrable tumor boundary, referred to as *gross target volume (GTV)*, CTVs, and OARs using planning CT images, and prescribing desired doses to these respective target and normal tissue volumes. Given these parameters, the computer optimizes the beam intensity pattern within each portal to generate the best dose distribution to fit the prescription.

Because of the physics of radiation beams (e.g., the scatter and penumbra), sometimes the prescriptions cannot be fully satisfied. In such cases, prioritization of doses to tumor versus normal structures can be modified. For example, a lower tumor dose might be acceptable if, for example, the brain

stem dose could not otherwise be kept below the specification. Conversely, an ideal low dose to the parotid gland may not be acceptable if the desired dose cannot be delivered to an adjacent large involved lymph node.

Once an IMRT plan is designed, several delivery methods are available. A common method for IMRT treatment delivery is to use multileaf collimator (MLC) at multiple (fixed) gantry positions (Fig. 3.9). The treatment mode can be either static (i.e., step-and-shoot method) or dynamic (i.e., dynamic multileaf collimator [DMLC]). In the step-and-shoot method, MLC leaves remain stationary during beam-on time and will move to the next set of leaf positions when the radiation beam is on hold. In the dynamic mode, MLC leaves can move during beam-on period, but the relation between leaf positions and the fractional dose delivered has to be maintained and synchronized. This will certainly call for a tighter specification on the MLC system.

Another system used clinically is a helical tomotherapy unit. Tomotherapy is an integrated three-dimensional (3-D) imaging and delivery system, in which the treatment couch advances continuously during the modulated arc beam delivery. In addition, there is a specially designed megavoltage CT scan imaging system, which can be used to perform a CT scan–guided treatment setup before treatment delivery. Other units with some specific features are also currently available.

VMAT is a more recent addition to the systems capable of providing IMRT-based therapy. As its name implies, it is arc therapy, with treatment delivered dynamically through a

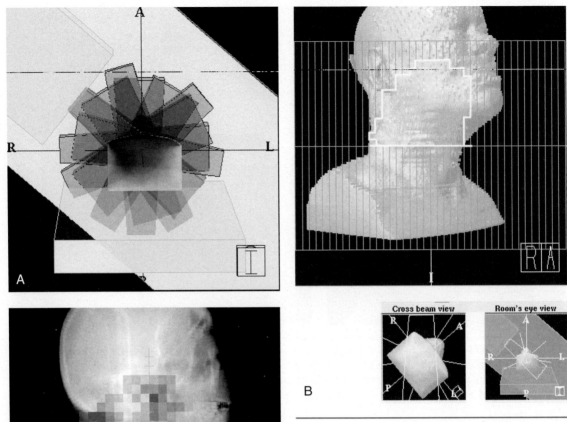

Figure 3.9 Intensity-modulated radiation therapy. **A:** Schematic of a nine-field beam orientation using DMLC–IMRT beams for the treatment of a patient with tonsillar carcinoma. **B:** Beam's eye view of one of nine fields used to deliver IMRT to the primary tumor and the upper neck nodes in a patient with tonsil carcinoma. The lower neck nodes receive radiation with an anterior portal through an isocentric match. **C:** The checkerboard-like pattern overlying the radiograph represents the fluence pattern of the field delivered with IMRT as seen through a beam's eye view.

continuing rotating gantry. The advance over classic arc therapy is the use of dynamic multileaf collimation throughout the rotation providing the intensity modulation. Treatment can be delivered in a single arc or multiple arcs with varying degrees of each arc size to a maximum of 360 degrees. The main advantage of VMAT is the speed of delivery of the entirety of the fraction. This allows for clinics to have improved throughput and is also better for the patient to lessen the time of immobilization. Similar to tomotherapy, a dynamic gantry approach may provide more conformality of treatment plans.

While proton therapy has been available for decades, there has been recent renewed interest in the use of this particle for therapy. The interest has been principally driven by improvements in the technology. One improvement has been in the decrease in space required to install and operate proton therapy machines, thus increasing the availability. Further improvements have been in the mode of delivery. Classic proton therapy (now commonly referred to as passive) relied

on delivering the beam and depending on the Bragg peak at the distal end to provide the conformality. However, the Bragg peak with a single energy is so narrow that to be clinically useful it must be spread out. To create this spread-out Bragg peak (SOBP), a modulating wheel is used. To further conform the shape of the beam to the patient's anatomy and tumor, individual compensators are designed.

The more modern approach is called active scanning, which allows for IMPT. Magnets deflect and steer the proton beams. The volume designed to receive the therapy is "painted" by delivering numerous narrow monoenergetic beams (pencil beams) voxel by voxel and then in successive layers. In addition to the improved conformality, scanning technology has less neutron contamination and so theoretically has a safety advantage.

Despite the advantage of improved conformality by capitalizing on the Bragg peak, there is some uncertainty regarding the precise location of the distal edge of the beam. This uncertainty needs to be taken under consideration. Similar to photon beam, one technique to overcome this problem is to rely on multiple fields. The disadvantage of multiple beams is larger volumes getting more of the low-dose bath, but as opposed to IMRT, this may be less since it is only in the proximal beam path.

Combining multiple scanned beams adds to the complexity. There are two basic approaches to planning when using multiple scanned beams. The first is referred to as "single-field optimization" (SFO). In this approach, each field is optimized separately, and then, the fields are combined and weighted to provide the desired dose distribution. The second technique, multifield optimization (MFO), has all the beams from all fields combined first and then optimized. MFO will typically provide a more optimal plan. However, the use of beams that rely on extreme precision but still have some uncertainty and adding even minute changes in anatomy and tumor size can lead to a decrease in the reproducibility of the desired dose to the targets. This requires repeated verification and frequent adaption.

Three-Dimensional Conformal Radiotherapy

Several conformal radiotherapy methods are presently available. Generally, using a 3-D planning system, the target volumes and structures for avoidance are defined on thin-section CT scans. Two-dimensional beam's eye views are used to visualize the targets and avoidance structures to select the optimal beam angles to best conform the radiation. In other words, the physician, physicist, and dosimetrist select what they believe are the ideal angles and number of beams and then, through an iterative process, select the appropriate weighting and, when desired, wedging. This type of procedure is referred to as *forward planning*. Beam arrangements can be either coplanar or noncoplanar. To derive a plan that is highly conformal, it often necessitates the use of a large number of beams. When only

custom-made cerrobend (Belmont Metal Inc., Brooklyn, NY) portal shaping is available, this can result in extremely long treatment sessions because therapists have to go in and out of the room to replace the blocks. The storage of these customized blocks inside a tight treatment vault can also be a problem.

The use of MLC facilitates treatment delivery by decreasing the time necessary for therapists to administer the multiple beams as described above. The ability to change the MLC-collimated field quickly adds further flexibility in designing treatment fields. For example, a field covering the target is designed and a smaller portal can be created within the first field to deliver additional dose to a portion of the target either to top up the regions receiving lower than the desired dose or to achieve dose escalation. This manual beam patching technique is called the *field-in-field* technique, a forward planning and treatment technique used to achieve a more desirable dose distribution.

PORTAL ARRANGEMENTS

Since IMRT portals are generated based on prescribed doses to predefined CTVs and OARs, this section is only applicable to three-dimensional conformal radiotherapy (3-D CRT) technique. However, we still find translating concepts from 3-D CRT applicable to our IMRT delivery. While continued improvement is ongoing in IMRT dosimetry, IMRT to the mid and lower neck can lead to unnecessary dose to the larynx and esophagus. A "split-field" technique (an IMRT variation of the classic three-field technique, Fig. 3.10) combines IMRT, delivered to the primary tumor and upper lymphatics while avoiding critical and salivary

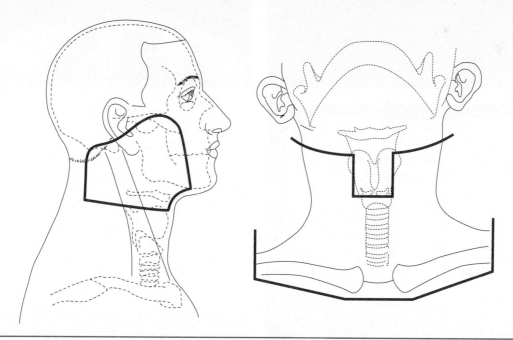

Figure 3.10 Schematic illustration of adjoining opposed lateral fields and appositional anterior field above the arytenoids.

structures, with anterior oriented beams (combined with posterior beams as needed) with the larynx, spinal cord, and esophagus shielded (Fig. 3.11).

Bilateral Irradiation

A three-field technique, with the patient immobilized in a supine position, is used for the treatment of most cancers of the oral cavity and pharynx (Fig. 3.10). The technique consists of two opposed lateral beams covering the primary tumor and upper draining lymphatics with an anterior field treating the lower neck lymphatics. The inferior border of the opposed fields matches the superior border of the anterior field. Because these fields match over the spinal cord, it is critical that care is taken to avoid overlap. The most common safety measure is a block over the spinal cord. If the tumor is not involving or adjacent to the larynx and hypopharynx, a larynx block is applied (see below) to the anterior field, and this block also serves as the spinal cord block.

The superior border is determined by the location of known disease and the likely spread pattern. Whenever possible, the optic pathways, part of the temporomandibular joints, temporal lobes, and auditory canals are excluded from the portals.

In the anterior border, a strip of anterior midline skin is shielded whenever possible to reduce lymph-drainage impairment after irradiation. This practice is not recommended when the primary tumor extends to the anterior subcutaneous tissues, large submandibular or jugular lymph nodes are present, the surgical scar (of neck dissection) approaches or crosses the midline, or histologic evidence of extracapsular nodal extension is present.

It is desirable to exclude the larynx proper from the lateral fields when this setup does not compromise the dose distribution to the primary tumor and/or involved neck nodes. Such a strategy is accomplished by placing the inferior border of the lateral fields just superior to the arytenoids. In patients who are able to hyperextend the head, it is preferable to use an asymmetric jaw (half beam), isocentric technique where the anterior lower neck field can be matched to the opposed lateral

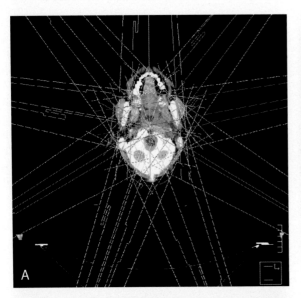

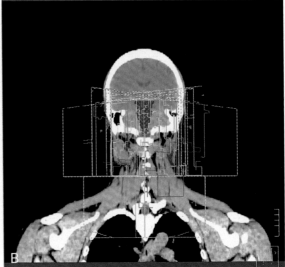

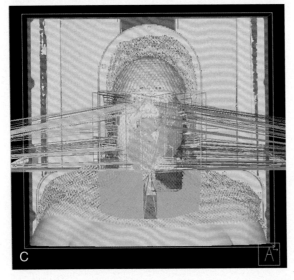

Figure 3.11 Demonstration of "split-field" IMRT technique. **A:** A nine-field static gantry approach is used for the IMRT component. The beam angles are roughly equidistant and shown on an axial view. (**B**) A coronal view, and (**C**) 3-D rendered view show all 12 beams, with the nine IMRT beams treating the primary tumor and upper neck and the three non-IMRT beams treating the lower neck. The nine IMRT beams are treated each fraction, while the non-IMRT beams are treated sequentially: first an anterior beam with a larynx block, then an anterior beam with a full midline block, and finally a posterior oriented beam that boosts the left mid neck just below gross adenopathy.

portals without collimator rotation. In patients who cannot hyperextend the head or when the primary tumor involves the vallecula, a slanted inferior border, at a maximal angle of 15 degrees (Fig. 3.10), can be used to avoid matching lateral portals and anterior lower neck field at the sloping submental area. A preferred option now is to use isocentric matching with collimator rotation for lateral portals and to turn the couch 90 degrees and angle the gantry (superior tilt) to correspond to the angle of collimator rotation for the matching anterior field. When the larynx cannot be excluded, the inferior border is usually placed at the neck–shoulder junction.

The location of the *posterior border* is dictated by the site of primary tumor and the extent of nodal disease.

- For N0 cases with low risk of subclinical spread to the posterior cervical nodes (e.g., carcinoma of the anterior floor of the mouth or oral tongue), the posterior border is placed just behind the insertion of the sternocleidomastoid muscle at the mastoid process.
- In N+ cases or primary tumors with substantial risk of subclinical spread to posterior cervical nodes (e.g., nasopharyngeal carcinoma), the posterior border is placed behind the spinous processes or even more posteriorly in the presence of large nodal masses. Once the spinal cord dose limit is reached, the posterior border is moved forward, usually to mid-vertebral body level. When the posterior pharyngeal wall or retropharyngeal nodes are part of the target volume, the border is placed closer to the posterior edge of the vertebral bodies. The posterior cervical strips that are no longer encompassed by the photon fields receive supplemental dose by lateral appositional electron fields. The electron beam energy is generally 9 MeV in the absence of a palpable node or higher (e.g., 12 MeV) in the presence of palpable nodes or in muscular patients. When electron energies of 12 MeV or greater are used to treat the posterior strips, CT scan dosimetry is crucial to compute the actual spinal cord dose.

After reaching the desired dose for the treatment of subclinical disease (most frequently 50 Gy/25 fractions), lateral fields are reduced to deliver the boost dose to the primary tumor and involved nodes. The field margins are determined by the extent of gross disease. Lateral or oblique photon fields, wedge-pair technique, or appositional electron fields can be used to deliver the boost dose, depending on the location and size of the primary lesion and nodes.

An anterior appositional photon field is usually used for irradiating the mid and lower neck nodes, supraclavicular nodes, and, when indicated, the tracheal stoma.

The *superior border* matches the inferior border of lateral portals by using asymmetric jaw (isocentric technique). The *inferior border* is located 1 cm below the clavicles. The *lateral borders* encompass the medial two thirds of the clavicles. A midline block is used to shield the larynx and esophageal inlet and also to prevent overlap at the spinal cord.

In some cases, the surgical scar may overlie the larynx and may be shielded by the midline block. In such cases, the prelaryngeal skin and subcutaneous tissues can be treated with a separate matching field, using low-energy (6 to 8 MeV) electrons. In postlaryngectomy patients requiring treatment of the stoma, no midline block is used. Overlap on the spinal cord is avoided by having a small spinal cord block placed in the lateral fields.

The combination of two lateral upper neck fields and a single anterior mid–lower neck field results in a somewhat lower dose to the midposterior cervical nodal region. Therefore, in the presence of posterior adenopathy, it is necessary to use anterior and posterior portals to irradiate the mid and lower neck. The most convenient setup in such situations is the monoisocentric (half-beam) match.

An alternative to the three-field approach is to use two primary beams, often caudally oriented to minimize the drastic change in tissue between beams going through the neck and shoulder. The advantage of this approach is to not have the concerns of the three-field technique of localizing an ideal match. The concerns of splitting a tumor bed and needing safety gaps or blocks to avoid overlap are obviated. The improvements in planning with dynamic wedging and field-in-field or patch fields to compensate for cold spots has made this approach for CRT more desirable. However, the orientation of the beams can lead to large amounts of normal tissue being irradiated, and while dosimetry has improved, in many situations it still may create undesired heterogeneity due to the sometimes steep changes in the anatomic contours.

Unilateral Irradiation

Well-lateralized tumors having a low risk of lymphatic spread to the contralateral neck nodes (e.g., retromolar trigone, buccal mucosa, salivary glands, and skin) receive treatment to the ipsilateral side only. In such cases, the patient can be immobilized in either a supine or an open neck position. However, using modern techniques (IMRT, VMAT, protons), the supine position allows for greater precision and reproducibility of setup.

The primary tumor and upper neck are encompassed and irradiated through an appositional lateral field using electrons or a combination of electrons and photons. The depth of the primary tumor determines the energy of the electron beam. When high-energy electrons are needed, approximately 20% of the dose is given with megavoltage photons to reduce the skin dose, thereby avoiding occurrence of moist skin desquamation.

The borders of the field are determined by the tumor location and extension (see Part II). The *inferior border* of the field is placed at or above the arytenoids whenever possible. The isodose constriction and greater-dose perturbation by tissue inhomogeneity associated with electron beams must be taken into account in determining margins. Therefore, these cases require CT scan–based dosimetry with heterogeneity corrections.

The mid and lower neck nodes are irradiated with a matching, slightly oblique (to exclude the larynx and spinal cord) ipsilateral photon portal when treatment is delivered in a supine position or with an adjoining appositional electron field in an open neck position. In the latter scenario, for a clinically negative neck, 9-MeV electrons are usually sufficient, except in patients with a large neck diameter. Palpable nodes may require higher energies, depending on their size and depth in the neck.

- *Superior border:* matches the inferior border of the primary field
- *Anterior border:* is just short of falloff
- *Posterior border:* is at the edge of the trapezius muscle
- *Inferior border:* is 1 cm below the clavicle

PORTAL SHAPING

Photon Beam

Modern linear accelerators have an integrated MLC system with a leaf width (at isocenter) of as small as 5 mm or even 3 mm. Combining the wide travel range (up to 40 × 40 cm field size) and the ultrahigh resolution and precision (usually <1 mm) in the leaf movement direction, the MLC has gradually replaced cerrobend blocks for portal shaping in the vast majority of cases. Within the primary rectangular shape field set by four collimator jaws, individual leaves can be adjusted to conform to the desired shape of the portal DMLC, which enables changing the beam shape while radiation is being delivered and provides the flexibility to achieve the desired dose distribution.

In most situations, MLC should produce shaped portals equivalent to those achieved with customized blocks. MLC also is useful because it can easily produce smaller fields within a larger portal (field-in-field technique) to compensate for underdosage to part of the target volumes because of differences in tissue thickness or heterogeneity. In rare occasions where millimeter precision is needed, the thickness of the leaves in most commercial systems may not be adequate. The use of cerrobend (Belmont Metal Inc., Brooklyn, NY) blocks is also preferable for shielding a nonlinear volume within the portal. Shielding the spinal cord from the anterior lower neck photon portal in a patient with scoliosis is an excellent example.

Cerrobend blocks are manufactured using a standard commercial block-cutter system (Clark Research and Development Inc., Folsom, LA). The quality control program includes evaluation of the accuracy of Styrofoam, cut out with a verification light, and assessment of the size, shape, and precision of mounting on the tray by projecting the light field on the outline on the simulation images with a block verification unit (Med-Tech Inc., Tulsa, OK). Deviations of 2 mm or less are uniformly considered acceptable.

Electron Beam

Shaping of electron field is done by secondary collimation. When necessary for treatment of tumors close to critical tissues, portal shaping can be accomplished by placing a customized lead shield or mask directly on the patient's skin (skin collimation). The construction of appropriate lead mask takes several steps (Figs. 3.12 and 3.13). First, the desired radiation field is drawn on the patient's skin. Then, an impression and mold are made (during this procedure,

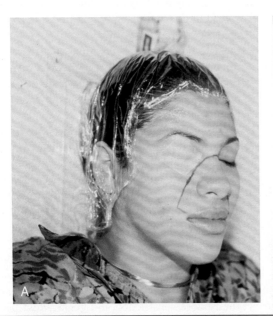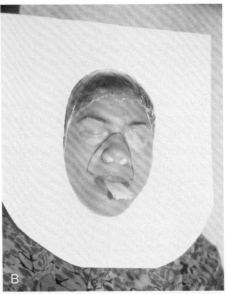

Figure 3.12 Procedure for manufacturing a lead mask for electron collimation and beeswax bolus. **A:** The field is outlined on the skin, and the patient is positioned on an appropriate head rest. Lubrication jelly is put around the hairline, and the hair is covered with Saran wrap and eyes with gauze dressings (lubricate the edges for extra protection). **B:** Cardboard, with patient's contour cut out, is placed at the desired position. The patient is informed that impression mixture will be poured over the face. Therefore, it is necessary to fill the nostrils with lubricated cotton to keep out the impression mixture and to keep straws in the mouth for breathing.

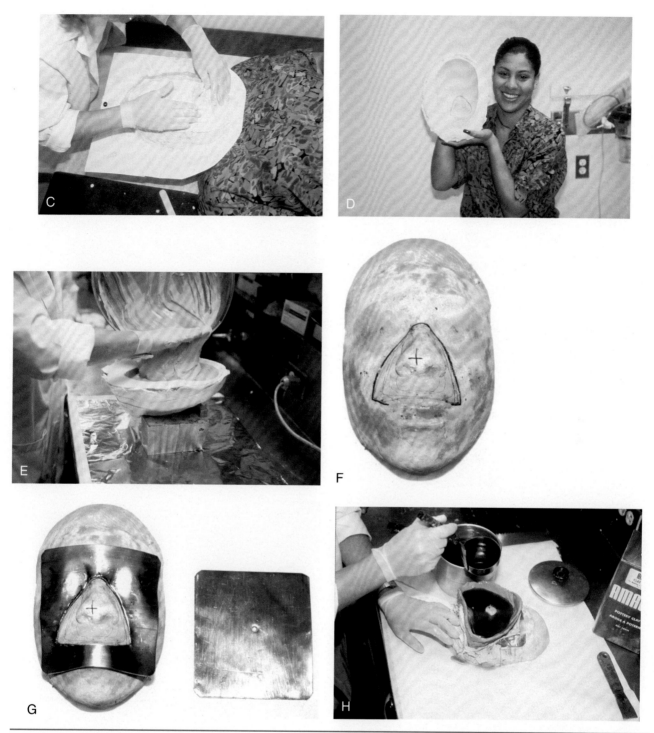

Figure 3.12 (*Continued*) **C:** Impression mixture is then poured over the area of interest and smoothed over until it sets. Plaster strips are placed over the impression to hold it together (2 to 3 layers). **D:** After hardening (2 to 4 minutes), the impression is removed. The field outline that has transferred to the impression is touched up. **E:** The impression is coated with lubricating jelly, and dental stone (Labstone or Denstone) is poured into it. The impression is vibrated for a few minutes for air bubbles to surface. **F:** The mold is removed the next day, and again the field outline is touched up. **G:** A thin sheet of lead is cut to the predetermined size. A hole is drilled through the center of the sheets. This is enlarged to approximate the radiation field. The sheets are then pounded onto the mold with rubber hammer. The shape of the hole is then further trimmed to fit the field outline. This procedure is repeated until the proper thickness is reached. A thin strip of foam is taped to the underside of the mask to improve wearer comfort. **H:** Customized beeswax bolus, when needed, is made directly on the mold. In this case, pottery clay is used to build a dam of the desired depth 1 cm beyond the field outline (to allow wax shrinkage by drying and cooling). The stone mold is lubricated generously, and a small amount of melted wax is poured into the dam; let it cool down before adding another layer of wax. This step is repeated until reaching the proper thickness. A hot knife is then used to trim the bolus to the final dimension. (Courtesy Robert Gastorf and Michelle Rittichier, Department of Radiation Physics. Described in detail by Gastorf, et al. Quality assurance in the fabrication of radiation treatment aids. In: Starkschall G, Horton JL, eds. *Proceedings of an American College of Medical Physics Symposium.* Madison, WI: Medical Physics Publishing, 1991:239–245.)

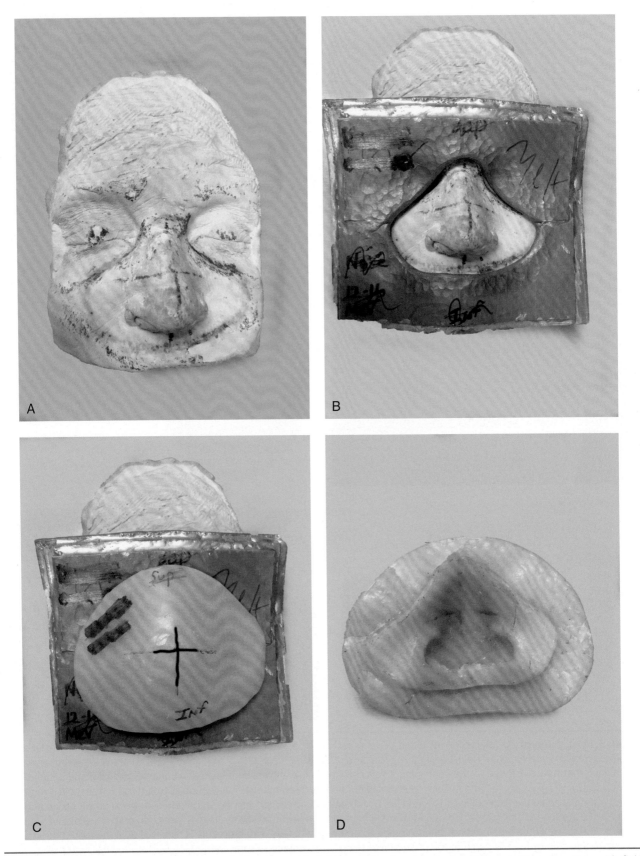

Figure 3.13 A: Impression of patient with nasal cancer, with field transferred to impression. **B:** Lead skin collimation with field open. Additional layers of lead are added over eyes. **C:** Entire setup including custom beeswax bolus that fits over nose within the lead collimation. **D:** Reverse view of custom bolus with nasal contour that fits over nose.

field borders are transferred automatically onto the impression). Subsequently, thin sheets of lead are cut, pounded into shape against the impression, and soldered together until the proper thickness is attained for the electron energy selected. The mask is then tried on the patient, and final adjustments are made. When a shrinking field technique is used, it is more practical to initiate treatment with the boost field because it is easier to enlarge the aperture of the mask by cutting out excess lead than to reduce its size.

DOSE SPECIFICATION

Intensity-Modulated Radiation Therapy

With IMRT, doses are prescribed to target volumes defined by clinicians. GTV, CTVs, and normal tissues of interest are delineated. The GTV encompasses all gross tumors (primary cancer and, when present, involved nodes) detectable by physical and endoscopic examination and by diagnostic imaging such as CT scan, magnetic resonance imaging (MRI), positron emission tomography (PET), etc. The high-dose CTV (CTV_{HD}) comprises the GTV and the immediate surrounding tissues judged to be at risk for harboring high density of tumor cells. Typical margins around the GTV are 0.5 to 1.5 cm depending on the nature of tumor border (well circumscribed vs. diffuse) and the proximity of critical organs (e.g., brain stem, optic chiasm), although exceptions exist, such as wider coverage for extensive perineural invasion.

GTV obviously does not exist after total surgical tumor resection. The CTV_{HD} in these cases include the tumor bed and margins as judged individually based on the presence of adverse surgical pathologic features such as extracapsular extension of nodal disease, positive section margins, extensive invasion of the neck soft tissue, etc. Additional CTVs are defined in undissected regions that are judged to have a sufficiently high probability of harboring microscopic disease to justify receiving elective irradiation. A patient may have several CTVs defined that differ in their assessment of risk and planned dose.

The planning target volumes (PTVs) are defined to provide an appropriate margin around each CTV, which accounts for variabilities in daily setup and, when applicable, organ motion and changes in anatomy due to tumor shrinkage. This margin is generally 4 to 5 mm, unless a center has studied and defined its own individual magnitude of uncertainty in setup or the tumor abuts a critical organ such as the spinal cord or the optic chiasm. Image guided radiation therapy (IGRT) using daily set up verification, particularly with CT imaging may allow for even tighter PTV margins.

The Radiation Therapy Oncology Group (RTOG) completed a phase II trial (RTOG 0022) assessing the feasibility of IMRT to provide adequate target coverage while sparing parotid glands for patients with early-stage oropharyngeal cancers (Eisbruch et al., 2010). The dose prescription is specified to an isodose that encompasses at least 95% of the

PTV_{HD}. Other requirements are that no more than 20% of the PTV will receive >110% of the prescribed dose and no more than 1% of the PTV will receive <93% of the prescribed dose. This regimen yielded a 2-year local–regional control rate of 91%. The incidence of grade 2 or higher xerostomia was 55% at 6 months but decreased to 25% at 12 months and 16% at 24 months.

Conventional Technique

For *photon* beam irradiation, the radiation dose is prescribed at the isocenter or an appropriate isodose line encompassing the target volume, maintaining dose heterogeneity within the target volume to no more than ±5%. The dose to the mid and lower neck given by an anterior appositional field is prescribed at D_{max} or 3 cm depth ($D_{3\,cm}$) depending on protocol specification.

For *electron* beam irradiation, the dose for elective treatment of nodal areas is prescribed at D_{max} and for therapeutic treatment of involved nodal areas is prescribed at 90% isodose line. The dose delivered through an appositional field for the treatment of cancer of the nasal vestibule or cavity, parotid gland, anterior faucial pillar, and retromolar trigone is prescribed at the desired isodose line (usually 90%). If medial coverage is inadequate, higher electron beam energy should be used, rather than specifying the dose to a lower isodose line. It is essential to obtain an isodose distribution with inhomogeneity corrections to ensure proper coverage of the target volume by the electron beam.

TECHNIQUES TO IMPROVE DOSE DISTRIBUTION

Compensating Filters

In situations where there is substantial variation in the tissue thickness within the treatment portals, photon beam dose homogeneity can be improved by the use of missing tissue compensating filters. The complexity of these filters in design and accuracy, and the improvements in technology with CT-based treatment planning to compensate not only for anatomic contour variations but also for changes in tissue density, as well as the capability of MLCs to improve dose distribution has made the use of compensating filters for photon therapy obsolete in most centers. IMRT and its variants have also decreased the need for compensating filters.

MLCs can create a large field designed to encompass the target. Within this field, one or more smaller fields can be created to deliver additional doses to portions of the target receiving lower than the desired dose (Fig. 3.14).

While compensating filters are rarely used nowadays for photon-based therapy, they are an important component of proton-based treatments. Passive scanning techniques remain an important tool in proton-based therapy,

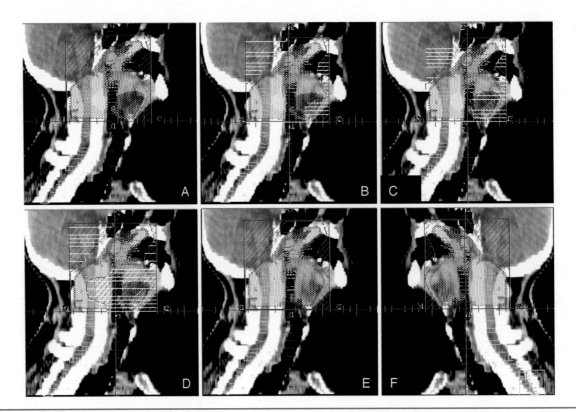

Figure 3.14 Distribution of radiation dose across the midsagittal plane, plotted in 5% gradients, of the initial large opposed lateral portals encompassing the primary tumor and upper cervical nodal basins. Without beam modulation, the dose distribution varies from 95% (*blue color wash*) to 115% at the tongue base region (*dark sky-blue color wash*) (**A**). Using MLC leaves (*white lines*) to shield the 115% isodose line from the right lateral field (**B**), the 110% line from the left lateral field (**C**), and finally the 105% line from the right portal (**D**) yield a dose distribution on the central plane to within 5% of the primary prescribed dose (**E,F**).

and proton compensating filters are critical for precise dose delivery to targets.

Electron Beam Bolus

Electron beam bolus may serve three functions. First, it can increase surface dose for low-energy beams when skin sparing is not warranted. Second, it can attenuate the beam to protect underlying tissues in cases where a different depth of penetration is desired in different parts of the portal. Finally, it can be useful to "smooth" irregular surface contours, which perturbs electron beam dosimetry through uneven scatter.

For a simple skin dose buildup on a reasonably flat surface, a layer of superflab of appropriate thickness is sufficient. For surface contour modification, a custom-made beeswax

bolus is preferred (Figs. 3.12 and 3.13). Care should be taken to ensure good contact between bolus material and the skin surface to minimize unintended perturbation of electron beam. Commercial systems, some with the use of 3-D printers are allowing for greater availability of custom bolus.

SUGGESTED READING

Eisbruch A, Harris J, Garden AS, et al. Multi-institutional trial of accelerated hypofractionated intensity-modulated radiation therapy for early-stage oropharyngeal cancer (RTOG 00-22). *Int J Radiat Oncol Biol Phys* 2010;76(5):1333–1338.

4

Practical Aspects of Endocavitary Beam Therapy, Intraoperative Radiation, and Brachytherapy

Key Points

- Endocavitary beam therapy can be an excellent method for delivering boost doses to selected patients presenting with accessible, well-circumscribed oral cancer.

- Brachytherapy, performed by an experienced team, either alone or as a supplement to external beam radiation, can yield high tumor control rates with low-toxicity profiles in selected patients.

- High-dose rate (HDR) intraoperative radiation therapy can be used to escalate dose to an operative bed, after the tumor resection, using a Harrison-Anderson-Mick (HAM) applicator.

- Most brachytherapy is currently delivered by using remote-controlled afterloaders that insert radioactive (^{192}Ir) sources.

- Currently available brachytherapy equipment and planning systems allow the flexibility to adjust radioactive source dwell time or intensity to optimize dose distribution.

- Primary treatment with both endocavitary beam and brachytherapy have largely fallen out of favor due to the greater availability of IMRT and stereotactic radiation therapy to provide heightened doses to limited areas.

For patients with accessible tumors, endocavitary beam therapy has historically been a valuable method of delivering boost doses to well-circumscribed lesions in the anterior oropharynx or oral cavity. As such, it is an alternative to brachytherapy or higher doses of external beam therapy. A common method of delivery is the use of orthovoltage x-ray beam of 125 to 250 kVp for this mode of therapy.

Traditionally, brachytherapy has had an important role in the radiotherapeutic management of cancers of the oral cavity since it allows escalation of dose to the tumor with minimal dose to adjacent critical structures. However, improvements in both techniques in reconstructive surgery, including use of free flaps, and radiation therapy, including the greater availability and comfort with IMRT, have resulted in significant decreases in the use of brachytherapy for these tumors. In addition, brachytherapy requires significant knowledge of appropriate technique, availability of the radioactive sources (typically ^{192}Ir using an afterloader), and operating room access.

Although intraoperative radiation therapy with a linear accelerator has largely fallen out of favor due to the difficulty in delivering treatment while the patient is undergoing surgery and questionable radiobiologic benefit, the availability of intraoperative radiation using a superficial HDR brachytherapy applicator does make it a potential method of boosting a tumor bed after resection.

While primary treatments are typically performed with external beam therapy using IMRT in the modern day, brachytherapy can still be used to deliver additional boost doses to residual infiltrative disease of the tongue base after external beam therapy or to treat selected lesions involving the buccal mucosa, lip, oral commissure, nasal vestibule and recurrent tumors of the nasopharynx. In addition, occasional patients with tumors of the oral tongue or floor of mouth who decline surgery are treated primarily with brachytherapy. Overall, the proportions of patients treated with brachytherapy for primary cancers (not recurrences) continue to decrease given the availability of alternative methods of dose escalation.

ENDOCAVITARY THERAPY INDICATIONS AND PROCEDURES

Ideal candidates for endocavitary beam therapy are those with a well-circumscribed lesion that is visible and accessible by cone through the mouth and does not involve the mucoperiosteum of the mandible (e.g., cancers of the soft palate or anterior faucial pillar). Patients with an exaggerated gag reflex are not suitable for this type of treatment.

A patient selected for endocavitary beam (intraoral cone) therapy generally receives this treatment component before external beam therapy for better tumor localization. Patients also tend to tolerate intraoral cone therapy better before the manifestation of mucositis induced by external beam irradiation. After a cone of appropriate size is selected, it is sometimes possible to manufacture a stent for automatic cone positioning (**Case Study 9.2**). After the cone is placed in the desired treatment position, the x-ray unit is docked to the cone. A periscope is then used to verify tumor location within the cone aperture.

For lateral lesions, the cone is angled to avoid irradiation of the spinal cord during the endocavitary beam therapy. This is not possible, however, when the tumor arises from the midline. In this case, the dose contribution to the spinal cord should be calculated and taken into account in planning the external beam therapy component of treatment.

BRACHYTHERAPY TYPES

Temporary Interstitial Brachytherapy

All temporary interstitial radiotherapy is given with iridium-192 (^{192}Ir) wires inserted into Teflon catheters or stainless steel needles, depending on the tumor site (**Case Study 12.3 through Case Study 12.5 and Case Study 18.8**).

Intraoperative HDR Brachytherapy

To boost a surgical bed at the time of resection, a Harrison-Anderson-Mick (HAM) applicator, which is a flat, malleable pad with HDR catheters spaced at 1 cm, is placed over the surgical bed, with margin. Adjacent normal tissues are displaced as much as possible. Doses of 10 to 20 Gy are typically given in a single fraction while the patient is still under anesthesia using a remote ^{192}Ir afterloader. Following the completion of this treatment, the surgical reconstruction is completed; external beam radiation can be used after that to treat other areas at risk (**Case Study 18.9**).

Endocavitary Brachytherapy

Either low-dose rate (LDR) or HDR brachytherapy can be used for the treatment of nasopharyngeal carcinoma. A high-activity ^{192}Ir stepping source is used for HDR. A remote-controlled HDR afterloader inserts the ^{192}Ir source into a flexible silicone applicator (e.g., the Rotterdam nasopharyngeal applicator).

Molds

A surface mold loaded with ^{192}Ir or ^{137}Cs is occasionally used, especially for lesions on the hard palate or the alveolar ridge.

DEFINITION OF THE IMPLANT TARGET VOLUME

The first step in preparation for brachytherapy is to determine the treatment volume so that the number, length, and intensity of radioactive sources can be appropriately planned in advance. When patients are to receive brachytherapy after completion of external beam therapy, the patient is examined, and the lesion is carefully documented before the tumor regresses or disappears.

PROTECTION OF NORMAL TISSUES

The most crucial aspect for reducing morbidity from brachytherapy is to provide separation between the radioactive sources and normal structures outside the target volume, because distance is the primary means of protection with this mode of irradiation. In certain cases, special stents can be constructed to increase the distance. Occasionally, the stents may include shielding material (e.g., 2 mm of lead reduces the dose to shielded structures up to 50%). When stents cannot be made, gauze, dental rolls, or other material may be used at the time of the procedure. Refinement of afterloading techniques and the availability of flexible radioactive wires have improved the accuracy of implants, thereby reducing the volume of normal tissues exposed to high radiation doses. Current brachytherapy equipment and planning systems also allow the flexibility to adjust radioactive source dwell time or intensity to reduce heterogeneity in dose distribution.

Care should be taken to place radioactive sources at least 0.5 cm away from the mucoperiosteum of the mandible, whenever possible, to minimize the risk of radiation-induced bone exposure and osteoradionecrosis. In the absence of bone involvement, one source can be placed in the vicinity of the mandibular periosteum, when necessary, without excessive risk of inducing osteonecrosis.

OPERATING ROOM PROCEDURE FOR IMPLANTATION

The patient should be under general anesthesia and should be positioned appropriately for the implant. Care should be taken to minimize the trauma associated with needle placement to avoid massive edema. However, even if little or no edema is apparent, patients receiving interstitial therapy to the tongue base may need a protective tracheotomy. Placement of needles or catheters is done primarily on the basis of disease extent rather than by attempting to follow prescribed geometric implant patterns. However, the basic concepts of source separation and active length must be kept in mind. In general, the higher the dose to be delivered with brachytherapy, the more closely the implantation rules need to be followed to prevent unwanted "hot" or "cold" spots.

Proper radiation protection measures should be applied in the operating room. Most temporary implants can be afterloaded, thereby obviating the risks to operating room personnel from radiation exposure. When active sources are being implanted permanently, the best protection for the operator and operating room personnel is to minimize the time of exposure. Everything should be kept in readiness before the implant is begun, and delays should be avoided. Personnel not actively involved in the implant should stand away from the sources.

DOSIMETRY

For afterloading techniques, catheters are loaded with dummy wires for obtaining orthogonal x-rays. The computer-generated dose distribution is then obtained on the basis of the specific activity of available interstitial sources, and a plan for afterloading is developed. Because of the decay of iridium sources, it is desirable to keep wires with varying linear intensities. Sources are chosen that will deliver dose rates of 30 to 50 cGy per hour at the periphery of the implant. As a general rule, for single-plane implants, the required activity is 0.5 to 0.7 mCi per cm radium equivalent for 1-cm-spaced sources. In choosing an isodose contour that will cover the tumor volume, care is taken to ensure that any "hot spots" around the sources are not too large.

Dosimetry for patients receiving permanent ^{198}Au seed implants is purely for the purpose of documentation because no adjustment is possible.

PATIENT CARE MANAGEMENT DURING IMPLANT

Most patients with head and neck implants in place require nasogastric or gastric tube feeding for the duration of the implant. Adequate analgesia is also provided, although pain is usually not a problem after the first day. Nursing care must be delivered in shielded rooms with restricted access.

REMOVAL OF INTERSTITIAL IMPLANTS

Most implants can be removed without the patient being under general anesthesia, except for implants for tumors of the posterior oral tongue and base of the tongue. Adequate provision is made for the possibility of hemorrhage when an interstitial implant is removed, especially from the tongue or pharynx. Upon removal of an implant, all sources must be accounted for and a radiation survey of the room performed after the sources are returned to the safe.

5

Patient Care Before, During, and After Radiotherapy

Key Points

- Dental assessment, supportive care, and rehabilitation are integral in the care of patients with head and neck neoplasms.

- Tooth restoration or, when indicated, extraction before commencement of radiotherapy is effective in preventing complications resulting from dental decay and infection.

- Stringent oral hygiene and systematic use of fluoride gel are essential to prevent dental hypersensitivity, caries, and osteoradionecrosis of the mandible following radiotherapy.

- Xerostomia is a common bothersome side effect of comprehensive head and neck irradiation, but, fortunately, its incidence and severity have decreased with the use of parotid-sparing intensity-modulated radiation therapy.

- Nutritional support and management of pain, nausea, and mucoid secretions are crucial for minimizing distress and facilitating completion of radiotherapy without interruption and recovery after treatment.

- Timely assessment and prescription of mouth-opening and swallowing exercises prescribed and supervised by speech pathologists facilitate preservation of functions and quality of life.

- Many unpleasant treatment-induced sequelae can be prevented or lessened by timely and proper interventions.

DENTAL CARE

Evaluation, treatment, and prevention of any preexisting oral or dental pathology are an integral part of management of patients with head and neck cancer because complications vary with dental condition, the type of malignancy, and the therapeutic approach. Underlying preexisting silent pathology can become prominent in a patient receiving radiation and particularly so in combined therapy. Mild problems of the oral cavity can develop into severe complications that can either compromise cancer therapy or cause considerable morbidity. Oral complications can be minimized and, in some cases, eliminated, if identified and addressed early by a dental team. It is, therefore, important to assess the patients' access to dental care and their commitment to daily oral hygiene procedures.

A comprehensive evaluation of patients presenting with head and neck tumors includes an oral and dental clinical examination supplemented by intraoral radiologic evaluation. Selected dental radiographs are essential in evaluating potential areas of infection that are not obvious on clinical examination (e.g., periodontal–periapical tooth pathology, residual cysts, and impacted or partially erupted exfoliating teeth). From this information, the dentist can plan oral treatment to bring the dental problem under control, thereby meeting immediate needs before radiation therapy. Oral treatment plans should be designed to correct restoration overhangs, rough or sharp edges in teeth, and any other defects that can cause soft tissue irritation. Patients should be instructed to avoid abrasive food that could traumatize soft tissues. Ill-fitting intraoral prostheses should not be worn during radiation therapy. Dental implants should be carefully assessed, and their removal should be considered if maintenance of peri-implant health cannot be reasonably anticipated or if integration is poor. Any potential source of oral infection should be identified and eliminated.

In general, patients with good dental status, including those who need routine restoration of a few cavities, are instructed to maintain oral hygiene and undergo brush training. They also receive custom-made carriers for fluoride prophylaxis to prevent caries and hypersensitivity of teeth. Mouth guards, made of flexible plastic material, may be necessary to prevent biting irradiated tissues that becomes edematous. Edentulous patients are instructed to maintain oral hygiene and to avoid trauma and premature use of prosthesis. In patients undergoing surgical therapy, the oral cavity should also be prepared for appropriate prosthetic rehabilitation to correct surgical deficits.

When there are findings of periapical pathosis, questionable periodontal status, unrestorable teeth with advanced caries, supererupted teeth, and, possibly, unopposed dentition, the teeth involved should be considered for extraction. Endodontic therapy is a viable alternative for pulpal necrosis, provided that the treatment can be expeditiously performed before the initiation of cancer therapy.

To ensure bone coverage and adequate wound healing, extractions should be performed 2 to 3 weeks before initiation of cancer therapy. Extractions and associated alveoloplasty should be performed with minimal trauma and should include smoothing of sharp surrounding hard tissue, appropriate irrigation, and primary closure in order to promote rapid healing. In general, periodontal surgical procedures should be avoided because prolonged healing and meticulous oral hygiene are needed to achieve the desired results.

The decrease in saliva production that often results from radiation to the head and neck region reduces the natural lavage of food and microbial debris from the oral cavity, which can lead to the development of dental caries. The change in the composition of saliva and reduced pH and buffering capacity also create a cariogenic oral environment, particularly in patients ingesting a diet high in carbohydrates or sucrose. Increased gingival recession may occur without signs or symptoms of periodontal inflammation. Therefore, special oral care is needed to prevent complications.

Good oral hygiene during and after therapy is essential for improving oral comfort and for reducing the risk of oral pathology. Bacterial and fungal superinfection can occur but are less likely to induce septicemia in patients undergoing radiotherapy alone than in those receiving concurrent chemotherapy, which causes bone marrow suppression. Oral rinsing with a solution of 1 teaspoon of sodium bicarbonate dissolved in 32 oz of water many times each day reduces oral microorganisms and aids in maintaining mucosal hydration. This measure, along with the elimination of secondary sources of irritation, such as alcohol, smoking, coarse or hot foods, alcohol- or phenol-containing mouth rinses, and sodium products, can help in minimizing mucositis.

The daily use of a fluoride gel can help minimize dental decay. The common formulations used are either 1.0% sodium fluoride gel or 0.4% stannous fluoride gel. Compared with sodium fluoride, stannous fluoride is slightly more acidic, but its uptake into the enamel matrices is four times greater. In adults with xerostomia, fluoride is released from the enamel within 24 hours; therefore, the fluoride regimen must be performed daily for optimal protection. The most efficient method of fluoride application is to use a custom-made polypropylene fluoride carrier that completely covers and extends slightly beyond the tooth surface. Patients fill the carriers with fluoride gel and place them onto the dentition daily for 10 minutes. Patients who receive low doses of radiation and are expected to have a slight degree of xerostomia can use a toothbrush to apply the fluoride gel. Sensitivity and pain are common side effects of fluoride and may necessitate a change in the fluoride concentration or the method of application. A daily fluoride program can decrease hypersensitivity, help mineralize cavitated enamel matrices, and, more important, inhibit caries-forming organisms.

Conventional oral physiotherapy is recommended during and after radiation, especially if the pterygoid muscles are within the radiation portals. Fibrosis of this musculature leads to trismus, which may be irreversible. Therefore, patients should be encouraged to perform mouth-stretching exercises before, during, and after radiation therapy. When needed, sophisticated means of mouth-opening exercises with opening devices (such as TheraBite, Jaw Dynasplint) may be recommended.

Radiation diminishes cellular elements of bone, thereby reducing its ability to heal after infection, trauma, or surgical procedure (e.g., dental extraction, alveoloplasty), which may result in osteoradionecrosis (ORN). Therefore, periodontal surgical intervention should be planned carefully, and the use of parenteral antibiotics and hyperbaric oxygen should be considered.

NUTRITIONAL SUPPORT

Assessment and Guidance

Nutritional care is crucial in the radiation treatment of patients with head and neck cancer. Patients receive dietary advice to help maintain their weight and nitrogen balance during the course of radiotherapy and the ensuing recovery period. Good nutritional support minimizes the need for therapy modifications (interruptions or dose reduction due to worsening of general condition and/or excessive reactions) that would compromise tumor cure probability.

It is essential that the dietician establishes a good rapport with the patient and provides basic instructions before the onset of acute reactions. It is prudent to counsel the patient's family members because the patient, who is under stress after learning the diagnosis and experiencing discomfort and pain, may not fully comprehend the instructions. Follow-up meetings are scheduled once a week or more often when interim problems occur, and data of weekly interviews are recorded along with the patient's initial and follow-up body weight. The attending physician and dietician should review the chart and recommend dietary adjustments when necessary.

Patients receiving radiation treatment of cancers of the oral cavity, oropharynx, nasopharynx, and hypopharynx are particularly prone to develop difficulties with food intake because of irradiation of a large area of mucous membranes and salivary glands. Therefore, they are encouraged to take supplemental calories at the beginning of treatment before the onset of reactions. The first problem encountered by this group of patients relates to alteration in salivary function, resulting in mucoid thick saliva. Moistened foods and increased fluid intake frequently facilitate mastication and deglutition during the first week.

Taste distortion (metallic flavor), loss of appetite, and burning sensation in the throat when swallowing citrus juices and acidic or spicy food become prominent during the second and third weeks. Helpful measures include the use of blander beverages, elimination of highly seasoned foods, addition of food aroma, and serving meals at room temperature.

Mucosal edema and denudation, resulting in dysphagia and pain, dominate the latter part of the treatment. At this time, the patient and family need constant support from the medical team. During this period, the diet should contain sufficient calories and supplementary protein to promote normal tissue regeneration. It is important to adjust the diet individually in terms of texture, consistency, and portion size. In general, soft diet (blended meat and vegetable) and frequent intake of small meals are recommended. Analgesics taken before meals can ease the pain.

Tube Feeding

Recommendations for feeding tube are individualized. The use of prophylactic placement of a feeding tube is controversial, but has not been our routine practice. Often percent weight loss from base line is used for decision making, with some suggesting a tube should be placed with 5% loss, and others using a 10% cutoff. In addition, though, the timing of oral challenge needs to be considered, as a patient having difficulties in week 2 may be more inclined to have tube placement than one who encounters difficulties in the final week of therapy. Additionally, other measures to correct intake challenges should be attempted, as simple remedies such as appropriate analgesia may obviate the need for tube placement. Occasionally, a Dobhoff nasogastric feeding tube is used. Nasogastric tubes are useful when either there is a contraindication for gastrostomy or the anticipated use is short term. Even when a gastrostomy is placed, continuation of swallowing exercises should be emphasized, to minimize risk of atrophy.

Several commercially prepared canned products are available for tube feeding. These formulas have a known nutritional composition and are convenient to use and store. Lactose-free and low-osmolarity products are also available to minimize diarrhea.

Examples of commonly used formulas include Isocal HN (1 cal/mL or 250 cal/can) and Protain XL (contains fiber and 237 cal/can). Isosource (contains fiber and 1.5 cal/mL or 375 cal/can) is more suitable for heavy patients. Tube feeding by gravity drip method begins with a half can on the day of gastric tube placement and increases gradually to six to eight cans per day, or more for heavier patients, generally divided into four or more sessions, depending on the estimated caloric requirement. Feedings are generally given over 1 hour for each session with a gravity drip and a bag. It is important to flush the gastric tube with 120 mL of water after feeding to prevent clogging. Depending on the fluid balance, supplemental water intake may be advised. It is important to encourage patients to continue to drink as much water and some liquid formula by mouth as possible to maintain swallowing motion.

In case patients or their family members wish to prepare the tube feeding formula at home, guidelines for adding minerals and vitamins are provided because these elements may be destroyed by food processing and by repeated heating. Patients receiving concurrent radiation and chemotherapy may need hospital admission for rehydration and feeding.

Diet after Completion of Radiotherapy

Instructions for future meal plans are provided at discharge. Generally, nutritional problems continue for 3 to 5 weeks after completion of radiotherapy. The recovery period is usually longer after combination of radiation with concurrent chemotherapy. Subsequently, the patient can progress gradually to a normal diet. Patients treated with parotid-sparing IMRT generally recover from acute xerostomia and swallowing dysfunction faster and better than those treated with the conventional technique. It is advantageous for patients to visit with their dieticians during follow-up visits to reassess their nutritional status and provide strategies to return to normal eating.

Swallowing Assessment and Rehabilitation

Both acute and late effects of radiation can disrupt a patient's ability to swallow. Early assessment by speech pathologists with expertise in swallowing rehabilitation is strongly recommended, preferably before initiation of radiation, for planning strategies for the prevention of chronic dependence on feeding tubes or swallowing dysfunction that can lead to aspiration.[1] Specific swallowing exercises designed to potentially prevent the debilitating effects of postradiation fibrosis, when recommended, need to be implemented as early as possible. Our work has demonstrated the importance of these exercises, as well as the challenges for patient adherence.[2]

Patients with postirradiation swallowing difficulties are also referred to speech pathologists for rehabilitation. A modified barium swallow, a study designed to examine the oropharyngeal movement while swallowing various food consistencies, provides information on bolus movement patterns, motility problems, and the cause of aspiration. A specific rehabilitation program can be implemented based on the findings.

SYMPTOMATIC MANAGEMENT OF REACTIONS

Careful management of acute reactions manifesting during treatment is important for decreasing discomfort and for avoiding interruption of radiotherapy, which is shown to compromise local–regional control of head and neck carcinoma.

Acute Mucositis

Treatment of acute mucositis is mainly symptomatic. In addition to pain management (see following text), patients receive instruction and encouragement to maintain good oral hygiene and to rinse and gargle with baking soda solution (1 teaspoon dissolved in 1 quart of water) after and between meals, at least five to six times a day, to minimize secondary infection. When oral candidiasis occurs, it is treated with nystatin suspension (100,000 U/mL, 4 to 6 mL, swish and swallow, four times per day) or clotrimazole troche (e.g., Mycelex, one troche orally, five times per day). Infections that do not respond to topical agents are treated with oral fluconazole.

Breakthroughs in mucositis prevention have been lacking. Phase III studies of palifermin, a truncated derivative of keratinocyte growth factor (KGF), were never completed, and while approved for mucositis prevention in patients receiving high-dose chemotherapy for hematologic malignancies, palifermin does not have a role in managing radiation-induced mucositis in patients with head and neck cancer. The data for efficacy of amifostine as a drug to diminish mucositis is controversial, and the cost and low benefit:risk ratio of the drug has led to this drug falling out of use for head and neck patients undergoing radiation or chemoradiation. Antibiotic therapy based on diminishing superinfection also has not been proven. A recent phase II study demonstrated that Caphosol, a high ionic electrolyte solution hypothesized to modulate the inflammatory response, did not reduce the incidence of mucositis.[3]

Analgesics

Almost all patients receiving head and neck radiotherapy need pain management to get through a period of acute radiation reactions. Various combinations of acetaminophen with hydrocodone, codeine, or oxycodone can be used. For easing mild-to-moderate pain starting to manifest 10 to 14 days into a course of radiotherapy, a frequently prescribed analgesic is acetaminophen 500 mg and hydrocodone bitartrate 7.5 mg tablets (Lortab 7.5/500) or elixir (15 mL contains about the same dose as one 500/7.5 tablet). The usual dosing is one to two tablets or 15 to 30 mL elixir every 4 to 6 hours. Other frequently used analgesics include acetaminophen 300 mg and codeine phosphate 30 mg (Tylenol with codeine No. 3), one to two tablets every 4 to 6 hours, and acetaminophen 325 mg and oxycodone hydrochloride 5 mg (Percocet).

Severe and refractory pain, which can occur during the second half of the radiotherapy regimen, may necessitate therapy with stronger opioids. Examples include morphine sulfate (10 or 20 mg/5 mL elixir, 10 to 30 mg orally every 4 to 6 hours), hydromorphone tablets (Dilaudid: 2 to 4 mg every 4 to 6 hours) or oral liquid (5 mg/5 mL every 4 to 6 hours), or suppositories (3 mg every 4 to 6 hours).

Sustained-release opioids may help in maintenance therapy for severe pain. Examples include morphine sulfate tablets (MS Contin: 30, 60 mg, or higher dose, every 12 hours) and fentanyl transdermal patch (Duragesic; 25, 50, 75, 100 µg/h every 3 days).

In general, topical anesthetics should be used cautiously because of their tendency to induce hypersensitivity reactions. When indicated, lidocaine gel 2% can be prescribed for topical application or swish and swallow/spit, up to four times a day. Frequently, minor oral or pharyngeal pain can be ameliorated with a solution of viscous lidocaine, diphenhydramine hydrochloride (Benadryl), and aluminum hydroxide/magnesium hydroxide (Maalox) (Xyloxylin: Magic Mouthwash).

Prevention and Treatment of Constipation

It is prudent to inform patients that analgesics tend to cause constipation and to prescribe sennoside tablets (Senokot: two tablets, up to four times a day) or docusate sodium capsules (Colace: 100 mg, one to two capsules everyday) to prevent this side effect. Patients receiving tube feeding can take docusate sodium syrup (15 mL, 20 mg/5 mL) plus sennoside syrup (Senokot: 5 mL, 8.8 mg/5 mL) two to three times per day via the gastric tube.

Antiemetics

Depending on the site and size of radiation portals, a variable proportion of patients experiences nausea and occasional vomiting. Useful medications include prochlorperazine maleate (Compazine: 5 or 10 mg tablets every 8 hours, 5 mg/5 mL syrup 1 to 2 teaspoons every 8 hours, or 25 mg suppositories twice daily) and metoclopramide hydrochloride (Reglan: 10 mg tablet or 1 to 2 teaspoons of syrup, 5 mg/5 mL, before meals and at bedtime). Capsules containing 0.34 mg lorazepam, 25 mg diphenhydramine, and 2 mg haloperidol (ABH capsules) or suppositories (containing 1 mg lorazepam, 12.5 mg diphenhydramine, and 2 mg haloperidol) are effective when given every 4 to 6 hours.

Serotonin 5-HT3 receptor antagonists such as ondansetron hydrochloride (Zofran: 8 mg tablets or sublingual preparation every 8 to 12 hours) are also effective, especially for patients receiving concurrent chemotherapy. However, nausea and vomiting are often secondary to poor oral fluid intake, resulting in dehydration, and therefore, intravenous fluids rather than antiemetics are required to correct the problem.

Skin Reactions

With megavoltage radiotherapy, skin care generally consists of prevention of local irritation by encouraging the use of soft clothing and avoiding sunlight exposure. Small areas of moist skin desquamation that occur occasionally require cleaning with a diluted 1% hydrogen peroxide solution to prevent secondary infection. Larger areas of moist skin desquamation can be managed with hydrogel sheet (e.g., CoolMagic) wound dressing.

Aquaphor ointment (a petroleum jelly based salve) is routinely prescribed for topical application after completion of radiotherapy. Radiation dermatitis management is similar to burn management, and there are numerous salves currently promoted for mild dermatitis including products containing hydrogels, aloe, lidocaine, and low-dose cortisone that helps alleviate the discomfort associated with dermatitis. More severe management is rarely needed, but wound/burn care salves such as biafine or silvadene can help patients with more severe dermal reactions. Patients are also instructed to use sunblock over the irradiated skin surface.

Prevention and Management of Xerostomia

The salivary glands are relatively radiosensitive. Determination of the specific dose that causes salivary gland damage has been challenging, and it is further recognized that there are differences between the radiosensitivity of the parotids that have a high percentage of serous cells, compared to the submandibular glands that have more mucous cells. Prevention of xerostomia has taken two directions: reducing radiation dose to the salivary glands and using chemical protectors. Advances in intensity-modulated radiation therapy technology enable sparing of the salivary gland even in patients not suitable for receiving unilateral irradiation. This approach has been studied in a number of centers[4,5] and by the Radiation Therapy Oncology Group[6,7] and is being implemented in many centers. The PARSPORT trial,[8] a phase 3 multicenter trial comparing IMRT to conventional radiation revealed fewer patients treated with IMRT had grade 2 or worse xerostomia than those treated with conventional therapy (38% vs. 74%, $P = 0.0027$). The median doses to the contralateral and ipsilateral parotid glands were 25.4

and 47.6 Gy, respectively, for patients treated with IMRT, compared to 61 and 61 Gy for patients treated with conventional therapy. It has generally been accepted that maintaining one gland to <26 Gy can minimize xerostomia, though it is further been shown that the TD50 (dose in which 50% complication is expected) of the parotid is roughly 39 Gy, but there is not threshold, and there is slow recovery beyond 1 year to even 5 years post treatment.[9] In addition to parotid sparing, there has been increased interest in lowering doses to the submandibular gland particularly if level 1b nodes are not at risk.

Amifostine has been studied extensively for prevention of various radiation side effects, particularly xerostomia. Despite a positive trial suggesting the drug reduces the incidence of xerostomia,[10] the necessity for daily injections, increase in nausea, and the efficacy of lower doses to salivary glands through conformal therapeutic radiation have severely reduced the use of this drug with head and neck radiation.

The role of pilocarpine (Salagen), a cholinergic agonist, in the treatment of xerostomia has been studied extensively. A large randomized trial compared 5 to 10 mg of pilocarpine, given three times a day, against placebo in patients with documented radiation-induced xerostomia. Both objective and subjective test endpoints demonstrated a benefit of the drug. A recently completed randomized trial of the Radiation Therapy Oncology Group revealed that pilocarpine administered during the course of radiotherapy resulted in significantly higher unstimulated salivary flows at the completion of radiotherapy and at 3 months after treatment. There was, however, no significant difference in unstimulated saliva production at 6 months after therapy or stimulated flow at any time points measured. In addition, no improvement in quality-of-life endpoints was detected.[11] Similar to amifostine, the use of these drugs has declined in practice.

Sialogogues and saliva substitutes are available and may benefit occasional patients. Caution is recommended regarding some sialogogues, particularly candies, because the limited subjective benefit can be countered by rapid dental decay.

Other Supportive Care

Moisturizing nasal spray (e.g., Ocean Spray, Nose Better) is recommended during the period of confluent mucositis occurring in the nasal cavity to prevent crusting and bleeding. Topical antibiotic (Neosporin ointment) is prescribed when infection develops.

Antitussive expectorant without suppressant (e.g., guaifenesin 600 mg, one to two tablets twice daily [Humibid-LA or Mucinex expectorant]) can relieve symptoms in a number of patients. Other options in lieu of hydrocodone bitartrate and aspirin include 5 mL syrup containing 10 mg hydrocodone bitartrate and 8 mg chlorpheniramine maleate (Tussionex), which can be a good cough suppressant for nighttime relief.

REFERENCES

1. Rosenthal DI, Lewin JS, Eisbruch A. Prevention and treatment of dysphagia and aspiration after chemoradiation for head and neck cancer. *J Clin Oncol* 2006;24:2636–2643.

2. Shinn EH, Base-Engquist K, Baum G, et al. Adherence to preventive exercises and self-reported swallowing outcomes in post-radiation head and neck cancer patients. *Head Neck* 2013;35:1707–1712.

3. Rao NG, Trotti A, Kim J, et al. Phase II multicenter trial of Caphosol for the reduction of mucositis in patients receiving radiation therapy for head and neck cancer. *Oral Oncol* 2014;50:765–769.

4. Eisbruch A, Ten Haken RK, Kim HM, et al. Dose, volume, and function relationships in parotid salivary glands following conformal and intensity-modulated irradiation of head and neck cancer. *Int J Radiat Oncol Biol Phys* 1999;45:577–587.

5. Garden A, Morrison W, Rosenthal D, et al. Intensity modulated radiation therapy (IMRT) for metastatic cervical adenopathy from oropharynx carcinomas. *Int J Radiat Oncol Biol Phys* 2004;60:S318.

6. Eisbruch A, Harris J, Garden AS, et al. Multi-institutional trial of accelerated hypofractionated intensity-modulated radiation therapy for early-stage oropharyngeal cancer (RTOG 00-22). *Int J Radiat Oncol Biol Phys* 2010;76:1333–1338.

7. Lee N, Harris J, Garden AS, et al. Intensity-modulated radiation therapy with or without chemotherapy for nasopharyngeal carcinoma: radiation therapy oncology group phase II trial 0225. *J Clin Oncol* 2009;27:3684–3690.

8. Nutting CM, Morden JP, Harrington KJ, et al. Parotid-sparing intensity modulated versus conventional radiotherapy in head and neck cancer (PARSPORT): a phase 3 multicentre randomised controlled trial. *Lancet Oncol* 2011;12:127–136.

9. Dijkema T, Raaijmakers CP, Ten Haken RK, et al. Parotid gland function after radiotherapy: the combined Michigan and Utrecht experience. *Int J Radiat Oncol Biol Phys* 2010;78:449–453.

10. Brizel DM, Wasserman TH, Henke M, et al. Phase III randomized trial of amifostine as a radioprotector in head and neck cancer. *J Clin Oncol* 2000;18:3339–3345.

11. Scarantino C, LeVeque F, Swann RS, et al. Effect of pilocarpine during radiation therapy: results of RTOG 97-09, a phase III randomized study in head and neck cancer patients. *J Support Oncol* 2006;4:252–258.

6

Target Delineation, Normal Tissue Contouring, and Normal Tissue Constraints

Key Points

- With 3D planning, contouring of individual tumor targets and normal tissue structures became a standard practice in radiation treatment for head and neck cancers.

- With IMRT, separate targets are delineated with differential dose specifications based on risk. These volumes all need to be individually drawn by the radiation oncologist.

- With the exception of a planning target volume (PTV) that accounts for uncertainty, standard margins and expansions are not utilized for head and neck radiation treatments.

- Delineation of normal tissues is just as important as delineation of tumor; planning algorithms use this information for avoidance, and the structures must be accurately drawn for optimal treatment plans.

- There are widely accepted, largely conservative, schema for dose constraints for normal tissues in the head and neck. As much as possible, these should be respected; however, for tumors that involve the critical structures themselves, limits may need to be pushed, with understanding by the patient and provider of the potential risks for toxicity.

TARGET DELINEATION

In the era of 3D planning based on simulation CT scans, contouring of the tumor targets and at-risk areas is the fundamental part of treatment planning for head and neck cancers. All pretreatment data, including physical examination, examination under anesthesia findings, diagnostic CT, PET, MRI, and ultrasound data, should be integrated in the creation of a target volume (**Case Study 6.1**).

If possible, multiple imaging techniques can be fused in the treatment planning software to help aid in target delineation. However, in some cases, this is challenging. Patients are often in very different positions in diagnostic scans (of any type) than in CT simulation scans for radiation planning. Deformable and rigid registration techniques can try to optimize alignment of diagnostic scans to simulation CT images; however, if this still is not optimal, then the radiation oncologist must extrapolate the findings onto the CT simulation scan (rather than having an automated solution). Alternatively, in some centers, it is possible to have patients undergo complementary imaging modalities in the treatment position, with the immobilization mask and devices (such as an oral stent). In these cases, the positioning should be the same as that at CT simulation; hence, it provides the best opportunity for multimodality treatment planning.

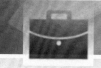

CASE STUDY 6.1

This 50-year-old man was diagnosed with HPV-associated right tonsillar carcinoma. He was clinically staged T2N2C, as the tumor was 3 cm, and there was bilateral adenopathy. He was simulated with a non-contrast CT scan (Fig. 6.1A), having just had a contrast-based CT scan (Fig. 6.1B) and PET/CT scan (Fig. 6.1C) for diagnostic purposes. He was also imaged with MRI (T1 with contrast, Fig. 6.1D) in the treatment position (on an in-house study). The 4 imaging studies were co-registered. Representative axial images at the same level through the tonsillar tumor are shown (Fig. 6.1A–D) with the drawn contours. GTV (*green*), CTV$_{HD}$ (*red*), and CTV$_{ID}$ (*blue*)

are shown. The contours on the non-contrast CT scan (Fig. 6.1A) that were ultimately used to plan the patient's treatment were propagated to the three coregistered diagnostic studies (Fig. 6.1B–D) as a tool to facilitate target accuracy. CTV$_{HD}$ added an approximate 10-mm margin to the GTV, and CTV$_{ID}$ added 0 to 5 mm to CTV$_{HD}$ as well as adding margin on the nodal CTV$_{HD}$ more inferiorly (not shown). The margin of CTV$_{ID}$ given to the primary CTV$_{HD}$ varied, being slightly more generous to cover the adjacent but uninvolved buccal space, a potential area for easy tumor extension, while minimizing unnecessary margin on the uninvolved vertebral body.

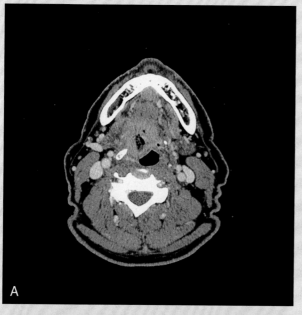

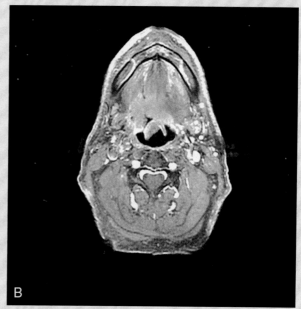

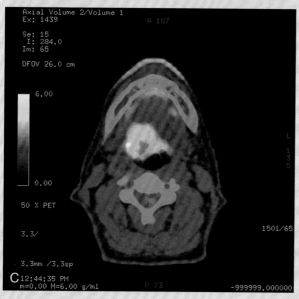

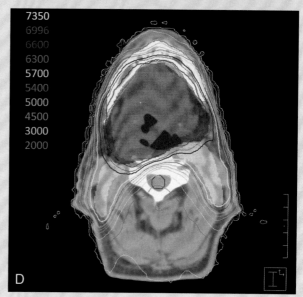

Case Figure 6.1A–D

Target Delineation for Intact, Previously Untreated Cancers

For patients who have gross disease that is previously untreated (no prior history of resection or induction chemotherapy), the entirety of the gross tumor should be contoured as the basis of the target volumes. The GTV of the primary tumor and nodal disease should be based on all cross-sectional imaging modalities available integrated with physical examination. Historically, CT has been used to delineate the extent of disease; outcomes of clinical studies reflect this practice. More recently, MRI has been utilized, which may demonstrate a disparate degree of soft tissue extension. Since outcomes of studies have been based on CT planning, the integral benefit of adding MRI is unclear. We recommend using CT, MRI, and physical examination findings to expand the GTV to include any potentially involved areas. PET scans have also been utilized to delineate gross disease; this technique is affected significantly by details of FDG administration, scan parameters, and windowing; hence, we recommend utilizing it only to determine involved regions (equivocal nodes on CT or MRI can be determined as FDG positive or negative); however, we do not recommend expanding cross-sectional contours to include all areas of FDG avidity (if these do not correspond to findings on CT or MRI).

Once the GTV has been determined, the clinical target volume (CTV) for the highest dose region (CTV$_{HD}$) is a geometric and anatomic expansion. Typically, we recommend an expansion of 8 to 10 mm circumferentially in all directions from the GTV. However, this should take into account natural barriers of tumor spread. For instance, a slightly smaller margin may be taken laterally for a tonsil tumor, since if the lateral musculature is intact it is unlikely that there is subclinical tumor involving the mandible.

The remaining targets are delineated to encompass subclinical disease. As guidelines for IMRT evolved it had become practice to delineate a CTV for an intermediate dose (CTV$_{ID}$) and a second CTV for a lower or "elective dose" CTV$_{ED}$. The rationale, which has been strictly empiric, was based on the concept that regions closer to GTV are more likely to harbor subclinical disease, and thus, more dose was necessary. Further, it has been argued, while conventional treatment most commonly made one dose reduction between the larger volumes that included subclinical disease and the boost volumes that only covered gross disease (with margin), the boost fields still frequently unintentionally included these higher risk subclinical sites. For example, in boosting a base of tongue cancer, parallel opposed fields would cover much of level II in the neck, even in the absence of gross nodal disease.

The absolute necessity of two separate targets to treat subclinical disease to differing doses (as opposed to one CTV for all subclinical disease) is a topic beyond the scope of this manual. We have chosen to give our guidelines for two subclinical targets as it has been our practice. CTV$_{ID}$ typically includes adjacent regions that may harbor microscopic disease. From CTV$_{HD}$, we recommend a 2- to 5 mm expansion to create CTV$_{ID}$. Furthermore, it is typical to cover the entire involved nodal level with CTV$_{ID}$. For instance, for a patient with nodal disease in level IIB, the gross nodes with an 8- to 10 mm margin would be delineated as CTV$_{HD}$, with the remainder of level II on that side being included in CTV$_{ID}$. The CTV for the elective dose (CTV$_{ED}$) should include all uninvolved, at risk regions. For patients with nodal disease, these will include at-risk nodal levels that are not involved or adjacent to gross disease. For instance, for a patient with nodal disease in level II, the gross nodes with an 8- to 10 mm margin would be delineated as CTV$_{HD}$, with the remainder of level II on that side being included in CTV$_{ID}$ and levels IB, III, IV, and V on the ipsilateral side and II to IV on the contralateral side being included in CTV$_{ED}$. For primary tumors that involve pharyngeal structures, the retropharyngeal nodes are also contoured as CTV$_{ED}$, if they are not involved. Principles of contouring intact cancers are demonstrated in **Case Study 6.2**.

Target Delineation for Patients Treated with Neoadjuvant (Induction) Chemotherapy

For patients who receive neoadjuvant or induction chemotherapy, there may be significant decrease in the extent of the primary or nodal disease. Nevertheless, there are no data supporting reduction of target volumes as a result of chemotherapy response. Hence, the initial extent of gross disease, with margin, is targeted, even in the setting of chemotherapy response.

Without a target, a "virtual" GTV must be created, which captures the extent of disease at presentation. After the virtual GTV is created, the expansions to create CTV$_{HD}$, CTV$_{ID}$, and CTV$_{ED}$ are the same as those described for definitive (intact) cases. In some centers, where there are available resources and appropriate logistics, patients are simulated for radiation treatment prior to acquisition of induction chemotherapy; they are then resimulated after chemotherapy for true radiation treatment planning. The benefits of this are the ability to delineate the initial prechemotherapy target volumes in the treatment position. The potential downfalls of this approach are that the patient may lose significant weight or have anatomic changes with chemotherapy, which requires a new mask after the induction chemotherapy, making the identification of the original disease more challenging since the pre- and post-chemotherapy setups are not identical. Most patients are simulated for radiation at the conclusion of the induction chemotherapy; thus the initial diagnostic imaging and examination are crucial to creation of the virtual GTV and subsequent expansions. **Case Study 6.3** describes optimal contouring of a patient who received induction chemotherapy.

CASE STUDY 6.2

A 40-year-old male presented with a left neck mass. Physical examination revealed left neck adenopathy as well as a left tonsil mass; biopsy was positive for squamous cell carcinoma (HPV positive). He was dispositioned to concurrent chemoradiation. The left tonsil mass is shown on CT imaging (Fig. 6.2A), delineated with arrows. To create a treatment plan, the tonsil primary was delineated based on CT imaging and physical examination. In Figure 6.2B, the GTV for the primary tumor is shown in green outline.

To create CTV$_{HD}$, an 8- to 10 mm margin was made around this area, with trimming laterally due to the proximity of the mandible (a natural barrier); the CTV$_{HD}$ is shown in red colorwash (Fig. 6.2C). To create CTV$_{ID}$, an additional 2 to 3 mm margin was made around the CTV$_{HD}$; this is shown in blue colorwash in Figure 6.2D. To create CTV$_{ED}$, elective regions (not involved) are contoured; on this axial slice, the contralateral retropharyngeal nodal region is CTV$_{ED}$, shown in yellow colorwash (also shown in Fig. 6.2D).

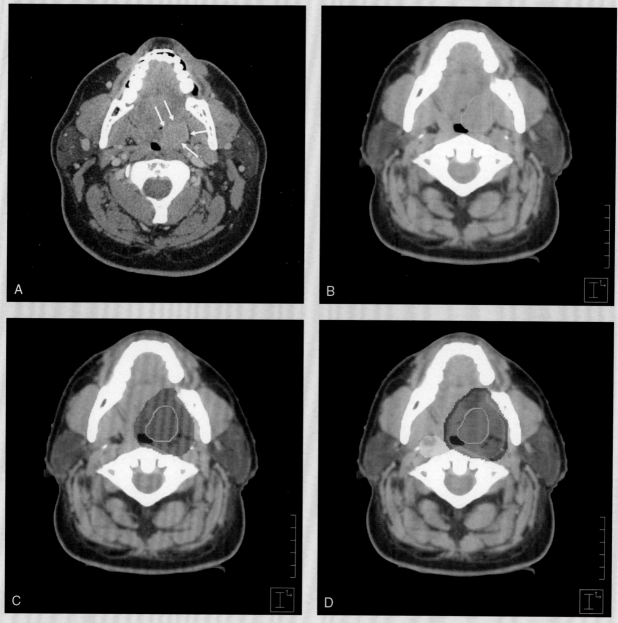

Case Figure 6.2A–D

Similarly, the nodal volumes are delineated using the same process. In Figure 6.2E, the left neck adenopathy is demonstrated on a diagnostic CT scan (delineated by *arrows*). In Figure 6.2F, the GTV for the nodal disease is shown in light green outline. To create CTV_{HD}, an 8- to 10 mm margin was made around this area; the CTV_{HD} is shown in red colorwash (Fig. 6.2G). Medially, the CTV_{HD} does include the pharyngeal wall and lateral base of tongue; this is the result of volu-

metric expansion of CTV_{HD} from the primary tonsil tumor more superiorly. To create CTV_{ID}, the entire involved nodal level is contoured around the involved nodal region; this is shown in blue colorwash in Figure 6.2H. To create CTV_{ED}, elective regions (not involved) are contoured; on this axial slice, the contralateral level II is CTV_{ED}, shown in yellow colorwash (Fig. 6.2H). The overall contouring schema is shown in the coronal view in Figure 6.2I.

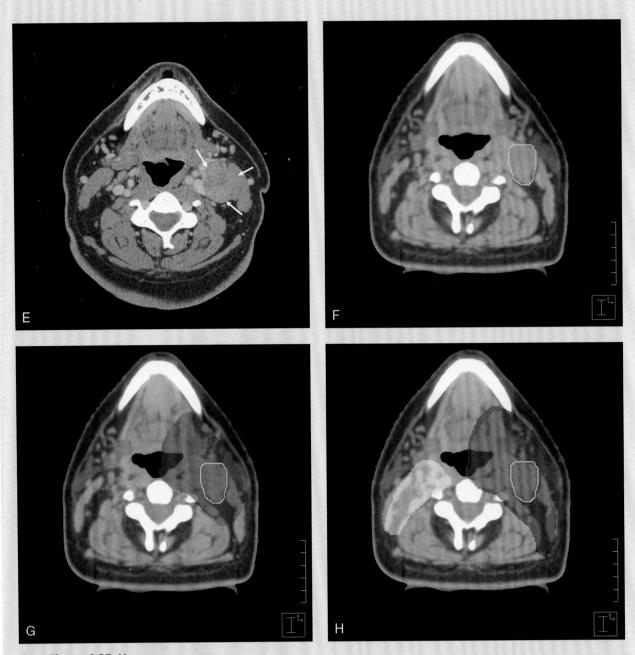

Case Figure 6.2E–H

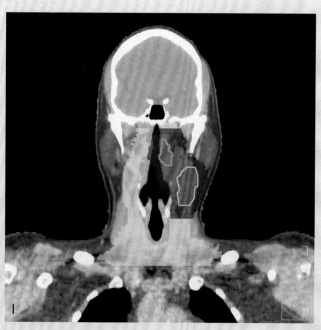

Case Figure 6.2I

 CASE STUDY 6.3

A 61-year-old male presented with a right neck mass and dysphagia. Physical examination revealed bilateral neck adenopathy as well as a large oropharynx mass, involving both the tonsil and base of tongue, with extension to the oral tongue; biopsy was positive for squamous cell carcinoma (HPV positive). The initial extent of disease is shown in Figure 6.3A. He was dispositioned to induction chemotherapy followed by chemoradiation; for induction, he received three cycles of docetaxel, cisplatin, and 5-fluorouracil (TPF). He had a response to chemotherapy, with regression of the oropharynx mass and the lymphadenopathy (Fig. 6.3B); the massive primary tumor had

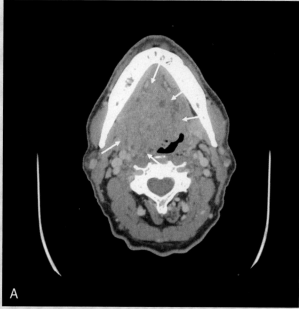

Case Figure 6.3A,B

shrunk considerably. He was dispositioned to concurrent chemoradiation. To create a treatment plan, the initial primary, prior to chemotherapy, was delineated based on CT imaging and physical examination. In Figure 6.3C, the virtual GTV for the primary tumor is shown in green outline; this is based on the prechemotherapy extent. To create CTV_{HD}, an 8- to 10 mm margin was made around this area, with trimming laterally due to the proximity of the mandible (a natural barrier); the CTV_{HD} is shown in red colorwash (Fig. 6.3D).

To create CTV_{ID}, an additional 2- to 3 mm margin was made around the CTV_{HD}; this is shown in blue colorwash in Figure 6.3E; the bilateral necks were also treated to this dose since there was involved adenopathy at this level on both sides (not shown). To create CTV_{ED}, elective regions (not involved) are contoured, including the bilateral retropharyngeal nodes and low neck. Similarly, the nodal volumes are delineated using the same process, based on the prechemotherapy extent of disease.

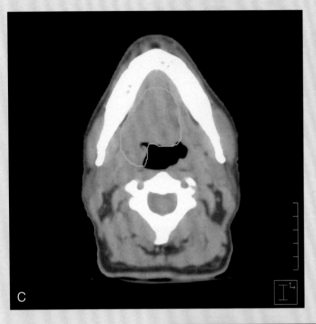

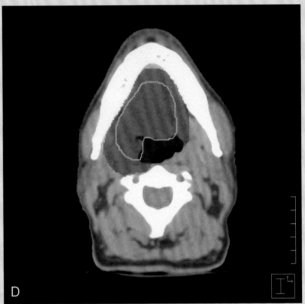

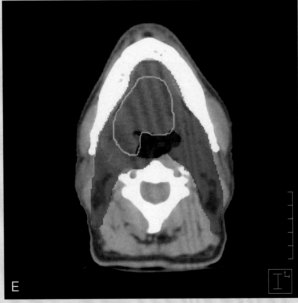

Case Figure 6.3C–E

Target Delineation for Patients Treated with Surgery

For patients who receive surgical resection followed by adjuvant radiation, there is no longer a visible target at the time of simulation for contouring. In fact, often times, there is a flap reconstruction and very different anatomy, even separate from the absence of the gross tumor. To create optimal treatment plans in postoperative cases, the initial extent of gross disease should be identified and reconstructed, to serve as the basis for target volumes.

Without a physical target, a "virtual" GTV must be created, which captures the extent of disease at presentation. After the virtual GTV is created, the expansions to create CTV_{HD}, CTV_{ID}, and CTV_{ED} are the same as those described for definitive (intact) cases. For patients who have a flap reconstruction, the entire flap is typically included in either CTV_{HD} or CTV_{ID}, depending on the size of the flap and proximity to the target. More important though than the coverage of the flap, is good coverage of the intact normal tissues that the flap abuts, as these represent the edge of the surgical bed and are more likely to harbor microscopic residual disease. Fundamentally, the suture lines for the resection (and reconstruction with the flap) is a high-risk area that should be widely covered. For patients who are found to have microscopic disease at the time of surgery that was not captured on pretreatment imaging or physical examination (for instance, pathologic adenopathy with no imaging correlate), the entire nodal level should be treated to CTV_{HD}. **Case Study 6.4** describes optimal contouring of a patient who received surgery and was dispositioned to adjuvant radiation therapy.

CASE STUDY 6.4

A 59-year-old female presented with an ulceration on the right anterolateral oral tongue. Physical examination revealed an ulcerated lesion in the right lateral oral tongue; biopsy was positive for squamous carcinoma with >4 mm depth of invasion. The initial extent of disease on diagnostic CT with contrast is shown in Figure 6.4A, with the primary tumor delineated by arrows. She had no suspicious adenopathy on imaging or physical examination. On clinical examination, she had a T1 N0 M0 right oral tongue lesion. She was dispositioned to surgery followed by assessment for radiation based on pathologic risk factors. At the time of surgery, she had a partial glossectomy with a reconstruction with an ulnar artery perforator flap; she also had a right neck dissection because of the depth of invasion of the primary tumor. On pathology, the primary lesion was a 2.3 cm moderately differentiated squamous carcinoma with perineural invasion and negative margins. In the right neck dissection, there were three nodes with microscopic disease (out of a total of 25 removed). These nodes were in levels IB and II. Given the adverse features of perineural invasion and multiple positive lymph nodes, she was dispositioned to adjuvant radiation therapy to the tongue and bilateral necks. To create a treatment plan, the initial primary, prior to surgery, was delineated based on CT imaging and physical examination. In Figure 6.4B, the virtual GTV for the

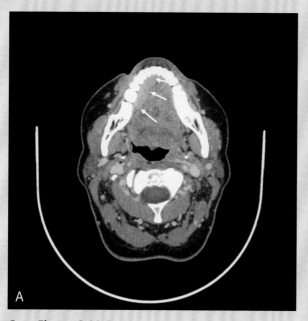
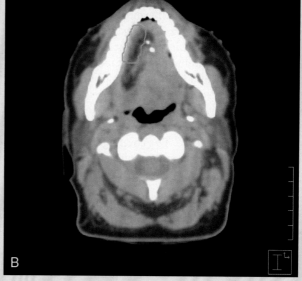

Case Figure 6.4A,B

primary tumor is shown in green outline; this is based on the presurgery extent. The flap reconstruction is visible on this axial slice. To create CTV$_{HD}$, an 8- to 10 mm margin was made around this area, with trimming laterally due to the proximity of the mandible (a natural barrier); the CTV$_{HD}$ is shown in red colorwash (Fig. 6.4C). In addition, the entire level IB and II were delineated as CTV$_{HD}$, since these had pathologically positive lymph nodes (with no pretreatment imaging showing suspicious adenopathy). To create CTV$_{ID}$, an additional 2- to 3 mm margin was made around the CTV$_{HD}$; this is shown in blue colorwash in Figure 6.4D. To create CTV$_{ED}$, elective regions (not involved) were contoured, including the contralateral levels I to IV (Fig. 6.4D).

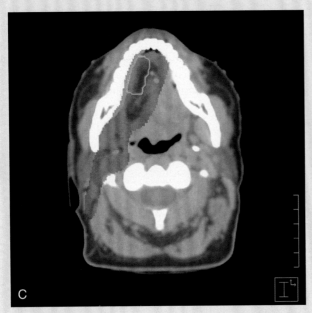
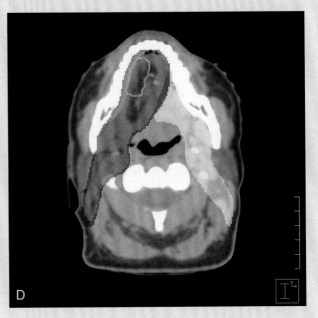

Case Figure 6.4C,D

Target Delineation for Patients with Cranial Nerve Involvement/Risk

To be discussed in subsequent chapters, inclusion of at risk cranial nerves in the target volume is recommended for certain neurotropic tumors. The most common scenarios to encounter perineural invasion are skin cancers and salivary gland cancers. Perineural invasion is also seen in oral tongue cancers and is an indication for radiation. However, it is unclear if perineural invasion in tongue cancer reflects true neurotropism.

Based on the above, the most common nerves to harbor disease are the trigeminal and facial nerves. The accompanying figures show representative CTVs covering these two cranial nerves and their pathways near the skull base (Figs. 6.5 to 6.8).

NORMAL TISSUE CONTOURING AND SUGGESTED DOSE CONSTRAINTS

Basic contoured normal structures for organs at risk (OAR) are represented in Figure 6.9.

Representative and commonly considered OARs are shown on noncontrast CT simulation datasets that were obtained for treatment planning purposes. In Figure 6.9A to N, axial CT images are shown, starting at the level of the eyes and ending in the lower neck (level IV). A sagittal view is shown in Figure 6.9O and coronal views at different depths in Figure 6.9P,Q. The pharyngeal constrictor muscle group is presented separately (Fig. 6.9R). An accurately registered T2-weighted MRI facilitates delineation of central nervous system and skull base OARs. In Figure 6.9A,B, a T2-weighted MRI image insert is shown to highlight the optic chiasm and brainstem. Likewise in Figure 6.9E, a T2-weighted MRI image insert shows detailed inner ear anatomy.

The lenses are hyperdense on CT imaging and easily contoured and should also be expanded 3 to 4 mm to create a surrogate structure in order to constrain dose to the corneas. The eyes/globes are shown here as a single OAR, but the posterior wall of the globe can be separately contoured to constrain dose to the retina. The lacrimal gland lies in the superior-lateral aspect of the bony orbit and should also be contoured and constrained when appropriate. Brain tissue and in particular temporal lobes should also be contoured when appropriate. In Figure 6.9C the right optic nerve is

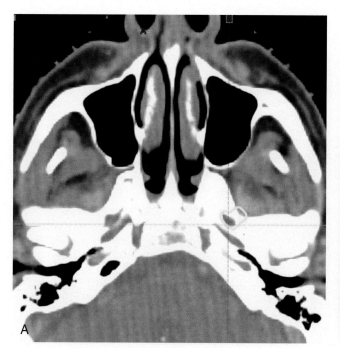

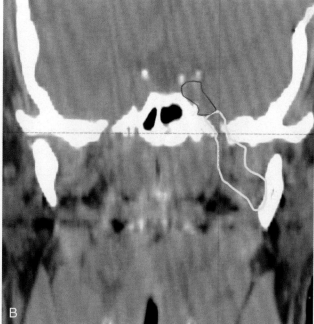

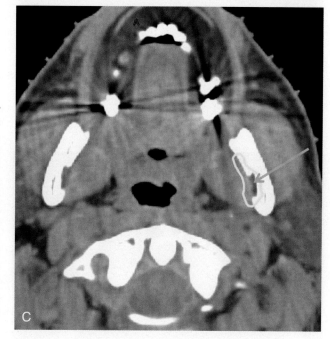

Figure 6.5 The mandibular division (V3) of the trigeminal nerve (*yellow contour*) at the level of foramen ovale in shown in **(A)**. V3 (*yellow contour*) coming off the fifth nerve just superior to foramen ovale, and then coursing through the masticator space toward the medial aspect of the mandible is shown in the coronal plane in **(B)**. For reference purposes the cavernous sinus is also shown (*red contour*). The inferior alveolar nerve (branch of V3) enters the mandible at the inferior alveolar foramen and supplies sensory innervation to the lower teeth/gum and sensory innervation to the skin of the chin (mental nerve). At the level of inferior alveolar foramen, the lingual nerve (branch of V3) travels slightly anterior to the inferior alveolar nerve. Representative CTV coverage of both the inferior alveolar nerve and lingual nerve (*yellow contour*) at the level of the inferior alveolar foramen (*blue arrow*) is shown in **(C)**.

visualized through the optic canal. The precise transition from nerve to chiasm is somewhat arbitrary and in this figure is at the posterior edge of the bony canal. The left nerve is seen just above the canal. For demonstration purposes, the nerve is split, as it does not go through the bone, but for planning purposes, it is safer to connect the contour through the bone, so the planning computer doesn't try to force dose in the gap.

We contoured and show the spinal cord proper, but for treatment planning purposes, the spinal cord should be expanded 5 mm in order to create a spinal cord planning volume at risk (PRV). Contouring of the spinal cord should start at the foramen magnum and extend at least 5 cm caudal to the most inferior aspect of the treatment volume.

The bilateral parotid glands should be contoured in a way that encompass the entirety of functional glandular tissue, including the deep lobe, which can encroach on the parapharyngeal space (see Fig. 6.9F,G) and the superficial aspect of the gland, or even accessory gland tissue, which can extend anteriorly over the masseter muscle (see Fig. 6.9F). Here, we also contoured the tail of the parotid gland (see Fig. 6.9H).

The oral cavity OAR shown in Figure 6.9F through 6.9I is broadly delineated to encompass the mucosal-bearing surfaces of the oral cavity, including the lips, hard palate,

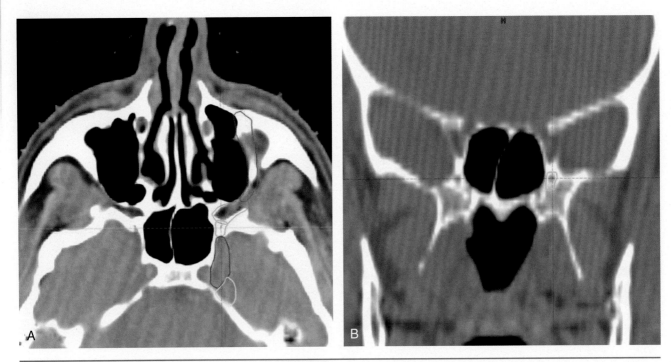

Figure 6.6 The infraorbital nerve, a branch of the maxillary division (V2) of the trigeminal nerve, provides sensory innervation to the midface and exits the maxilla through the infraorbital foramen. The course of the infraorbital nerve (*purple contour*) and V2 at the level of foramen rotundum (*green contour*) and the cavernous sinus (*red contour*) are shown in **(A)**. The infraorbital nerve travels in the roof of the maxilla and through the pterygopalatine fossa (*orange contour*). V2 exits the skull base though foramen rotundum. The trigeminal ganglion resides in Meckel's cave (*light blue contour* in **A**). V2 in foramen rotundum (*green contour*) is shown in the coronal plane in **(B)**.

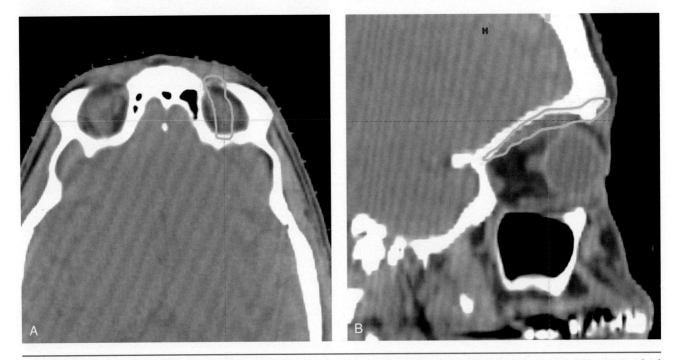

Figure 6.7 Sensory innervation to the forehead skin is provided by the frontal nerve (a branch of the ophthalmic division [V1] of the trigeminal nerve) and its two branches, the supraorbital and supratrochlear nerve. The course of the frontal nerve (*green contour*) in the roof of the orbit toward the superior orbital fissure is shown in axial **(A)** and sagittal **(B)** views.

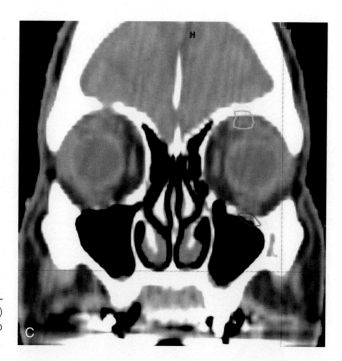

Figure 6.7 (*Continued*) Both the frontal nerve (*green contour*) and the infraorbital nerve (*purple contour*) and their relationship to the orbit in the coronal plane, are shown in **(C)**.

buccal surfaces, gingiva, oral tongue, and floor of mouth. An extended oral cavity structure may also be contoured, which includes the aforementioned structures, plus the base of tongue. However, contoured, the purpose of this structure is to limit the unnecessary irradiation to any nontarget upper aerodigestive tract mucosa.

Likewise, the larynx OAR as delineated here includes the entirety of the mucosal-covered aspects of the organ, from the tip of the epiglottis through the subglottic region, excluding the external cartilaginous framework. Smaller, functionally important subunits may be separately contoured, including the arytenoids and cricopharyngeal inlet.

Multiple brachial plexus contouring aids and guidelines are available, and it should be contoured when the prescription dose exceeds 60 Gy in the lower neck. It is generally contoured from then neural foramina into the axilla. The brachial plexus lies initially between the anterior and middle scalene muscles, which are contoured in Figure 6.9L.

The pharyngeal constrictor muscle OAR is shown in Figure 6.9R. While it is composed of three muscle groups (superior, middle, and inferior), for simplicity, recent guidelines have recommended contouring these as a single OAR.

Table 6.1 lists three common fractionation and dosing schedules used for IMRT in the most common treatment scenarios. These schedules will be reinforced throughout the text for each specific site. Table 6.2 lists normal tissue constraints.

Many of the constraints listed in Table 6.2 are empiric in nature and are commonly accepted constraints that do not

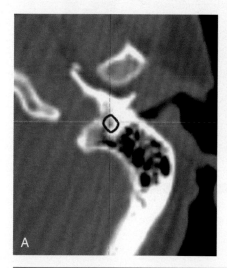
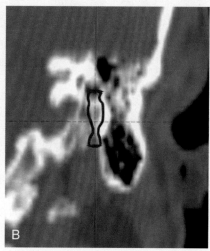
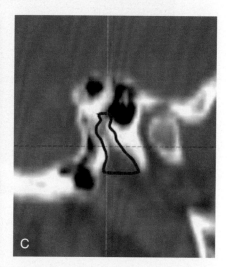

Figure 6.8 The facial nerve travels in the facial canal of the temporal bone and exits the skull base at the stylomastoid foramen. The course of the vertical segment of the facial nerve (*blue contour*) is shown the axial **(A)**, coronal **(B)**, and sagittal **(C)** figures.

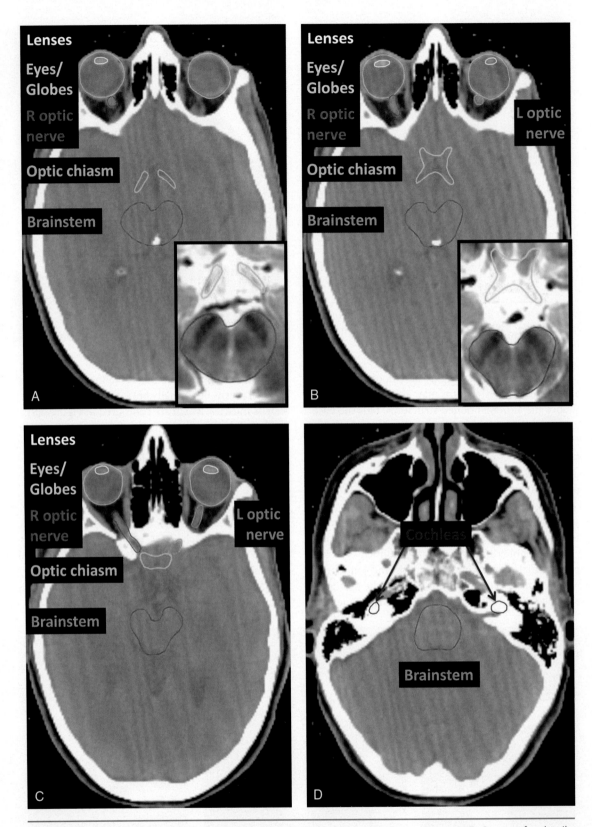

Figure 6.9 Representative contours of organs at risk (OARs) or normal tissue contours. **A–R:** See text for details.

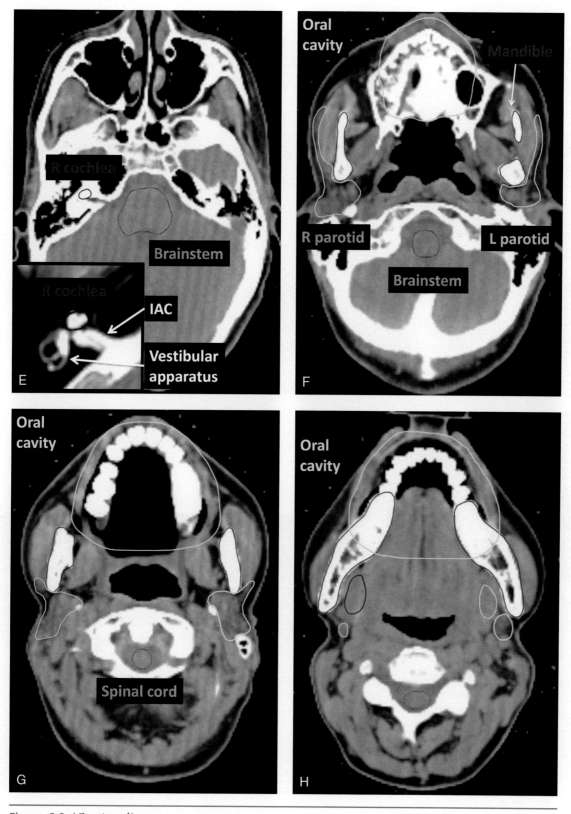

Figure 6.9 (*Continued*)

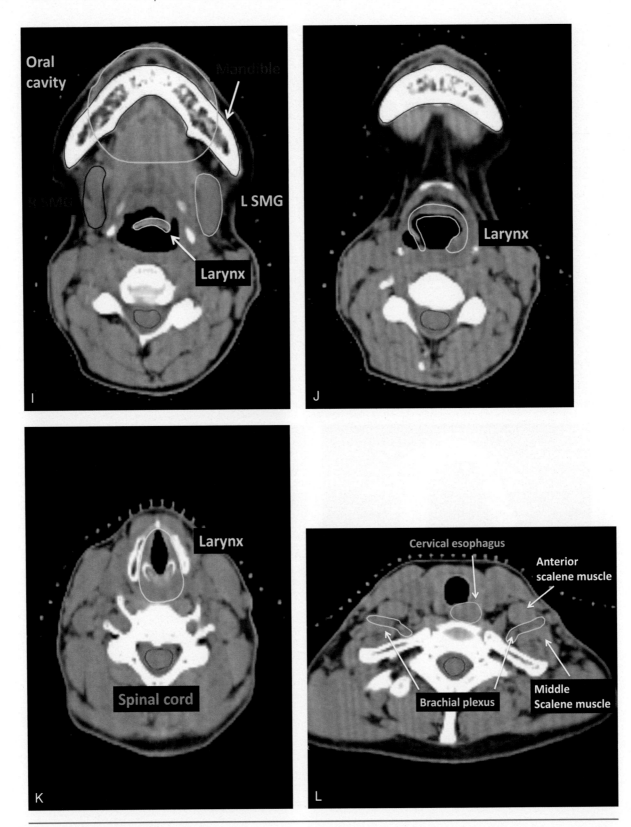

Figure 6.9 (*Continued*)

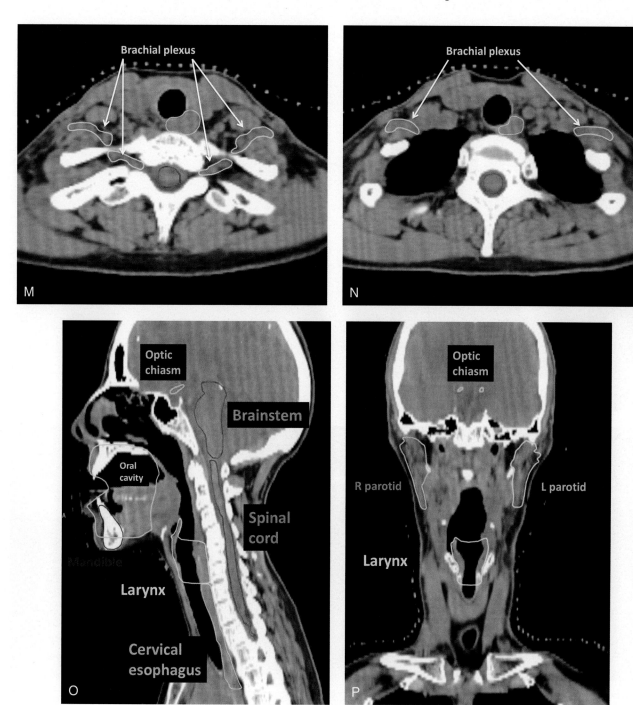

Figure 6.9 (*Continued*)

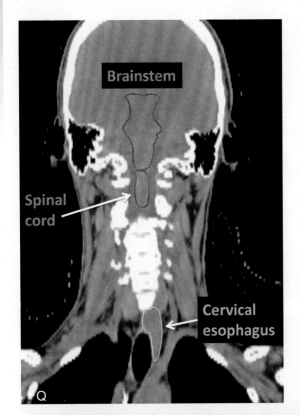

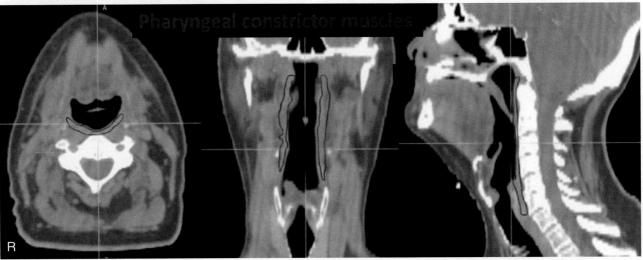

Figure 6.9 (*Continued*)

TABLE 6.1 Common Fractionation/Dosing Schema for the Different Target Volumes for IMRT

	CTV$_{HD}$	CTV$_{ID}$	CTV$_{ED}$	Total Fractions
Radiation alone (small tumor volume)	66 Gy (2.2 Gy/fraction)	60 Gy (2 Gy/fraction)	54 Gy (1.8 Gy/fraction)	30
Concurrent chemoradiation or radiation alone for large volume disease	70 Gy (2.12 Gy/fraction)	63 Gy (1.9 Gy/fraction)	57 Gy 1.7 Gy/fraction)	33
Postoperative radiation or chemoradiation[a]	60 Gy (2 Gy/fraction)	57 Gy (1.9 Gy/fraction)	54 Gy (1.8 Gy/fraction)	30

[a]Consider fourth volume of 63–66 Gy to small high-risk volumes.

TABLE 6.2 Dose Constraints for Normal Tissues using IMRT with Conventional Fractionation

	Traditional/Anecdotal	RTOG(NRG)	QUANTEC/Emami
Spinal cord	Dmax < 45 Gy	PRV cord 50 Gy ≤ 0.01 mL	Dmax < 54 Gy (rate <1%)
Brainstem	Dmax < 54 Gy	PRV brainstem 52 Gy ≤ 0.03 mL	D 1–10 mL < 59 Gy Dmax < 64 Gy (point dose <1 mL)
Parotid glands	Mean dose < 26 Gy	1 parotid: mean dose < 26 Gy	1 parotid: mean dose < 20 Gy Both: mean < 25 Gy
Submandibular glands	ALARA	Contralateral: mean dose < 39 Gy	Mean < 35 Gy
Cervical esophagus	ALARA	ALARA Mean dose < 30 Gy	V35 < 50% V50 < 40% V70 < 20% Mean dose < 34 Gy
Mandible	Dmax < 70 Gy	ALARA Dmax < 66 Gy	Dmax < 70 Gy
Cochlea/inner ear	Mean dose < 35 Gy	V55 < 5%	Mean dose < 35–45 Gy
Larynx	ALARA	ALARA Mean dose < 20 Gy	V50 < 27% Mean dose < 44 Gy Dmax < 66 Gy

(Continued)

TABLE 6.2 Dose Constraints for Normal Tissues using IMRT with Conventional Fractionation *(Continued)*

	Traditional/Anecdotal	RTOG(NRG)	QUANTEC/Emami
Pharyngeal constrictors	Mean dose < 50 Gy	OAR pharynx ALARA V50 < 33% V60 < 15% Mean dose < 45 Gy	Mean dose < 50 Gy
Uninvolved oral cavity	ALARA	ALARA Mean dose < 30 Gy	Not specified
Brachial plexus	Dmax < 66 Gy	Dmax < 66 Gy	Dmax < 60 Gy
Lens	Dmax < 10 Gy	Dmax < 50 Gy	Not specified
Globe	Dmax < 50 Gy	Dmax < 50 Gy	Not specified
Optic nerves and chiasm	Dmax < 54 Gy	Dmax < 50 Gy PRV < 54 Gy	Dmax < 55 Gy (rate <3%) Dmax 55–60 Gy (rate 3%–7%) Dmax > 60 Gy (rate >7%)

ALARA, as low as reasonably achievable; PRV, planning volume at risk; Dmax, maximal dose; OAR, organ at risk.

have strong literature support. In fact, data are so sparse for some organs that the acronym ALARA, as low as reasonable achievable, is used.

The lack of strong data for the tolerance of many tissues within the head and neck has led to the creation of expert consensus groups for opinion pieces on tissue constraints and reliance on the leadership of the Radiation Therapy Oncology Group (RTOG) to establish guidelines. Table 2 summarizes these, along with more tradition/anecdotal constraints, and the reader is referred to the Suggested Readings for more details. It is important to highlight that the total dose constraints in Table 2 are principally based on fraction sizes of 1.8 to 2 Gy. It is important to also consider with IMRT that it is the fraction size of the dose to the normal tissue and not the prescription dose to the CTV.

While the dose tolerance to many structures remains unclear, the current capabilities of our planning systems to more accurately capture the dose delivered to structures has led to better efforts to quantify the relationship of dose and volume to toxicity. Details are beyond the scope of the manual, but the interested reader is referred to the Suggested Readings for studies related to salivary glands, mandible, swallowing muscles and the brachial plexus for examples.

The principle focus on organ avoidance has been to establish thresholds to avoid sequelae of treatment, particularly severe effects. However our research has demonstrated that even "acceptable doses" can result in toxicities. Therefore,

ALARA is a good principle to follow even for those organs with defined constraints.

One of our current research goals is to determine if by decreasing the intermediate and lower "safe" doses to normal tissue that are a by-product of IMRT with IMPT, patients can experience less acute and late toxicity.

SUGGESTED READINGS

Chen AM, Wang PC, Daly ME, et al. Dose—volume modeling of brachial plexus-associated neuropathy after radiation therapy for head-and-neck cancer: findings from a prospective screening protocol. *Int J Radiat Oncol Biol Phys* 2014;88:771–777.

Dijkema T, Raaijmakers CP, Ten Haken RK. Parotid gland function after radiotherapy: the combined Michigan and Utrecht experience. *Int J Radiat Oncol Biol Phys* 2010;78:449–453.

Emami B. Tolerance of normal tissue to therapeutic radiation. *Reports Radiother Oncol* 2013;1(1):35–48.

Henk JM, et al. Radiation dose to the lens and cataract formation. *Int J Radiat Oncol Biol Phys* 1993;25(5):815–820.

Quantitative Analyses of Normal Tissue Effects in the Clinic (QUANTEC). *Int J Radiat Oncol Biol Phys* 2010;76(3):S1–S160.

Quantitative Analyses of Normal Tissue Effects in the Clinic (QUANTEC). *Int J Radiat Oncol Biol Phys* 2010;76(3):S1–S160.

Rosenthal DI, Chambers MS, Fuller CD, et al. Beam path toxicities to non-target structures during intensity-modulated radiation therapy for head and neck cancer. *Int J Radiat Oncol Biol Phys* 2008;72:747–755.

RTOG Foundation. RTOG 1016 protocol documents. Phase III trial of radiotherapy plus cetuximab versus chemoradiotherapy in HPV-associated oropharynx cancer. Available at www.rtog.org

RTOG Foundation. RTOG 0615 protocol documents. A phase II study of concurrent chemoradiotherapy using 3-dimensional conformal radiotherapy (3D-CRT) or intensity-modulated radiation therapy (IMRT) + Bevacizumab (BV) for locally or regionally advanced nasopharyngeal cancer. Available at www.rtog.org

Schwartz DL, Hutcheson K, Barringer D, et al. Candidate dosimetric predictors of long-term swallowing dysfunction after oropharyngeal intensity-modulated radiotherapy. *Int J Radiat Oncol Biol Phys* 2010;78:1356–1365.

Tsai CJ, Hofstede TM, Sturgis EM, et al. Osteoradionecrosis and radiation dose to the mandible in patients with oropharyngeal cancer. *Int J Radiat Oncol Biol Phys* 2013;85:415–420.

Wang X, Eisbruch A. IMRT for head and neck cancer: reducing xerostomia and dysphagia. *J Radiat Res* 2016;57 Suppl 1:i69–i75.

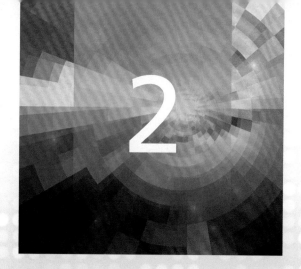

Site-Specific Indications and Techniques

The second part of this manual systematically presents the treatment approach and technique of radiotherapy applied in each disease site. A uniform presentation format is followed to facilitate review. First, the treatment strategies for various tumor stages are summarized. A large number of clinical studies, including most of those cited in the previous edition, have been completed in the interim, and some have yielded data that change our standard of care. Therefore, the treatment strategy and recommendations for a number of cancers have been updated. The staging system used for treatment recommendations for individual sites is based on the 7th edition manual of the American Joint Committee on Cancer, published in 2010, unless otherwise specified.

Subsequently, the technical details of radiation treatment (target volumes, field setup and arrangements, and dose prescription and fractionation) are described. Case studies (i.e., history, treatment modality, simulation, target volumes, and other relevant materials) are presented for common disease varieties. This is intended to allow readers to follow each step of treatment planning and delivery in day-to-day practice. Historically, patients with head and neck cancer were treated with conventional radiation portals, based either on bony landmarks (2-D) or on target delineation of at-risk areas on cross-sectional simulation (3-D). In the United States, conventional treatment has almost universally been replaced with intensity-modulated radiation therapy (IMRT), due to increasing availability and data from multiple trials suggesting benefits in terms of toxicity reduction and outcomes (see Part 1). Nevertheless, the principles of modern radiation therapy, even with IMRT, are largely based on the foundations of conventional therapy. In addition, in large portions of the world, IMRT is unavailable; hence, the conventional treatment fields and discussions have remained in the book to serve as historic perspective and as guidance for centers that are still using conventional treatment or are just now beginning the transition to IMRT. Proton therapy is emerging as a more widely available technique throughout the world; prospective trials are ongoing to determine its potential benefit. In disease sites in which data exist, sample cases treated with proton therapy are included.

Finally, background clinical data are referenced. It is not the intention to provide a comprehensive review of the literature but rather to present data that have contributed to the development of our institutional standards and the results that have been obtained by applying such strategies. It should be noted that the stages presented in the clinical background data sections are obviously according to the staging system used by the authors during the respective study periods. Therefore, it is not prudent to make a direct comparison between data of different series because the characteristics of the study populations are not equivalent among most series.

7

Oral Cavity

LIP

Treatment Strategy

Surgery is generally preferred in medically operable patients in the following situations:

- T1 lesions (up to 2 cm in diameter) that do not involve the oral commissure. Excision of such lesions is generally simple (V or W excision with primary closure or flap reconstruction), and the functional and cosmetic outcome is satisfactory.
- Younger patients who will have prolonged sunlight exposure (e.g., those engaged in outdoor work).
- Diffuse superficial lesions of the vermilion or the presence of severe actinic keratosis adjacent to the carcinoma. A lip shave with oral mucosa advancement closure generally yields a good control rate with satisfactory cosmetic outcome.

Radiation is an option for lesions larger than 2 cm or those involving the commissure, in which surgical resection results in microstomia or oral incontinence. Radiotherapy can be delivered by external beam irradiation, brachytherapy, or a combination of both, depending on the location and size of the lesion.

A combination of surgery and radiotherapy is frequently required for advanced destructive lesions, such as those invading the bone or nerve or tumors with nodal involvement.

Primary Radiotherapy

Target Volume

Initial Target Volume

- T2 N0: Primary tumor with 2-cm margins. Elective neck irradiation is not given routinely for well-differentiated carcinomas.
- T3 N0: Primary tumor with 2-cm margins and level 1–2 nodes.
- T2–T3 N+: Primary tumor with 2-cm margins and level 1–4 nodes.

A boost volume encompasses the primary lesion with 1-cm margins and, when present, involved nodes.

Setup and Field Arrangement for External Beam Irradiation

An intraoral stent containing Cerrobend is used to displace the tongue posteriorly and, if feasible, shield the alveolar ridge. The patient is immobilized in a supine position. An appositional field is used to treat the primary tumor. Field borders are determined clinically by bimanual palpation. Treatment can be given with orthovoltage x-rays or electrons. Electron energy is chosen on the basis of the thickness of the lesion. The upper neck nodes are treated with parallel-opposed lateral photon fields:

- *Anterior border:* 1 cm in front of the mandibular arch.
- *Superior border:* Splitting the horizontal ramus of the mandible.
- *Posterior border:* Midvertebral body.
- *Inferior border:* Just above the arytenoids.

Mustache field for upper lip lesion: appositional electron fields (usually approximately 15-degree gantry angle) are used to treat the facial lymphatics.

- *Medial border:* Matches the lateral border of the anterior field (primary tumor).
- *Anterior border:* Extends down from oral commissure to midmandible.
- *Posterior border:* From the upper edge of the anterior field to just above the angle of the mandible.
- *Inferior border:* Splitting the horizontal ramus of the mandible and adjoining the upper neck field.

This field is set up clinically after designing the primary tumor and upper neck portals.

Patients with clinical node(s) receive irradiation to mid- and lower neck nodes through an anterior portal. The primary lesion receives boost dose through an appositional field with orthovoltage x-rays or electrons. Nodal metastases receive boost dose with appositional electrons or glancing photon fields.

Brachytherapy

Brachytherapy is usually accomplished by afterloading iridium 192 (^{192}Ir) wire implants. Whenever possible, a custom-made plastic device is placed between the lip and gum to increase the distance between the radioactive sources and alveolar structures to decrease radiation exposure to normal tissues. Occasionally, Cerrobend can be incorporated in the device to provide additional protection.

Dosage

- *Small lesions (<1.5 cm):* 50 Gy in 25 fractions followed by 10 Gy in five fractions boost dose by external irradiation or 60 to 65 Gy over 5 to 7 days by implants.
- *Larger lesions:* 50 Gy in 25 fractions followed by 16 Gy in eight fractions boost by external beam or 20- to 25-Gy boost by implants.
- *Elective treatment of facial (mustache area) and upper neck nodes:* 50 Gy in 25 fractions.

Clinically involved nodes receive boost dose to a total dose of 66 to 70 Gy depending on the size.

Dose Specification

In external beam irradiation, the dose to the primary lesion is administered at D_{max} for orthovoltage x-rays and at 90% for electrons. This accounts for the difference in relative biologic effectiveness between the two beam modalities.

For brachytherapy, the dose is administered at the isodose line encompassing the lesion.

Mustache fields are irradiated with 6-MeV electrons, and the dose is prescribed at D_{max}.

Postoperative Radiotherapy

The majority of advanced stage cancers of the lip are treated with surgery and adjuvant radiation. Indications for postoperative irradiation include bone involvement, perineural invasion, or multiple lymph nodes and for postoperative chemoradiation are positive margins or extracapsular extension (ECE).

In general, the radiation setup is the same as that for primary radiotherapy but should be tailored individually depending on the location of the primary lesion (upper lip vs. lower lip) and on the extent of nerve and lymphatic coverage. The dose prescription is 60 Gy in 30 fractions to areas with high-risk features, 56 Gy per 28 fractions to the surgical bed, and 50 Gy in 25 fractions to electively irradiated regions.

In the modern era, radiation is most commonly performed using IMRT, which is especially helpful given the ability to track the at-risk nerves for patients with perineural invasion. The dose prescription is 60 Gy in 30 fractions to areas with high-risk features (CTV_{HD}) with 57 Gy to the operative bed (CTV_{ID}) and 54 Gy to the undissected at-risk areas, including the perineural tracts (CTV_{ED}).

FLOOR OF MOUTH, ORAL TONGUE, AND MANDIBULAR GINGIVA

Treatment Strategy

Surgical resection is generally preferred in medically operable patients. Depending on the size, depth of invasion, and grade of differentiation of the primary tumor and nodal status, surgery may include a modified neck dissection.

Postoperative radiotherapy is recommended in the following situations: large primary tumor (e.g., T3 or T4); close or positive surgical margins; presence of perineural spread, vascular invasion, or both; or presence of multiple positive nodes or ECE **(Case Study 7.1 through Case Study 7.8)**. Patients considered at high risk, such as those having positive margins or ECE are recommended to receive concurrent postoperative chemoradiation.

Primary radiotherapy is generally reserved for patients who refuse surgery and believed to produce inferior results.

Postoperative Radiotherapy

Target Volume

Initial Target Volume

The initial target volume includes the resected primary tumor bed and dissected neck(s). Elective nodal irradiation is given in conjunction with postoperative radiotherapy to the primary tumor bed in N0 patients who did not have a nodal dissection.

Boost Volume

In areas of original tumor and involved nodes, a second cone down may be made to deliver additional boost dose to the region carrying the highest risk of recurrence (e.g., sites of extracapsular nodal disease or positive margins).

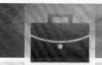

CASE STUDY 7.1

A 59-year-old man presented with a 1-month history of sore mouth. Physical examination revealed a 2.5-cm ulcerative, mobile lesion in the right anterior part of the floor of the mouth. The tumor involved the frenulum of the tongue, but did not cross the midline. The mobility of the tongue was normal. A 1.5-cm mobile lymph node was palpated at the right submandibular area. Biopsy of the primary tumor showed moderately differentiated squamous cell carcinoma (SCC). Stage: T2 N1 M0. This patient underwent a wide local excision of the primary tumor and bilateral supraomohyoid neck dissections. The defect in the floor of the mouth was repaired with a split-thickness skin graft. At the time of surgery, the tumor was found to involve the sublingual gland and the deep musculature. The initial deep margin was positive, but was converted to negative by further excision of the muscle. Of the five nodes recovered from the right neck specimen, one submandibular node measuring 2 cm was involved with carcinoma without evidence of ECE. Seven lymph nodes recovered from the left side were all free of tumor. Pathologic stage: p T4 N1. The patient received postoperative radiotherapy. The primary site and upper neck were treated with parallel-opposed lateral photon fields (Fig. 7.1). By using a tongue depressor, the hard palate and part of the soft palate and upper gums could be excluded from the radiation field. The mid- and lower neck nodes were treated with an anterior appositional photon field with a midline block to shield the larynx.

This block was placed just above the surgical scar in the neck, which is marked with a wire. The primary tumor bed and uninvolved nodal areas received 56 Gy in 28 fractions. The involved nodal area was boosted to 60 Gy in 30 fractions. The boost dose to the right upper neck was delivered with an appositional electron field. He had no evidence of disease and was free of complications 2 years after treatment.

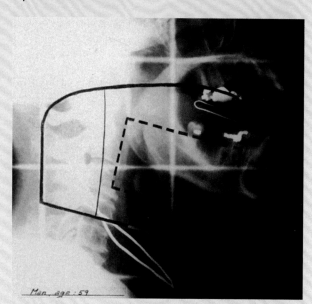

Case Figure 7.1

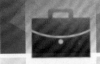

CASE STUDY 7.2

A 65-year-old man presented with ill-fitting dentures and oral pain. Physical examination revealed a 4-cm tumor on the right lateral tongue, an enlarged submandibular gland, and a 3.5-cm conglomerate of right level II nodal mass. Stage T2 N2b M0. He underwent a partial glossectomy and selective right neck dissection. Histologic examination showed an SCC of the tongue with negative section margins but presence of perineural invasion. Five of 40 dissected nodes were positive and there was ECE. He received adjunctive postoperative radiotherapy delivered with 6 MV photons for the entire treatment using an isocentric technique. A 3-mm tissue equivalent bolus was placed over the scar. A digitally reconstructed radiograph with the fields is shown (Fig. 7.2A). An off–spinal cord reduction was made at 42 Gy and a boost cone down at 56 Gy. The posterior cervical strips were supplemented with 9-MeV electrons, 18 Gy to the right strip, and 8 Gy to the left strip. Figure 7.2B,C shows axial and sagittal isodose distributions through the tongue. The supraclavicular field had a larynx (and spinal cord safety) block. Both sides of the lower neck received 50 Gy. The right mid- and lower neck received 6 Gy boost dose. These fields were further reduced off the inferior border to take the right neck at risk to 60 Gy.

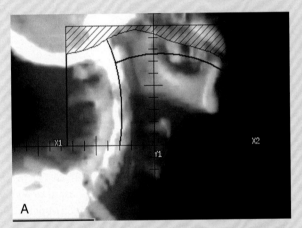

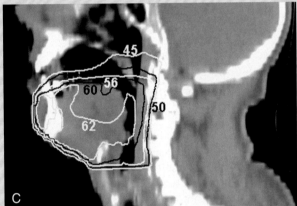

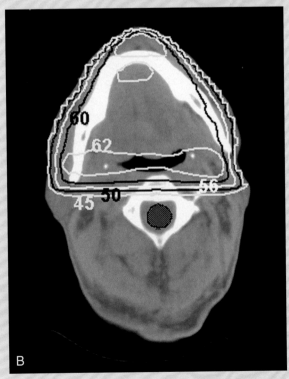

Case Figure 7.2A–C

CASE STUDY 7.3

A 59-year-old woman developed a clinical T1 N0 M0 (stage I) right oral tongue SCC. She presented with irritation of the right lateral tongue. A biopsy was positive for well-differentiated squamous carcinoma. A computed tomography (CT) scan (Fig. 7.3A) demonstrated an enhancing lesion in the right lateral oral tongue (delineated with *arrows*) and no pathologic adenopathy. She was taken for a right partial glossectomy and free ulnar flap reconstruction; a right neck dissection was performed because the depth of invasion was >4 mm. Final pathology revealed a 2.3-cm primary, moderately differentiated squamous carcinoma with focal perineural invasion and two of seven positive lymph nodes in right level IB and one of five in right level II; there was ECE as well. She was dispositioned to adjuvant radiation due to the perineural invasion and multiple positive lymph nodes, with concurrent cisplatin due to the presence of perineural invasion. Figure 7.3B shows an axial view with contours of target volumes at approximately the level of the resected

primary tumor. The red color wash depicts the volume targeted to 60 Gy (CTV_{HD}), encompassing the resected disease in the tongue and right neck levels IB and II, with margin. The blue color wash represents the remaining operative bed (including a wired scar) planned to 57 Gy (CTV_{ID}). The yellow color wash represents the remaining tongue, perineural tracts of V3 and XII, and contralateral neck nodes planned to 54 Gy (CTV_{ED}). Figure 7.3C demonstrates a lower axial slice, demonstrating that the high dose is taken to the level of the hyoid, due to the propensity of oral tongue tumors recurring deep and caudal to the primary volume. Figure 7.3D demonstrates an axial slice of the low neck, treated with CTV_{ED}; since the patient had postsurgical changes extending anterior to the larynx, the treatment was delivered as a single VMAT plan. Figure 7.3E demonstrates a coronal slice demonstrating coverage of V3 to the foramen ovale (*arrow*) in CTV_{ED}. The patient remains well 1 year from treatment with excellent speech and oral comfort.

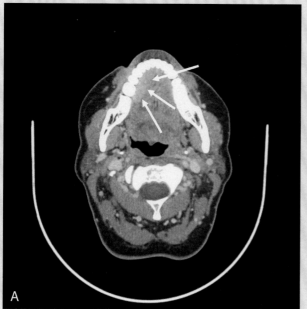

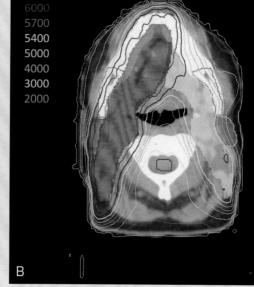

6300
6000
5700
5400
5000
4000
3000
2000

Case Figure 7.3A,B

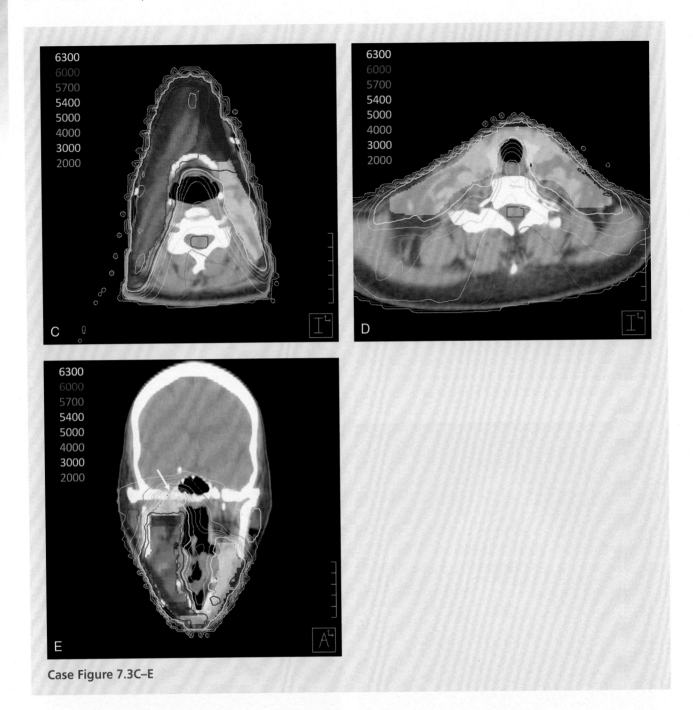

Case Figure 7.3C–E

Setup and Field Arrangement for Conventional Radiotherapy Technique

The patient is immobilized in a supine position with a thermoplastic mask. For tumors of the oral tongue or floor of the mouth that extend close to or into the tongue, an intraoral stent is used to open the mouth and depress the tongue. This device allows exclusion of a large area of the buccal mucosa, lower lip, and oral commissure from the radiation portals. For tumors of the floor of the mouth not extending into the oral tongue, a stent that opens the mouth

and elevates the tip of the tongue beyond the field is used to exclude as much of the tongue (tip, dorsum) from the radiation portal as possible. Marking of surgical scar and oral commissures before obtaining a simulation film may facilitate portal design.

Tumors of the mandibular gingiva or small tumors of the oral tongue that are well lateralized without histologic evidence of lymph node involvement can be treated ipsilaterally. This can be accomplished with a wedged-pair of photon beams designed to encompass the operative bed with 1- to 2-cm surrounding margins.

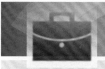

CASE STUDY 7.4

A 47-year-old man presented with biopsy proven SCC of the left oral tongue. He underwent a partial glossectomy with selective left neck dissection. The primary tumor was 1.2 cm in size and had negative margins. The neck dissection yielded three positive nodes in levels II and III without ECE. He was treated with postoperative radiation. The tumor bed, consisting of the left lateral tongue and left upper neck, with margin was identified as CTV$_{HD}$ (60 Gy). The undissected right neck and right hemitongue was contoured as CTV$_{ED}$ (54 Gy—*blue*). Figure 7.4 shows CTV$_{HD}$ (*red*) and CTV$_{ED}$ (*blue*) paired with isodose distributions at the level of the tongue (Fig. 7.4A,B) and upper neck (Fig. 7.4C,D). Figure 7.4E,F shows isodose distributions on a sagittal view through the midtongue and a coronal view, respectively. An intraoral stent opens the mouth and separates the palate from the tongue (Fig. 7.4E). The isocenter was placed just above the thyroid notch. IMRT was delivered to fields above the isocenter. Level III and IV nodes were treated with an anterior beam with a larynx block to 40 Gy and with a full midline block to 50 Gy. Right level III was boosted to a total of 60 Gy with glancing photon beams. The patient remains without disease 5 years later.

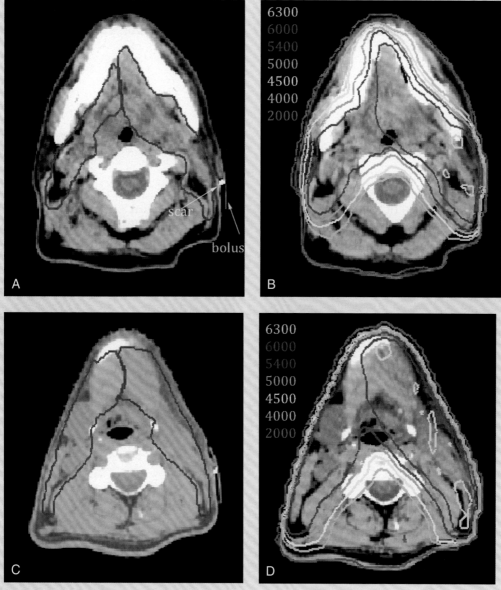

Case Figure 7.4A–D

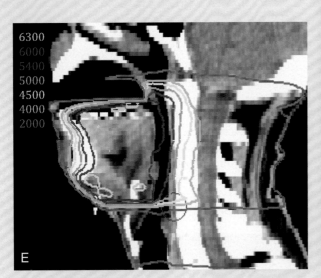

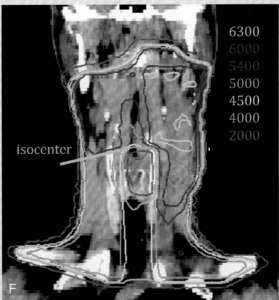

Case Figure 7.4E,F

CASE STUDY 7.5

A 78-year-old man presented with an anterior oral tongue tumor and a palpable left level IB node, also detected on the staging CT scan (Fig. 7.5A). Biopsy of the primary tumor was positive for SCC. He underwent a partial glossectomy and left selective neck dissection. Histologic examination revealed a 2.5-cm carcinoma with negative margins. The neck dissection revealed only one positive lymph node, 2.5 cm in size consistent with the clinical

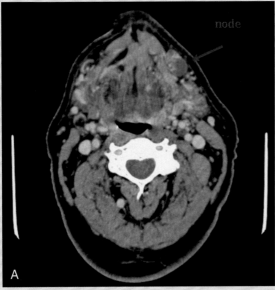

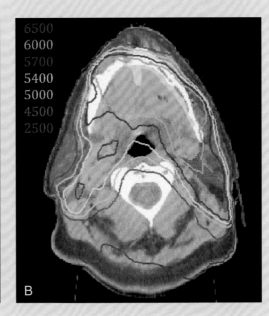

Case Figure 7.5A,B

findings. There was ECE. He was treated with postoperative IMRT. Concurrent chemotherapy was indicated but not given due to concern about tolerance secondary to overall performance status and age.

The tumor bed, consisting of the anterior tongue and left upper neck, with margin was identified as CTV$_{HD}$ (60 Gy—*orange*). Dissected ipsilateral level IIb node was contoured as CTV$_{ID}$ (57 Gy—*blue*). The undissected right neck and an additional 0.5 to 1 cm on the tongue were identified as CTV$_{ED}$ (54 Gy—*yellow*). The region of the positive node at left level IB was delineated to give a simultaneous integrated boost to a total dose of 65 Gy (*red*).

Representative axial slices of the isodose distribution from the level of the midtongue to inferior level II of the neck are shown (Fig. 7.5B–D). The isocenter was placed just above the thyroid notch. IMRT was delivered to fields above the isocenter. Level III and IV nodes were treated with an anterior beam with a larynx block to 40 Gy and with a full midline block to 50 Gy. Right level III was boosted to 60 Gy with glancing photon beams. Also shown are isodose distributions through the isocenter in sagittal (Fig. 7.5E) and coronal (Fig. 7.5F) view and through the midtongue and level IB in coronal view (Fig. 7.5G). The patient remains without disease 3 years later.

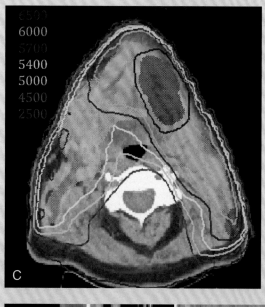
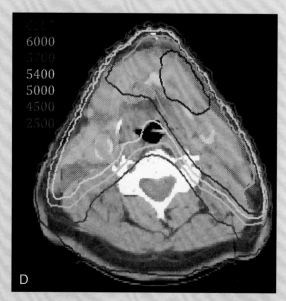
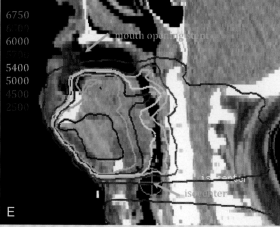
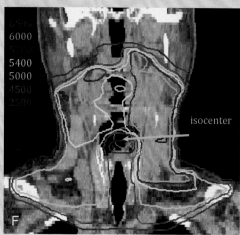

Case Figure 7.5C–F

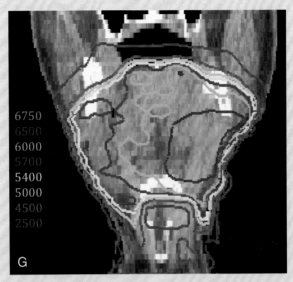

Case Figure 7.5G

CASE STUDY 7.6

A 66-year-old man presented with a 2.5-cm anterior floor of mouth tumor with extension onto the ventral tongue without palpable lymph adenopathy (T2 N0). He underwent a partial glossectomy and bilateral supraomohyoid neck dissections. Histologic examination revealed a 1.8-cm SCC with negative margins. The neck dissection specimen contained five positive nodes, two in left level III, two in right level I, and one in right level II compartments. There was no ECE. He received postoperative radiation using IMRT to the primary tumor bed and upper neck and a matching anterior portal for lower neck as described in **Case Study 7.7.**

Since the positive nodes were scattered through the neck, and were not well identified on preoperative imaging, bilateral level I and II nodes, the floor of the mouth and anterior tongue, and the musculature that inserts onto the hyoid bone were defined as CTV_{ED} (60 Gy). Figure 7.6 shows target volumes on two axial images at the levels of the mandible (Fig. 7.6A) and upper neck (Fig. 7.6B) and sagittal image (Fig. 7.6C) along with isodose distributions on axial (Fig. 7.6D), sagittal (Fig. 7.6E), and coronal (Fig. 7.6F) views. The patient is without disease 2 years later.

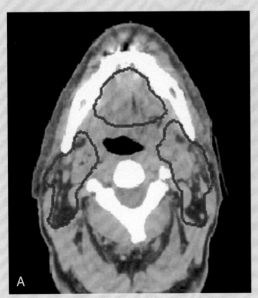
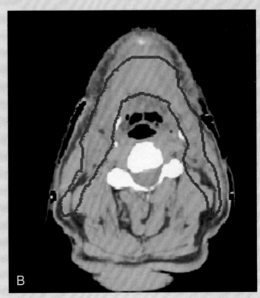

Case Figure 7.6A,B

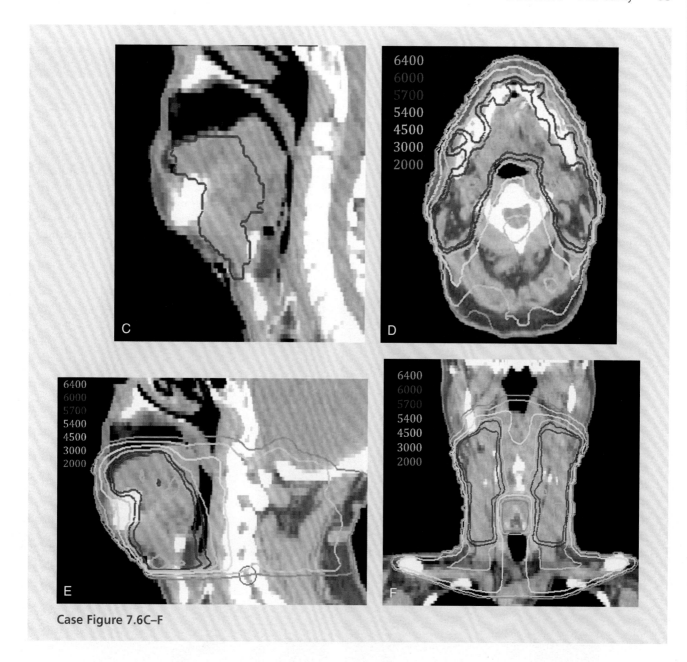

Case Figure 7.6C–F

The remaining tumors that require bilateral radiation are treated with parallel-opposed lateral photon fields encompassing the primary tumor bed and upper neck nodes.

- *Anterior border:* Just in front of the mandible for anterior tumors or 2 cm in front of the scar for posterior oral cavity lesions. The lower lip is shielded whenever possible.
- *Superior border:* 1 to 1.5 cm superior to the dorsum of the tongue or the scar if part of the oral tongue can be spared. In the event of positive nodes, this border should encompass the high jugular nodes to the jugular fossa.
- *Posterior border:* Usually is dictated by the surgical scar. The level II nodes are systematically irradiated.

Therefore, the posterior border is placed behind the spinous processes or farther back to cover an extended scar.

- *Inferior border:* Just superior to the arytenoids.

An anterior appositional field is used to treat the mid- and lower neck nodes. Field borders are indicated in the section "General Principles."

To deliver the boost dose to the primary tumor and upper neck nodes, the size of lateral fields is reduced to encompass the known disease locations. It is also prudent to cover the root of tongue or deep floor of the mouth muscles to the insertion at the hyoid bone in the boost volume since recurrence tends to occur in these regions even for relatively superficial tumors.

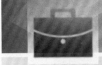

CASE STUDY 7.7

A 67-year-old man presented with oral pain and was found to have a tumor of the anterior floor of the mouth that spilled over the anterior gingiva. CT scan revealed a lesion in the floor of the mouth eroding the mandible (Fig. 7.7A). He underwent surgical resection including an anterior mandibulectomy and bilateral supraomohyoid neck dissections followed by reconstruction with a fibula free flap. Histologic examination revealed SCC, poorly differentiated, invading the bone. There was carcinoma in situ at the tongue margin.

He received postoperative IMRT to the primary tumor bed and upper neck. The tumor bed, consisting of the floor of the mouth, resected right mandibular bed, and anterior tongue with margin, was identified as CTV_HD (60 Gy). The dissected necks that did not harbor disease were contoured as CTV_ID (57 Gy). Figure 7.7 shows isodose distributions on axial images at the level of the reconstructed mandible and flap (Fig. 7.7B) and upper neck (Fig. 7.7C) and a sagittal view through the midplane (Fig. 7.7D).

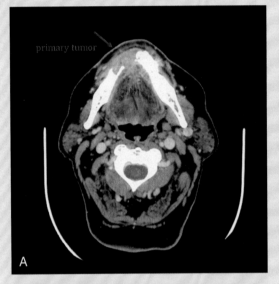

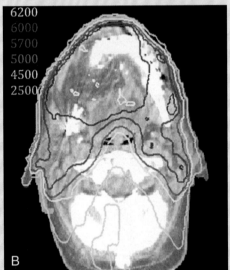

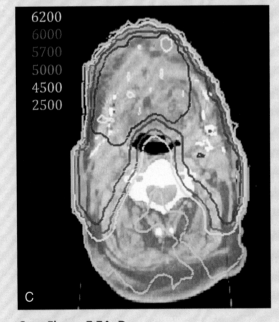

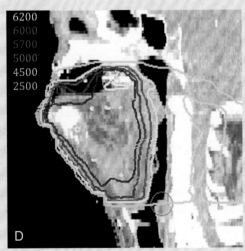

Case Figure 7.7A–D

The IMRT beams were matched at an isocenter, placed above the thyroid notch, to an anterior portal for treating the lower nodal stations. The initial anterior beam had a larynx block and was treated to 40 Gy (Fig. 7.7E). A full midline block was added and the fields treated to 50 Gy (Fig. 7.7F). Bilateral level III, part of the operative bed, was boosted to 56 Gy with an anterior beam (Fig. 7.7G). The patient remains without disease 3 years later.

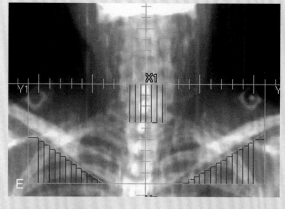

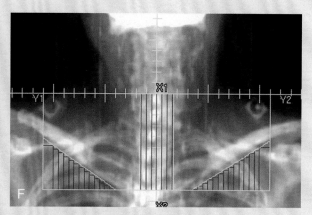

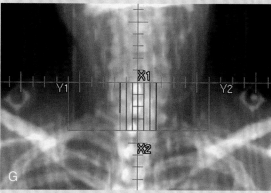

Case Figure 7.7E–G

CASE STUDY 7.8

A 49-year-old man presented to his dentist with left-sided oral pain and was found to have a lesion of the left alveolar ridge. A biopsy was positive for SCC. A diagnostic CT scan revealed an invasive primary tumor eroding the left mandible as shown in Figure 7.8A (*green arrows*). Treatment began with a wide local resection, including left mandibulectomy, and left neck dissection followed by reconstruction using an osteocutaneous free fibular flap and skin graft. The fibula replaced the horizontal ramus, whereas the soft tissue filled in the space of the resected left ascending ramus. Histologic examination revealed a 2.9-cm poorly differentiated SCC with bone invasion, but margins were negative. None of the 28 nodes were positive for disease. Stage pT4 N0.

He was treated with adjuvant ipsilateral IMRT because the tumor was well lateralized and there was no nodal involvement. Figure 7.8B shows a coronal view through the right ascending ramus of the mandible with CTV$_{HD}$ (*red*) and CTV$_{ID}$ (*blue*) outlined. CTV$_{HD}$ encompasses the preoperative tumor volume with generous margins, and CTV$_{ID}$ covers the operative bed with including generous coverage of the masticator space. The absence of the left ascending mandibular ramus can be appreciated on this coronal view. Figure 7.8C–F shows axial isodose distributions along with CTV$_{HD}$ (*red*) and CTV$_{ID}$ (*blue*) at the level of the inferior maxilla and masticator space, the superior aspect of the horizontal ramus of the mandible, the fibula graft and epicenter of the original tumor, and level II nodal region, respectively. Note that CTV$_{HD}$ includes 1 cm of the residual mandible across the midline and the upper neck to encompass soft tissues of the inferior lateral portion of the floor of the mouth musculature and tissues inferior to the angle of the mandible. The left level III and IV nodes were treated with a matching anterior beam to a dose of 50 Gy in 25 fractions. The patient had no evidence of disease 2 years after treatment.

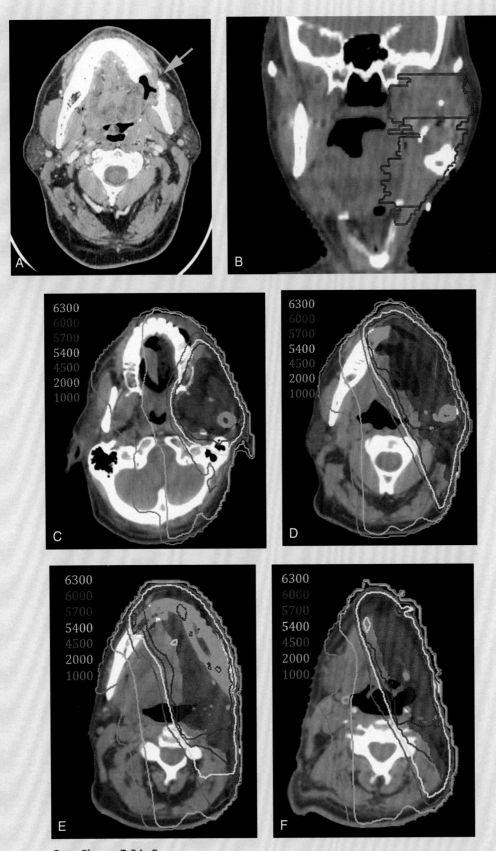

Case Figure 7.8A–F

To boost the upper neck without the primary site, a lateral appositional electron field is used. To deliver the boost to the mid- or lower neck, a lateral appositional electron field or glancing photon fields are used.

Dose

- A dose of 60 Gy in 30 fractions is administered to areas with high-risk features, which are close or microscopically positive margins, perineural extension, vascular invasion, positive nodes, or extranodal extension. An additional boost dose of 6 Gy in three fractions may be given when indicated, such as when multiple adverse features are present or when the interval between surgery and radiation is much longer than 6 weeks.
- A dose of 56 Gy in 28 fractions to the surgical bed.
- A dose of 50 Gy of elective irradiation in 25 fractions to undissected regions.

Intensity-Modulated Radiation Therapy

IMRT is considered standard of care in the treatment of postoperative oral cavity cases in modern times, allowing optimal dosing to the targets while protecting normal tissues. Treatment is typically given in 30 fractions, as illustrated in **Case Study 7.4 through Case Study 7.8**. Postoperative dose to fully resected (R0) tumors is 60 Gy; however, in the case of positive margins, ECE of identified lymph nodes, or small areas of heightened concern by the surgeon, smaller target volumes can be escalated to a total dose of 64 to 66 Gy.

The patient is immobilized in a supine position, with an extended thermoplastic mask covering the head and shoulders. Oral stents can be used to help depress the tongue, open the mouth, and immobilize the anatomy. Thin-cut CT images are obtained in treatment position and target volumes are outlined for dosimetric planning. The gross target volume (GTV), clinical target volumes (CTVs), and planning target volumes (PTVs) are outlined for dosimetric planning.

Virtual Gross Target Volume

There is no actual GTV after complete surgical tumor resection. However, it can be useful to formulate a virtual GTV (vGTV) to facilitate target volume definition. The vGTV is a best approximation of the tissues having high likelihood of harboring microscopic tumor reconstructed based on findings of preoperative clinical examination, imaging studies, and surgical–pathologic assessment. Bulky flaps can cause substantial distortions in the tumor bed and should, therefore, be taken into account in reconstructing the vGTV.

Clinical Target Volumes

Three CTVs are generally delineated.

- CTV1 delineates volumes to receive the highest dose (therefore also referred to as CTV_{HD}). This includes the primary and nodal vGTVs with 8- to 10-mm margins. For larger primary tumors, CTV_{HD} often covers the entire tongue and floor of the mouth.
- CTV2 delineates volumes to receive an intermediate dose (therefore also referred to as CTV_{ID}). For the primary tumor bed, CTV_{ID} encompasses a 5- to 10-mm additional margin beyond CTV_{HD}. For the neck, it covers the dissected neck not harboring involved nodes.
- CTV3 delineates volumes to receive an elective dose for subclinical disease (therefore also referred to as CTV_{ED}). In the N0 neck, nodal levels I to IV are included in CTV_{ED}. When microscopic perineural invasion is present, CTV_{ED} includes the lingual nerve and/or inferior alveolar nerve to approximately the distal end of the mandibular nerve (V3) either ipsilaterally or, for tumors extending to or crossing midline, bilaterally. For extensive perineural extension (involvement of large nerve or presence of clinical signs), CTV_{ED} includes proximal V3 up to the skull base or even the trigeminal ganglion.

The isocenter is generally placed above the arytenoids. Level III and IV nodes are preferentially treated with a matching anterior beam similar to conventional techniques. With this technique, the larynx can be shielded for the initial 40 Gy and then a full midline block can be used up to 50 Gy. The dissected uninvolved nodal levels are boosted to 56 Gy, and an additional 4 Gy is added if these lower neck nodes harbored disease.

Some patients have extensive reconstruction with large flaps that extend to the level of the larynx or a body habitus with a short neck, making matching a low neck beam complicated or nonoptimal geometrically. In these cases, treating all the targets with a single IMRT plan may be more effective, though additional attention should be paid to delineating the larynx and esophagus as avoidance structures for minimizing the dose to these organs. In this scenario, volumetric modulated arc therapy (VMAT), when available, often provides more homogeneous dose distributions than step-and-shoot IMRT, with an enhanced ability to spare the larynx. VMAT also reduces the treatment time, which may be beneficial in patients with bulky flaps who often have difficulty lying flat.

Timing of Postoperative Radiotherapy

Ideally, postoperative radiotherapy should begin as soon as possible after the healing of surgical wounds. With good communication between surgical, radiation, and dental oncologists, simulation should be planned approximately 3 to 4 weeks after surgery, and radiotherapy can start within a week following simulation in most patients. When delayed wound healing postpones the start of postoperative radiation beyond 6 to 8 weeks, treatment escalation with accelerated fractionation, such as concomitant boost, should be considered. In this scenario, the treatment can be delivered twice a day for 5 treatment days, either once a week or toward the end of the radiation course, to reduce the potential hazard of prolonged cumulative treatment time.

Primary Radiotherapy

Primary radiation therapy has been the subject of intensive study for oral cavity cancers. Multiple studies suggest that outcomes are significantly improved in patients that can have surgery followed by adjuvant radiation, rather than nonsurgical techniques, especially for advanced disease. The discussion of primary radiation is included for guidance on treatment for patients that are not surgical candidates.

Target Volume

Initial Target Volume

- *A well-differentiated, superficial lesion of 1 cm or less with no palpable lymphadenopathy (T1 N0):* primary tumor with 2-cm margins.
- *Floor of the mouth (mostly anterior) lesion of 1- to 4-cm maximal diameter without palpable lymphadenopathy (T1–T2 N0):* primary tumor with at least 2-cm margins and level I (submental and submandibular) and level II nodes.
- *Oral tongue tumor >1 cm thick with no palpable lymphadenopathy:* primary tumor with at least 2-cm margins and level I to IV nodes.
- Presence of lymphadenopathy (N+) at diagnosis calls for irradiation of the entire cervical nodal basins.

A boost volume encompasses the primary tumor (1- to 2-cm margins) and involves lymph nodes.

Setup and Field Arrangement

For small T1 N0 lesions, the entire treatment is given with an intraoral cone or by implant (if the risk for anesthesia is low).

For all other stages, treatment is given with external beam irradiation by conventional technique or IMRT as described above for postoperative radiotherapy. Use of stent, insertion of a seed at the anterior border of the tumor, and marking the oral commissures before obtaining simulation images facilitate shaping of the target volumes.

The boost dose to the primary tumor is preferably delivered by interstitial implant. If the patient cannot undergo anesthesia, boost dose is given with orthovoltage x-rays through an intraoral cone when accessible; in this case, the boost is delivered before the start of the external beam therapy while the tumor is clearly visible and palpable. In rare cases when neither implant nor intraoral cone is feasible, the boost is delivered using an external beam encompassing the tumor with 1- to 2-cm margins.

The technique for delivering the boost dose to palpable nodes depends on the strategy selected for the treatment of the primary lesion. It could be an interstitial implant, electron beams, or photons (included in the primary boost field or with separate fields, depending on the location).

Dose

Initial Target Volume

This volume receives 40 Gy in 20 fractions if this is followed by an interstitial implant, or 50 Gy in 25 fractions if the boost is delivered by intraoral cone or external beam.

Boost

The boost dose to the primary lesion delivered by an interstitial implant is 40 Gy, specified at an isodose line approximately 0.5 cm from the tumor margin; the boost dose by intraoral cone is 15 Gy in 3-Gy fractions or 20 to 25 Gy in 2.5-Gy fractions and by external beam is 20 Gy in 10-Gy fractions for T1 lesions or 20 to 24 Gy in 2-Gy fractions for T2 to T3 lesions.

The dose to involved lymph nodes is in general 66 to 70 Gy for <3 cm nodes, or even higher for larger nodes if neck dissection is not contemplated because of anesthesia risk.

Small (<1 cm), superficial lesions may be treated with the intraoral cone (40 Gy in 10 fractions) or by an implant only (60 Gy in approximately 6 days).

Background Data

See Tables 7.1 to 7.5.

TABLE 7.1 Oral Cavity Cancers Treated with Surgery and Postoperative Irradiation: Influence of Margin Status on Local Control (Literature Review)

Margin Status	Oral Tongue		Floor of the Mouth	
	No. Controlled/Total (%)		No. Controlled/Total (%)	
	MSKCC	U of FL[a]	MSKCC	U of FL[a]
Negative	7/9 (78%)	9/12 (75%)	9/9 (100%)	10/13 (77%)
Close	10/16 (62%)	7/11 (64%)[b]	6/8 (75%)	8/9 (89%)[b]
Positive	2/4 (50%)	1/4 (25%)	4/5 (80%)	8/13 (62%)
Total	19/29 (66%)	17/27 (63%)	19/22 (86%)	26/35 (74%)

[a]Local–regional control.
[b]Includes close and initially positive margins.
MSKCC, Memorial Sloan Kettering Cancer Center (Zelefsky MJ, Harrison LB, Fass DE, et al., 1993); University of Florida (Parsons JT, Mendenhall WM, Springer SP, et al., 1997).

TABLE 7.2 Oral Cavity Cancers Treated with Surgery and Postoperative Radiation: Disease Control by Site, Margin Status, and Nodal Extent

	Patients Number	5-Year Actuarial Control Rate			
		Local Control	Nodal Control	Above Clavicles	Distant Metastases
Oral tongue	137	78%	74%	65%	23%
Floor of the mouth	107	70%	82%	60%	27%
Mandibular gingiva	28	81%	77%	63%	21%
Positive margin	32	73%	80%	58%	38%
Nodal ECE	110	72%	62%	48%	35%
Multiple nodes	158	67%	69%	51%	35%
Overall results	272	75%	77%	63%	27%

Data from MD Anderson Cancer Center, 1970–1995.
ECE, extracapsular extension.

TABLE 7.3 Results of Postoperative IMRT in Cancer of the Oral Cavity

First Author	Year	Patient Number	Median Follow-Up (Months)	Disease Control
Feng	2006	36	36	69% (LRC—crude)
Yao	2007	49	24	82% (LRC, 2 yr)
Studer	2007	28	19	92% (LC, 2 yr)
Chen	2009	22	44	64% (DFS, 3 yr)
Gomez	2009	35	29	77% (LRC, 3 yr)
Daly	2009	30	38	60% (LRC, 3 yr)
Sher	2011	30	25	91% (LRC, 2 yr)
Chan	2013	180	34	78% (LRC, 2 yr)
Quinlan-Davidson	2016 (submitted)	289	35	76% (LRC, 5 yr)

LRC, locoregional control; LC, local control; DFS, disease-free survival.
Adapted from Feng M, et al. Predictive factors of local-regional recurrences following parotid sparing intensity modulated or 3D conformal radiotherapy for head and neck cancer. *Radiat Oncol* 2005;77:32–38; Yao M, et al. The failure patterns of oral cavity squamous cell carcinoma after intensity-modulated radiotherapy—the University of Iowa experience. *Int J Radiat Oncol Biol Phys* 2007;67:1332–1341; Studer G, et al. IMRT in oral cavity cancer. *Radiat Oncol* 2007;2:16; Chen WC, et al. Comparison between conventional and intensity-modulated post-operative radiotherapy for stage III and IV oral cavity cancer in terms of treatment results and toxicity. *Oral Oncol* 2009;45:505–510; Gomez DR, et al. Intensity-modulated radiotherapy in postoperative treatment of oral cavity cancers. *Int J Radiat Oncol Biol Phys* 2009;73:1096–1103; Daly ME, et al. Intensity-modulated radiotherapy for oral cavity squamous cell carcinoma: patterns of failure and predictors of local control. *Int J Radiat Oncol Biol Phys* 2011;80(5):1412–1422; Sher DJ, et al. Treatment of oral cavity squamous cell carcinoma with adjuvant or definitive intensity-modulated radiation therapy. *Int J Radiat Oncol Biol Phys* 2011;81:e215–e222; Chan AK, et al. Postoperative intensity-modulated radiotherapy following surgery for oral cavity squamous cell carcinoma: patterns of failure. *Oral Oncol* 2013;49;255–260; Quinlan-Davidson SR, et al. Oral cavity carcinoma: outcomes of patients treated with surgery followed by postoperative intensity modulated radiation therapy. *Personal Communication of submitted manuscript*, 2016.

TABLE 7.4 Primary Control of Oral Tongue Carcinoma by T-Stage and Mode of Radiotherapy

Method of Treatment	T1	T2	Total
Interstitial only	7/8 (88%)	4/9 (44%)	11/17 (65%)
Interstitial + external <40 Gy	2/2 (100%)	21/23 (92%)	23/25 (92%)
Interstitial + external = 40 Gy	4/6 (66%)	25/39 (64%)	29/45 (64%)
External only	—	2/7 (29%)	2/7 (29%)
Total	13/16 (81%)	52/78 (67%)	65/94 (69%)

Data from MD Anderson Cancer Center.
Modified from Wendt CD, Peters LJ, Delclos L, et al. Primary radiotherapy in the treatment of stage I and II oral tongue cancers: importance of the proportion of therapy delivered with interstitial therapy. *Int J Radiat Oncol Biol Phys* 1990;18:1287–1292.

TABLE 7.5 Primary Failure Rate by Treatment Method: Stage T1 N0 and T2 N0 Squamous Cell Carcinomas of the Oral Tongue

Method of Treatment	Number	At Risk <24 Months	Primary Failure	Salvage (Salv/ Attempted)	Ultimate Primary Control
Interstitial only	18	1	6	5/6	16/17 (94%)
Interstitial + external <40 Gy	31	6	2	0/2	23/25 (92%)
Interstitial + external = 40 Gy	46	1	16	9/16	38/45 (84%)
External only	8	1	5	2/4	4/7 (57%)

Data from MD Anderson Cancer Center.
Modified from Wendt CD, Peters LJ, Delclos L, et al. Primary radiotherapy in the treatment of stage I and II oral tongue cancers: importance of the proportion of therapy delivered with interstitial therapy. *Int J Radiat Oncol Biol Phys* 1990;18:1287–1292, with permission.

RETROMOLAR TRIGONE

Treatment Strategy

Like oral tongue cancers, optimal treatment for retromolar trigone cancers is surgery with adjuvant radiation therapy, when indicated by pathologic assessment; adjuvant chemoradiation is used in the presence of ECE or positive margins. Primary radiotherapy is considered less effective, so it is reserved for patients who are not surgical candidates. In the modern era, IMRT is widely accepted for retromolar trigone cancers; conventional treatment may be used when IMRT is not available.

Primary Radiotherapy

Target Volume

Initial Target Volume

- *A well-lateralized tumor without lymphadenopathy:* primary lesion (at least 2-cm margins) and ipsilateral level IB and II nodes.
- *A well-lateralized tumor with a single small ipsilateral node (N1):* primary lesion and the entire ipsilateral neck (including supraclavicular nodes).
- *Other cases (larger tumors and/or more advanced N-stage):* primary lesion and bilateral neck.

Boost Volume

The coned-down boost volume encompasses the primary tumor (1- to 2-cm margins) and, when present, the involved node. A limited planned neck dissection is carried out in rare occasions where a residual neck mass is present 6 weeks after completion of radiotherapy.

Setup and Field Arrangement for Conventional Radiotherapy Technique

For unilateral treatment only, generally, a combination of electrons and photons, in a ratio of 4:1, is used. Insertion of metal seed(s) at tumor border(s), when feasible, and marking of ipsilateral oral commissure may facilitate portal design. An intraoral stent is used to shield the tongue and to displace it to the contralateral side (see Chapter 3). The patient is immobilized in an open-neck position. An appositional lateral field encompasses the primary tumor and upper neck nodes:

- *Anterior border:* at least 2 cm anterior to the tumor.
- *Superior border:* includes the pterygoid plates when the tonsillar fossa is involved (this border is at least 1 to 1.5 cm rostral to the hard palate).
- *Posterior border:* just behind the mastoid process (N0) or behind the spinous processes (N+).
- *Inferior border:* just above the arytenoids.

When indicated, an adjoining appositional electron field is added to irradiate the mid- and lower neck (see "General Principles"). To deliver the boost dose to the primary tumor and, if necessary, upper neck, the field size is reduced to encompass the known disease locations with 1- to 2-cm margins.

For bilateral treatment, metal seeds are inserted, when feasible, to help delineate the primary lesion, and oral commissures are wired to aid in shaping the portal. The patient is immobilized in a supine position. Parallel-opposed lateral photon fields are used to treat the primary tumor and upper neck. Field borders are similar to that of ipsilateral treatment. An anterior appositional photon field is used to treat the mid- and lower neck borders (see "General Principles"). The lateral portals are reduced to deliver the boost dose to the primary tumor and the upper neck node(s).

The boost dose to the involved mid- or lower neck nodes can be given through an appositional electron field or anterior photon portal.

Dose

The initial target volume receives 50 Gy in 25 fractions or 54 Gy in 30 fractions when a concomitant boost regimen is prescribed.

The external beam boost is 16 Gy in eight fractions for T1 and small, superficial T2 lesions and 18 Gy in 12 fractions (given as second daily fractions according to concomitant boost regimen) for large T2 tumors.

Setup and Field Arrangement for IMRT

IMRT has become the preferred treatment for patients with indications for radiation therapy for oral cavity cancer, when available. For patients in whom unilateral therapy is sufficient, IMRT is beneficial if the depth dose profiles of the electron beam are insufficient for tumor coverage. Dose heterogeneity (hotspots) on the mandible can also be minimized to reduce the risk for osteoradionecrosis in these patients. In those patients requiring bilateral treatment, IMRT can spare a large portion of the contralateral parotid gland from the high-dose volume without compromising the coverage of the primary tumor and draining lymphatics.

The patient is immobilized in a supine position with an extended thermoplastic mask covering the head and shoulder. Thin-cut CT images are obtained in treatment position. The GTV and CTVs are outlined for dosimetric planning. As described above and in Part I, CTV_{HD} encompasses the primary and nodal GTVs with 8- to 10-mm margins. CTV_{HD} should include the adjacent inner cortex of the mandible, since retromolar trigone tumors abut the bone, and the involved nodal region. CTV_{ID} adds additional approximately 1-cm margin to CTV_{HD}, and CTV_{ED} delineates volumes to receive an elective dose for subclinical disease.

For patients in which the anatomy allows a match, optimal dosimetry can be achieved by matching an IMRT field above the arytenoids to a conventional low neck portal for the low neck. If this is not feasible, the entire treatment may be delivered with a single IMRT or VMAT plan. Typically, we prescribe a dose of 66 Gy in 30 fractions for T1–T2 tumors or N1 node. A dose 70 Gy in 33 fractions is prescribed for larger lesions or N2–N3 nodes. The uninvolved nodal regions receive 54 Gy in 30 fractions or approximately 56 Gy in 33 fractions.

Postoperative Radiotherapy

Target Volume

The initial target volume is the entire surgical bed **(Case Study 7.9 and Case Study 7.10)**. Guidelines for ipsilateral versus bilateral treatment and for treatment of nodal areas are the same as those for primary radiotherapy. Extension of the surgical scar well over the midline is another indication for bilateral irradiation.

For the boost volume, the same principle applies as for postoperative radiotherapy for the oral tongue and floor of the mouth.

Setup and Field

The same principles described for primary radiotherapy apply to postoperative treatment. Marking the external surgical scar may facilitate portal design. The *anterior* and *superior field borders* are determined by the local spread of the primary tumor as well as by the extent of surgery (guided by the scar).

Dose

- A dose of 60 Gy in 30 fractions to areas with high-risk features: close or microscopically positive margins, perineural extension, vascular invasion, positive nodes, or extranodal extension. An additional boost dose of 6 Gy in three fractions may be given when indicated, such as when multiple adverse features are present or when the interval between surgery and radiation is much longer than 6 weeks.
- A dose of 56 Gy in 28 fractions is given to the surgical bed.
- A dose of 50 Gy of elective irradiation in 25 fractions is given to undissected regions.

Intensity-Modulated Radiation Therapy

When using IMRT in the postoperative setting, the treatment is typically delivered in 30 fractions. The target volumes to receive various levels of doses are delineated and dosimetric plans are generated by iterative process.

The patient is immobilized in a supine position with an extended thermoplastic mask covering the head and shoulder. Thin-cut CT images are obtained in treatment position, and target volumes are outlined for dosimetric planning.

Virtual Gross Target Volume

There is no actual GTV after complete surgical tumor resection. However, it can be useful to formulate a vGTV to facilitate target volume definition. The vGTV is a best approximation of the tissues having high likelihood of harboring microscopic tumor reconstructed based on findings of preoperative clinical examination, imaging studies, and surgical–pathologic assessment. Bulky flap can cause substantial distortions in the tumor bed and should, therefore, be taken into account in reconstructing the vGTV.

Clinical Target Volume

Three CTVs are generally delineated **(Case Study 7.11)**.

- CTV_{HD} delineates volumes to receive the highest dose, which includes the primary and nodal vGTVs with 8- to 10-cm margins.
- CTV_{ID} delineates volumes to receive an intermediate dose. For the primary tumor bed, CTV_{ID} encompasses a 0.5- to 1-cm additional margin beyond $vCTV_{HD}$.

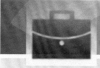

CASE STUDY 7.9

A 59-year-old man presented with toothache, dysphagia, 30-pound weight loss, and right otalgia. A tumor in the right retromolar trigone region was found, and a biopsy showed SCC. CT scan revealed the lesion with invasion of the mandible as well as upper jugular adenopathy. He underwent resection of the tumor, including partial glossectomy, pharyngectomy, palatectomy, hemimandibulectomy, and a right modified radical neck dissection. The defect was repaired with a pectoralis major rotational flap. Histologic examination showed negative section margins and revealed involvement of 6 of 26 nodes with ECE. Stage: p T4 N2b. He had a Zubrod performance status 2 with nutritional support through a percutaneous gastrostomy tube. Adjunctive postoperative radiotherapy was delivered to a dose of 60 Gy in 30 fractions. Chemotherapy was not recommended because of the rather poor general condition.

Figure 7.9 shows digitally reconstructed radiograph with portal design (Fig. 7.9A) and an axial isodose distribution (Fig. 7.9B) (note the missing portion of the mandible secondary to the surgery). The patient began his therapy with large opposed photon beam portals to 42 Gy followed by off–spinal cord and boost photon fields (16 and 4 Gy, respectively). The posterior cervical strips were treated with 9-MeV electrons, 18 Gy to the right side and 8 Gy to the clinically uninvolved left side. A matching anterior supraclavicular field with larynx block was treated to 50 Gy. Because the neck dissection scar was in close proximity to the larynx block, the skin over the larynx was treated with 6-MeV electrons to a dose of 42 Gy in 14 fractions. The right neck received additional irradiation with cone down portal with an appositional 9-MeV electron beam to a total of 60 Gy.

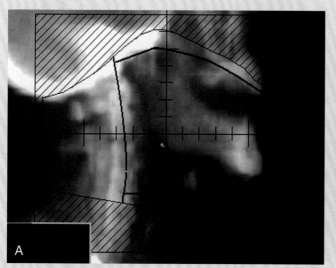

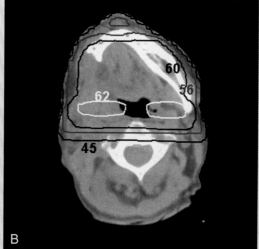

Case Figure 7.9A,B

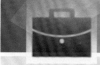

CASE STUDY 7.10

A 53-year-old male presented with soreness of the mouth and a right upper neck mass. Examination revealed a right retromolar trigone tumor and a 4-cm upper jugular node. Figure 7.10 shows axial CT images of the primary tumor (*green arrow*) extending into the posterior buccal space (Fig. 7.10A) and a node (*red arrow*) anterior to the right submandibular gland (Fig. 7.10B). He underwent

resection of the primary tumor, which included a marginal mandibulectomy with free flap reconstruction along with a selective right neck dissection. Histologic examination revealed SCC and negative margins. The neck dissection specimen revealed a 3.5-cm carcinoma in the level Ib soft tissue, consistent with completely replaced lymph node.

He was enrolled on protocol and treated with postoperative radiation with concurrent chemotherapy (weekly cetuximab and docetaxel). A stent was constructed to move the tongue away from the beams, which encompassed the retromolar trigone—buccal operative bed and right neck. Figure 7.10C shows the orientation of the beams on an axial image (Fig. 7.10C) through the operative bed. Initial beams consisted of an anterior and right posterior oblique beams (*red*). After 44 Gy, the anterior beam was rotated to miss the spinal cord (*green*) and treated to 50 Gy. A small field reduction was made off the superior and inferior borders (*blue*). A left anterior oblique beam (*orange*) was used to supplement the superior aspect of the volume that would otherwise have been underdosed due to the increased depth. These fields were matched to a field that covered the right lower neck using a left anterior oblique beam (Fig. 7.10D). Isodose distributions on axial slices through the superior masticator space (Fig. 7.10E) and operative bed (Fig. 7.10F) are shown. He did well for 4 years, but then developed a second primary carcinoma of the oral tongue. This second primary cancer was managed surgically, and he is without disease.

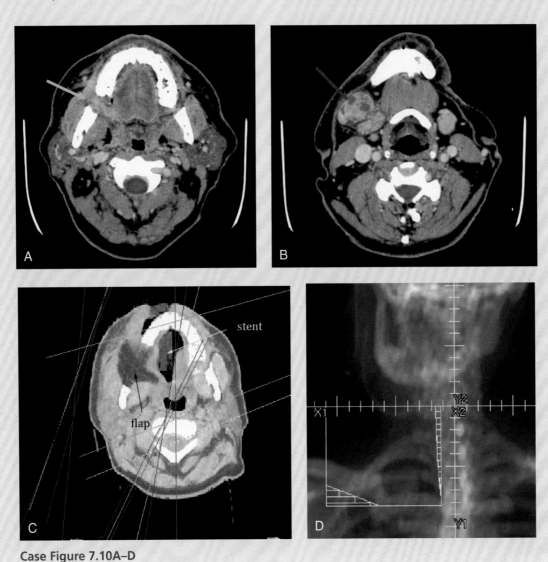

Case Figure 7.10A–D

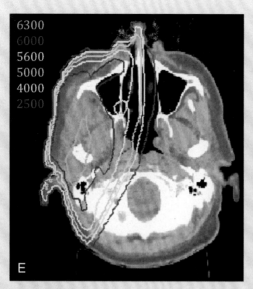

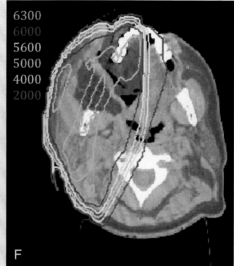

Case Figure 7.10E,F

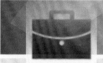

CASE STUDY 7.11

An 87-year-old woman presented a painful mass of the left jaw. Staging PET–CT scan revealed a retromolar trigone tumor extending into the masticator space including the infratemporal fossa. Figure 7.11 shows the primary tumor (*green arrow*) in representative coronal (Fig. 7.11A) and axial (Fig. 7.11B) images. She underwent a resection including partial mandibulectomy, parotidectomy, infratemporal fossa dissection, and left neck dissection, with a soft tissue free flap reconstruction. Histologic

examination revealed SCC with perineural, muscle, and bone invasion. Two nodes were positive in levels Ib and IIa with ECE.

She was treated with postoperative radiation. Her performance status prohibited concurrent chemotherapy despite the multiple adverse features. It was elected to treat ipsilaterally with IMRT. A tongue-displacing stent was used. The tumor bed with margin was identified as CTV$_{HD}$ (60 Gy) and the remaining operative bed

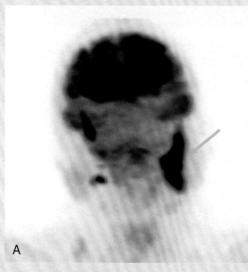

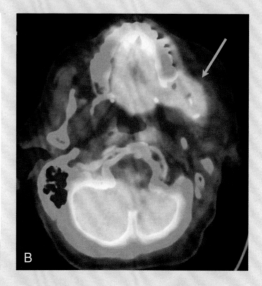

Case Figure 7.11A,B

as CTV$_{ID}$ (57 Gy). The undissected left supraclavicular nodes were contoured as CTV$_{ED}$ (54 Gy). Axial images with the contours of CTV$_{HD}$ (*red*), CTV$_{ID}$ (*blue*), and CTV$_{ED}$ (*yellow*) are paired with isodose distributions at the same level (Fig. 7.11C–J). A coronal view of the isodose distribution is also shown (Fig. 7.11K) with the targets color washed. She remains without disease 2 years out from treatment.

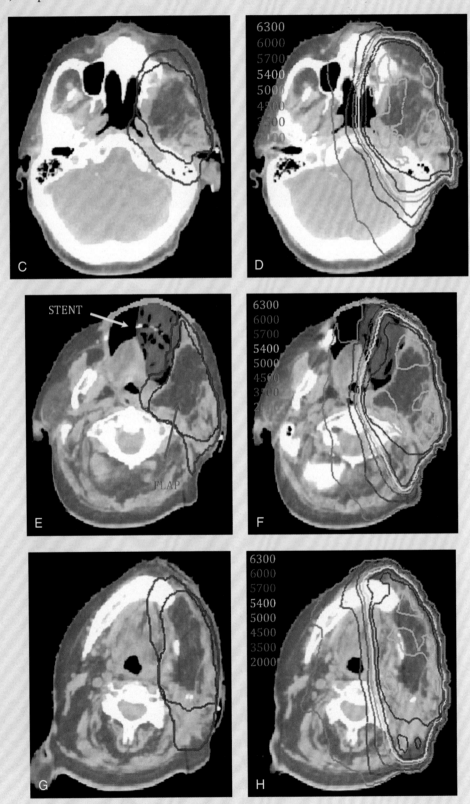

Case Figure 7.11C–H

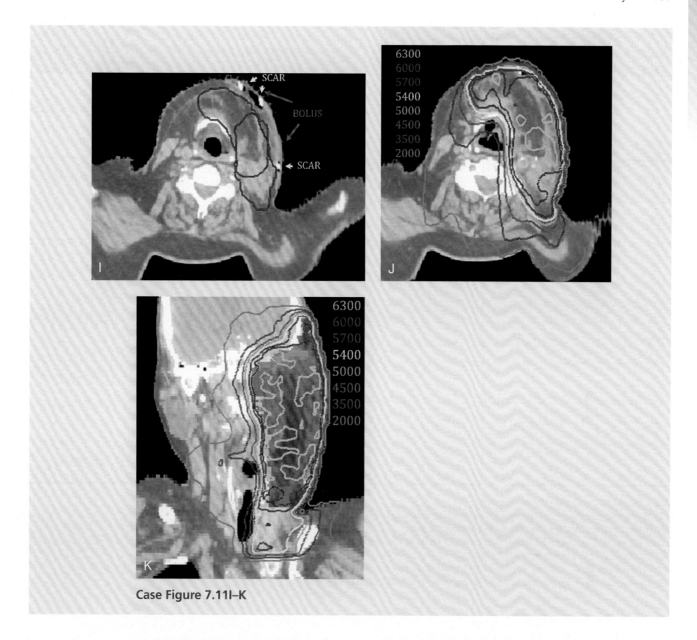

Case Figure 7.11I–K

For the neck, CTV_{ID} covers the dissected neck beyond CTV_{HD}. For patients with a flap reconstruction, the entire flap and suture lines are typically covered in at least CTV_{ID} or CTV_{HD}, when indicated.

- CTV_{ED} delineates volumes to receive an elective dose for subclinical disease. CTV_{ED} encompasses ipsilateral nodal levels I to IV in patients with a clinically negative neck who do not undergo neck dissection. In the presence of large ipsilateral nodal mass (N2–N3) or when the primary tumor is not well lateralized, CTV_{ED} includes the clinically uninvolved contralateral level I to IV neck nodes.

Doses prescribed are generally 60 Gy to CTV_{HD}, 57 Gy to CTV_{ID}, and 54 Gy to CTV_{ED}. Smaller volumes considered to be at extra high risk, often determined in collaboration with the surgeon and based on pathologic findings, are to receive 64 to 66 Gy.

Timing of Postoperative Radiotherapy

It is desirable to commence postoperative radiotherapy as soon as possible after healing of surgical wounds. With good communication between surgical, radiation, and dental oncologists, simulation can usually take place 3 to 4 weeks after surgery, and radiotherapy can start within a week in most patients. When delayed wound healing postpones commencement of postoperative radiation to beyond 6 to 8 weeks, we administer accelerated fractionation, such as concomitant boost, by delivering twice-a-day irradiations for 5 treatment days, either once a week or toward the end of the radiation course, to reduce the potential hazard of prolonged cumulative treatment time.

Background Data

See Table 7.6.

TABLE 7.6 Local Control Rates in Evaluable Patients (Anterior Faucial Pillar–Retromolar Trigone): January 1966–August 1981 (Analysis January 1986)

Stage	All Patients Under Local Control	Evaluable Patients[a]			
		Local Control (%)	Treatment of Primary Failure	No. of Patients Salvaged	Ultimate Control Rate No. (%)
T1	15/20 (75%)	12/17 (71%)	Surgery (5)[b]	5/5	17/17 (100%)
T2	69/93 (74%)	57/81 (70%)	No treatment (2)		
			Surgery (21)		
			Surgery + XRT (1)	19/24[c]	76/81 (94%)
T3	30/36 (83%)	19/25 (76%)	Surgery (5)		
			Surgery + Chemo (1)	4/6[c]	23/25 (92%)
T4	8/10 (80%)	3/5	Surgery (1)		
			Chemo (1)	1/2[c]	4/5 (80%)

Data from MD Anderson Cancer Center.
[a]31 patients who died in <2 years with no evidence of local disease are not evaluable.
[b]Numbers in parentheses indicate number of patients.
[c]Five T2, one T3, and one T4 patients died in <2 years with no evidence of local disease.
XRT, radiotherapy; Chemo, chemotherapy.
Modified from Lo K, Fletcher GH, Byers RM, et al. Results of irradiation in the squamous cell carcinomas of the anterior faucial pillar—retromolar trigone. *Int J Radiat Oncol Biol Phys* 1987;13:969–974.

BUCCAL MUCOSA

Treatment Strategy

Regardless of size, data suggest that patients have optimal outcomes with surgical resection and adjuvant radiation therapy when indicated.

In theory, for T1 to T2 lesions, either surgery or primary radiotherapy may be appropriate as primary treatment, depending on the thickness and location of the lesion, anticipated functional/cosmetic outcome, and patient preference **(Case Study 7.12)**.

For T3 to T4 lesions, surgery followed by postoperative radiotherapy is recommended.

Primary Radiotherapy

Target Volume

Initial Target Volume

- *T1 to T2 N0:* primary tumor and ipsilateral level IB (submandibular) and level II (subdigastric) nodes.
- *T1 to T2 N1:* primary tumor and entire ipsilateral neck.
- *N2 to N3:* bilateral irradiation.

CASE STUDY 7.12

A 50-year-old woman presented with a tumor of the left buccal mucosa. She had no associated symptoms. A biopsy was positive for moderately differentiated SCC. Examination revealed a 2.5-cm, superficial tumor in the left buccal mucosa, with extension posteriorly toward the mucosa overlying the ascending ramus of the mandible. There was a 2-cm level IB lymph node palpable. Stage T2 N1 M0. It was elected to treat her with chemoradiation consisting of conventional fractionation with cisplatin (100 mg/m^2 i.v. on days 1, 22, and 43). An appositional field was used with the patient in an open-neck position to deliver a dose of 50 Gy specified to the 90% isodose line using a combination of 16-MeV electrons and 6-MV photons, loaded 4:1. A boost was delivered to both the primary tumor and gross nodal disease with 12-MeV electrons to an additional 18 Gy also specified at the 90% line. Figure 7.12 shows a digitally reconstructed radiograph of the initial field covering the primary tumor and upper neck (Fig. 7.12A) along with the axial isodoses through the primary tumor (Fig. 7.12B) and neck node (Fig. 7.12C). The low neck was treated to 50 Gy, at D_{max}, with a matching appositional 9-MeV electron portal.

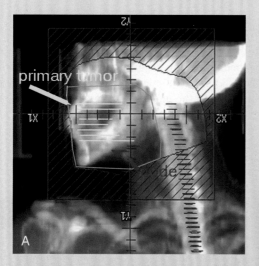

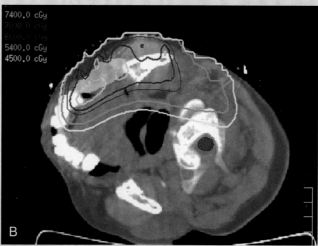

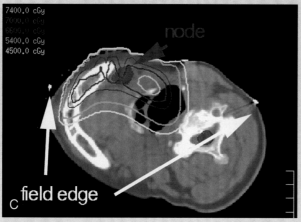

Case Figure 7.12A–C

Boost volume encompasses the primary tumor and, when present, involves lymph nodes.

Setup and Field Arrangement for Conventional Technique

Tumor borders are marked by seeds or wires, whenever possible, along with the ipsilateral oral commissure to help shape the field. An intraoral stent is used to displace the tongue toward the contralateral side and to shield it (see Chapter 3). The patient is generally placed in an open-neck position for ipsilateral irradiation with combination of electrons and photons (usually in a ratio of 4:1).

An appositional field is used to irradiate the primary lesion and upper neck nodes.

- *Anterior and superior borders*: at least 2-cm margins from the visible–palpable tumor borders.
- *Posterior and inferior borders*: same as for those for retromolar trigone primary.

The commissure and lips are shielded whenever possible to reduce morbidity. Care should be taken to exclude the eyes from the radiation field.

An appositional electron field is used (see "General Principles") to irradiate mid- and lower neck when indicated.

For delivering the boost dose with external beam, the field is reduced to encompass the tumor with at least 1-cm margins and, when present, involved upper neck nodes. Superficial, circumscribed lesions receive boost dose with brachytherapy. Field borders for bilateral treatment are the same as those for unilateral irradiation; however, the patient is immobilized in a supine position.

Dose

The initial target volume receives 50 Gy in 25 fractions. The boost dose depends on the size of the primary tumor and on the technique used. For external beam technique, 16 Gy in 8 fractions for T1 and 20 Gy in 10 fractions for T2 lesions are administered. For brachytherapy, 25 to 30 Gy is administered.

Postoperative Radiotherapy

Target Volume

The initial target volume **(Case Study 7.13)** is the entire surgical bed, including primary site and ipsilateral levels IB to IV. The boost volume encompasses areas of known disease locations. In the modern era, IMRT is preferred, when available.

CASE STUDY 7.13

A 33-year-old man, who had a long history of chewing tobacco and betel nuts, sought medical attention because of a persistent ulcer in the left buccal mucosa. Biopsy of this lesion showed an infiltrating, poorly differentiated carcinoma. Physical examination revealed a 5- × 3-cm ulcerative lesion extending from the left oral commissure back and downward to the gingivobuccal sulcus. The lesion infiltrated the subcutaneous tissues of the cheek, but there was no palpable lymphadenopathy. Further head and neck exam was unremarkable (stage: T3 N0 M0). He underwent a wide excision of the primary lesion that involved a through-and-through removal of a large part of the left cheek and a small part of the upper and lower lips, a left supraomohyoid neck dissection, and reconstruction of the cheek with a free myocutaneous flap. Histologic examination showed negative section margins, except the inferior border had a close margin of 2 mm, and involvement of one of seven submental–submandibular lymph nodes without ECE (stage p T3 N1 M0). Postoperative radiotherapy was recommended because of these findings. It was initially planned to treat the primary tumor bed and

ipsilateral neck nodes. However, physical examination after surgery showed that the graft was 4 to 5 cm thick. Irradiating the primary tumor bed with electrons would have required the use of the 20-MeV beam. This would have resulted in delivering high doses to the lips and part of the oral and nasal cavities. Therefore, it was decided to treat the patient with photons. Parallel-opposed oblique fields were used to irradiate the primary tumor bed and ipsilateral upper neck nodes. Figure 7.13 shows the right anterior oblique (Fig. 7.13A) and left posterior oblique (Fig. 7.13B) radiation fields relative to the facial structures. The thin wire taped on the cheek indicated the size of the graft. One end of the thick wire was inserted in the oral cavity and brought in contact with the surface of the reconstructed mucosa and the other end was twisted at the commissure and taped on the skin to define the thickness of the graft and to facilitate portal design. This setup prevented irradiation of most of the lips and oral and nasal cavities. A total dose of 60 Gy was given in 30 fractions through the oblique fields. The ipsilateral lower neck received 50 Gy in 25 fractions through an abutting anterior appositional field.

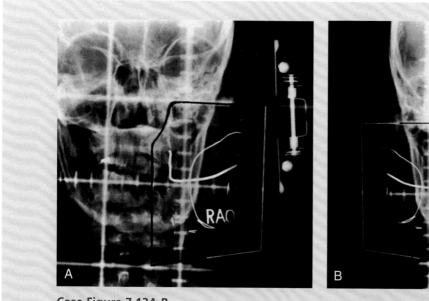

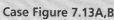

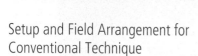

Case Figure 7.13A,B

Setup and Field Arrangement for Conventional Technique

This is similar to that of primary radiotherapy. Marking the external surgical scar facilitates portal design. The anterior and superior field borders are determined by the contiguous spread pattern of the primary tumor and by the extent of surgery (scar, flap).

Dose

- A dose of 60 Gy in 30 fractions is given to areas with high-risk features, that is, close or microscopically positive margins, perineural extension, vascular invasion, positive nodes, or extranodal extension. An additional boost dose of 6 Gy in three fractions may be given when indicated, such as when multiple adverse features are present or when the interval between surgery and radiation is much longer than 6 weeks.
- A dose of 56 Gy in 28 fractions is given to the surgical bed.
- A dose of 50 Gy of elective irradiation in 25 fractions is given to undissected regions.

Intensity-Modulated Radiation Therapy

When using IMRT in the postoperative setting, treatment is given in 30 fractions. The target volumes to receive various levels of doses are delineated and dosimetric plans are generated by iterative process.

Three CTVs are generally delineated **(Case Study 7.14 and Case Study 7.15)**.

- CTV_{HD} delineates volumes to receive the highest dose, which includes the primary and nodal vGTVs with 8- to 10-mm margins.

- CTV_{ID} delineates volumes to receive an intermediate dose. For the primary tumor bed, CTV_{ID} encompasses a 0.5- to 1-cm additional margin beyond CTV_{HD}. For the neck, it covers the dissected neck not harboring involved nodes. The buccal space should be included in this volume, and for bulky primary tumors, or tumors involving the posterior buccal mucosa, CTV_{ID} should include the adjacent masticator space.
- CTV_{ED} delineates volumes to receive an elective dose for subclinical disease. CTV_{ED} encompasses ipsilateral nodal levels I to IV in patients with clinically negative neck who do not undergo neck dissection. In the presence of large ipsilateral nodal mass (N2–N3) or when the primary tumor is not well lateralized, CTV_{ED} includes the clinically uninvolved contralateral level I to IV neck nodes.

Generally, CTV_{HD} receives 60 Gy, CTV_{ID} 57 Gy, and CTV_{ED} 54 Gy. Smaller volumes considered to be at extra high risk, often determined in collaboration with the surgeon and based on pathologic findings, are to receive 64 to 66 Gy.

The patient is immobilized in a supine position with an extended thermoplastic mask covering the head and shoulder. Thin-cut CT images are obtained in treatment position, and target volumes are outlined for dosimetric planning.

Timing of Postoperative Radiotherapy

It is desirable to begin postoperative radiotherapy as soon as possible after healing of surgical wounds. With good communication between surgical, radiation, and dental oncologists, simulation can usually take place 3 to 4 weeks after surgery, and radiotherapy can start within a week in most patients. When delayed wound healing postpones commencement of

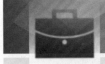

CASE STUDY 7.14

A 54-year-old male presented with a left buccal mucosa lesion after suffering bite trauma. A biopsy was positive for SCC. Staging CT scan of the head and neck revealed the lesion (Fig. 7.14A, *green arrow*). He underwent a wide local excision with free flap reconstruction and a left selective neck dissection. Histologic examination revealed a 1-cm tumor, moderately differentiated SCC. Surgical margins and nodes were negative, but there was perineural invasion of large nerves.

He was treated with postoperative IMRT. The tumor bed with margin was identified as CTV$_{HD}$ (60 Gy), the remaining operative bed was identified as CTV$_{ID}$ (57 Gy), and the perineural pathways to the base of skull were contoured as CTV$_{ED}$ (54 Gy). A tongue-displacing stent was used to move the tongue to the right. Seven beams were used. The beam orientation and color-washed target volumes (CTV$_{HD}$, *khaki*; CTV$_{ID}$, *blue*; and CTV$_{ED}$, *yellow*) are shown on an axial CT image at the approximate location of the tumor (Fig. 7.14B). Figure 7.14C–G shows axial images of the isodose distributions from the skull base superiorly to the top of the hyoid inferiorly. The patient remains well 3 years later.

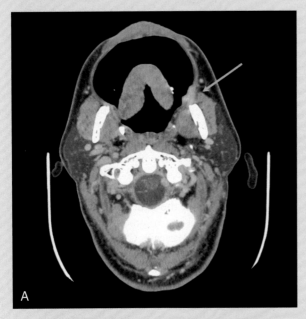

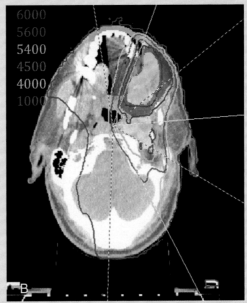

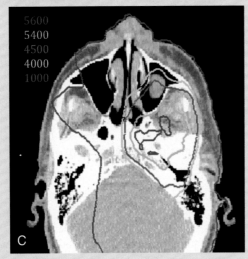

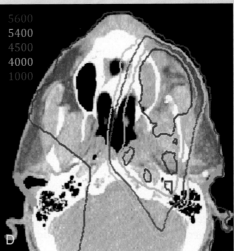

Case Figure 7.14A–D

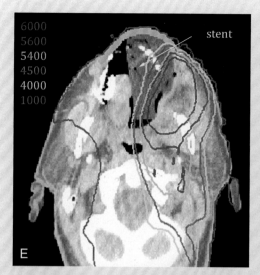
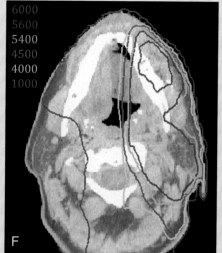
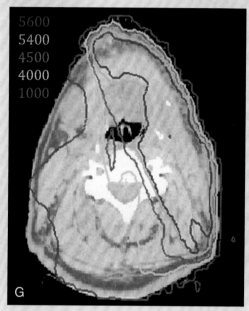

Case Figure 7.14E–G

CASE STUDY 7.15

A 67-year-old male with a long history of left buccal mucosa pain presented with left neck adenopathy. Physical examination and staging CT scan of the head and neck revealed multiple nodes. Figure 7.15A shows a representative axial slice demonstrating numerous level IB nodes (*red arrows*). He underwent a wide local excision of the buccal lesion and a neck dissection. Histologic examination of the primary tumor revealed SCC with dysplasia at the margins. The neck dissection specimens contained 15 nodes harboring carcinoma, with nodes positive within all levels (I to V), and numerous nodes with ECE.

He was treated with postoperative chemoradiation on protocol. The chemotherapy consisted of weekly cisplatin and cetuximab per protocol. Radiation was delivered with IMRT in 30 fractions. A tongue-displacing stent was used. The tumor bed with margin was identified as CTV_{HD} (60 Gy) and the remaining operative bed as CTV_{ID} (57 Gy). The undissected right neck was contoured as CTV_{ED} (54 Gy). The treatment plan is shown on representative axial images (Fig. 7.15B–E) from the level of the buccal space to inferior level II nodes. Two months after completion of radiation, he developed distant disease.

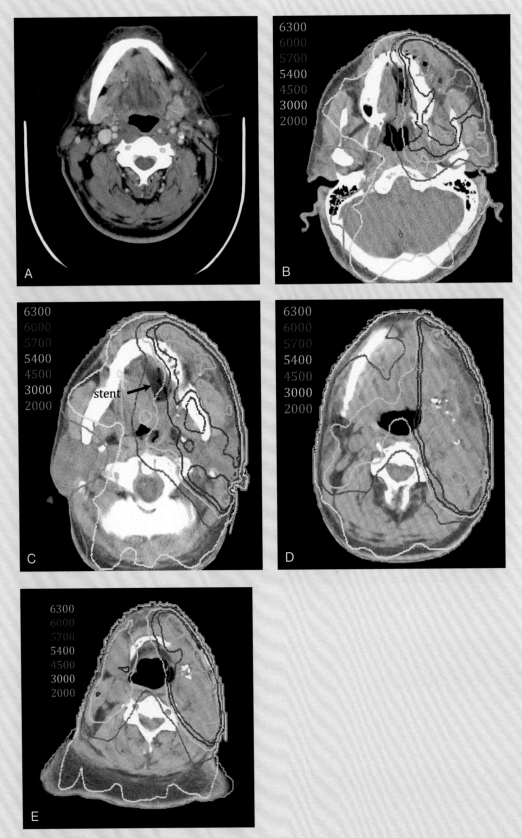

Case Figure 7.15A–E

TABLE 7.7 Results of Radiotherapy in Cancer of the Buccal Mucosa: Site of Failure by UICC, T and N Stages

Stage	Primary Failure No. (%)	Nodal Failure No. (%)	Total Failure No. (%)
T1 N0	0/13 (0%)	0/13 (0%)	0/13 (0%)
T2 N0	13/49 (27%)	7/49 (14%)	18/49 (37%)
T3 N0	15/49 (31%)	1/49 (2%)	15/49 (31%)
T4 N0	6/12 (50%)	1/12 (8%)	7/12 (58%)
Any T and N1	51/94 (54%)	48/94 (51%)	55/94 (59%)
Any T and N3	12/17 (71%)	15/17 (88%)	14/17 (82%)

Modified from Nair MK, Sankaranarayanan R, Padmanabhan TK. Evaluation of the role of radiotherapy in the management of carcinoma of the buccal mucosa. *Cancer* 1988;61:1326.

TABLE 7.8 Five-Year Survival Rates in 119 Patients with Squamous Cell Carcinoma of the Buccal Mucosa

Variable	5-Year Survival Rate (%)
AJCC stage I	78
AJCC stage II	66
AJCC stage III	62
AJCC stage IV	50
Node negative	70
Node positive	49
No extracapsular spread	69
Extracapsular spread	24

Data from MD Anderson Cancer Center.
AJCC, American Joint Committee on Cancer.
Modified from Diaz EM Jr, Holsinger FC, Zuniga ER, et al. Squamous cell carcinoma of the buccal mucosa: one institution's experience with 119 previously untreated patients. *Head Neck* 2003;25:267–273.

postoperative radiation to beyond 6 to 8 weeks, we administer accelerated fractionation, such as concomitant boost, by delivering twice-a-day irradiations for 5 treatment days, either once a week or toward the end of the radiation course, to reduce the potential hazard of prolonged cumulative treatment time.

Background Data

See Tables 7.7 and 7.8.

HARD PALATE AND UPPER ALVEOLAR RIDGE

This section deals with true hard palate and alveolar ridge cancers. Most hard palate and alveolar ridge tumors are manifestations of maxillary sinus cancers.

Treatment Strategy

Surgery is the treatment of choice in most cases. Postoperative radiotherapy is delivered when indicated (see "Floor of Mouth and Oral Tongue" section).

Primary radiotherapy may be used for small, superficial SCCs.

Postoperative Radiotherapy

Target Volume

Initial Target Volume

The entire surgical bed is encompassed **(Case Study 7.16)**. In most cases, the location of the primary lesion, the extent of surgery, or both necessitate treatment with opposed lateral fields. Ipsilateral irradiation (wedge pair) may suffice in well-lateralized lesions of the alveolar ridge.

Elective irradiation of upper neck nodes is given to patients with SCC. All cervical nodal areas are irradiated in patients with positive lymph nodes, regardless of histologic type. Boost volume encompasses areas of known disease.

Setup and Field Arrangement for Conventional Technique

For bilateral irradiation, an intraoral stent is used to open the mouth and, for an anterior lesion, to protrude the upper lip. If the surgical defect is large enough, a water-containing

CASE STUDY 7.16

A 42-year-old woman noticed a tumor on the palate. Physical examination revealed a 4- × 3-cm exophytic tumor on the left side of the hard palate. The lesion extended posteriorly to involve the anterior part of the soft palate, laterally onto the left upper alveolar ridge, medially approaching the midline, and anteriorly to the level of the first premolar. There was no palpable adenopathy in the neck. A CT scan confirmed the physical findings and also showed involvement of the floor of the maxillary sinus with bone destruction. A biopsy showed moderately differentiated SCC. Stage: T4 N0 M0. She underwent a left intraoral palatectomy and maxillectomy. Histologic examination showed involvement of bone and extension to the mucosa of the floor of the maxillary sinus and floor of the left nasal cavity. There was perineural spread along the greater palatine nerve. All margins of resection were negative. She received postoperative radiotherapy with lateral parallel-opposed photon fields (Fig. 7.16) encompassing the surgical bed and the course of the palatine and maxillary nerves to the gasserian ganglion, to a dose of 54 Gy in 30 fractions. The tumor bed was then boosted to a total dose of 63 Gy.

Ten months after completion of radiotherapy, she started to experience left-sided back pain. Physical examination showed no evidence of local–regional disease. However, chest x-rays revealed a paravertebral mass at the level of the third intercostal space. A fluoroscopic-guided

fine-needle aspiration showed SCC consistent with metastatic deposit from the palate lesion. Palliative radiotherapy was given, which diminished the back pain. She expired a month later.

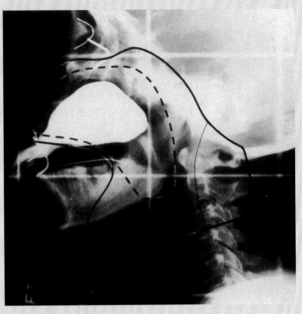

Case Figure 7.16

balloon is used to fill the surgical defect (see Chapter 3). Most surgical defects are now filled with a free flap reconstruction. Otherwise, the mouth-opening stent is fabricated with the palatal prosthesis in place. Marking the external surgical scar, oral commissures, and lateral canthi may facilitate portal design. The patient is immobilized in a supine position.

The initial target volume encompasses parallel-opposed fields to treat the primary tumor bed and, when indicated, the upper neck nodes.

- *Anterior and superior borders:* at least 2 cm beyond the surgical bed. If disease extended into the maxillary sinus, the entire sinus is included up to the floor of the orbit.
- *Posterior border:* at midvertebral bodies for non-SCC and N0; behind the mastoid process for SCC and N0; behind the spinous processes for N+ (or more posteriorly to cover large surgical bed).
- *Inferior border:* just above the arytenoids for SCC with no nodal involvement, or 2 cm below the surgical margin for low-grade minor salivary gland tumors.

In the presence of positive nodes, an anterior photon field is used for irradiation of the mid- and low cervical nodes.

For boost volume, the fields are reduced to encompass the tumor bed with at least 1-cm margins; involved upper neck nodes are included in the lateral fields or in a separate appositional electron field; involved mid- and lower neck nodes are irradiated with an appositional electron field or glancing photon fields.

For ipsilateral irradiation, the patient is immobilized in a supine position. Anterior and ipsilateral wedge-pair photon fields are used to treat the primary tumor bed (usually with 45-degree wedges).

- *Lateral field: borders* are the same as those for bilateral treatment.
- *Anterior field: medial border* is 2 cm beyond the surgical margin; *lateral border* is short of falling off; and *superior* and *inferior borders* correspond to those of the lateral field.

A lateral appositional electron field is used for elective treatment of the submandibular and subdigastric nodes when ipsilateral treatment is adopted for SCCs.

- *Superior border:* matches the inferior border of the photon fields (a small triangle over the cheek may be spared).

- *Anterior border:* just short of falloff.
- *Posterior border:* behind the mastoid process.
- *Inferior border:* at the thyroid notch.

For boost irradiation, photon fields are reduced to encompass the tumor volume with at least a 1-cm margin.

Dose

- A dose of 60 Gy in 30 fractions given to areas with high-risk features, that is, close or microscopically positive margins, perineural extension, vascular invasion, positive nodes, or extranodal extension. An additional boost dose of 6 Gy in three fractions may be given when indicated, such as when multiple adverse features are present or when the interval

between surgery and radiation is much longer than 6 weeks.

- 56 Gy in 28 fractions given to the surgical bed.
- 50 Gy of elective irradiation in 25 fractions given to undissected regions.

Intensity-Modulated Radiation Therapy Planning

IMRT is the treatment of choice for lesions of the hard palate and upper alveolar ridge **(Case Study 7.17)**, when available. Adjuvant IMRT is given in 30 fractions.

Three CTVs are generally delineated.

- CTV_{HD} delineates volumes to receive the highest dose, which includes the primary and nodal vGTVs with 8- to 10-mm margins.

CASE STUDY 7.17

An 82-year-old male underwent an extraction of a left maxillary molar tooth. The extraction site did not heal and eventually a biopsy was performed, which revealed an SCC. A diagnostic CT scan revealed a focal destructive lesion at the inner table of the alveolar ridge of the left maxilla adjacent to the last two molar teeth. Figure 7.17A shows the primary tumor (*green arrows*) on a representative axial slice.

The patient underwent a left infrastructure maxillectomy. Histologic examination revealed a 1.4-cm tumor, moderately differentiated SCC, invading bone. Margins were negative.

He was staged as having a pT4 N0 tumor and treated with postoperative IMRT. As the lesion was well lateralized, and the nodes clinically negative, it was elected to treat the ipsilateral side only. Figure 7.17B,C shows a

coronal view through the orbits and maxillary sinuses and axial slice through the infrastructure, respectively, with contours of CTV_{HD} (*red*), CTV_{ID} (*blue*), and CTV_{ED} (*yellow*). The remaining panels show axial isodose distributions along with CTV_{HD} (*red*), CTV_{ID} (*blue*), and CTV_{ED} (*yellow*) at the level of the infrastructure (Fig. 7.17D), midmaxillary sinus (Fig. 7.17E), inferior to the palate (Fig. 7.17F), and nodal stations IB and II (Fig. 7.17G).

CTV_{HD} encompasses the residual tissues surrounding the resection cavity that is clearly seen in Figure 7.17B,C. CTV_{ID} covers the remaining operative bed, the residual left maxillary sinus to the floor of the orbit (Fig. 7.17B), the medial 1 cm of the remaining hard palate (Fig. 7.17B), and the left soft palate and masticator space (Fig. 7.17C,F). CTV_{ED} covers levels IB and II of the undissected left neck (Fig. 7.17G). The patient remains well 2 years following treatment.

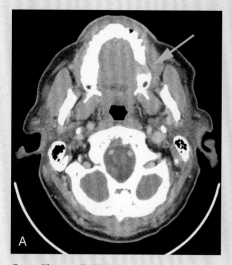
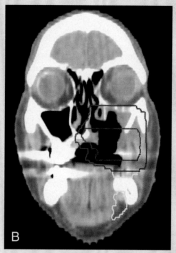

Case Figure 7.17A,B

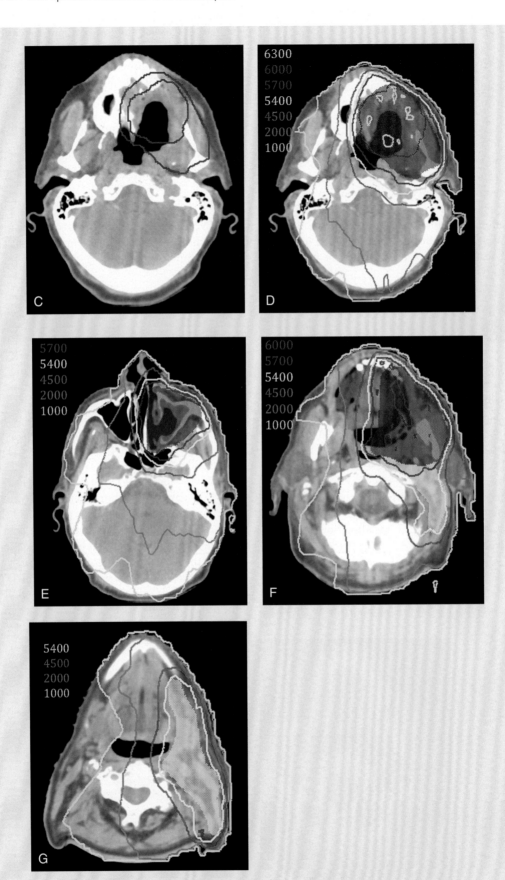

Case Figure 7.17C–G

- CTV$_{ID}$ delineates volumes to receive an intermediate dose. For the primary tumor bed, CTV$_{ID}$ encompasses a 5- to 10-mm additional margin beyond CTV$_{HD}$. For the neck, it covers the dissected neck not harboring involved nodes. The buccal space should be included in this volume, and for bulky primary tumors, or tumors involving the posterior buccal mucosa, CTV$_{ID}$ should include the adjacent masticator space.
- CTV$_{ED}$ delineates volumes to receive an elective dose for subclinical disease. CTV$_{ED}$ encompasses ipsilateral nodal levels I to IV in patients with clinically negative neck who do not undergo neck dissection. In the presence of large ipsilateral nodal mass (N2–N3) or when the primary tumor is not well lateralized, CTV$_{ED}$ includes the clinically uninvolved contralateral level I to IV neck nodes.

Generally, CTV$_{HD}$ receives 60 Gy, CTV$_{ID}$ 57 Gy, and CTV$_{ED}$ 54 Gy. Smaller volumes considered to be at extra high risk, often determined in collaboration with the surgeon and based on pathologic findings, are to receive 64 to 66 Gy.

Timing of Postoperative Radiotherapy

It is desirable to begin postoperative radiotherapy as soon as possible after healing of surgical wounds. With good communication between surgical, radiation, and dental oncologists, simulation can usually take place 3 to 4 weeks after surgery, and radiotherapy can start within a week in most patients. When delayed wound healing postpones commencement of postoperative radiation to beyond 6 to 8 weeks, we administer accelerated fractionation, such as concomitant boost, by delivering twice-a-day irradiations for 5 treatment days, either once a week or toward the end of the radiation course, to reduce the potential hazard of prolonged cumulative treatment time.

Primary Radiotherapy

Target Volume

- *Initial target volume:* primary tumor with 2-cm margins (no elective neck irradiation for small, superficial lesions).
- *Boost volume:* primary tumor with 1-cm margins.

Setup and Field Arrangement

This is similar to that of postoperative radiotherapy. The boost dose is preferably delivered with a surface mold.

Dose

The initial target volume receives 50 Gy in 25 fractions.

The boost dose is 15 to 20 Gy at 0.5-cm depth when delivered by surface mold and 16 Gy in 8 fractions (T1) or 20 Gy in 10 fractions (T2) when delivered by external beam.

The dose delivered by intraoral cone is specified at D_{max}.

Intensity-Modulated Radiation Therapy

Similar to that of postoperative setting.

Background Data

See Table 7.9.

TABLE 7.9 Hard Palate Carcinoma Treated with Radiotherapy

	Number of Patients	5-Year Actuarial Survival Rate (%)	Crude Local Recurrence Rate (%)
T1 and T2	17	54	18
T3 and T4	14	55	57
Node negative	24	65	37
Node positive	7	19	29
Squamous cell carcinoma	19	48	32
Salivary gland carcinoma	12	63	42

Data from Christie Hospital, Manchester, UK.
Modified from Yorozu A, Sykes AJ, Slevin NJ. Carcinoma of the hard palate treated with radiotherapy: a retrospective review of 31 cases. *Oral Oncol* 2001;37:493–497.

SUGGESTED READINGS

Akine Y, Tokita N, Ogino T, et al. Stage I–II carcinoma of the anterior two-thirds of the tongue treated with different modalities: a retrospective analysis of 244 patients. *Radiother Oncol* 1991;21:24.

Beauvois S, Hoffstetter S, Peiffert D, et al. Brachytherapy for lower lip epidermoid cancer: tumoral and treatment factors influencing recurrences and complications. *Radiother Oncol* 1994;33:195.

Benk V, Mazeron JJ, Grimard L, et al. Comparison of curietherapy versus external irradiation combined with curietherapy in stage II squamous cell carcinomas of the mobile tongue. *Radiother Oncol* 1990;18:339.

Byers RM, Anderson B, Schwarz EA, et al. Treatment of squamous carcinoma of the retromolar trigone. *Am J Clin Oncol* 1984;7:647.

Chan AK, Huang SH, Le LW, et al. Postoperative intensity-modulated radiotherapy following surgery for oral cavity squamous cell carcinoma: patterns of failure. *Oral Oncol* 2013;49:255–260.

Chaudhary AJ, Pande SC, Sharma V, et al. Radiotherapy of carcinoma of the buccal mucosa. *Semin Surg Oncol* 1989;5:322.

Chung CK, Johns ME, Cantrell RW, et al. Radiotherapy in the management of primary malignancies of the hard palate. *Laryngoscope* 1980;90:576.

D'Cruz AK, Vaish R, Kapre N, et al. Elective versus therapeutic neck dissection in node-negative oral cancer. *N Engl J Med* 2015;373:521.

Dearnaly DP, Dardoufas C, A'Hearn RP, et al. Interstitial irradiation for carcinoma of the tongue and floor of mouth: Royal Marsden Hospital experience. *Radiother Oncol* 1991;21:183.

Delclos L. Afterloading interstitial irradiation techniques. In: Levitt SH, Khan FM, Potish RA, eds. *Technological basis of radiation therapy*, 2nd ed. Philadelphia, PA: Lea & Febiger, 1992.

Diaz EM Jr, Holsinger FC, Zuniga ER, et al. Squamous cell carcinoma of the buccal mucosa: one institution's experience with 119 previously untreated patients. *Head Neck* 2003;25:267.

Dixit S, Vyas RK, Toparani RB, et al. Surgery versus surgery and postoperative radiotherapy in squamous cell carcinoma of the buccal mucosa: a comparative study. *Ann Surg Oncol* 1998;5:502–510.

Eicher SA, Overholt SM, el-Naggar AK, et al. Lower gingival carcinoma. Clinical and pathologic determinants of regional metastases. *Arch Otolaryngol Head Neck Surg* 1996;122:634.

Fletcher GH. Oral cavity and oropharynx. In: Fletcher GH, ed. *Textbook of radiotherapy*, 3rd ed. Philadelphia, PA: Lea & Febiger, 1980.

Genden EM, Ferlito A, Shaha AR, et al. Management of cancer of the retromolar trigone. *Oral Oncol* 2003;39:633.

Greenberg JS, El Naggar AK, Mo V, et al. Disparity in pathologic and clinical lymph node staging in oral tongue carcinoma. Implication for therapeutic decision making. *Cancer* 2003;98:508.

Guibert M, David I, Vergez S, et al. Brachytherapy in lip carcinoma: long-term results. *Int J Radiat Oncol Biol Phys* 2011;81:e839.

Hicks WL Jr, Loree TR, Garcia RI, et al. Squamous cell carcinoma of the floor of mouth: a 20-year review. *Head Neck* 1997;19:400.

Hinerman RW, Mendenhall WM, Morris CG, et al. Postoperative irradiation for squamous cell carcinoma of the oral cavity: 35-year experience. *Head Neck* 2004;26:984.

Lefebvre JL, Coche-Dequeant B, Castelain B, et al. Interstitial brachytherapy and early tongue squamous cell carcinoma management. *Head Neck* 1990;12:232.

Lo K, Fletcher GH, Byers RM, et al. Results of irradiation in the squamous cell carcinomas of the anterior faucial pillar—retromolar trigone. *Int J Radiat Oncol Biol Phys* 1987;13:969.

Lydiatt DD, Robbins KT, Byers RM, et al. Treatment of stage I and II oral tongue cancer. *Head Neck* 1993;15:308.

Maciejewsky B, Withers HR, Taylor JM, et al. Dose fractionation and regeneration in radiotherapy for cancer of the oral cavity and oropharynx. Part 1. Tumor dose-response and repopulation. *Int J Radiat Oncol Biol Phys* 1989;16:831.

Mazeron JJ, Grimard L, Raynal M, et al. Iridium-192 curietherapy for T1 and T2 epidermoid carcinomas of the floor of the mouth. *Int J Radiat Oncol Biol Phys* 1990;18:1299.

Mazeron JJ, Simon JM, Le Pechoux C, et al. Effect of dose rate on local control and complications in definitive irradiation of T1–2 squamous cell carcinomas of mobile tongue and floor of mouth with interstitial iridium-192. *Radiother Oncol* 1991;21:39.

Meoz RT, Fletcher GH, Lindberg RD. Anatomic coverage in elective irradiation of the neck for squamous cell carcinoma of the oral tongue. *Int J Radiat Oncol Biol Phys* 1982;8:1881.

Nair MK, Sankaranarayanan R, Padmanabhan TK. Evaluation of the role of radiotherapy in the management of carcinoma of the buccal mucosa. *Cancer* 1988;61:1326.

Pederson AW, Salama JK, Witt ME, et al. Concurrent chemotherapy and intensity-modulated radiotherapy for organ preservation of locoregionally advanced oral cavity cancer. *Am J Clin Oncol* 2011;34:356-61.

Pernot M, Hoffstetter S, Peiffert D, et al. Epidermoid carcinomas of the floor of mouth treated by exclusive irradiation: statistical study of a series of 207 cases. *Radiother Oncol* 1995;35:177.

Pernot M, Malissard L, Aletti P, et al. Iridium-192 in the management of 147 T2N0 oral tongue carcinomas treated with irradiation alone: comparison of two treatment techniques. *Radiother Oncol* 1992;23:223.

Pierquin B, Wilson JF, Chassagne D, eds. *Modern brachytherapy.* New York, NY: Masson Publishing, 1987.

Pop L, Eijkenboom WM, de Boer MF, et al. Evaluation of treatment results of squamous cell carcinoma of the buccal mucosa. *Int J Radiat Oncol Biol Phys* 1989;16:483.

Rodgers LW Jr, Stringer SP, Mendenhall WM, et al. Management of squamous cell carcinoma of the floor of mouth. *Head Neck* 1993;15:16.

Scher ED, Romesser PB, Chen C, et al. Definitive chemoradiation for primary oral cavity carcinoma: a single institution experience. *Oral Oncol* 2015;51:709–715.

Shah JP, Candela FC, Poddar AK. The patterns of cervical lymph node metastases from squamous cell carcinoma of the oral cavity. *Cancer* 1990;66:109.

Shaha AR, Spiro RH, Shah JP, et al. Squamous carcinoma of the floor of the mouth. *Am J Surg* 1984;148:455.

Sher DJ, Thotakura V, Balboni TA, et al. Treatment of oral cavity squamous cell carcinoma with adjuvant or definitive intensity-modulated radiation therapy. *Int J Radiat Oncol Biol Phys* 2011:81;e215–e222.

Smith GI, O'Brien CJ, Clark J, et al. Management of the neck in patients with T1 and T2 cancer in the mouth. *Br J Oral Maxillofac Surg* 2004;42:494.

Thanh Pham T, Cross S, Gebski V, et al. Squamous carcinoma of the lip in Australian patients: definitive radiotherapy is an efficacious option to surgery in select patients. *Dermatol Surg* 2015;41:219.

Wang CC, Kelly J, August M, et al. Early carcinoma of the oral cavity: a conservative approach with radiation therapy. *J Oral Maxillofac Surg* 1995;53:687.

Wendt CD, Peters LJ, Delclos L, et al. Primary radiotherapy in the treatment of stage I and II oral tongue cancers: importance of the proportion of therapy delivered with interstitial therapy. *Int J Radiat Oncol Biol Phys* 1990;18:1287.

Yorozu A, Sykes AJ, Slevin NJ. Carcinoma of the hard palate treated with radiotherapy: a retrospective review of 31 cases. *Oral Oncol* 2001;37:493.

Zelefsky MJ, Harrison LB, Fass DE, et al. Postoperative radiation therapy for squamous cell carcinomas of the oral cavity and oropharynx: impact of therapy on patients with positive surgical margins. *Int J Radiat Oncol Biol Phys* 1993;25:17.

8

Nasopharynx

Key Points

- Nasopharyngeal carcinoma (NPC) is uncommon in the United States but is endemic in many areas in Asia, particularly southeastern China.

- In endemic regions, NPC is strongly associated with Epstein-Barr virus (EBV).

- Radiation is the mainstay of treatment. The addition of chemotherapy has been demonstrated to improve disease control rates in locally advanced NPC.

- Because NPC is located in a horseshoe-shaped region in the proximity of critical normal structures, IMRT is used to improve conformality of dose distribution to the tumor and to reduce dose to the brainstem, optic nerve and chiasm, temporal lobes, parotid glands, etc.

- An increasing body of data indicates that IMRT improves geographic coverage of NPC resulting in high disease control rate while reducing toxicity, particularly xerostomia.

- Intensity-modulated proton therapy (IMPT) has promise to potentially improve outcomes through reduction of integral dose to nontarget structures.

TREATMENT STRATEGY

The current standard treatment for stage I NPC is radiotherapy, though consideration for concurrent chemoradiation can be given for patients with bulky T1 disease. It is important to note that the American Joint Committee on Cancer (AJCC) staging system has downstaged the T Category through several iterations, making trial comparisons complex. As an example, a bulky T1 tumor may have been considered T3 a decade ago.

The standard treatment for stage II to IV NPC is a combination of radiation and chemotherapy. Outside protocol study setting, the recommended chemotherapeutic regimen in the United States was established through an intergroup phase III trial. This regimen consists of 100 mg/m^2 of cisplatin given during weeks 1, 4, and 7 of radiation and followed 3 to 4 weeks later by three courses of adjuvant therapy comprising 80 mg/m^2 of cisplatin given on day 1 and 1,000 mg/m^2/d of fluorouracil on days 1 to 4 and repeated every 4 weeks. More recent studies, including randomized trials and meta-analyses, confirm the importance of the concurrent component and continue to question the need for adjuvant (or neoadjuvant) therapy.

Neck dissection is indicated in a very small number of patients who have a residual neck mass 6 to 10 weeks after completion of radiotherapy.

DETAILS OF RADIOTHERAPY

Target Volume

Initial Target Volume

The initial portals encompass the primary tumor and contiguous routes of spread and the retropharyngeal and cervical nodes. For T1 lesions, the following structures are to be treated: nasopharynx, floor of sphenoid sinus, clivus, pterygoid fossa, parapharyngeal space, retropharyngeal nodes, and bilateral cervical nodes, including level V (spinal accessory) nodes. The extent of nasal cavity and/or oropharynx coverage depends on the contiguous spread of the primary tumor.

For T2 lesions, adjust the target volume to encompass the disease extension in the parapharyngeal space. For T3 to T4 tumors, adjust the target volume to encompass the disease extension in the clivus, cranial fossa, infratemporal fossa, or hypopharynx. It is important to have generous coverage of the base of skull and known intracranial extension up to the tolerance dose of normal tissues. Intensity-modulated radiation therapy (IMRT) allows better coverage of the primary tumor or retropharyngeal nodes while maintaining normal tissues below unacceptable dose levels. IMPT has promise to further improve outcomes through reduction of integral dose to nontarget structures.

Boost Volume

The boost portals cover gross disease sites with 0.5- to 1-cm margins, depending on the type of adjacent normal tissues. In case of tumor extension through the clivus, the margin on the brainstem can be only a few millimeters to avoid delivery of >60 Gy to this critical structure.

Dose

With the conventional technique, 50 Gy is given in 25 fractions to regions at risk for harboring subclinical disease, followed by a boost dose of 16 to 20 Gy in 8 to 10 fractions to the primary tumor and involved node(s), depending on the size.

With IMRT, 66 to 70 Gy is given to CTV_{HD} and 60 Gy to CTV_{ID} in 33 fractions. The fraction size varies from 1.8 Gy to the CTV_{ID} to 2.12 Gy to the CTV_{HD}.

Setup and Field Arrangement for Conventional Radiotherapy Technique

The patient is immobilized in a supine position. Marking of lateral canthi, external auditory canals, and palpable nodes may facilitate portal design. With conventional technique, the primary tumor and upper neck nodes are irradiated with lateral–opposed photon fields (**Case Study 8.1 and Case Study 8.2**).

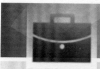

CASE STUDY 8.1

A 46-year-old man presented with a 3-week history of sinusitis, nasal congestion, and a left neck mass. An excisional biopsy of this neck mass showed squamous cell carcinoma. He was referred to our institution for workup and treatment. Physical examination revealed an erythematous mass in the nasopharynx centered on the right posterolateral wall and extending across the midline. The left posterior oropharyngeal wall was swollen consistent with enlarged retropharyngeal nodes. The nasal cavities were unremarkable. Neck examination showed a well-healed scar in the left subdigastric region with underlying residual adenopathy. A 3.5 × 2.5-cm node and a 2-cm node were palpated in the right subdigastric area. A CT scan confirmed the physical findings and showed that the base of skull was uninvolved. A biopsy from the nasopharyngeal lesion showed poorly differentiated squamous cell carcinoma (stage: T1, N2, M0). This patient received primary radiotherapy according to the concomitant boost schedule.

The primary tumor and upper neck nodes were treated with lateral–opposed photon fields (Fig. 8.1). The lateral orbital canthi and external auditory canals were marked along with the upper neck scar and palpable neck nodes.

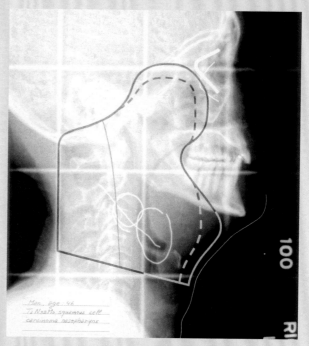

Case Figure 8.1

The mid and lower neck nodes were treated through an anterior appositional photon field with a midline block to shield the larynx and spinal cord. The dose to the primary tumor and involved neck nodes was taken to 72 Gy in 42 fractions over 6 weeks. Areas of subclinical disease received 54 Gy in 30 fractions over 6 weeks. Because the

nodal biopsy site on the palpable left and the nodes on the right side were partly in the electron fields supplementing the posterior cervical areas, these fields were also taken to a total dose of 72 Gy. To deliver an adequate dose to the involved nodal areas, 12-MeV electrons were used and the dose was specified at the 90% isodose line.

CASE STUDY 8.2

A 52-year-old woman presented with pressure-like sensation in her left ear. Further workup revealed a polypoid mass centered and confined to the roof of the nasopharynx. A biopsy was positive for World Health Organization (WHO) type 3 NPC. There was no adenopathy. Staging workup included MRI, which confirmed that the lesion was confined to the nasopharynx (stage: T1, N0, M0).

This patient received primary radiotherapy according to the concomitant boost schedule. The primary tumor and upper neck nodes were treated with lateral–opposed photon fields using 6 MV photons.

Figure 8.2A shows a digitally reconstructed sagittal view through the nasopharyngeal mass shown overlaid by a

representation of the lateral primary, off–spinal cord, and boost portals. The initial fields were reduced off the spinal cord at 41.4 Gy. The off–spinal cord fields continued to 54 Gy. The posterior cervical strips were treated with 9-MeV electrons to 54 Gy. The boost was delivered as second daily fractions with 18-MV photons to 18 Gy in 12 fractions, bringing the total dose to the tumor to 72 Gy. Isodose distributions of the lateral photon fields through the nasopharynx are shown in both axial (Fig. 8.2B) and sagittal (Fig. 8.2C) views. The mid and lower neck nodes were treated through an anterior appositional photon field with a midline block to shield the larynx and spinal cord. Areas of subclinical disease received 54 Gy in 30 fractions over 6 weeks.

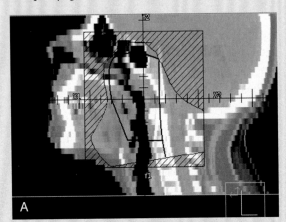

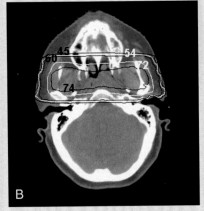

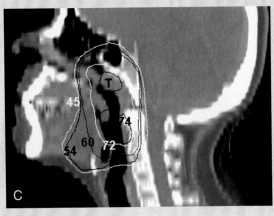

Case Figure 8.2 A–C

- *Anterior border:* Posterior one third to one half of the nasal cavities, depending on the size of the lesion (or 2 cm beyond tumor extension). Usually, most of the oral cavity can be shielded by shaping the field with a notch below the soft palate.
- *Superior border:* At the floor of the pituitary fossa and just above the clivus for T1 to T2 lesions. An initial margin of 2 cm is taken beyond tumor extension into the clivus or intracranially for T3 to T4 disease.
- *Posterior border:* Just behind the spinous processes or more posteriorly when large spinal accessory nodes are present.
- *Inferior border:* The inferior border is placed just above the arytenoids. When more advanced neck disease is present, it is preferred to junction therapy through the nodes above the larynx.
- After an off-spinal cord reduction continue with the *posterior border* placed over the posterior one third of the vertebral bodies to ensure adequate coverage of the posterior pharyngeal wall and retropharyngeal nodes. It may be necessary to use oblique lateral fields in the presence of retrostyloid parapharyngeal extension of primary disease or large retropharyngeal node(s). Patients with bilateral retrostyloid parapharyngeal extension present a particularly difficult technical problem in covering the extent of the disease without overdosing the medulla and upper cervical spinal cord. This obstacle of conventional technique can be overcome with the use of conformal techniques.

An anterior appositional portal is used for the mid neck and lower neck. If there is nodal disease in the posterior mid-cervical chain, a posterior field is added to supplement the dose to this area (see "General Principles").

For the *boost volume*, lateral fields are reduced to include the primary tumor and involved upper neck nodes:

- *Superior border:* adjusted to exclude the optic nerves, chiasm, and tracts after a dose of 54 Gy.
- *Anterior border:* 1 to 1.5 cm beyond gross disease.
- *Posterior border:* over the posterior one third of the vertebral bodies. Proper margins for the boost volumes are taken to encompass all clinically or radiologically apparent disease extension. These margins may be extremely tight posteriorly for tumors invading through the skull base or brain to avoid brain stem injury.
- *Inferior border:* depends on the nodal status. If N0, the inferior border is at the level of the midtonsillar fossa (more inferior if the oropharynx is involved). If upper neck nodes are involved, the border is above the arytenoids.
- As with the initial off-cord reduction, it may be necessary to use oblique lateral fields to cover retropharyngeal or parapharyngeal disease.
- Electron fields or glancing photon fields are used to boost the nodes in the mid and lower neck. In cases where both the posterior strip and the mid neck need to be boosted, a single L-shaped electron field is typically used.

Intensity-Modulated Radiation Therapy

IMRT has become an established and preferred technique for NPC. Careful target volume delineation is crucial with this technique, which requires acquisition of thin-cut planning computed tomography (CT) scans for outlining the gross target volume (GTV), clinical target volumes (CTVs), and planning target volumes (PTVs), for dosimetric planning (Case Study 8.3 through Case Study 8.10). Because magnetic resonance imaging (MRI) is generally better for delineating the disease extent, particularly at the skull base region, it is crucial to incorporate diagnostic MRI findings into the planning process, preferably by image coregistration within treatments planning systems.

Gross Target Volume

GTV represents all areas determined from clinical examination and imaging studies to contain macroscopic disease. Any cervical lymph node >1 cm or retropharyngeal lymph node >0.5 cm is considered to contain a tumor.

Clinical Target Volume

Two CTVs are generally delineated.

- CTV_{HD} or CTV_1 delineates volumes to receive the highest dose, usually 70 Gy, which includes the primary tumor and involved nodes with 0.5- to 1.0-cm margins. Protection of neural structures may necessitate tighter margins on the GTV. The entire nasopharynx is encompassed unless the tumor is well lateralized.
- CTV_{ID} or CTV_2 delineates volumes to receive an intermediate dose, usually around 60 Gy. The general guidelines for delineating CTV_{ID} to provide additional margin on the primary tumor are as follows:

  - *Anterior:* posterior third of the nasal cavity and maxillary sinuses or 1 cm beyond CTV_{HD} if these structures are encompassed by CTV_{HD}
  - *Posterior:* retropharyngeal regions and clivus
  - *Lateral:* parapharyngeal regions extending to the middle of the pterygoid muscles or more laterally as dictated by the extent of the tumor
  - *Superior:* inferior half of the sphenoid sinus, and adjacent skull base, or 1 cm superior to CTV_{HD} for T3 to T4 tumors
  - *Inferior:* 1-cm margin beyond the nasopharynx or inferior to CTV_{HD}

- Additional targets can be delineated. In situations where 70 Gy may create concerns of neural toxicity, a target with a 2 to 4 Gy reduction may be painted in within CTV_{HD}. Additionally, nodes ≤ can be place in a 66 Gy target. Similarly, a CTV_{ED} can be applied of 54 to 57 Gy, if the elective volume approximates neural or optic structures or the uninvolved nodal echelons covered are deemed low risk (i.e., levels 3 to 4 in an N0 patient)

Elective Nodal Irradiation

In the absence of clinical nodal involvement, levels II to V receive elective irradiation. These levels are generally included in CTV$_{ID}$ as radiation is given in 33 to 35 fractions over 6.5 to 7 weeks. In the presence of involved nodes, CTV$_{ID}$ includes levels IB to V outside CTV$_{HD}$. In situations where IMRT is used only for the primary tumor and upper neck nodes, the lower neck lymphatics are irradiated with a matched anterior portal. However, a opposed posterior beam is often required to achieve adequate dosing to positive posterior cervical, level V nodes.

CASE STUDY 8.3

A 58-year-old man presented with a right upper neck mass. Examination revealed a 3-cm upper jugular node and a lesion in the right fossa of Rosenmüller. An axial MRI image demonstrated a small tumor on the right torus tubarius ablating the fossa of Rosenmüller (Fig. 8.3A). Biopsy of the primary tumor showed an undifferentiated carcinoma, WHO type 3. He was staged T1, N1, M0 and treated with IMRT and three cycles of high-dose cisplatin.

Gross tumor in the nasopharynx and neck with margin was identified as CTV$_{HD}$ (70 Gy). Additional margin was added to cover the inferior sphenoid sinus, clivus, posterior ethmoid and maxillary sinuses, posterior nasal cavity, and medial masticator space and defined as CTV$_{ID}$ (60 Gy). In addition, the upper neck and retropharyngeal nodes outside the CTV$_{HD}$ were included in CTV$_{ID}$. Isocenter was placed above the thyroid notch, and the low neck was treated with a matching anterior beam. A larynx block was used for the first 40 Gy, and then a full midline block was added for the remaining 10 Gy. The right lower neck received an additional 10 Gy, to a total of 60 Gy, with glancing photon fields. Figure 8.3B to F show isodose distributions of the treatment plan. Axial isodose distributions are demonstrated through the nasopharynx (Fig. 8.3B), retropharyngeal region at C1 (Fig. 8.3C), and upper neck (Fig. 8.3D). CTV$_{HD}$ (70 Gy) is shown in red colorwash and CTV$_{ID}$ (60 Gy) in *blue* colorwash. Sagittal (Fig. 8.3E) and coronal (Fig. 8.3F) distributions are shown through midline and gross disease, respectively. He also received adjuvant chemotherapy with cisplatin and fluorouracil.

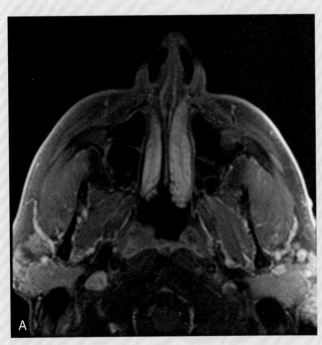

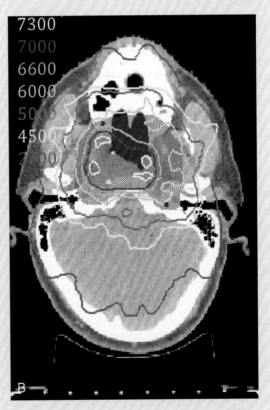

Case Figure 8.3 A,B

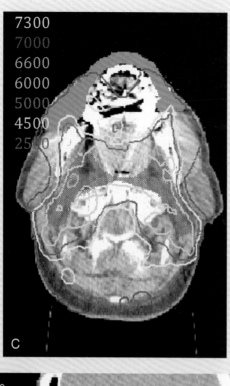

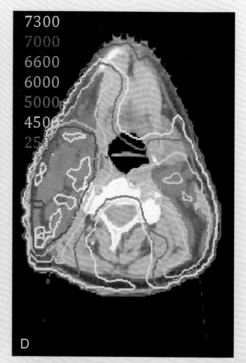

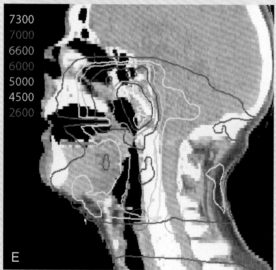

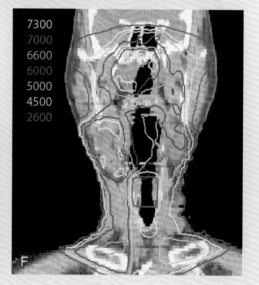

Case Figure 8.3 C–F

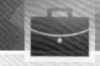

CASE STUDY 8.4

A 46-year-old Middle-Eastern woman presented with right ear fullness and a right upper neck lump. On physical examination, a right middle ear effusion and a mostly right-sided nasopharyngeal mass were evident. There were no cranial neuropathies on exam. MRI demonstrated a nasopharyngeal mass with extension into the apex of the right fossa of Rosenmüller (Fig. 8.4A, *white arrow*) and a positive right node of Rouvière (Fig. 8.4B, *white arrow*) lying just medial to the internal carotid artery. There was no parapharyngeal extension, clival involvement, or intracranial extension seen on imaging. Biopsy of the nasopharyngeal mass showed nasopharyngeal undifferentiated carcinoma, positive for Epstein-Barr virus by *in situ* hybridization. PET/CT showed the primary mass (Fig. 8.4C) and right level II adenopathy (Fig. 8.4D). Clinical stage: T1, N1, M0.

She was treated with induction TPF chemotherapy × 3 cycles, with a complete response on restaging MRI obtained after cycle 2. She then received definitive radiation therapy alone using IMRT. Four dose levels were treated in a single integrated IMRT plan. The initial prechemotherapy extent of gross disease with margin (CTV_HD) was treated to 66 to 70 Gy in 33 daily fractions. Thus, 2 CTVsHD were created; the 70 Gy volume covered the original primary site disease and bulkier

nodes, while the 66 Gy volume covered subcentimeter nodal disease noted on the pre-chemotherapy imaging. The surrounding soft tissue and boney regions at the skull base were treated to 63 Gy (CTV_ID). The at-risk upper neck lymphatics (CTV_ED) were treated to 57 Gy. Split-field IMRT technique was used, with 50 Gy in 25 fractions delivered to the bilateral lower neck and supraclavicular regions from a 6-MV anterior field. A tapered 3 × 4 cm larynx block was used for the initial

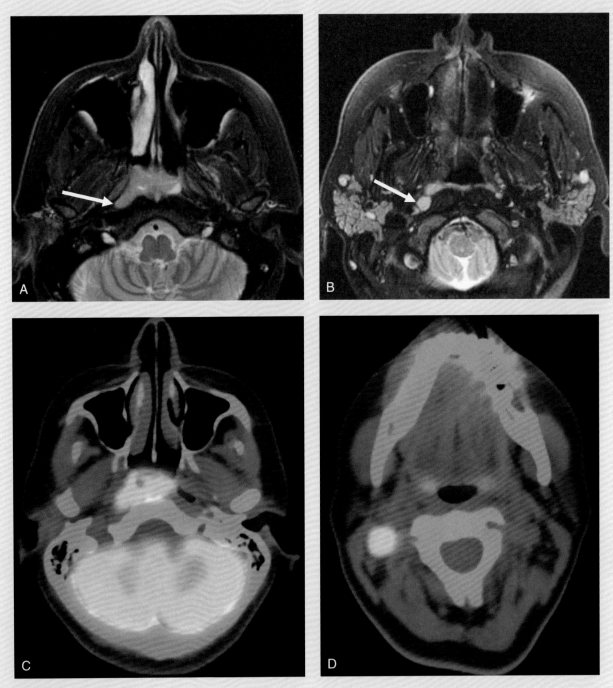

Case Figure 8.4 A–D

40 Gy (Fig. 8.4E) and was extended to a full midline block for final 10 Gy.

The CTVs and corresponding IMRT dose distributions are shown in the axial plane at the level of the nasopharynx (Fig. 8.4F,G) and upper neck (Fig. 8.4H,I). Right nodal levels Ib and V were included in CTV_ED.

The postchemotherapy nodal remnant (white arrow) is shown in Figure 8.4H. Figure 8.4J and K shows the posttherapy PET/CT obtained 12 weeks after treatment completion. She remains without evidence disease or serious treatment-related toxicity 4 years since treatment completion.

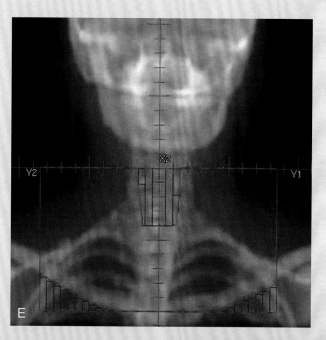

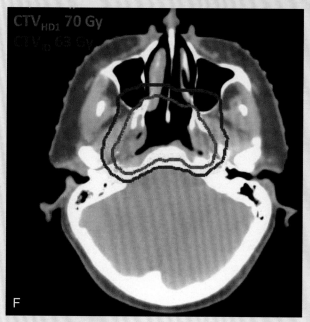

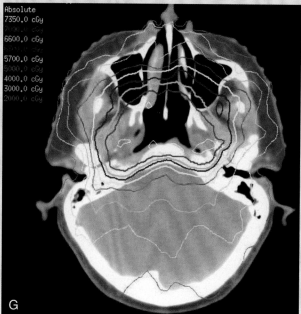

Case Figure 8.4 E–G

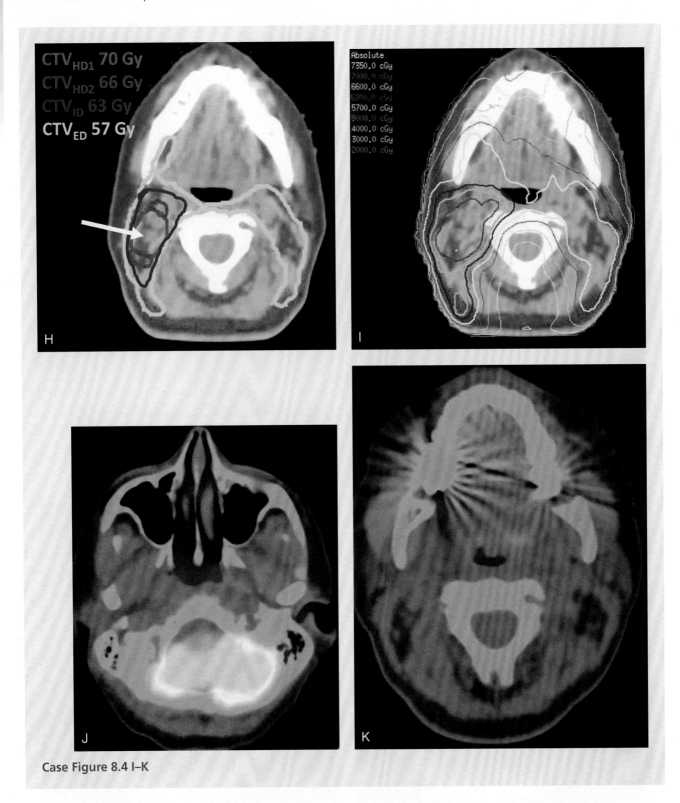

CTV~HD1~ 70 Gy
CTV~HD2~ 66 Gy
CTV~ID~ 63 Gy
CTV~ED~ 57 Gy

Case Figure 8.4 I–K

CASE STUDY 8.5

A 53-year-old woman presented with a left upper neck mass, otalgia, and sore throat. Fine-needle aspiration was nondiagnostic, so an incisional nodal biopsy was performed, which revealed poorly differentiated squamous cell carcinoma. Examination revealed fullness in the left neck and a lesion in the left side of the nasopharynx, obliterating the fossa of Rosenmüller and eustachian tube.

A PET-CT scan demonstrated the tumor in the left nasopharynx (Fig. 8.5A) and, on a more inferior axial view (Fig. 8.5B), left-sided adenopathy in the upper neck, including a left retropharyngeal node anterior to the vertebral body. Imaging further demonstrated the primary tumor extending into the retropharyngeal space, bilateral retropharyngeal adenopathy, and a small right level II node. She was staged T2, N2, M0 and treated with IMRT and three cycles of high-dose cisplatin.

CTV$_{HD}$ (70 Gy, *red*) and CTV$_{ID}$ (60 Gy, *blue*) were delineated (Fig. 8.5C–G); the isocenter was placed above the thyroid notch, and the low neck was treated with a matching anterior portal. A larynx block was used for the first 40 Gy, and then a full midline block was added for 10 Gy. The left lower neck nodes received a 10-Gy boost dose with glancing photon fields. Superiorly (Fig. 8.5C), CTV$_{ID}$ encompassed the posterior maxillary sinuses, posterior nasal cavity, and the sphenoid sinus.

At the level of the nasopharynx (Fig. 8.5D), gross disease with margin was designated CTV$_{HD}$. In addition to the sinus and nasal cavity, the medial masticator space and clivus were encompassed in CTV$_{ID}$. At the level of C1 (Fig. 8.5E), the involved retropharyngeal nodes were covered by CTV$_{HD}$, and CTV$_{ID}$ provided more margin. At the level of C2 and the upper neck (Fig. 8.5F), the left-sided adenopathy with an approximate 1-cm margin was covered by CTV$_{HD}$. CTV$_{ID}$ provided more margin in the left neck, as well as covering the inferior retropharyngeal nodal bed and superior right level II nodes. At the level of the hyoid (Fig. 8.5G), just above the isocenter, CTV$_{HD}$ included involved nodes with margin including a small right-sided node, and CTV$_{ID}$ covered the remaining nodal basins. Note that whether level IB nodes should be treated is controversial. In most situations, we do cover level IB if level II nodes are involved.

Figure 8.5H to J shows axial, sagittal, and coronal isodose distributions through the nasopharynx, respectively. As per regimen of the intergroup protocol, she received adjuvant chemotherapy. She developed mild necrosis in the right ear canal, responded well to conservative treatment, and had bilateral high-frequency sensorineural hearing loss. She remained without disease and with good overall function 3 years later.

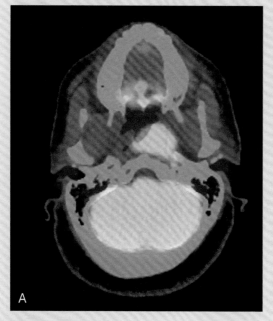
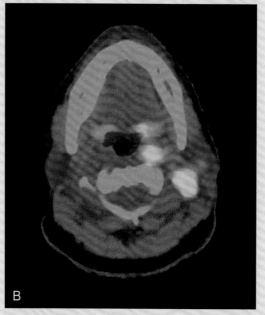

Case Figure 8.5 A,B

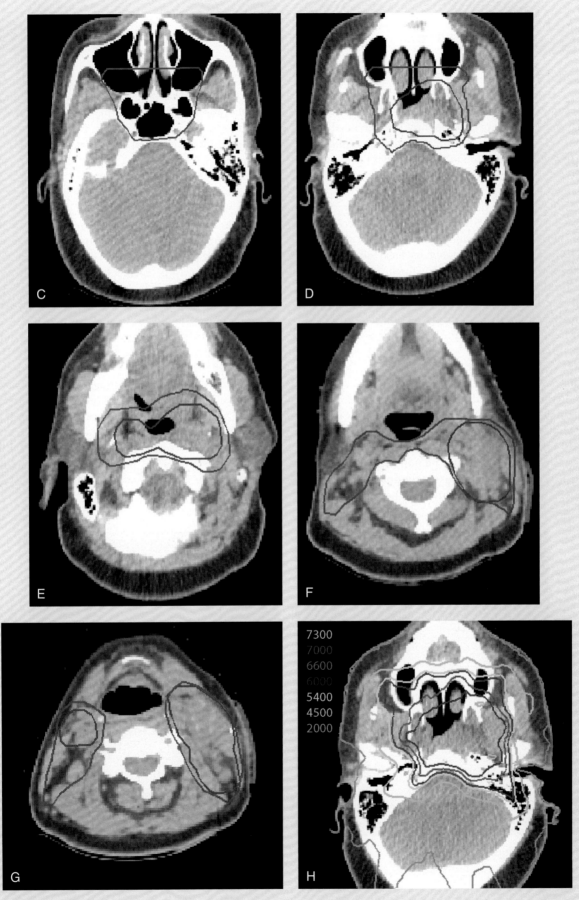

Case Figure 8.5 C–H

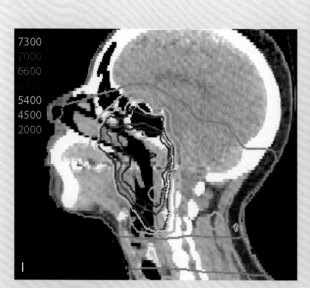
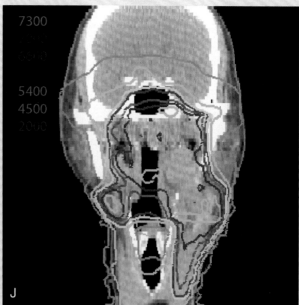

Case Figure 8.5 I,J

CASE STUDY 8.6

A 50-year-old woman presented with a left upper neck mass and decreased hearing. Examination revealed multiple nodes in the left neck including level V region and a tumor in the nasopharynx. Biopsy of the primary tumor showed non-keratinizing poorly differentiated squamous cell carcinoma.

A lateral view of the PET scan (Fig. 8.6A) shows the primary tumor and extensive adenopathy including level V nodes, and an axial image of PET-CT scan (Fig. 8.6B) demonstrates the extent of the adenopathy in the posterior neck. Not shown are bilateral retropharyngeal and contralateral neck nodes. An MRI was also performed and demonstrated erosion of the clivus. Clinical stage T3,N2,M0. Given the extent of the disease with skull base involvement, she was dispositioned for induction cisplatin and

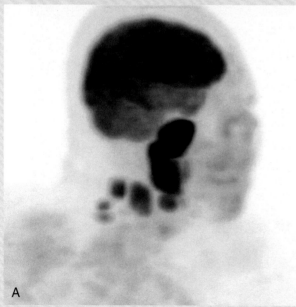
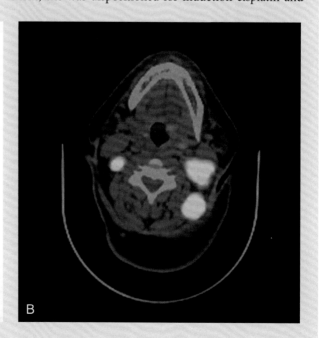

Case Figure 8.6 A,B

docetaxel, which caused renal function impairment after one cycle. Therefore, cisplatin was replaced by carboplatin for two additional cycles. Chemotherapy yielded a complete response of the primary tumor and partial response of the neck nodes. She was then treated with IMRT and concurrent carboplatin.

Prechemotherapy gross disease in the nasopharynx and neck with margin were outlined as CTV_{HD} (70 Gy), and CTV_{ID} (60 Gy) added additional margins. Isocenter was placed above the thyroid notch, and the low neck was treated with parallel opposed anterior and posterior portals. A larynx block was used for the first 40 Gy, and then

a full midline block was added for 10 Gy. The fields were reduced off level IV and 10 Gy was given to level III nodes bilaterally, and then, an additional 10 Gy was administered to the right mid neck. Isodose distributions on axial images of the treatment plan are shown (Fig. 8.6C–G). Views of the roof of the nasopharynx (Fig. 8.6C), mid-nasopharynx (Fig. 8.6D), retropharyngeal region anterior to C1 (Fig. 8.6E), in addition to the upper (Fig. 8.6F) and mid neck (Fig. 8.6G) are shown. The nodal disease that did not completely respond to induction chemotherapy can be seen in Figure 8.6F and G (*black arrow*). The patient was without disease 2 years from therapy.

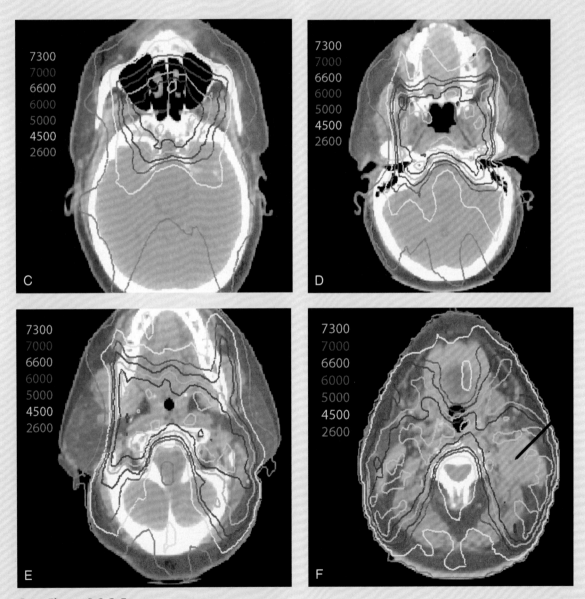

Case Figure 8.6 C–F

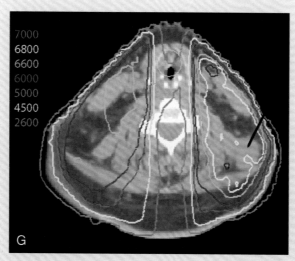

Case Figure 8.6 G

CASE STUDY 8.7

A 40-year-old man was diagnosed with poorly differenti-ated carcinoma of the nasopharynx, stage T3, N2, M0. He received concurrent radiation and chemotherapy.

The sagittal and axial images (Fig. 8.7A,B) demon-strate the full-thickness destruction of the clivus (note the absence of bone). The isodose distribution demonstrates

the ability of IMRT to provide conformal coverage in this difficult case. The tumor extent necessitated taking the surface of the brainstem to 60 Gy to yield reasonable tumor coverage. The patient was without disease at the follow-up visit 3 years out from therapy without neuro-logic deficit.

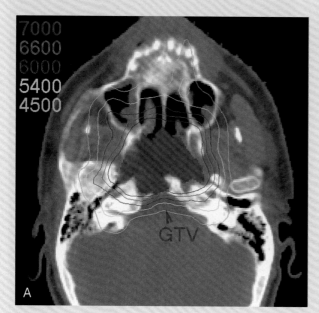
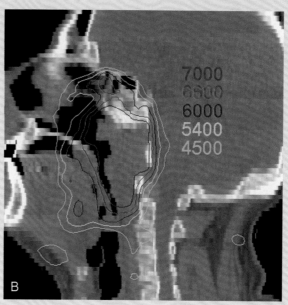

Case Figure 8.7 A,B

CASE STUDY 8.8

A 52-year-old man who was a former smoker presented with left ear fullness and headache. Initial workup revealed a left nasopharyngeal mass. Biopsy of the mass showed nonkeratinizing squamous carcinoma, positive for Epstein-Barr virus by *in situ* hybridization. On physical examination, there were no cranial neuropathies evident. A 2.5-cm left upper neck node was palpable below the angle of the jaw. The initial T1-weighted MRI with gadolinium image in Figure 8.8A shows the posterior–lateral extension of tumor and involvement of the left aspect of the clivus (*white arrows*). PET/CT showed the primary mass (Fig. 8.8B) and left level II adenopathy (Fig. 8.8C). Clinical stage: T3, N1, M0.

He was treated with induction chemotherapy × 3 cycles (cisplatin and paclitaxel), with a partial response observed on restaging MRI obtained after the second cycle. He then received definitive concurrent chemoradiation therapy using IMRT. He received weekly chemotherapy during radiation, initially with cisplatin, but was later switched to carboplatin due to tinnitus.

Three dose levels were treated in a single integrated IMRT plan. The initial prechemotherapy extent of gross disease with margin (CTV$_{HD}$) was treated to 70 Gy, delivered in 33 daily fractions. The surrounding soft tissue and bone regions at the skull base were treated to 59.4 Gy (CTV$_{ID}$). The at-risk but uninvolved cervical lymphatics (CTV$_{ED}$) were treated to 57 Gy. The bilateral retropharyngeal, bilateral neck levels II–IV, and left neck levels Ib and V were targeted.

The CTVs and corresponding IMRT dose distributions are shown in paired axial images at the level of the upper nasopharynx (Fig. 8.8D,E), mid clivus (Fig. 8.8F,G), and neck just below the hyoid level (Fig. 8.8H,I). Figure 8.8J shows the before- and Figure 8.8K the after-therapy coronal MRI with complete resolution of tumor. He remains without evidence disease or serious treatment-related toxicity now 6 years since completing treatment. He does have some left eustachian tube dysfunction and associated conductive hearing loss.

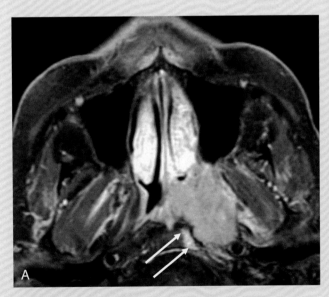

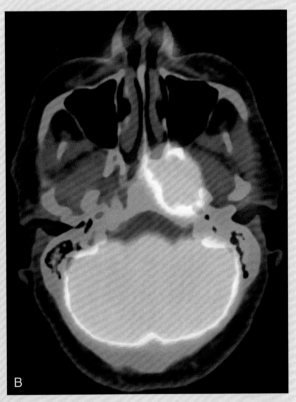

Case Figure 8.8 A,B
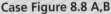

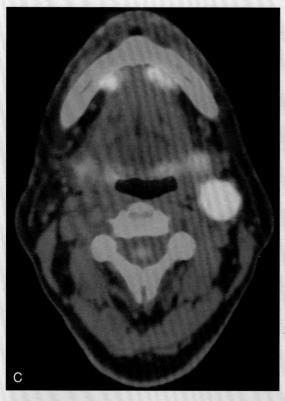

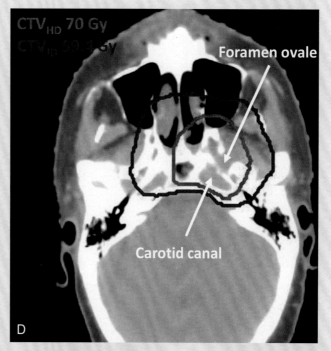

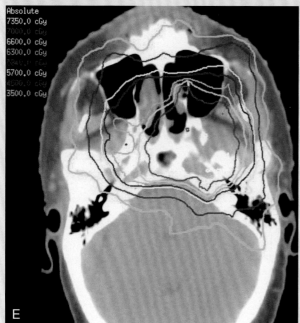

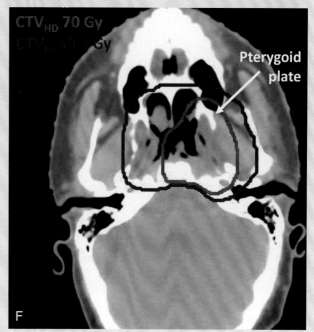

Case Figure 8.8 C–F

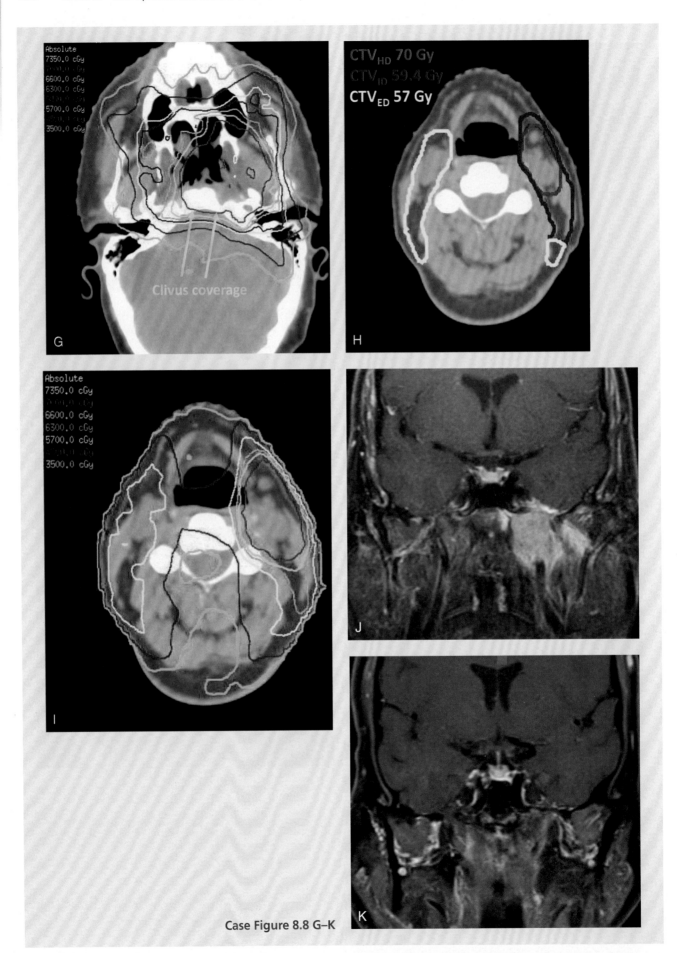

Case Figure 8.8 G–K

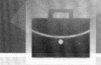

CASE STUDY 8.9

A 30-year-old Asian man presented with a left neck mass and headaches. Examination revealed a 4-cm left neck node and a nasopharyngeal mass that involved the left torus tubarius, fossa of Rosenmüller, posterior wall, and roof. A biopsy was positive for undifferentiated NPC, WHO type 3. MRI revealed a large, left-sided nasopharyngeal tumor with destruction of the ipsilateral clivus, floor of the sella, and floor of the medial portion of middle fossa, with tumor extending into the adjacent sphenoid sinus. There was minimal asymmetrical plaquelike thickening along the left parasellar dura suggesting intracranial tumor invasion. The left petrous apex was irregularly eroded. The tumor infiltrated the left prevertebral muscle and was associated with large left lateral retropharyngeal lymphadenopathy. The clinically apparent 4-cm lymph node in the upper jugular region was seen along with multiple additional nodes suspicious for metastatic lymphadenopathy (stage: T4, N1, M0). The treatment consisted of a combination of concurrent cisplatin and radiation. IMRT with nine separate beam angles was delivered with "step-and-shoot" collimation. A separate isocentrically matched anterior field treated the low neck and supraclavicular fossa to 50 Gy.

Figure 8.9 shows isodoses on a coronal (Fig. 8.9A) and axial (Fig. 8.9B) image through the primary tumor and neck. The primary nasopharynx tumor and involved neck nodes received 70 Gy, and subclinical disease in the contralateral neck received 57 Gy. The brainstem and optic chiasm doses were limited to 54 Gy and the spinal cord to 45 Gy. He is without disease more than 10 years out from treatment with only grade-1 xerostomia.

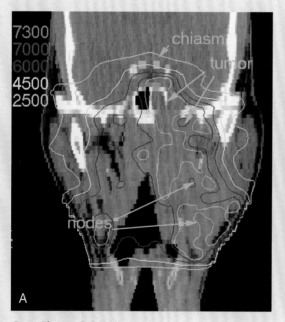
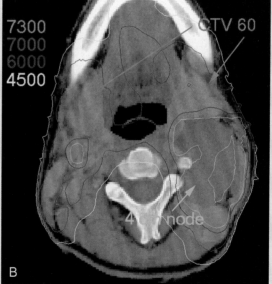

Case Figure 8.9 A,B

CASE STUDY 8.10

A 47-year-old man presented with epistaxis and hearing loss for nearly a year. Examination revealed right neck adenopathy and a tumor filling the nasopharynx. He also had atrophy of the right tongue and diminished elevation of the right palate. A biopsy of the primary tumor was positive for moderately differentiated squamous cell carcinoma. An axial MRI image (Fig. 8.10A) demonstrates tumor extension adjacent to Meckel's cave, and a coronal image (Fig. 8.10B) demonstrates the bulky disease with extension through the middle cranial fossa. He was staged T4, N1, M0 and treated with IMRT and three cycles of high-dose cisplatin.

CTV$_{HD}$ (70 Gy) and CTV$_{ID}$ (60 Gy) were delineated, isocenter was placed above the thyroid notch, and the low neck

was treated with an anterior beam. A larynx block was used for the first 40 Gy; then a full midline block was added for 10 Gy. Figure 8.10C to E shows axial (Fig. 8.10C), sagittal (Fig. 8.10D), and coronal (Fig. 8.10E) isodose distributions through the nasopharynx. The black arrows show the disease along the middle cranial fossa floor. An axial isodose (Fig. 8.10F) at the level of intracranial extension is also shown. To respect the temporal lobe tolerance, a dose of 66 Gy was accepted for coverage of the high dose PTV covering CTVHD (70 Gy). He was restaged and found to have a partial response. He received adjuvant chemotherapy, which was poorly tolerated, and died due to complications from therapy.

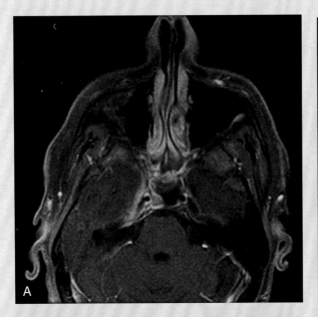

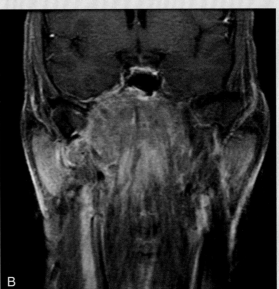

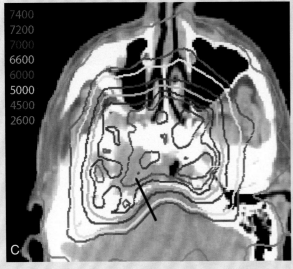

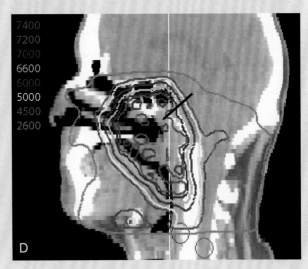

Case Figure 8.10 A–D

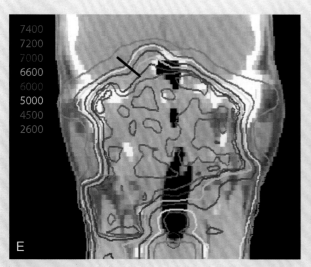 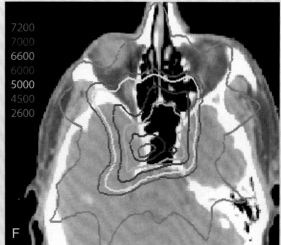

Case Figure 8.10 E,F

Intensity-Modulated Proton Therapy

Advances in spot-scanning IMPT techniques have provided the ability to treat geometrically complex NPC target volumes. IMPT reduces integral dose to nontarget structures compared to IMRT, particularly those anterior and posterior to the target volumes. However, there is a somewhat greater dose heterogeneity within the targets.

The same principles of therapy described in the IMRT section apply to IMPT. Representative IMPT dose distributions for NPC are shown in **Case Study 8.11 and Case Study 8.12**.

Background Data

See Tables 8.1 to 8.8.

CASE STUDY 8.11

A 20-year-old female was initially evaluated for nasal obstruction, epistaxis, and right ear fullness. A nasopharyngeal mass filling the nasopharynx and bilateral neck adenopathy was evident on physical examination. Biopsy of the nasopharynx mass showed nasopharyngeal carcinoma, undifferentiated, which was positive for Epstein-Barr virus by *in situ* hybridization.

MRI of the skull base and neck showed a 4.3-cm nasopharyngeal mass with parapharyngeal extension but no invasion of clivus or intracranial extension, with bilateral retropharyngeal and bilateral level IIa/b adenopathy. The largest lymph node was 3.2 cm. PET/CT was confirmatory and showed no distant disease. Final staging was T2, N2, M0. She was treated with induction chemotherapy (TPF × 3 cycles) with a near-complete clinical response after two cycles as determined by clinical exam and MRI.

She was then treated with definitive concurrent chemoradiation (initially weekly cisplatin for two cycles and subsequently weekly carboplatin). Active scanning IMPT-MFO technique (see Chapter 2) was used. Beam arrangement consisted of two anterior obliques and a posterior field. The patient was immobilized with a custom posterior head, neck, and shoulder mold and a full length head and neck mask. A mouth-opening tongue-depressing oral stent with an integrated bite block was used for CT simulation and treatment.

The pre- and postchemotherapy MRIs were fused with the CT simulation data set in order to contour targets and avoidance structures at the skull base. Four dose levels were treated in a single integrated plan. The initial prechemotherapy extent of gross disease with margin was treated to 70 Gy (radiobiologic equivalent [RBE] in 33 daily fractions). The clivus was targeted to 57 to 70 Gy (RBE), depending on proximity to initial tumor, but dose distributions were optimized to respect critical structure tolerance. CTVs and corresponding dose distributions are shown in the paired axial (Fig. 8.11A,B), sagittal (Fig. 8.11C,D), and coronal (Fig. 8.11E,F) planes. Surrounding soft tissue and bony regions at risk and the bilateral neck (levels Ib–V) were treated to 57 to 59.4 Gy (RBE). CTVs and dose distributions in the neck are shown in Figure 8.11G,H and H (at the level of hyoid bone).

She remains free of disease or substantial toxicity now 4 years after treatment completion. Pre- and post-treatment axial MRI (T1 with gadolinium) images are shown in Figure 8.11I and J, respectively. The white arrow in Figure 8.11I indicates the enhancing tumor in right fossa of Rosenmüller and the red arrow the nasal cavity extension. The corresponding posttherapy image shows resolution of disease and restoration of normal anatomy.

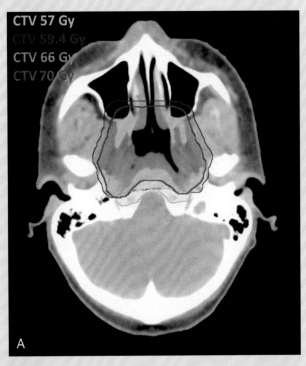

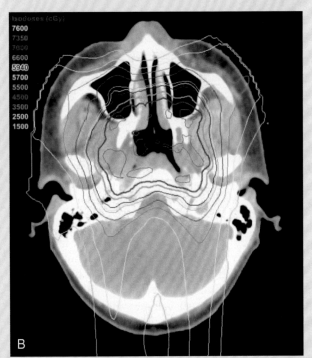

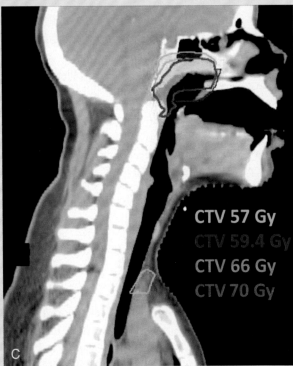

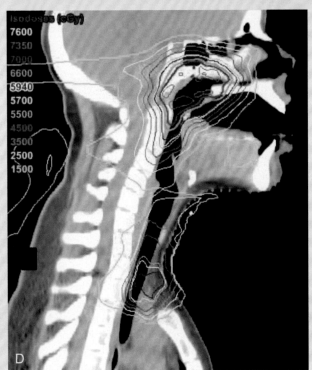

Case Figure 8.11 A–D

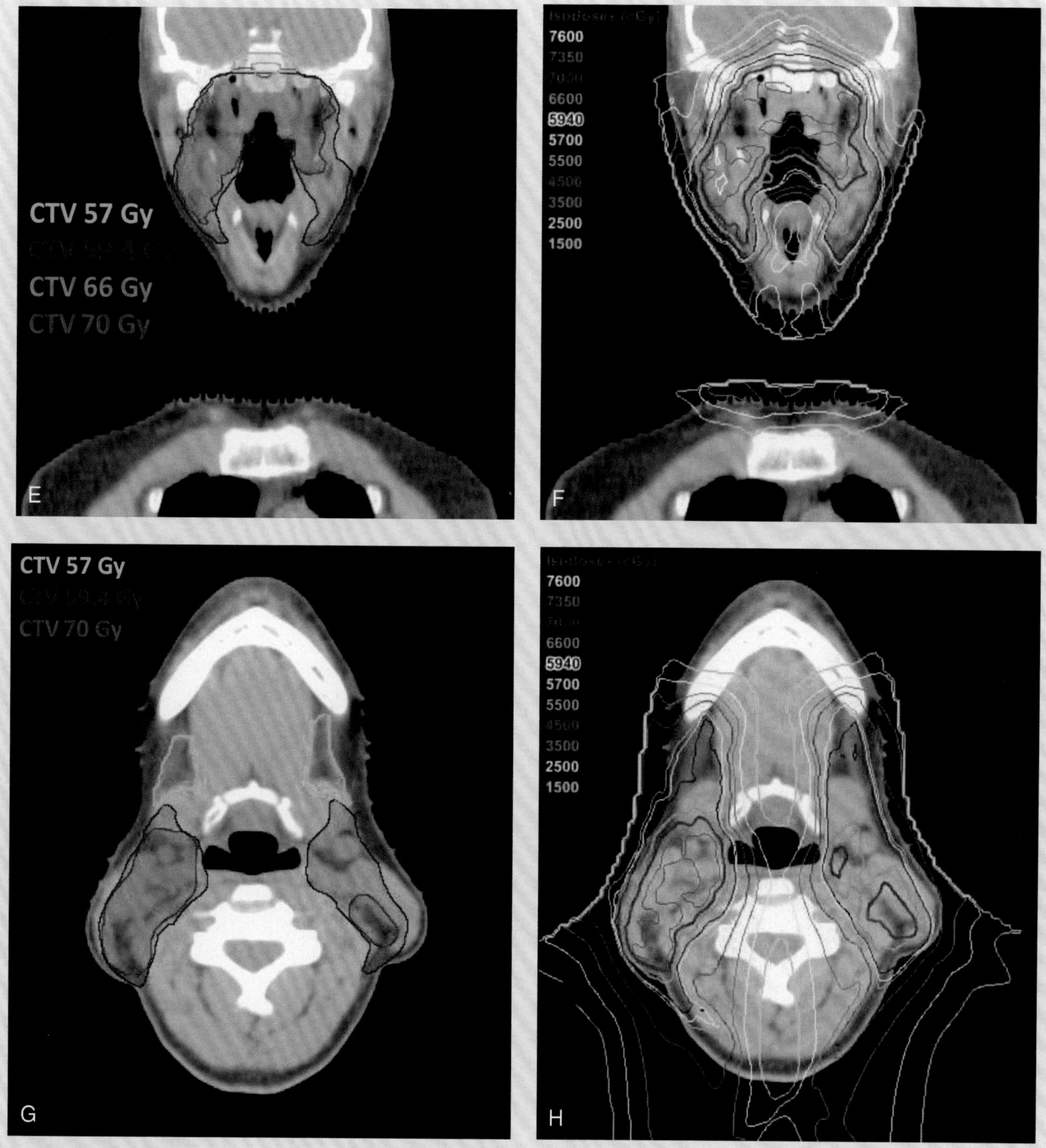

Case Figure 8.11 E–H

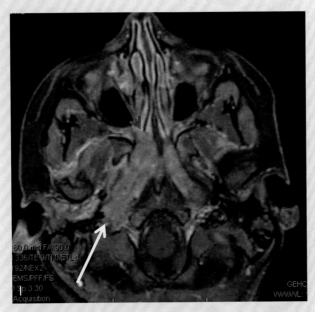
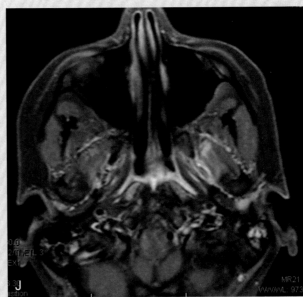

Case Figure 8.11 I,J

CASE STUDY 8.12

A 35-year-old Caucasian man presented to the emergency center with headache, left ear fullness, left face numbness, and slurred speech. Initial examination showed left midface hypesthesia, paralysis of the left side of the tongue, and tongue deviation. MRI face and neck demonstrated a destructive nasopharyngeal mass with intracranial extension along multiple routes. Figure 8.12A shows the tumor involving the left pterygopalantine fossa (white arrow) with spread through foramen rotundum (red arrow), cavernous sinus involvement on the right (green arrow). Figure 8.12B shows spread along the carotid canals (white arrows) and tumor in the roof of the nasopharynx with infiltration of the clivus. Figure 8.12C demonstrates posterior–lateral extension of tumor on the left (white arrows) and involvement of the left hypoglossal canal (red arrow). PET/CT additionally showed bilateral level II adenopathy. Biopsy of the mass showed nasopharyngeal undifferentiated carcinoma, positive for Epstein-Barr virus by *in situ* hybridization. Clinical stage: T4, N2, M0.

He was treated with induction TPF chemotherapy × 3 cycles, with rapid improvement in his symptoms and near-complete response on restaging MRI obtained after cycle 2. He then received definitive concurrent chemoradiation (weekly carboplatin), and active scanning IMPT-MFO technique (see Chapter 2) was used.

Three dose levels were treated in a single integrated IMPT plan. The initial prechemotherapy extent of gross disease with margin (CTV$_{HD}$) was treated to 70 Gy (radiobiologic equivalent[RBE] in 33 daily fractions). The prechemotherapy intracranial extent of disease was largely targeted to 66 Gy(RBE) (CTV$_{ID}$) but dose distributions were optimized to respect optic, brain, and brainstem tolerance. Bilateral levels Ib through V and bilateral retropharygeal regions were included in the treatment volume. Elective regions were treated to 57 Gy(RBE).

The CTVs and corresponding proton therapy dose distributions are shown in the axial plane at the level of the sphenoid sinus and optic chiasm (Fig 8.12D,E), cavernous sinus and pterygopalantine fossa (Fig 8.12F,G), roof of the nasopharynx, carotid canal and foramen ovale (Fig 8.12H,I), C1 vertebral body (Fig 8.12J,K), upper neck (Fig 8.12L,M), midneck and larynx (Fig 8.12N,O), and lower neck (Fig 8.12P,Q). Figure 8.12R shows the pretherapy MRI in the coronal plane showing disease at foramen rotundum (white arrow) and tumor in the roof of the nasopharynx (red arrows). Dose distributions in the coronal plane are shown in Figure 8.12S. He remains without evidence disease or serious treatment-related toxicity 3 years since treatment completion.

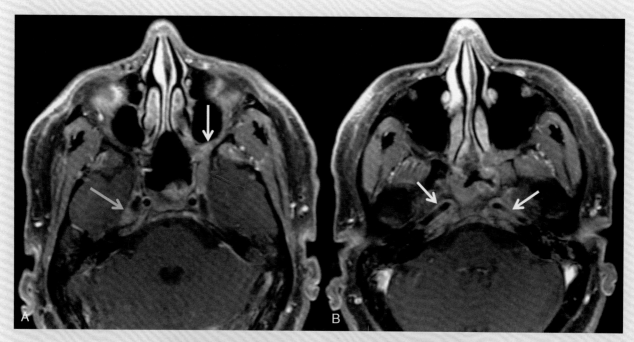

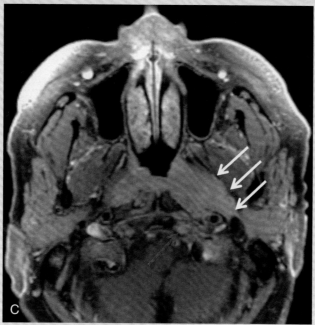

Case Figure 8.12 A–C

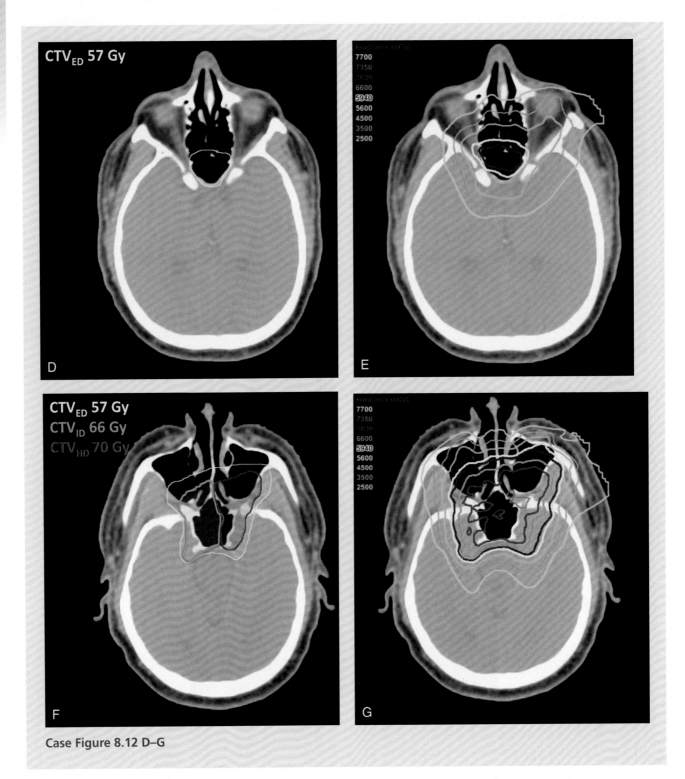

Case Figure 8.12 D–G

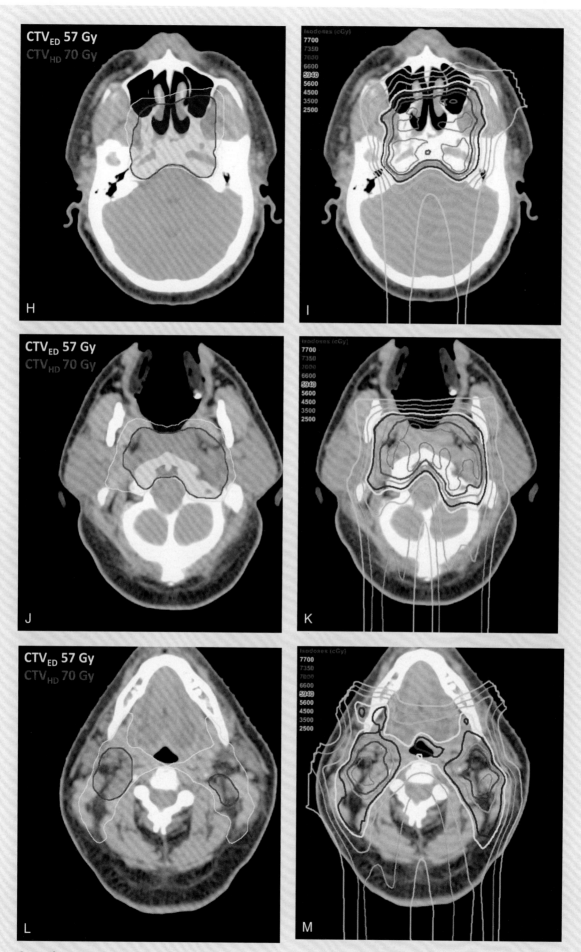

Case Figure 8.12 H–M

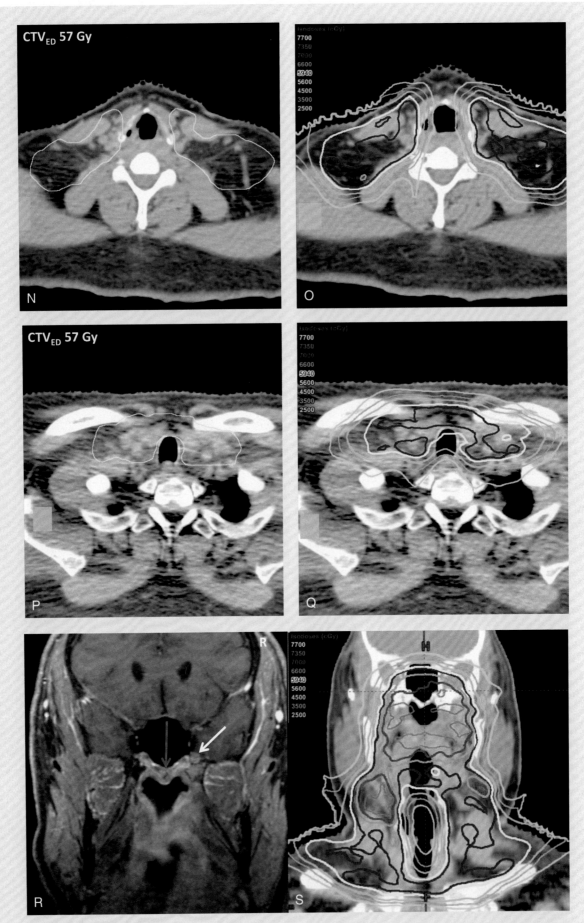

Case Figure 8.12 N–S

TABLE 8.1 Failures at the Primary Site in Tumors of the Nasopharynx

Stage (1992 AJCC System)	No. of Patients	10-yr Actuarial Local Control (%)
T1	55	87
T2	138	75
T3	67	63
T4	118	45
Total	378	66

AJCC, American Joint Committee on Cancer.
Data from M.D. Anderson Cancer Center.
Adapted from Sanguineti G, Geara FB, Garden A, et al.
Carcinoma of the nasopharynx treated by radiotherapy alone: determinants of local and regional control. *Int J Radiat Oncol Biol Phys* 1997;37:985–996, with permission.

TABLE 8.2 Nodal Recurrence by Lymph Node Stage and Histology

Stage (1992 AJCC System)	No. of Patients	10-yr Actuarial Regional Control (%)
N0	80	95
N1	32	94
N2a	38	91
N2b	50	80
N2c	80	77
N3	70	71

AJCC, American Joint Committee on Cancer.
Data from M.D. Anderson Cancer Center.
Adapted from Sanguineti G, Geara FB, Garden AS, et al.
Carcinoma of the nasopharynx treated by radiotherapy alone: determinants of local and regional control. *Int J Radiat Oncol Biol Phys* 1997;37:985–996, with permission.

TABLE 8.3 Results of Adjuvant and Neoadjuvant Chemotherapy and Radiation: Randomized Trials[a] (Literature Review)

First Author	Chemotherapy: No. of Cycles	Radiation (Gy)	No. of Patients Randomized	Overall survival HR [95% CI][b]
Chua	CE: ×2–3 before RT	66–74	334	0.99 [0.68, 1.44]
INCSG	BEC: ×3 before RT	65–70	339	1.00 [0.75, 1.33]
Hui	DC: ×2 before CRT	66	65	0.64 [0.29, 1.40]
Fountzilas	PCE: ×2 before CRT	66–70	144	0.99 [0.59, 1.66]
Tan	GCP: ×3 before CRT	70	172	1.05 [0, 2.19]
Chen	CF: ×3 after CRT	70	508	0.79 [0.47, 1.30]

[a]All trials randomized patients to radiation alone or radiation and chemotherapy.
[b]HR are computed using updated data from the MAC-NPC meta-analysis (Blanchard P, Lee A, Marguet S, et al. *Lancet Oncol.* 2015;16:645.), except for Tan trial.
INCSG, International Nasopharynx Cancer Study Group; CF, cisplatin, 5-FU; CE, cisplatin, epirubicin; BEC, bleomycin, epirubicin, cisplatin; CRT: concurrent chemoradiotherapy; DC, docetaxel, cisplatin; GCP, gemcitabine, carboplatin, and paclitaxel; PCE, paclitaxel, cisplatin, and epirubicin; RT, radiation alone; CRT, radiation and chemotherapy. CI, confidence interval; HR, hazard ratio.
Data from Chua DT, Sham JS, Choy D, et al. *Cancer* 1998;83:2270; INCSG. *Int J Radiat Oncol Biol Phys* 1996;35:463; Hui EP, Ma BB, Leung SF, et al. *J Clin Oncol* 2009;27:242; Fountzilas G, Ciuleanu E, Bobos M, et al. *Ann Oncol* 2012;23:427; Tan T, Lim WT, Fong KW, et al. *Int J Radiat Oncol Biol Phys* 2015;91:952; Chen L, Hu CS, Chen XZ, et al. *Lancet Oncol* 2012;13:163.

TABLE 8.4 Results of IMRT in the Treatment of Nasopharyngeal Carcinoma (Literature Review)

Authors	Patient Number	Median Follow-Up	% Local Control	% Nodal Control
Tham et al.	195	37 mo	90% (3 yr)	ND
Lee et al.	68	2.6 yr	93% (2 yr)	91%
Lin et al.	370	31 mo	95% (3 yr)	97%
Han et al.	305	35 mo	94% (3 yr)	98%
Ng et al.	193	31 mo	95% (2 yr)	96%
Sun et al.	868	50 mo	95% (3 yr) local–regional control	
Peng et al.	306	42 mo	91%	92%
Wu et al.	249	54 mo	87%	88%
Zhang et al.	2245	47 mo (mean)	96%	96%
Setton et al.	177	52 mo	83%	91%

IMRT, intensity-modulated radiation therapy; ND, not described; mo, months.
Data from Tham IW, et al. *Int J Radiat Oncol Biol Phys* 2009;75:1481; Lee N, et al. *J Clin Oncol* 2009;27:3684; Lin S, et al. *BMC Cancer* 2010;10:39; Han L, et al. *Chin J Cancer* 2010;29:145; Ng WT, et al. *Int J Radiat Oncol Biol Phys* 2011;79:420; Sun X, et al. *Radiother Oncol* 2014;110:398; Peng G, et al. *Radiother Oncol* 2012;104:286; Wu F, et al. *Radiother Oncol* 2014;112:106; Zhang MX, et al. *Eur J Cancer* 2015;51:2587; Setton J. *Oral Oncol* 2016;53:67.

TABLE 8.5 Results of IMRT in the Treatment of T4 Nasopharyngeal Carcinoma (Literature Review)

Authors	Patient Number	Median Follow-Up	% Local Control
Peng et al.	103	42 mo	82% (5 yr)
Cao et al.	70	27 mo	82% (2 yr)
Chen et al.	154	53 mo	81% (5 yr) local–regional control
Kong et al.	81	37 mo	84% (3 yr)
Sun et al.	164	50 mo	83% (5 yr) local–regional control
Takiar et al.	66	38 mo.	89% (2 yr) local–regional control

IMRT, intensity-modulated radiation therapy; mo, months.
Data from Peng G, et al. *Radiother Oncol* 2012;104:286; Cao C, et al. *Oral Oncol* 2013;49:175; Chen JL, et al. *Strahlenther Onkol* 2013;189:1001; Kong FF, et al. *PLoS One* 2014;9:e91362; Sun X, et al. *Radiother Oncol* 2014;110:398; Takiar V, et al. *Head Neck* 2015.

TABLE 8.6 Randomized Trials of Concurrent Chemotherapy and Radiation for Nasopharyngeal Cancer

First Author, Year	Pt Number	Concurrent Approach	Adjuvant Chemotherapy	Overall Survival HR[a] [95% CI]
Al-Sarraf, 1998	147	CDDP wk 1, 4, and 7	Yes	0.50 [0.36,0.70]
Chan, 2005	350	CDDP every week	No	0.81 [0.61, 1.07]
Zhang, 2005	115	Oxaliplatin every week	No	0.54 [0.31, 0.94]
Wee, 2005	221	CDDP wk 1, 4, and 7	Yes	0.68 [0.48, 0.96]
Lee, 2005	348	CDDP wk 1, 4, and 7	Yes	0.73 [0.54, 0.99]
Chen, 2013	316	CDDP every week	Yes	0.69 [0.48, 0.99]

[a]HR are computed using updated data from the MAC-NPC meta-analysis (Blanchard P, Lee A, Marguet S, et al. Chemotherapy and radiotherapy in nasopharyngeal carcinoma: an update of the MAC-NPC meta-analysis. *Lancet Oncol* 2015;16:645–655).
CDDP, cisplatin; CI, confidence interval; HR, hazard ratio.
Data from Al-Sarraf M, LeBlanc M, Giri PG, et al. *J Clin Oncol* 1998;16:1310; Chan AT, Leung SF, Ngan RK, et al. *J Natl Cancer Inst* 2005;97:536; Zhang L, Zhao C, Peng P, et al. *J Clin Oncol* 2005;23:8461; Wee J, Tan EH, Tai BC, et al. *J Clin Oncol* 2005;23:6730; Lee AW, Lau WH, Tung SY, et al. *J Clin Oncol* 2005;23:6966; Chen Y, Sun Y, Liang S-B, et al. *Cancer* 2013;119:2230.

TABLE 8.7 Summary of the Results, Overall and by Chemotherapy Timing for all Endpoints

	Overall Survival	Progression-Free Survival	Loco-regional Control	Distant control
Induction[a]	0.96 [0.80;1.16]	0.81 [0.69;0.95]	0.84 [0.66;1.07]	0.62 [0.48;0.79]
Adjuvant[a]	0.87 [0.68;1.12]	0.80 [0.64;1.00]	0.61 [0.41;0.92]	0.80 [0.59;1.09]
Concomitant[a]	0.80 [0.70;0.93]	0.81 [0.71;0.92]	0.82 [0.67;1.01]	0.74 [0.61;0.90]
Concomitant plus adjuvant[a]	0.65 [0.56;0.76]	0.62 [0.53;0.72]	0.54 [0.41;0.71]	0.56 [0.45;0.70]
Overall[a]	0.79 [0.73;0.86]	0.75 [0.69;0.81]	0.73 [0.64;0.83]	0.67 [0.59;0.75]
Overall test[b]	$P < 0.0001$	$P < 0.0001$	$P < 0.0001$	$P < 0.0001$
Interaction test[b] (timing × treatment effect)	$P = 0.01$	$P = 0.04$	$P = 0.05$	$P = 0.18$
Residual heterogeneity test[b]	$P = 0.36$	$P = 0.62$	$P = 0.78$	$P = 0.03$

[a]Hazard ratio [95% confidence interval]
[b]P value
Reproduced from Blanchard P, Lee A, Marguet S, et al.; MAC-NPC Collaborative Group. Chemotherapy and radiotherapy in nasopharyngeal carcinoma: an update of the MAC-NPC meta-analysis, *Lancet Oncol* 2015;16(6):645–655, with permission.

TABLE 8.8 Outcomes of Patients with Nasopharyngeal Carcinoma Treated with Intensity-Modulated Proton Therapy at M.D. Anderson Cancer Center

No. of Patients	No. of Stage III/IV	Median Follow-up (Months)	No. with Gastrostomy Placed During or After Therapy	% Local–Regional Control (2 Years)	% OS (2 Years)
10	7	24.5	3[a]	100	89

[a]No patient had a feeding tube at last follow-up.
Data from Lewis GD, Holliday EB, Kocak-Uzel E, et al. Intensity-modulated proton therapy for nasopharyngeal carcinoma: decreased radiation dose to normal structures and encouraging clinical outcomes. *Head Neck* 2016;38(Suppl 1):E1886–1895.

SUGGESTED READINGS

Al-Sarraf M, LeBlanc M, Giri PG, et al. Chemoradiotherapy versus radiotherapy in patients with advanced nasopharyngeal cancer: phase III randomized intergroup study 0099. *J Clin Oncol* 1998;16:1310.

Blanchard P, Lee A, Marguet S, et al.; MAC-NPC Collaborative Group. Chemotherapy and radiotherapy in nasopharyngeal carcinoma: an update of the MAC-NPC meta-analysis. *Lancet Oncol* 2015;16:645.

Chan AT, Teo P, Huang DP. Pathogenesis and treatment of nasopharyngeal carcinoma. *Semin Oncol* 2004;31:794.

Chua DT, Ma J, Sham JS, et al. Long-term survival after cisplatin-based induction chemotherapy and radiotherapy for nasopharyngeal carcinoma: a pooled data analysis of two phase III trials. *J Clin Oncol* 2005;23:1118.

Delclos L, Moore BE, Sampiere VA. A disposable "afterloadable" nasopharyngeal applicator for radioactive point sources. *Endocur Hypertherm Oncol* 1994;10:43.

Jiang W, Chamberlain PD, Garden AS, et al. Prognostic value of p16 expression in Epstein-Barr virus-positive nasopharyngeal carcinomas. *Head Neck* 2016;38(Suppl 1):E1459.

Kam MK, Teo PM, Chau RM, et al. Treatment of nasopharyngeal carcinoma with intensity-modulated radiotherapy: the Hong Kong experience. *Int J Radiat Oncol Biol Phys* 2004;60:1440.

Le QT, Tate D, Koong A, et al. Improved local control with stereotactic radiosurgical boost in patients with nasopharyngeal carcinoma. *Int J Radiat Oncol Biol Phys* 2003;56:1046.

Lee N, Harris J, Garden AS, et al. Intensity-modulated radiation therapy with or without chemotherapy for nasopharyngeal carcinoma: radiation therapy oncology group phase II trial 0225. *J Clin Oncol* 2009;27:3684.

Lee AW, Tung SY, Chan AT, et al. Preliminary results of a randomized study (NPC-9902 Trial) on therapeutic gain by concurrent chemotherapy and/or accelerated fractionation for locally advanced nasopharyngeal carcinoma. *Int J Radiat Oncol Biol Phys* 2006;66:142.

Lee AW, Tung SY, Chua DTT et al. Randomized trial of radiotherapy plus concurrent-adjuvant chemotherapy vs radiotherapy alone for regionally advanced nasopharyngeal cancer. *J Natl Cancer Inst* 2010;102:1188.

Lee AW, Tung SY, Ngan RK, et al. Factors contributing to the efficacy of concurrent-adjuvant chemotherapy for locoregionally advanced nasopharyngeal carcinoma: combined analyses of NPC-9901 and NPC-9902 trials. *Eur J Cancer* 2011;47:656.

Lee N, Xia P, Quivey JM, et al. Intensity-modulated radiotherapy in the treatment of nasopharyngeal carcinoma: an update of the UCSF experience. *Int J Radiat Oncol Biol Phys* 2002;53:12.

Levendag PC, Keskin-Cambray F, de Pan C, et al. Local control in advanced cancer of the nasopharynx: is a boost dose by endocavitary brachytherapy of prognostic significance?. *Brachytherapy* 2013;12:84.

Lewis GD, Holliday EB, Kocak-Uzel E, et al. Intensity-modulated proton therapy for nasopharyngeal carcinoma: decreased radiation dose to normal structures and encouraging clinical outcomes. *Head Neck* 2016; 38(Suppl 1):E1886–1895.

Pow EHN, Kwong DLW, McMillan AS, et al. Xerostomia and quality of life after intensity-modulated radiotherapy vs. conventional radiotherapy for early-stage nasopharyngeal carcinoma: initial report on a randomized controlled clinical trial. *Int J Radiat Oncol Biol Phys* 2006;66:981.

Sanguineti G, Geara FB, Garden AS, et al. Carcinoma of the nasopharynx treated by radiotherapy alone: determinants of local and regional control. *Int J Radiat Oncol Biol Phys* 1997;37:985.

Setton J, Han J, Kannarunimit D, et al. Long-term patterns of relapse and survival following definitive intensity-modulated radiotherapy for non-endemic nasopharyngeal carcinoma. *Oral Oncol* 2016;53:67.

Sun Y, Li W-F, Chen N-Y, et al. Induction chemotherapy plus concurrent chemoradiotherapy versus concurrent chemoradiotherapy alone in locoregionally advanced nasopharyngeal carcinoma: a phase 3, multicentre, randomised controlled trial. *Lancet Oncol* 2016;17:1509–1520.

Takiar V, Ma D, Garden AS, et al. Disease control and toxicity outcomes for T4 carcinoma of the nasopharynx treated with intensity-modulated radiotherapy. *Head Neck* 2016;38(Suppl 1):E925–933.

Teo PM, Leung SF, Chan AT, et al. Final report of a randomized trial on altered-fractionated radiotherapy in nasopharyngeal carcinoma prematurely terminated by significant increase in neurologic complications. *Int J Radiat Oncol Biol Phys* 2000;48:1311.

9

Oropharynx

Key Points

- The oropharynx is comprised of the soft palate, tonsillar (faucial) pillars, tonsillar fossa, base of tongue, and pharyngeal walls.

- The majority of oropharyngeal squamous cell carcinomas arise in the lymphoid-bearing areas of the tonsil and base of tongue, particularly those that are associated with human papillomavirus (HPV).

- The incidence of oropharyngeal carcinoma is rising in North America and Europe particularly due to the increase in HPV-associated carcinoma, afflicting mainly younger individuals (40 to 60 years of age), who may have minimal to no history of tobacco use (see Chapter 1). Patients with HPV-positive oropharyngeal carcinoma treated with established therapy regimens have a largely favorable prognosis.

- Radiation alone is often the preferred modality of therapy for early-stage oropharyngeal carcinomas. Ipsilateral radiotherapy is highly successful in controlling tonsillar carcinomas confined to the fossa.

- Combinations of radiation with systemic therapy represent standard approaches for patients with locally advanced oropharyngeal carcinoma. The primary tumor and nodal volume, the general condition of the patients, and preference determine the specific choices.

- A planned neck dissection following (chemo)radiation for patients with advanced nodal disease is not mandatory. Only patients with residual nodal disease after radiation or combined therapy are managed with neck dissection.

- Intensity-modulated radiation therapy (IMRT) is commonly used to spare normal tissues. IMRT can reduce the incidence of xerostomia, dysphagia, and osteoradionecrosis.

- Advances in spot-scanning intensity-modulated proton therapy (IMPT) techniques have provided the ability to treat geometrically complex oropharyngeal carcinoma target volumes. IMPT reduces integral dose to nontarget structures compared to IMRT, particularly those anterior and posterior to the target volumes.

BACKGROUND DATA

- Although the detail of radiation planning and delivery may differ among cancers arising from different anatomical subsites within the oropharynx, the treatment outcomes have been usually reported in aggregate. Therefore, this chapter begins by summarizing the general background outcome data before addressing individual oropharyngeal subsites.

See Tables 9.1 to 9.4.

TABLE 9.1 Outcomes of 1,042 Patients with Squamous Carcinoma of the Oropharynx Treated with Radiotherapy at the M.D. Anderson Cancer Center 2000 to 2007

	No. of Patients	5-yr Local–Regional Control (%)	5-yr Overall Survival (%)
Primary site			
Tonsillar fossa	460	91	83
Base of tongue	511	86	80
Other[a]	75	65	43
T stage			
T1–T2	640	94	90
T3–T4	406	75	60
N stage			
N0	57	74	65
N1–N2a	317	93	86
N2b–N2c	573	86	79
N3	99	80	59
Total	1,046	87	78

[a]Soft palate and pharyngeal wall.
Data from Garden AS, Kies MS, Morrison WH, et al. Outcomes and patterns of care of patients with locally advanced oropharyngeal carcinoma treated in the early 21st century. *Radiat Oncol* 2013;8:21.

TABLE 9.2 First Site of Failure Distribution for Stage I and II Oropharynx Cancer Treated with Radiation at the M.D. Anderson Cancer Center (1970 to 1998)

		First Site of Failure							
		None	L	R	LR	DM	L and DM	R and DM	Total
T stage	T1 and Tx	45	3	1	1	1	0	0	51
	T2	87	21	5	1	8	1	1	124
Total		132	24	6	2	9	1	1	175

L, local recurrence; R, regional recurrence; LR, loco-regional recurrence; DM, distant metastases; L and DM, synchronous local recurrence and distant metastases; R and DM, synchronous regional recurrence and distant metastases.
Modified from Selek U, Garden AS, Morrison WH, et al. Radiation therapy for early-stage carcinoma of the oropharynx. *Int J Radiat Oncol Biol Phys* 2004;59:743–775.

TABLE 9.3 Survival of Patients with Oropharyngeal Carcinoma Based on Tumor HPV Status

First Author	Patient Number	Marker	Overall Survival Rates (Positive vs. Negative)
Ang	223	p16^{INK4A}	84% vs. 51% (3-yr)
Fahkry	62	HPV	84% vs. 50% (3-yr)
Lassen	815	p16^{INK4A}	80% vs. 37% (5-yr)
Rischin	185	p16^{INK4A}	91% vs. 74% (2-yr)
Shi	111	HPV	88% vs. 67% (3-yr)
Rosenthal	84[a]	p16^{INK4A}	88% vs. 42% (3-yr)
O'Sullivan	2,603	HPV or p16	80% vs. 48% (5-yr)

[a]Those receiving cetuximab and radiation therapy.
Data from Ang KK, et al. *N Engl J Med* 2010;363:24–35; Fahkry C, et al. *J Natl Cancer Inst Phys* 2008;100:261–269; Lassen P, et al. *Radiother Oncol* 2014;113:310–316; Rischin D, et al. *J Clin Oncol* 2010;28:4142–4148; Shi W, et al. *J Clin Oncol* 2009;27:6213–6221; Rosenthal DI, et al. *J Clin Oncol* 2016;34(12):1300–1308; O'Sullivan B, et al. *Lancet Oncol* 2016;17(4):440–451.

TABLE 9.4 Results of Intensity-Modulated Radiation Therapy for Cancer of the Oropharynx

First Author	Year	Patient Number	Median Follow-Up (mo)	Disease Control Rate (%)
Feng	2005	94	36	94 (LRC–crude)
Yao	2006	66[a]	27	99 (LRC, 3-yr)
Studer	2007	105[a]	ND	88 (LC, 2-yr)
Huang	2008	71	29	90 (LRC, 3-yr)
Sanguineti	2008	38	33	94 (LC, 3-yr)
Eisbruch	2010	69	32	91 (LRC, 2-yr)
Mendenhall	2010	130	42	84 (LRC, 5-yr)
Daly	2010	107[a]	29	92 (LRC, 3-yr)

(Continued)

TABLE 9.4 Results of Intensity-Modulated Radiation Therapy for Cancer of the Oropharynx *(Continued)*

First Author	Year	Patient Number	Median Follow-Up (mo)	Disease Control Rate (%)
Setton	2012	442	37	85 (OS, 3-yr)
May	2013	170	33	91 (LRC, 3-yr)
Garden	2013	776	54	90 (LRC, 5-yr)

[a]Included patients treated with definitive and postoperative radiation.

LRC, locoregional control; LC local control; ND, not described.

Data from Feng M, et al. *Radiother Oncol* 2005;77:32–38; 64:363–373; Yao M, et al. *Am J Clin Oncol* 2006;29:606–612; Studer G, et al. *Strahlenther Onkol* 2007;183:417–423; Huang K, et al. *Cancer* 2008;113:497–507; Sanguineti G, et al. *Int J Radiat Oncol Biol Phys* 2008;72:737–746; Eisbruch A, et al. *Int J Radiat Oncol Biol Phys* 2010;76:1333–1338; Mendenhall WM, et al. *Laryngoscope* 2010;120:2218–2222; Daly ME, et al. *Int J Radiat Oncol Biol Phys* 2010;76:1339–1346; Setton J, et al. *Int J Radiat Oncol Biol Phys* 2012;82:291; May JT, et al. *Head Neck* 2013;35:1796; and Garden AS, et al. *Int J Radiat Oncol Biol Phys* 2013;85:941.

SOFT PALATE

Treatment Strategy

Primary radiotherapy is preferred for T1 to T2 N0 to N1 carcinomas. Superficial T1 lesions without lymphadenopathy may be amenable to local excision only.

Combination of radiation with systemic therapy is the treatment of choice for T3 and selected T4 or N2 to N3 tumors. As presented in Chapter 1, outside the protocol study setting, radiation with concurrent cisplatin is the favored treatment. Radiation with concurrent high-dose cisplatin (100 mg/m², given every 3 weeks) has the longest track record and the strongest evidence basis, but the clinical use of weekly cisplatin (40 mg/m²) has increased. Cetuximab is recommended concurrent with radiation in patients for whom cisplatin is contraindicated.

Patients presenting with N2 or N3 nodal disease achieving a complete clinical and radiographic response do not require a planned neck dissection.

T4a tumors with bone invasion or extensive normal tissue destruction resulting in deformation and/or impaired functions are best treated with surgery and postoperative radiotherapy and, in the presence of pathologic evidence of extracapsular extension or positive margin, radiation is combined with concurrent chemotherapy.

Primary Radiotherapy

Target Volume

The initial target volume is primary tumor with at least 2-cm margins and bilateral neck nodes, including the retropharyngeal and level II, III, and IV nodes (plus level V nodes in the node positive hemineck). The target volume also includes ipsilateral level IB in the presence of level II node(s). For lateralized tumors, the target volume includes the ipsilateral tonsillar pillars, parapharyngeal space, and lateral aspect of the pterygoid muscle. The boost volume encompasses the primary tumor and involved node(s) with 1- to 2-cm margins.

Setup and Field Arrangement for Conventional Radiotherapy Technique

Insertion of metal seeds at the borders of the tumor, when feasible, facilitates portal shaping. The patient is immobilized in a supine position with thermoplastic mask. An extended head and shoulder mask is used for conformal radiotherapy. With conventional technique, lateral parallel–opposed photon fields are used to treat the primary tumor and upper neck nodes **(Case Study 9.1)**.

- *Anterior border*: at least 2 cm anterior to the tumor.
- *Superior border*: at least 1.5 cm above the soft palate. If the primary tumor spreads into the tonsillar fossa, this border is extended superiorly to encompass the medial pterygoid muscle to the pterygoid plate.
- *Posterior border*: behind the mastoid tip when N0, behind the spinous processes when N+, or even more posteriorly if needed to cover a large nodal mass.
- *Inferior border*: just above the arytenoids except when the extent of nodal disease requires a lower inferior border.

Boost Volume

- Lateral fields are reduced to cover the primary tumor with 1- to 2-cm margins. For selected T1 and small, superficial T2 tumors, it may be preferable to administer the boost dose with an intraoral cone when feasible (i.e., the lesion is accessible and the patient can

CASE STUDY 9.1

A 55-year-old man sought medical attention for a 6-month history of sore throat. Physical examination revealed a 3.5-cm exophytic tumor of the uvula and soft palate with minimal extension to the right anterior tonsillar pillar. The hard palate was not involved. There were no palpable neck nodes. Biopsy showed a moderately differentiated squamous cell carcinoma (SCC). Stage: T2 N0 M0. This patient was treated with primary radiotherapy according to the concomitant boost regimen. The fields were designed to encompass the primary tumor and upper neck nodes (Fig. 9.1). The boost volume covered the primary tumor with generous margins. The seed indicated the superior and anterior border of the tumor on the palate. The mid and lower neck nodes were treated through a matching anterior photon field with a midline block to shield the larynx. The dose to the primary tumor was 70.5 Gy in 41 fractions over 6 weeks. Areas of subclinical disease in the upper neck received 54 Gy in 30 fractions over 6 weeks. The mid and lower neck received 50 Gy in 25 fractions over 5 weeks. He had no evidence of disease 5 years after therapy. However, there was a slight retraction of the soft palate without functional repercussion.

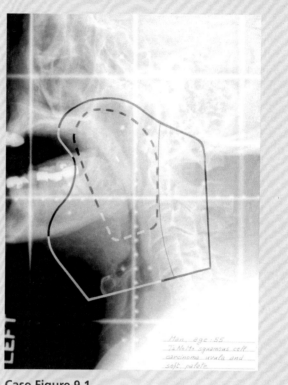

Case Figure 9.1

tolerate an intraoral cone without gagging) to reduce treatment morbidity by limiting the dose to the mandible and soft tissues. In such cases, it is desirable to administer the boost dose first while the tumor is clearly visible and palpable.

Nodal metastases in the upper neck are encompassed in the lateral portals. Nodes in the mid or lower neck can receive boost dose with a glancing photon field or appositional electron portal.

Dose

For patients with T1 N0 and superficial T2 N0 tumors: conventional fractionation delivering 50 Gy in 25 fractions to the initial target volume followed by a boost dose of 16 Gy in 8 fractions by external beam or 15 Gy in 5 to 6 fractions given by intraoral cone.

For patients with larger T2 N0 to N1 tumors or T3 to T4 tumors who do not receive systemic treatment: concomitant boost schedule to total doses of 72 Gy in 42 fractions. The initial volume receives 1.8-Gy fractions to 54 Gy in 6 weeks. The boost volume receives an additional 1.5 Gy to a dose of 18 Gy given as second daily fractions during the last 2.5 weeks of the wide-field irradiations. The spinal cord dose is limited to 45 Gy or less.

For patients with T3 to T4 or N2 to N3 tumors who receive systemic therapy: conventional fractionation (70 Gy in 35 fractions over 7 weeks) with concurrent cisplatin. The benefit of acceleration (similar to patients who do not receive systemic therapy) for patients who receive cetuximab is controversial.

Intensity-Modulated Radiation Therapy

IMRT has now been widely adopted for the treatment of patients with oropharyngeal carcinomas. The patient is immobilized in a supine position with an extended head and shoulder thermoplastic mask. Thin-cut CT scans are obtained in treatment position. The gross target volume (GTV), and clinical target volumes (CTVs), are delineated by the radiation oncologist, and planning target volumes (PTVs) are generated for dosimetric planning **(Case Study 9.2)**.

Gross Target Volume

GTV represents all areas determined from clinical examination and imaging studies to contain gross disease. It is very important to integrate the latest physical examination findings (including in-office fiberoptic endoscopy) in treatment planning, as CT scan alone may not detect superficial mucosal tumor extension.

CASE STUDY 9.2

A 79-year-old woman presented with nasal voice, mild bilateral otalgia, and a globus sensation. Physical examination revealed a 2.5-cm exophytic lesion on the posterior aspect of the soft palate. A biopsy revealed moderately differentiated SCC. Staging workup included a CT scan of the head and neck, which showed a thickened soft palate and a 1.5-cm left level II node. She was treated with IMRT delivered in 30 fractions.

CTV_{HD} (66 Gy) encompassed the soft palate and left upper jugular involved node with margin. The remainder of left level II not included in CTV_{HD} and left level IB nodes were defined as CTV_{ID}. The retropharyngeal nodes and right level II nodal bed were delineated as CTV_{ED} (54 Gy).

Figure 9.2A–D shows CTV_{HD} (*red*), CTV_{ID} (*blue*), and CTV_{ED} (*yellow*) on representative axial cuts from the level of the retropharyngeal nodes and soft palate superiorly and to the hyoid inferiorly. Figure 9.2E,F shows the isodose distributions on two axial images through the palate.

Figure 9.2A shows the medial and lateral retropharyngeal nodes contoured in CTV_{ED}. Because the medial

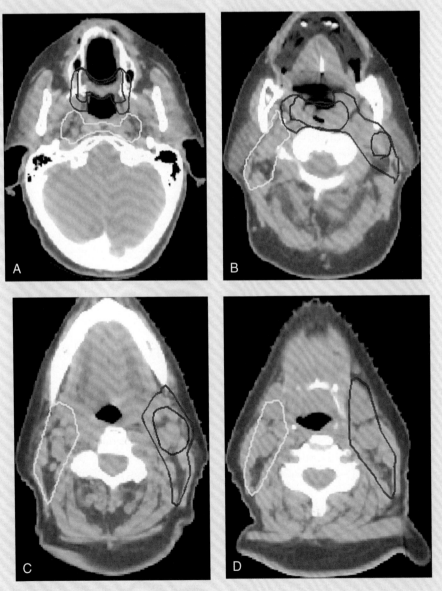

Case Figure 9.2 A–D

nodes are at very low risk, we no longer include them in CTV$_{ED}$, creating two separate contours for the lateral nodes that lie medial to the carotid and lateral to the prevertebral muscles.

Figure 9.2C,D shows CTV$_{ED}$ covering the node-negative right neck. To ensure coverage of anterior 2A, we covered the posterior half of the submandibular gland. As interest in sparing this gland has increased, along with improvements in dosimetry, we currently contour to the posterior edge of the gland rather than bisect it for delineation of CTV$_{ED}$.

The isocenter was placed above the thyroid notch, and the low neck was treated with a matching anterior beam. A larynx block was used for the first 40 Gy (Fig. 9.2G), and then a full midline block was added for 10 Gy. The left mid neck (level III) was boosted to 60 Gy with glancing photon fields. The patient remained well without disease 5 years later.

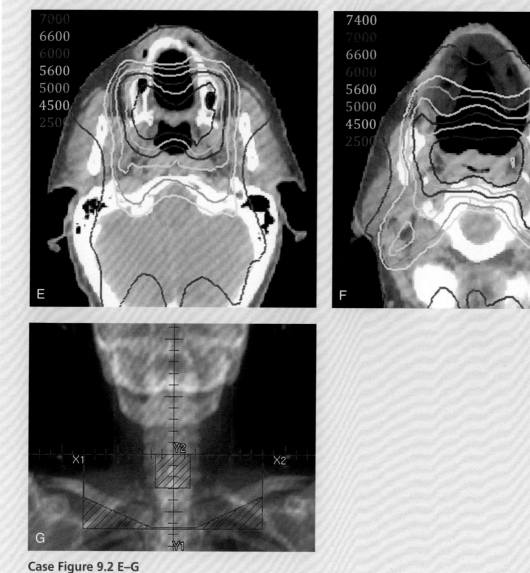

Case Figure 9.2 E–G

Clinical Target Volumes

Three CTVs are generally delineated.

- CTV$_{HD}$ delineates volumes to receive the highest dose, which includes the primary and nodal GTVs with 0.5- to 1-cm margins. Margins should be more generous if the tumor borders are less well defined.

- CTV$_{ID}$ delineates volumes to receive an intermediate dose, which includes the remaining soft palate and the adjacent parapharyngeal space. CTV$_{ID}$ covers the superior aspect of the tonsillar pillars for lateral tumors and, in the presence of positive node(s), the involved and adjoining nodal compartment(s).

- CTV$_{ED}$ delineates volumes to receive an elective dose for potential subclinical disease. In the N0 neck, CTV$_{ED}$ includes bilateral nodal levels II to IV and retropharyngeal nodes (plus level V in the node positive heminuk). When level II node is involved, CTV$_{ED}$ also includes clinically uninvolved ipsilateral level IB nodes.

Dose

For patients with T1 N0 and superficial T2 N0 tumors: 66 Gy to CTV$_{HD}$, 60 Gy to CTV$_{ID}$, and 54 Gy to CTV$_{ED}$, given in 30 fractions over 6 weeks.

For patients with larger tumors who do not receive systemic therapy: options are (1) 70 Gy to CTV$_{HD}$, 63 Gy to CTV$_{ID}$, and 56 Gy to CTV$_{ED}$ given in 35 fractions over 6 weeks (1 day a week of twice-a-day irradiation), (2) 70 Gy to CTV$_{HD}$, 60 Gy to CTV$_{ID}$, and 57 Gy to CTV$_{ED}$ given in 33 fractions over 6.5 weeks, or (3) a concomitant boost-type regimen, which requires two IMRT plans (see IMRT Section of Chapter 1).

For patients with T3 to T4 or N2 to N3 tumors who receive systemic therapy: options are (1) 70 Gy to CTV$_{HD}$, 60 to 63 Gy to CTV$_{ID}$, and 57 Gy to CTV$_{ED}$ given in 33 fractions over 6.5 weeks or (2) 70 Gy to CTV$_{HD}$, 63 Gy to CTV$_{ID}$, and 56 Gy to CTV$_{ED}$ given in 35 fractions over 6 weeks (1 day a week of twice-a-day irradiation) when combined with two cycles of high-dose cisplatin or weekly cetuximab.

Postoperative Radiotherapy

Adjuvant radiotherapy is indicated in occasional patients treated with upfront surgery. The principles are similar to those for the treatment of retromolar trigone or posterior oral cavity tumors as presented in detail, in Chapter 7.

Target Volume

With conventional techniques, the initial target volume encompasses the entire surgical bed and all nodal areas of the neck. The boost volume encompasses areas of known disease location with 1- to 2-cm margins. If IMRT is used, the delineation of CTV$_{HD}$, CTV$_{ID}$, and CTV$_{ED}$ as described for oral cavity cancers (Chapter 7) is applied. If a small area of high risk is identified (such as a positive margin or the area of extracapsular extension), an addition high-dose target of 6 Gy can be delineated. Depending on the volume of this high-dose CTV, and the patient's condition, this can be treated as a simultaneous integrated boost, receiving 2.2 Gy per fraction (as treatment is typically 30 fractions), or treated as a sequential boost in 3 additional fractions.

Setup and Field Arrangement

The general technique is the same as that described under "Primary Radiotherapy." Marking of the external surgical scar facilitates portal design. The *anterior* and *superior field borders* or CTVs are mainly determined by the local spread of the primary tumor and the extent of surgery (scar/flap). It is prudent to include 1- to 2-cm margins beyond the mucosal scar.

Dose

- A dose of 60 Gy in 30 fractions to areas with high-risk features, that is, close or microscopically positive margins, perineural extension, vascular invasion, positive nodes, or extranodal extension. An additional boost dose of 6 Gy may be given when indicated, such as when multiple adverse features are present or when the interval between surgery and radiation is much longer than 6 weeks. Patients who had no evidence of disease after diagnostic tonsillectomy are treated similarly as those having T1 disease.
- A dose of 56 Gy in 28 fractions to the surgical bed.
- A dose of 50 Gy in 25 fractions to undissected regions to receive elective irradiation.

Similar dosing is applied if IMRT is used with treatment typically delivered in 30 fractions. CTV$_{HD}$, CTV$_{ID}$, and CTV$_{ED}$ are prescribed 60 Gy, 57 Gy, and 54 Gy, respectively.

Timing of Postoperative Radiotherapy

It is desirable to commence postoperative radiotherapy as soon as possible after healing of surgical wounds. With good communication between surgical, radiation, and dental oncologists, simulation can usually take place 3 to 4 weeks after surgery, and radiotherapy can start within a week in most patients. When delayed wound healing postpones commencement of postoperative radiation to beyond 5 to 6 weeks, we administer accelerated fractionation, such as concomitant boost, by delivering twice-a-day irradiations for 5 treatment days, either once a week or daily toward the end of the radiation course, to reduce the potential hazard of prolonged cumulative treatment time.

However, commencing treatment too soon after tonsillectomy or intraoral surgery prior to the wound healing can lead to soft tissue necrosis. Wound healing may require 4 to 6 weeks, but as the majority of these patients have favorable prognoses, and many get concurrent chemotherapy, the need to accelerate radiation in the event of delay is moot.

TABLE 9.5 Local Control of Soft Palate Tumors by T Stage

Stage	No. of Patients	5 yr (%)
T1	53	90–92
T2	111	67–90
T3	93	58–67
T4	34	37–57

Adapted from Keus RB, Pontvert D, Brunin F, et al. Results of irradiation in squamous cell carcinoma of the soft palate and uvula. *Radiother Oncol* 1988;11:311–317; and Chera BS, Amdur RJ, Hinerman RW, et al. Definitive radiation therapy for squamous cell carcinoma of the soft palate. *Head Neck* 2008;30:1114–1119.

Background Data

See Table 9.5.

TONSILLAR FOSSA

Treatment Strategy

Primary radiotherapy is an excellent treatment option for T1 to T2 N0 to N1 carcinomas. With the increasing popularity of minimally invasive intraoral approaches, surgery is being performed more frequently for tonsillar carcinomas at many centers. Surgery may be preferred if there is a high probability that single-modality therapy will suffice. Combination of radiation with systemic therapy is the treatment of choice for T3 and selected T4 or N2 to N3 tumors. As presented in Chapter 1, concurrent cisplatin is favored, and concurrent cetuximab is considered second-line therapy for patients who cannot receive cisplatin.

Patients presenting with N2 to N3 nodal disease achieving a complete clinical and radiographic response do not require a planned neck dissection.

T4a tumors with bone invasion, laryngeal dysfunction, or severe trismus are best treated with surgery followed by adjuvant radiotherapy and, in the presence of extracapsular extension or positive margin, combined with concurrent cisplatin.

Primary Radiotherapy

Target Volume

For the initial target volume:

- *T1 and T2 (confined to the tonsillar fossa), N0 to N2b (nodal disease confined to upper neck) tumors:* primary lesion with 2-cm margins and ipsilateral retropharyngeal and level II to IV nodes **(Case Study 9.3)**. The target volume also includes ipsilateral level V in node positive cases and ipsilateral level IB in the presence of level II node(s).
- *T2 (with base of tongue or soft palate involvement), T3, and selected T4 or N2 to N3 tumors:* tonsillar fossa, faucial pillars, soft palate, base of tongue, medial pterygoid muscle, and bilateral neck nodes (parapharyngeal–retropharyngeal, level II to IV/V, and ipsilateral level IB).

For the boost volume: primary tumor and involved node(s) with 1- to 2-cm margins.

Conventional Radiation Planning for Ipsilateral Treatment (for T1 to T2 Confined to Tonsillar Fossa, N0 to N2b Tumors)

Insertion of metal seeds at the borders of the tumor, when feasible, facilitates portal shaping. The patient is immobilized in a supine position with thermoplastic mask for irradiation of the primary tumor and upper neck nodes with wedge-pair photon portals.

Field borders for the initial target volume:

- *Anterior border:* at least 2 cm anterior to the tumor.
- *Superior border:* encompasses the insertion of the medial pterygoid muscle at the pterygoid plate.
- *Posterior border:* 2 cm behind the mastoid tip and behind the edge of the sternocleidomastoid muscle.
- *Inferior border:* just above the arytenoids.

A matching anterior photon portal is used to irradiate the mid and lower neck nodes.

For the boost volume, the field is reduced to cover initial gross disease with 1- to 2-cm margins.

Intensity-Modulated Radiation Therapy Planning for Ipsilateral Treatment (for T1 to T2 Confined to Tonsillar Fossa, N0 to N2b Tumors)

Clinical Target Volume

Three CTVs are generally delineated **(Case Study 9.4 through Case Study 9.6)**.

- CTV$_{HD}$ delineates volumes to receive the highest dose, which includes the primary and nodal GTVs with 0.5- to 1-cm margins. The entire tonsillar fossa is generally encompassed from the maxillary tuberosity (superior) to the hyoid bone (inferior). An additional 1 cm is added if the GTV is at the edges of or beyond these cranial and caudal landmarks. CTV$_{HD}$ also encompasses the adjacent glossopharyngeal sulcus and 1 cm of the ipsilateral adjacent base of tongue. Laterally, CTV$_{HD}$ covers the parapharyngeal space and 1 cm of the pterygoid muscle. Many patients present after tonsillectomy for small-volume tonsillar disease. In this situation, the medial pterygoid muscle should have 1 to 2 cm of coverage.

- CTV$_{ID}$ delineates volumes to receive an intermediate dose, which includes an additional 1-cm margin of coverage beyond the CTV$_{HD}$ toward the pterygoid musculature laterally, and superiorly, the retromolar trigone, soft palate, and base of tongue. In the presence of positive node(s), CTV$_{ID}$ encompasses the involved and adjoining nodal compartment(s).

- CTV$_{ED}$ delineates volumes to receive an elective dose for subclinical disease. It is prudent to cover the medial pterygoid musculature to the pterygoid plates. In the N0 neck, CTV$_{ED}$ includes nodal levels II to IV and lateral retropharyngeal nodes. When level II node is involved, CTV$_{ED}$ also includes clinically uninvolved ipsilateral level IB nodes. Level V is typically targeted in the node positive hemineck.

Conventional Radiation Planning for Bilateral Treatment

Insertion of metal seeds at the borders of the tumor, when feasible, and marking of oral commissures facilitate portal shaping. The patient is immobilized in a supine position.

Field borders for the initial target volume **(Case Study 9.7)**:

- *Anterior border:* at least 2 cm anterior to the tumor or more anteriorly if necessary to encompass level IB nodes.
- *Superior border:* encompasses pterygoid plates and retropharyngeal nodes.
- *Posterior border:* just behind the spinous processes or more posteriorly in the presence of large posterior cervical nodal masses.
- *Inferior border:* just above the arytenoids. In the presence of large nodal disease below this level, the border can be extended more inferiorly.

An anterior appositional photon field is used for elective treatment of the mid and lower neck nodes bilaterally.

For the boost volume, the lateral portals are reduced to include the primary tumor with 1- to 2-cm margins and the involved upper neck nodes. In the presence of trismus, the ipsilateral medial pterygoid muscle is included in the boost fields. Nodal disease outside the primary boost field is generally treated with anterior–posterior glancing photon fields.

CASE STUDY 9.3

A 47-year-old woman presented with a swollen right tonsil and underwent tonsillectomy. Histologic examination revealed invasive poorly differentiated SCC with lymphatic and perineural invasion. The final margins after additional resection were free. On presentation to our center, she had postsurgical changes without evidence of residual disease and was, therefore, staged as having a Tx (pT1) N0 tonsil carcinoma. We elected to treat this patient ipsilaterally with a wedged-pair technique, using "field-in-field" compensation (see Chapter 3). The total dose was 66 Gy in 33 fractions.

Figure 9.3 shows that the initial volume encompassed the tonsillar bed and upper neck, and was reduced after 50 Gy. This target (*red*) included the pterygoid muscle, parapharyngeal space, the lateral base of tongue, the lateral soft palate, and the ipsilateral retropharyngeal nodes. The boost volume encompassed the tonsillar bed only (*green*). An axial isodose distribution through the superior tonsillar region is shown. The initial wedged-pair fields were matched above the arytenoids to an anterior field that covered ipsilateral levels III and IV nodes to 50 Gy. She had no evidence of disease and had no sequelae 2 years after therapy.

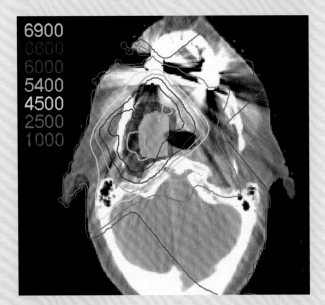

6900
6600
6000
5400
4500
2500
1000

Case Figure 9.3

CASE STUDY 9.4

A 40-year-old woman presented after an excisional biopsy of an asymptomatic left neck mass. Histologic examination revealed SCC in a 2.3-cm lymph node. Staging workup did not reveal any residual nodal disease, but the left tonsil was firm. A biopsy of the tonsil done during examination under anesthesia revealed SCC. Stage was T1Nx (pN1). It was elected to treat her with ipsilateral IMRT.

Figure 9.4 shows axial isodose distributions through the superior tonsillar fossa and upper neck. The tonsillar region (CTV$_{HD}$, *red*) received 66 Gy (Fig. 9.4A), and an additional rim of surrounding tissues (CTV$_{ID}$, *green*) along with ipsilateral levels IB and II nodes received 60 Gy. The involved nodal bed defined from the prebiopsy imaging (a second CTV$_{HD}$, *blue*) was prescribed a minimum dose of 63 Gy (Fig. 9.4B). The excision scar was wired for planning, and a 2-mm bolus was applied over the scar. The left low neck was treated with an appositional anterior field to 50 Gy, matched with an isocentric technique to the IMRT fields. She had no evidence of disease and had no sequelae 2 years after therapy.

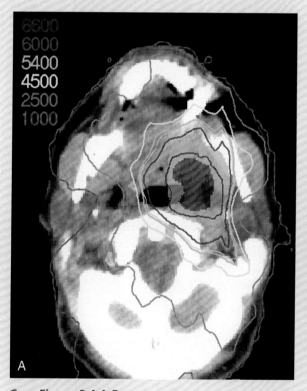

Case Figure 9.4 A,B

CASE STUDY 9.5

A 43-year-old man presented with a right upper neck mass. Excisional biopsy revealed SCC without obvious extracapsular extension. Postexcision CT scan did not reveal obvious disease. He underwent an examination under anesthesia and a right tonsillectomy. The right tonsil was found to contain SCC. Stage T1 Nx (1) M0. As the primary disease was confined to the tonsil, it was elected to prescribe ipsilateral IMRT.

CTV$_{HD}$ (66 Gy) encompassed the tonsillar and nodal excision beds, CTV$_{ID}$ (60 Gy) covered the remainder of level II and level IB nodes, and CTV$_{ED}$ (54 Gy) delineated the ipsilateral retropharyngeal nodes, superior parapharyngeal space, and the medial pterygoid muscle up to the pterygoid plate.

Figure 9.5 shows CTV$_{HD}$ (*aqua*), CTV$_{ID}$ (*khaki*), and CTV$_{ED}$ (*maroon*) along with the isodose distributions on representative axial images at the level of the high retropharyngeal nodes (Fig. 9.5A), mid-tonsillar fossa (Fig. 9.5B), and inferior tonsillar fossa (Fig. 9.5C), respectively.

The primary tumor and nodal regions above the thyroid notch were irradiated with IMRT. A matching left anterior–oblique beam, angled 5 to 10 degrees to be parallel to the right wing of the thyroid cartilage, was used to treat the ipsilateral lower neck nodes to 50 Gy. This portal was reduced to bring the total dose to the level III region to 60 Gy. Treatment was delivered in 30 fractions. Figure 9.5D shows the isodose distribution on a coronal view through the pharynx. The patient is doing well without disease 3 years later.

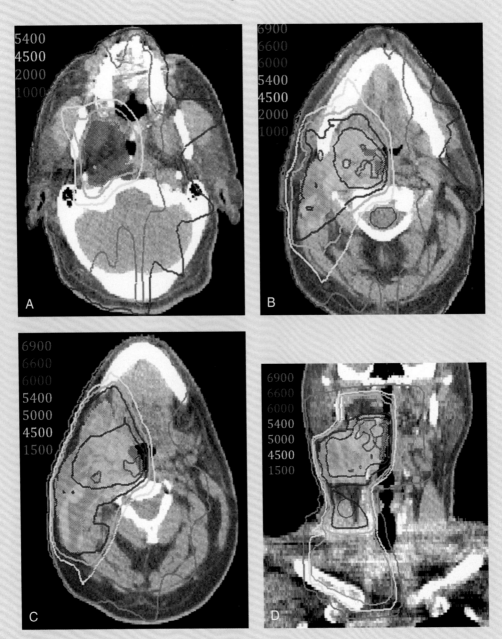

Case Figure 9.5 A–D

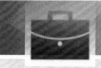

CASE STUDY 9.6

A 48-year-old man presented with "tonsillitis" and right neck adenopathy. A core biopsy of the node was positive for squamous cell carcinoma, HPV and p16 positive. His exam findings included a 2- to 3-cm right level II neck mass and a <2-cm lesion in the mid right tonsil. His staging included a PET/CT scan which revealed the tonsillar primary tumor and adenopathy, which can be appreciated on a coronal image (Fig. 9.6A). The palpated nodal mass can be appreciated on an axial image from a contrast CT scan (Fig. 9.6B, *red arrow*), along with a second small cystic node (*green arrow*) just posterior to the right jugular vein. There was no clinical or radiographic evidence of left sided disease. Clinical stage: T1N2b.

He was treated with single-modality radiation. The radiation plan was designed with IMRT, using seven beams. Only the right side was targeted. Three targets were defined: CTV_{HD} covered gross disease with margin, CTV_{ID} added additional margin to CTV_{HD} and also covered level II, while CTV_{ED} covered the right retropharyngeal nodes and the remaining uninvolved right upper nodal levels. Doses prescribed to CTV_{HD}, CTV_{ID}, and CTV_{ED} were 66 Gy, 60 Gy, and 54 Gy, respectively, and delivered in 30 fractions. Figure 9.6C–H are paired images showing the delineated contours with the associated isodose lines. Figure 9.6C is at the level of the maxillary tuberosity, where typically the superior aspect of CTV_{HD} for a tonsillar tumor is defined. Figure 9.6E shows the target delineation

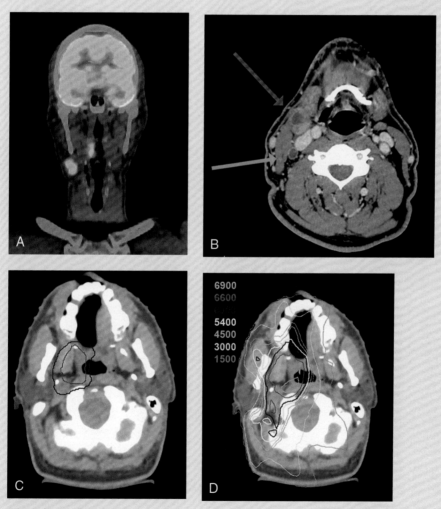

Case Figure 9.6 A–D

through the tonsillar tumor, and Figure 9.6G demonstrates the target delineation through the level II adenopathy.

An isocenter was placed just above the larynx, and a left anterior oblique field treated the lower neck nodes to 50 Gy. Figure 9.6I shows the lower neck field, and Figure 9.6J the associated isodose distribution.

He was last seen over 2 years out of therapy, doing well without disease.

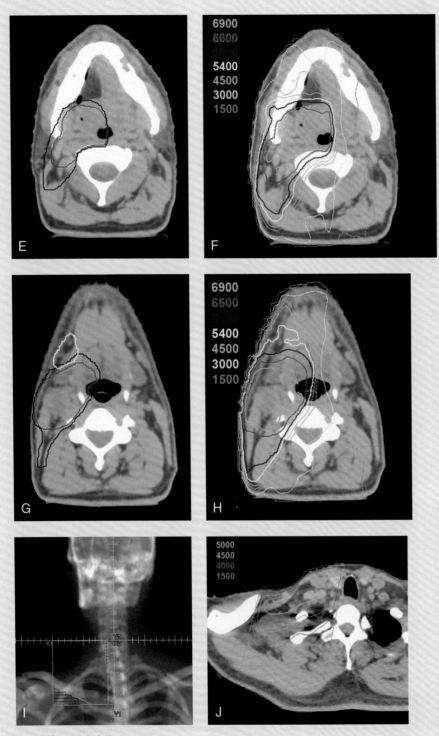

Case Figure 9.6 E–J

CASE STUDY 9.7

A 49-year-old man presented with several months of otalgia and sore throat. Examination revealed a right neck mass. A fine needle aspirate specimen of this mass was positive for poorly differentiated SCC. Physical examination revealed a 3-cm primary tumor located in the superior aspect of the right tonsil and extending onto the soft palate. There was no trismus. The neck examination revealed a 5-cm mass of matted lymph nodes. Stage T2 N2b M0. He was treated with radiation alone using concomitant boost regimen.

Treatment started with two lateral portals and an anterior portal matched at a single isocenter above the arytenoids as shown in Figure 9.7A,B. The large lateral portals received 41.4 Gy. To encompass the gross disease in the photon fields, for the off–spinal cord reduction and boost fields, parallel–opposed oblique fields were used. The posterior cervical strips were treated with 9 MeV electrons to 54 Gy. The boost was delivered concomitantly, 18 Gy in 12 fractions. The anterior field continued to 54 Gy with a full midline block inserted at 45 Gy to shield the spinal cord. The gross nodal disease in the mid neck was boosted with a posterior photon beam, matched at the single isocenter. Figure 9.7C,D shows digital reconstructions of the blocks for the boost fields with the GTV contoured.

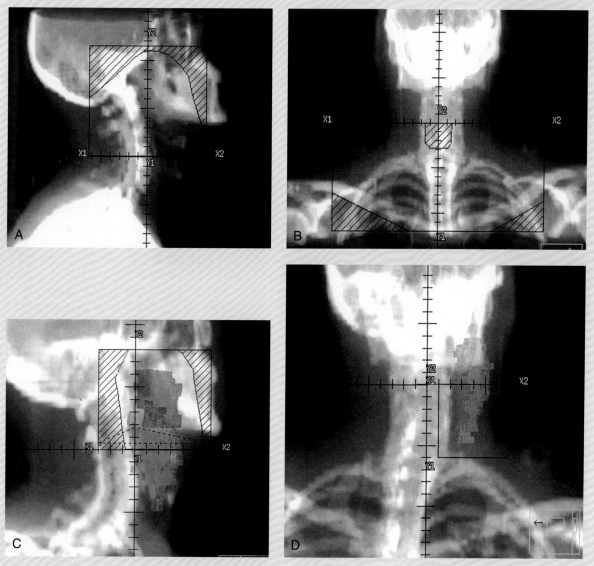

Case Figure 9.7 A–D

Axial views of the isodoses through the primary target (*T*) and through the mid neck are shown in Figure 9.7E,F. A selective right neck dissection was performed because a residual neck mass remained 6 weeks after completion of radiotherapy. Ten lymph nodes were removed from levels II and III, but none contained viable tumor.

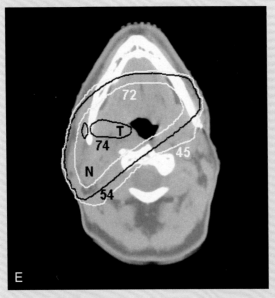

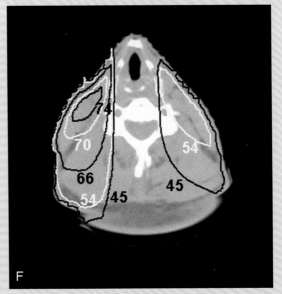

Case Figure 9.7 E,F

Intensity-Modulated Radiation Therapy Planning for Bilateral Treatment

IMRT has now been widely adopted for the treatment of patients requiring bilateral irradiation because of its potential for exclusion of a large portion of at least one of the parotid glands from the high-dose volume, thereby reducing xerostomia without compromising coverage of the primary tumor and draining lymphatics. The patient is immobilized in a supine position with an extended head and shoulder thermoplastic mask. Thin-cut CT scans are obtained in treatment position. The GTV, CTVs, and PTVs are outlined for dosimetric planning **(Case Study 9.8 through Case Study 9.11)**.

As for ipsilateral treatment, CTV_{HD} delineates the primary and nodal GTVs with 0.5- to 1-cm margins. CTV_{ID} extends an additional 1 cm beyond CTV_{HD} to include, for example, at least the retromolar trigone anteriorly, 1 cm of the adjacent base of tongue medially, and the remaining pterygoid muscle between CTV_{HD} and the mandible laterally. Margins are defined by the nature of tumor invasion and may include the inner cortex of the ascending ramus of the mandible and larger volume of tongue base, soft palate, or medial pterygoid muscle, etc. In the presence of positive node(s), CTV_{ID} encompasses the involved and adjoining nodal compartment(s).

CTV_{ED} delineates volumes to receive an elective dose for subclinical disease. In the N0 neck, CTV_{ED} includes nodal levels II to IV and retropharyngeal nodes. When level II node is involved, CTV_{ED} also includes clinically uninvolved ipsilateral level IB nodes. Level V is typically targeted in the node positive hemineck.

The primary tumor and nodal regions above the thyroid notch are irradiated with IMRT, and the lower neck nodes are irradiated with a matching anterior portal to allow shielding of the larynx. The presence of bulky level III nodes may necessitate treating all target volumes (primary tumor and neck nodes including level IV/V regions) using IMRT. With this technique, it is important to outline the larynx and esophagus (at least the arytenoids and esophageal inlet) as avoidance structures to minimize the dose to these organs, thus reducing the risk for long-term swallowing dysfunction and esophageal stricture.

Dose

Dose fractionation regimens used are similar to those presented in detail above in the "Soft Palate" Section. Briefly, for patients with T1 and superficial T2 N0: conventional technique delivering 50 Gy in 25 fractions to the initial target volume followed by 16 Gy in 8 fractions to the boost volume or IMRT administering 66 Gy to CTV_{HD} given in 30 fractions over 6 weeks.

For patients with larger tumors who do not receive systemic therapy: concomitant boost schedule to total doses of 72 Gy in 42 fractions or IMRT delivering 70 Gy to CTV_{HD} in 35 fractions over 6 weeks (1 day a week of twice-a-day irradiation) or a concomitant-type regimen (72 Gy in 42 fractions over 6 weeks), which requires two IMRT plans.

For patients with T3 to T4 or N2 to N3 tumors who receive systemic therapy: 70 Gy in 35 fractions over 7 weeks (when combined with three cycles of concurrent) or either 70 Gy given in 35 fractions over 6 weeks (1 day a week of twice-a-day irradiation) or 70 Gy to CTV_{HD} given in 33 fractions over 6.5 weeks

CASE STUDY 9.8

A 60-year-old man presented with an asymptomatic left neck mass. A fine needle aspiration showed metastatic SCC. Physical examination revealed a 3-cm exophytic left tonsillar mass and a 3-cm mobile left level II node. He received treatment with IMRT to a dose of 66 Gy in 30 fractions.

Figure 9.8 shows the GTVs (primary tonsillar tumor and solitary lymph node) contoured in colorwash along with axial isodose distributions at the levels of the pterygoids (Fig. 9.8A), mid-tonsil (Fig. 9.8B), inferior oropharyngeal wall and midlevel II (Fig. 9.8C), and a coronal isodose distribution through the tonsil tumor and involved lymph node (Fig. 9.8D). The IMRT fields were matched above the arytenoids to an anterior supraclavicular field with a larynx block, which delivered 50 Gy in 25 fractions. Left level III received additional irradiation to a total of 60 Gy (low neck dosimetry not shown). A selective neck dissection performed after radiotherapy revealed no residual disease. He had no evidence of disease at the last follow-up for over 2 years after treatment. He has been able to eat all types of foods including bread.

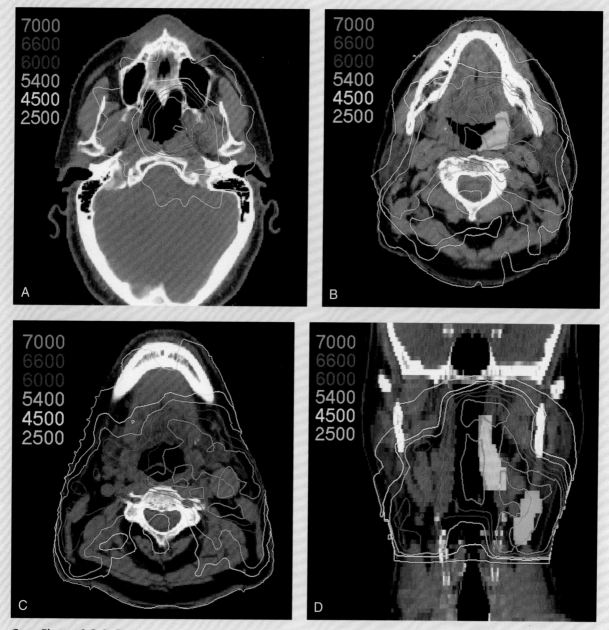

Case Figure 9.8 A–D

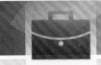

CASE STUDY 9.9

A 49-year-old male presented with excessive snoring and was found to have a right tonsillar mass. A biopsy was performed, and pathology revealed nonkeratinizing squamous cell carcinoma, HPV and p16 positive. A PET/CT was performed and demonstrated the bulky primary tumor as well as ipsilateral adenopathy (Fig. 9.9A). Small but avid nodes were detected in right levels II and III, and a 9-mm right retropharyngeal (RP) node was also thought to be suspicious. A coronal view of the patient's contrast CT scan demonstrates the bulky primary tumor

impinging into the parapharyngeal space and extending from the soft palate superiorly, to the level of the suprahyoid epiglottis inferiorly (Fig. 9.9B, *red arrows*). On physical examination, a 5-cm tumor was observed, and on palpation the tumor extended onto the lateral soft palate and glossopharyngeal sulcus. Clinical stage: T3N2b.

He was treated with IMRT using nine coplanar beams that encompassed the primary tumor and upper lymphatics. Figure 9.9C–H shows paired images of the contours and isodose distribution. The contour delineation

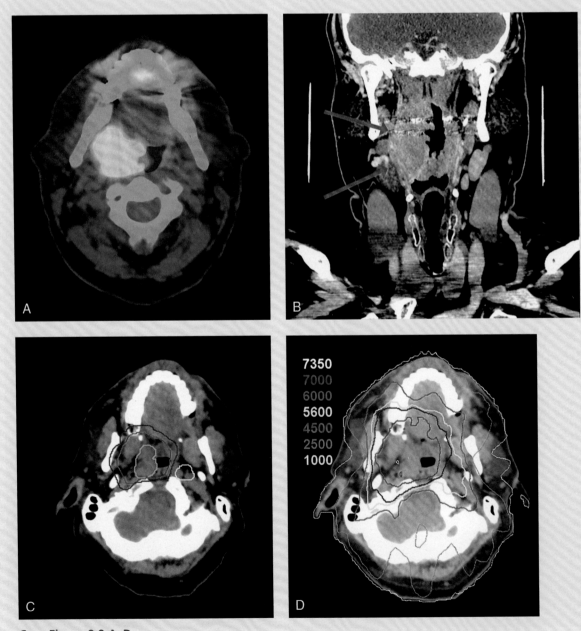

Case Figure 9.9 A–D

is as follows: vGTV, *green*, CTV$_{HD}$, *red*, CTV$_{ID}$, *blue*, and CTV$_{ED}$, *yellow*. CTV$_{HD}$ was defined as vGTV with 8- to 10-mm margin, CTV$_{ID}$ gave CTV$_{HD}$ an additional 3- to 5-mm margin and covered the upper right neck levels, and CTV$_{ED}$ covered the left-sided nodes including the left RP nodes and left level II. The doses prescribed to CTV$_{HD}$, CTV$_{ID}$, and CTV$_{ED}$ were 70 Gy, 60 Gy, and 56 Gy, respectively. Three axial views are shown: (1) a view through the superior aspect of the tonsil just posterior to the maxillary tuberosity (Fig. 9.9C,D). CTV$_{HD}$ covers not only the primary tumor but also the small RP node detected on pretreatment imaging, (2) a view at the middle of the tonsil, where the bulky tumor adjacent to the right ascending ramus of the right mandible can be seen (Fig. 9.9E,F), and (3) a view through the inferior aspect of the tumor,

just superior to the tip of the epiglottis (not shown), and medial to the upper neck levels (Fig. 9.9G,H). A coronal view of the isodose distribution through the tumor and adjacent tissues is shown in Figure 9.9I.

The IMRT treatment was matched above the level of the arytenoids with an anterior beam that treated level III and IV nodes. A larynx block was used for the first 40 Gy, and then a full midline block was used for an additional 10 Gy, to bring the total dose to both sides of the neck to 50 Gy. A glancing posterior photon beam boosted the right level III node an additional 10 Gy in 5 fractions. This was followed by an appositional 9 MeV beam to give a final boost to the right level III node of 6 Gy in 3 fractions.

The patient remains well without disease and minimal symptom burden nearly 3 years from treatment.

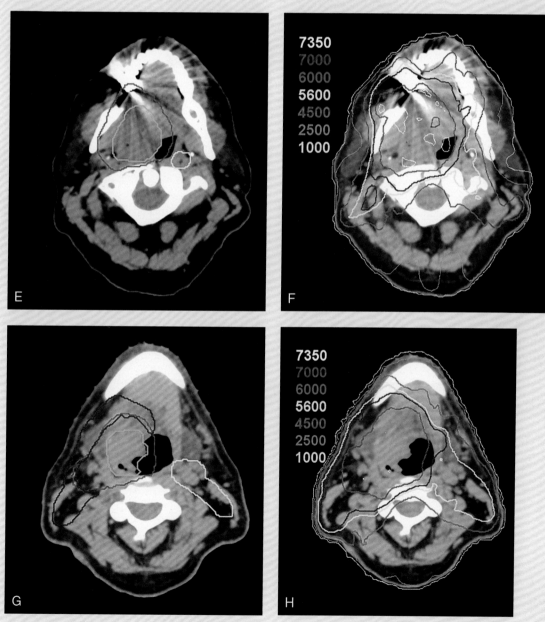

Case Figure 9.9 E–H

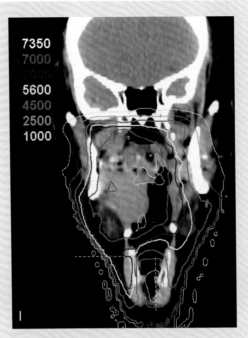

Case Figure 9.9 I

CASE STUDY 9.10

A 66-year-old male presented with a right upper neck mass without any associated symptoms. A fine needle aspiration of the mass was positive for SCC. Examination revealed a 4-cm neck mass and a 2.5-cm exophytic tumor of the inferior aspect of the right tonsil.

Figure 9.10A shows a representative slice of diagnostic CT scan, which confirmed the physical exam findings, demonstrating the involved node (*red arrow*) and the primary tonsillar tumor (*green arrow*). Stage: T2 N2a M0. As the primary tumor was relatively small (albeit T2) and

exophytic, he was treated with radiation alone. The pros and cons of ipsilateral versus bilateral irradiation were discussed with the treatment team and the patient, and it was decided to treat bilaterally.

GTV (primary, orange; node, magenta), CTV_{HD} (66 Gy), and CTV_{ID} (60 Gy), which encompassed additional 0.5- to 1-cm margins beyond CTV_{HD}, level IB, and the remainder of ipsilateral level II nodes, respectively, were delineated along with CTV_{ED} (54 Gy) that covered the retropharyngeal and left level II nodes. Figure 9.10B,C

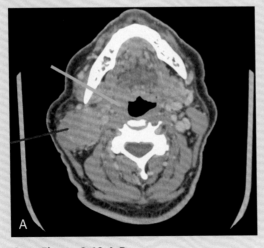
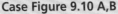
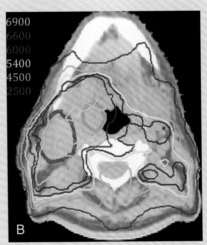

Case Figure 9.10 A,B

shows representative axial isodose distributions at the level of the mid-tonsil (Fig. 9.10B) and hyoid (Fig. 9.10C). The tumor and nodal GTVs are shown with thick orange and magenta lines, respectively.

The isocenter was placed above the thyroid notch, and the low neck was treated with an anterior beam. A larynx block was used for the first 40 Gy, and then a full midline block was added for 10 Gy. The ipsilateral level III node was boosted to 60 Gy with glancing photon fields and to 69 Gy with 9 MeV electrons as the inferior aspect of the node was split at isocenter. The electron treatments were delivered as second daily doses. Figure 9.10D shows the low neck photon field, the location of the match between the IMRT fields, and mid neck boost fields and the isodose distribution on a coronal view. The primary tumor and neck node had a complete response, so a neck dissection was not performed. The patient remains without disease over 5 years out from treatment.

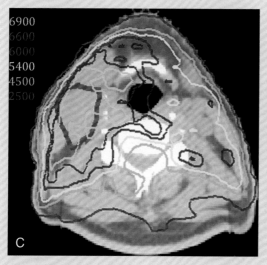
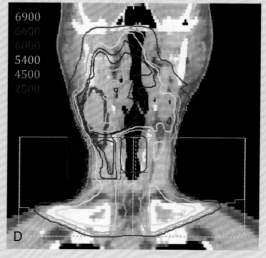

Case Figure 9.10 C,D

CASE STUDY 9.11

A 43-year-old woman presented with a right neck mass, right otalgia, and odynophagia. Physical examination revealed a bulky right tonsillar mass extending to the right lateral soft palate superiorly and to just above the pharyngoepiglottic fold inferiorly. Biopsy of the primary tumor revealed squamous cell cancer, positive for HPV.

Figure 9.11 shows slices of staging head and neck CT scan at the level of the ascending ramus of the mandible (Fig. 9.11A) and level II region (Fig. 9.11B) demonstrating the bulky primary tumor (*green arrow*) and the lymphadenopathy just posterior to the jugular vein (*red arrow*). She was treated with IMRT given in 33 fractions with concurrent high-dose cisplatin delivered on weeks 1, 4, and 7.

GTV, CTV_{HD} (70 Gy), and CTV_{ID} (62 Gy), which encompassed additional 0.5- to 1-cm margins beyond CTV_{HD} and the remainder of ipsilateral level II nodes, were delineated along with CTV_{ED} (57 Gy) that covered the retropharyngeal, level IB, and left level II nodes. Figure 9.11 also shows representative axial isodose distributions at the level of the pterygoid plates (Fig. 9.11C), epicenter of the primary tumor (Fig. 9.11D), and level II neck (Fig. 9.11E), and a coronal view with the tumor GTV outlined in thick red line (Fig. 9.11F).

The isocenter was placed above the thyroid notch, and the low neck was treated with an anterior beam. A larynx block was used for the first 40 Gy, and then a full midline block was added for 10 Gy. The right level III node was boosted to 60 Gy with glancing photon fields. An axial view of the isodose distribution at the level of the mid neck is shown in Figure 9.11G. The patient did well and is without disease 6 years later.

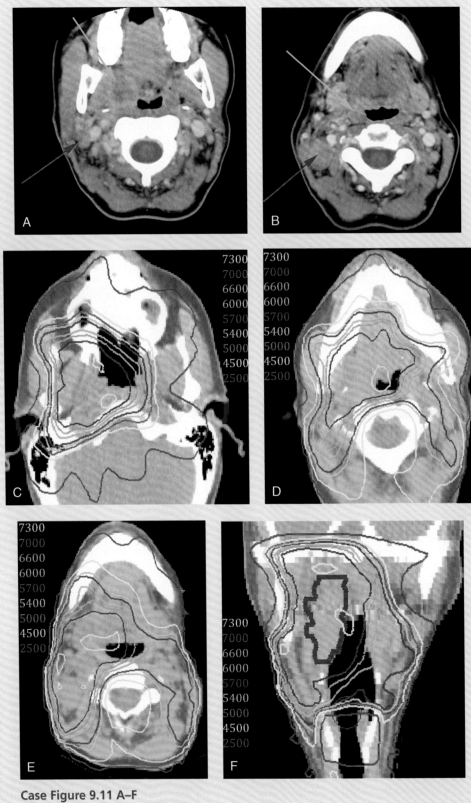

Case Figure 9.11 A–F

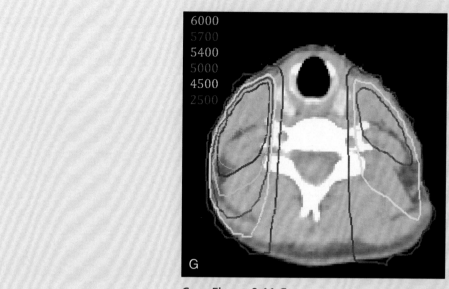

Case Figure 9.11 G

when combined with two cycles of high-dose cisplatin or weekly cetuximab.

Postoperative Radiotherapy

Adjuvant radiotherapy is indicated in occasional patients treated with upfront surgery. There are two distinct scenarios. The first is patients who are operated for locally advanced tumors, typically with open procedures, and often with reconstruction. In this setting, the principles of postoperative radiation are similar to those for the treatment of retromolar trigone or posterior oral cavity tumors as presented in detail in Chapter 7.

The second scenario is in patients who are operated using minimally invasive techniques with intraoral approaches for small tumors. If the indication for therapy is based on adverse features of the primary tumor, and the neck dissection is negative, treatment can be delivered to the primary site only. If the indication for therapy is due to adverse features discovered in the neck pathology, our current approach is to treat the primary site and neck. Investigations are ongoing to determine if the primary site is excised without concerning findings, whether treatment can be directed to the neck only.

Target Volume

With conventional techniques, the initial target volume encompasses the entire surgical bed and all nodal areas of the neck. The boost volume encompasses areas of known disease location with 1- to 2-cm margins. If IMRT is used, the delineation of CTV_{HD}, CTV_{ID} and CTV_{ED} as described for oral cavity cancers (Chapter 7) is applied. If postoperative radiation is planned after minimally invasive surgery, a vGTV (virtual gross target volume) based on the clinical, radiographic, and surgical/pathologic findings is defined. CTV_{HD} is delineated by adding an additional 5 to 10 mm to the vGTV. CTV_{ID} covers the CTV_{HD} with an additional 3 to 5 mm margin, and the remainder of the tonsillar region. CTV_{ID} also covers the operated neck, not delineated as CTV_{HD}. CTV_{ED} is defined as the remaining tissues at risk not defined in the higher dose volumes, in particular lymph node–bearing areas not operated. Decisions regarding ipsilateral versus bilateral neck treatment post minimally invasive surgery are based on disease extent similar to the definitive setting.

Setup and Field Arrangement

The general technique is the same as that described under Primary Radiotherapy. Marking of the external surgical scar facilitates portal design.

Dose

- A dose of 60 Gy in 30 fractions to areas with high-risk features; that is, close or microscopically positive margins, perineural extension, vascular invasion, positive nodes, or extranodal extension. An additional boost dose of 6 Gy may be given when indicated, such as when multiple adverse features are present or when the interval between surgery and radiation is much longer than 6 weeks.
- A dose of 56 Gy in 28 fractions to the surgical bed.
- A dose of 50 Gy in 25 fractions to undissected regions to receive elective irradiation.

Similar dosing is applied if IMRT is used with treatment typically delivered in 30 fractions. CTV_{HD}, CTV_{ID}, and CTV_{ED} are prescribed 60 Gy, 57Gy, and 54 Gy, respectively. The ECOG-ACRIN Cancer Research Group is currently randomizing patients who are deemed to require postoperative radiation following transoral robotic surgery for HPV-associated oropharyngeal cancers and do not have high-risk features (positive margins or extracapsular extension) to 50 Gy versus 60 Gy. Patients with high-risk features are treated to 60 Gy with concurrent chemotherapy. Whether

TABLE 9.6 Local Control Analysis in 150 Patients with Tonsil Carcinoma Treated at the M.D. Anderson Cancer Center

Tumor Stage	All Patients	Evaluable Patients[a]			
	Local Control After XRT (%)	Local Control After XRT (%)	Salvage Surgery	Local Control After Surgery	Ultimate Local Control (%)
T1	16/17 (94)	15/16 (94)	1	1/1	16/16 (100)
T2	48/59 (81)	41/52 (79)	6	3/6	44/52 (85)
T3	44/66 (67)	30/52 (58)	10	1/10	31/52 (60)
T4	5/8 (63)	3/6 (50)	1	0/1	3/6 (50)
Total	113/150 (75)	89/126 (71)	18	5/18	94/126 (75)

Note: July 1968 to December 1983; Analysis, December 1986.
XRT, radiation therapy.
[a]Twenty-four patients who died within 2 years from date of irradiation without local failure are excluded from analysis of local control. Length of follow-up after salvage ranges from 26 to 162 months.
From Wong CS, Ang KK, Fletcher GH, et al. Primary radiotherapy for squamous cell carcinoma of the tonsillar fossa. *Int J Radiat Oncol Biol Phys* 1989;16:657–662, with permission.

patients with high-risk features require chemotherapy is subject to debate, and many now quantify ECE; nodes with ECE < 1 mm from the capsule are not considered high risk.

Timing of Postoperative Radiotherapy

It is desirable to commence postoperative radiotherapy as soon as possible after healing of surgical wounds. With good communication between surgical, radiation, and dental oncologists, simulation can usually take place 3 to 4 weeks after surgery, and radiotherapy can start within a week in most patients. When minimally invasive surgery is performed on a tonsillar cancer, sufficient time must be allowed for the wound to heal to avoid chronic soft tissue necrosis.

Background Data

See Tables 9.6 to 9.8.

TABLE 9.7 Patterns of Failure in Patients Irradiated for Tonsillar Carcinoma from 2003 to 2012

		HPV+ (n = 325)							
		Pattern of Failure							
	Total	None	L	R	D	LR	LD	RD	LRD
T1	104	97	1	1	3	1	0	0	1
T2	123	112	1	2	5	0	1	1	1
T3	58	47	1	0	3	2	1	3	1
T4A	38	29	4	1	0	1	1	1	1
T4B	2	0	0	0	2	0	0	0	0

TABLE 9.7 Patterns of Failure in Patients Irradiated for Tonsillar Carcinoma from 2003 to 2012 *(Continued)*

	Total	All (n = 755)							
		None	L	R	D	LR	LD	RD	LRD
T1	228	210	3	5	7	2	0	0	1
T2	260	228	8	3	15	2	1	1	2
T3	129	98	8	1	10	6	2	3	1
T4A	132	87	12	3	9	10	4	4	3
T4B	6	1	0	0	2	1	0	0	2

HPV+, Human papillomavirus related; All, HPV status not tested; None, No evidence of recurrence; L, Local; R, Regional; D, Distant. Adapted from raw data from Dahlstrom KR, Garden AS, William WN Jr, et al. Proposed staging system for patients with HPV-related oropharyngeal cancer based on nasopharyngeal cancer N categories. *J Clin Oncol* 2016;34(16):1848–1854.

TABLE 9.8 Contralateral Neck Failure in Patients with Tonsillar Carcinoma Treated with Ipsilateral Radiation

First Author	Patient Number	Patients with T3–T4 Disease (%)	Patients Node Negative (%)	Contralateral Neck Recurrences
Jackson	178	38	58	4
O'Sullivan	228	16	57	5
Rusthoven	20	10	0	0
Chronowski	102	0	32	2
Liu	58	32	25	0

Data from Jackson SM, et al. *Radiother Oncol* 1999;51:123; O'Sullivan B, et al. *Int J Radiat Oncol Biol Phys* 2001;51:332; Rusthoven KE, et al. *Int J Radiat Oncol Biol Phys* 2009;74:1365; Chronowski GM, et al. *Int J Radiat Oncol Biol Phys* 2012;83:204; Liu C, et al. *Head Neck* 2014;36:317.

BASE OF TONGUE

Treatment Strategy

Similar to carcinoma of the tonsil, primary radiotherapy is a very effective treatment for T1 to T2 N0 to N1 carcinomas. With the increasing popularity of minimally invasive intraoral approaches, surgery for base of tongue carcinomas is being performed more frequently at many centers. Surgery may be preferred if there is a high probability that single-modality therapy will suffice. Combination of radiation with systemic therapy is the treatment of choice for T3 and selected T4 or N2 to N3 tumors. As presented in Chapter 1, concurrent cisplatin is favored, and cetuximab is approved for patients who cannot receive cisplatin.

Patients presenting with N2 to N3 nodal disease achieving a complete clinical and radiographic response do not require a planned neck dissection.

T4a tumors extending into the deep muscles of the tongue or soft tissue of the neck or those causing swallowing or laryngeal dysfunction, for example, can be considered for surgery followed by adjuvant radiotherapy and, in the presence of extracapsular extension or positive margin, combined with concurrent cisplatin. However, surgery for these advanced tumors is often prohibitively morbid, so particularly for HPV-positive tumors, definitive concurrent chemotherapy and radiation is often preferred.

Primary Radiotherapy

Target Volume

The margins of tongue-base carcinomas are frequently less well defined due to the presence of lymphoid tissues. Therefore, the initial target volume encompasses the base of tongue with a generous margin toward oral tongue, vallecula, epiglottis, superior preepiglottic space, lateral oropharyngeal walls, and bilateral neck nodes, including the retropharyngeal nodes, and level II, III, and IV nodes. The target volume also includes ipsilateral level IB in the presence of level II node. Level V is often included in the node positive hemineck. The margins are more generous in infiltrative lesions.

The boost volume encompasses the primary tumor and involved nodes with 1- to 2-cm margins.

Setup and Field Arrangement for Conventional Radiation Technique (Case Study 9.12)

An intraoral stent is frequently used to open the mouth and to depress and immobilize the tongue. The patient is immobilized in a supine position with a thermoplastic mask. Lateral

CASE STUDY 9.12

A 67-year-old man presented with mild sore throat. Physical examination revealed a 5-cm exophytic mass occupying the left base of tongue with extension to the vallecula and crossing the midline. The tongue mobility was normal, and there was no adenopathy. A biopsy was positive for invasive grade 2 SCC. Stage T3 N0 M0. He was treated with radiation alone using concomitant boost fractionation.

Treatment started with two lateral (Fig. 9.12A) and an anterior (Fig. 9.12B) portals matched at a single isocenter localized at the top of the arytenoids. A spinal cord

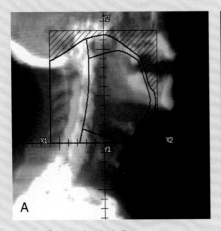
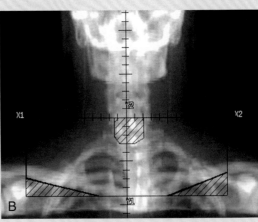

Case Figure 9.12 A,B

reduction was made at 41.4 Gy, and the boost dose was delivered through parallel–opposed fields. All portals received radiation with 6 MV photons, except that the right lateral boost portal was irradiated with 18 MV pho-

tons to minimize hot spot in the right mandible and soft tissues. Representative isodose distribution through the tumor (*T*) irradiated to 72 Gy is shown in (Fig. 9.12C) and that of the low neck field to 54 Gy in (Fig. 9.12D).

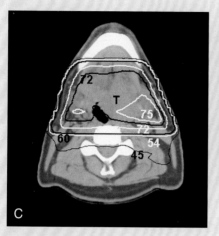
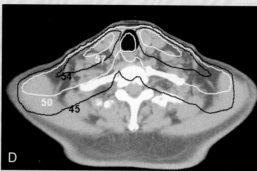

Case Figure 9.12 C,D

parallel–opposed photon fields are used for treatment of the primary tumor and upper neck nodes.

- *Anterior border:* at least 2 cm anterior to the palpable tumor border.
- *Superior border:* to include the retropharyngeal and level II nodes.
- *Posterior border:* just behind the spinous processes or more posteriorly in the presence of a large nodal mass.
- *Inferior border:* just above the arytenoids or lower in the presence of vallecula or preepiglottic space involvement.

A matching anterior appositional photon field is used for elective treatment of the mid and lower neck nodes.

For the boost volume, the lateral portals are reduced to include the primary tumor with 1- to 2-cm margin and involved upper neck nodes. Nodal disease outside the primary boost field is treated with appositional electron field or anterior–posterior glancing photon fields.

Intensity-Modulated Radiation Therapy

IMRT has now been widely adopted for treatment of base of tongue cancer. With careful planning, it can exclude many normal structures, allowing for less late toxicity.

The patient is immobilized in a supine position with an extended head and shoulder thermoplastic mask. For patients in whom disease does not extend into the tonsillar fossa, the use of a mouth opening, tongue depressing stent can help in reducing the dose to the palate and maxilla. Thin-cut CT scans are obtained in treatment position. The GTV, CTVs, and PTVs are outlined for dosimetric planning **(Case Study 9.13 through Case Study 9.16).**

Clinical Target Volume

Three CTVs are generally delineated.

- CTV_{HD} delineates volumes to receive the highest dose, which includes the primary tumor GTV with 1- to 2-cm margins and nodal GTV with 0.5- to 1-cm margins. For T1 tumors where GTV is difficult to visualize on imaging, 2-cm thickness of the base of tongue from the posterior edge is included.
- CTV_{ID} delineates volumes to receive an intermediate dose, which includes an additional 1-cm margin beyond the CTV_{HD} coverage. Except for very small volume primary tumors that are well lateralized or only involving the most superior or inferior aspects of the base of tongue, CTV_{ID} includes the remaining base of tongue. When tumor extends close to or into the vallecula or involves the pharyngoepiglottic fold, CTV_{ID} includes the superior preepiglottic space or the lateral supraglottic larynx and vestibule of the pyriform sinus. In the presence of positive node(s), CTV_{ID} encompasses the positive and adjoining nodal compartment(s).
- CTV_{ED} delineates volumes to receive an elective dose for subclinical disease. In the N0 neck, CTV_{ED} includes nodal levels II to IV and retropharyngeal nodes. When level II node is involved, CTV_{ED} also includes clinically uninvolved ipsilateral level IB nodes. Level V is often included in the node positive hemineck.

Dose

Dose fractionation regimens used are similar to those presented in detail above in the "Soft Palate" Section. Briefly, for patients with T1 and superficial T2 N0: conventional technique delivering 50 Gy in 25 fractions to the initial target volume followed by

CASE STUDY 9.13

A 51-year-old man presented with a left upper neck mass. Mistaken for a branchial cleft cyst, the mass was excised, but histologic examination revealed SCC, without obvious extracapsular extension. Postexcision CT scan did not reveal obvious disease. He underwent an examination under anesthesia and a small tumor was found in the base of tongue and was biopsy positive for SCC. Stage: T1 Nx (1) M0.

He received primary IMRT. The GTV was determined based on the clinical exam, as it was not appreciated on imaging. CTV_{HD} (66 Gy) covered GTV with generous margin and the nodal excision bed. CTV_{ID} (60 Gy) encompassed additional 0.5- to 1.5-cm margins beyond CTV_{HD} and also included level IB and the remainder of level II nodes ipsilaterally. CTV_{ED} (54 Gy) covered the retropharyngeal and contralateral level II nodes. Isocenter was placed above the thyroid notch, and the low neck was treated with an anterior beam. A larynx block was used for the first 40 Gy, and then a full midline block was added for 10 Gy. The ipsilateral level III node was boosted to 60 Gy with glancing photon fields.

Figure 9.13 shows in colorwash the CTV_{HD} (base of tongue, *orange*; neck, *aqua*), CTV_{ID} (*forest green*), and CTV_{ED} (*purple*) on the CT images along with isodose distributions in representative axial (Fig. 9.13A), sagittal (Fig. 9.13B), and coronal (Fig. 9.13C,D) views. Treatment was delivered in 30 fractions. He remained without disease 4 years from treatment with only mild xerostomia.

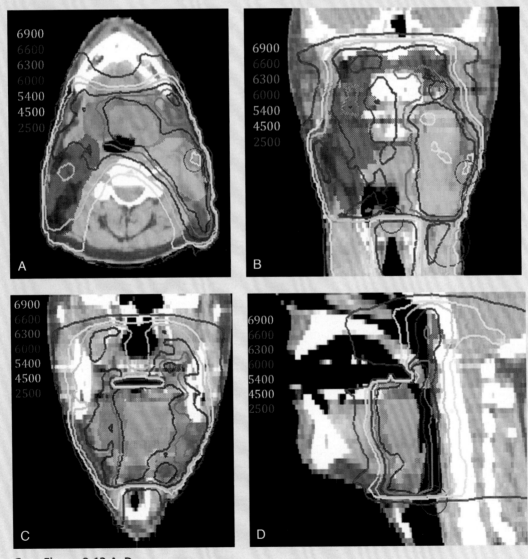

Case Figure 9.13 A–D

CASE STUDY 9.14

A 53-year-old man presented with complaints of spitting up blood, food getting stuck in his throat on swallowing, and right otalgia. He was found to have a base of tongue mass, which was biopsied. Pathology revealed squamous cell carcinoma, HPV and P16 positive.

A CT scan was performed, and revealed the bulky primary tumor, 4.3 cm in greatest dimension (Fig. 9.14A,B, *red arrows*), and bilateral adenopathy with cystic nodes (Fig. 9.14A, *green arrows*).

Clinical Stage: T3N2c.

He was treated with IMRT using VMAT, with 2 arcs. Figure 9.14C–N shows paired images of the contours and isodose distribution. The contour delineation is as follows: vGTV, *green* (primary tumor, *dark green* and nodes, *light green*), CTV$_{HD}$, *red*, CTV$_{ID}$, *blue*, and CTV$_{ED}$, *yellow*. CTV$_{HD}$ was defined as vGTV with 8- to 10-mm margin, CTV$_{ID}$ gave CTV$_{HD}$ an additional 3- to 5-mm margin and covered the involved and adjacent neck levels not included in CTV$_{HD}$, and CTV$_{ED}$ covered the retropharyngeal nodes and the uninvolved nodes in left

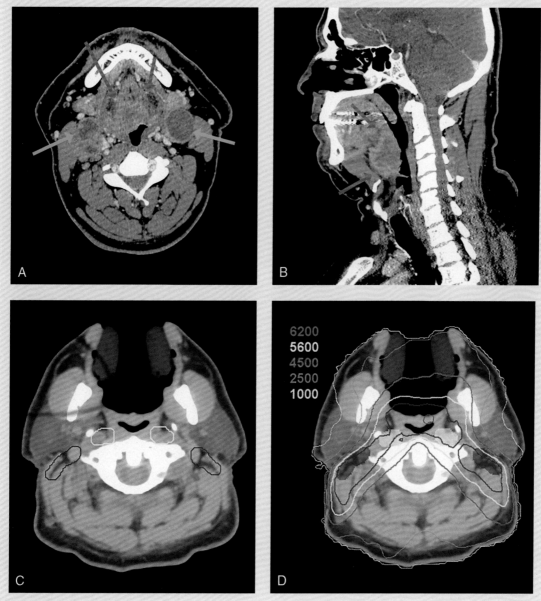

Case Figure 9.14 A–D

levels III and IV and right level IV. The doses prescribed to CTV_{HD}, CTV_{ID}, and CTV_{ED} were 70 Gy, 62 Gy, and 56 Gy, respectively. Four axial views are shown: (1) a view at C1 (Fig. 9.14C,D), at the level of the retropharyngeal nodes and parotid glands, (2) a view at the middle of the base of tongue, where the bulky tumor and bilateral neck nodes can be seen (Fig. 9.14E,F), (3) a view through the inferior aspect of the tumor, just superior to the vallecula. The primary tumor can be seen abutting the epiglottis (Fig. 9.14G,H), and (4) a view at the level of the larynx and level III. The small right level III node is seen, while left level III is uninvolved (Fig. 9.14I,J). In Figure 9.14J, the isodose lines are shown. As the right neck node was small, and this level approximates the superior aspect of the brachial plexus, the plan was accepted even though coverage of the entirety of the CTV (and PTV) was pinched. Often, with small nodes in level III and IV, particularly in patients with HPV-associated disease, we will create a 4th CTV that prescribes 65 to 66 Gy to lower the dose to the brachial plexus.

Coronal and sagittal views of the contours and isodose distribution through the tumor and adjacent tissues are shown in Figure 9.14K–M. On the sagittal view, the benefit of the mouth opening stent displacing the majority of the superior oral cavity can be appreciated.

The patient is doing well 2 years after treatment.

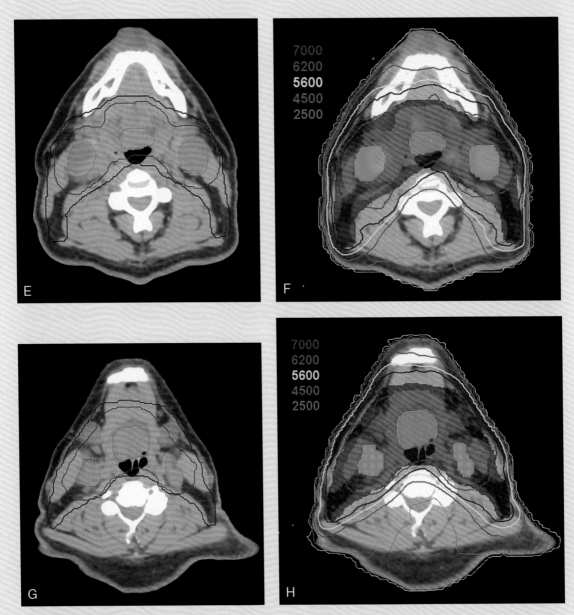

Case Figure 9.14 E–H

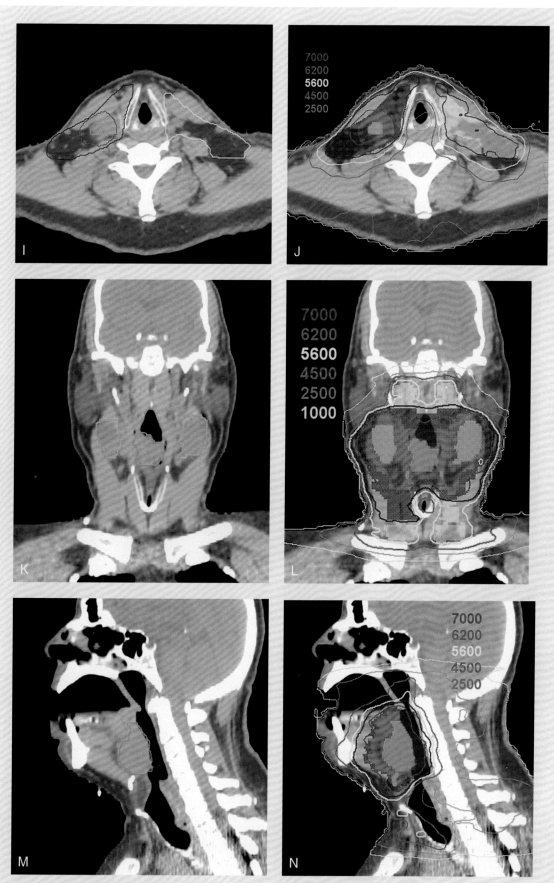

Case Figure 9.14 I–N

CASE STUDY 9.15

A 58-year-old woman presented with an asymptomatic right neck mass. Examination revealed an exophytic mass, over 4 cm, in the middle of base of tongue, involving both sides and extending to the valleculae. Biopsy was positive for SCC. Neck examination revealed bilateral adenopathy, a 5-cm level II and III right neck mass and a 3-cm left level II node. Stage T3 N2c M0. She was treated with concurrent cisplatin and conventional radiation (70 Gy in 35 fractions). IMRT was chosen because it was anticipated to provide a better distribution to the bilateral adenopathy that was located deep in the neck in additional to sparing salivary glands.

Figure 9.15 shows representative axial isodose distribution (Fig. 9.15A) through the base of tongue tumor (*T*) and bilateral nodes (*N*) along with a sagittal isodose (Fig. 9.15B) through the midplane including the primary (*T*). The patient had residual bilateral masses 6 weeks after treatment. She underwent bilateral neck dissections and examination under anesthesia. No residual primary tumor was detected. All 29 dissected nodes had fibrosis and treatment effects with no detectable viable tumor cells. She remained without disease 4 years from posttreatment.

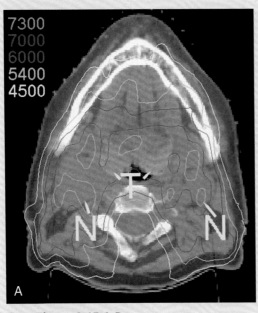
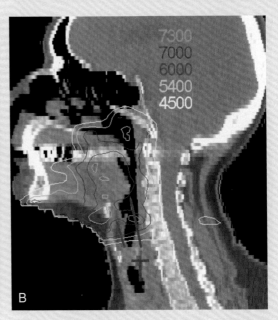

Case Figure 9.15 A,B

CASE STUDY 9.16

A 66-year-old man presented with a right upper neck mass. Examination revealed a 3-cm level II node and a base of tongue tumor, >4 cm. Fine needle aspiration of the node showed SCC.

Figure 9.16A,B shows representative diagnostic CT scan slices demonstrating an exophytic right base of tongue tumor (*green arrow*) extending across midline (Fig. 9.16A), to the valleculae (Fig. 9.16B), and to the lingual surface of the epiglottis. These images also revealed

nodal disease (*red arrow*) just anterior to the right jugular vein (Fig. 9.16A) and, at the level of the hyoid, in between the vein and the submandibular salivary gland.

He was treated with IMRT with three cycles of concurrent high-dose cisplatin. Because of the laryngeal involvement, it was decided to treat all target volumes with IMRT, rather than matching IMRT to an anterior lower neck portal above the thyroid notch. Figure 9.16C–L shows axial CTVs paired with corresponding isodose distributions from the retropharyngeal region to the level IV nodal region. Prescribed doses were 70 Gy to CTV$_{HD}$ (*red*), 63 Gy to CTV$_{ID}$ (*blue*), and 56 Gy to CTV$_{ED}$ (*yellow*) given in 35 fractions over 7 weeks.

Figure 9.16M,N shows sagittal and coronal isodose distributions through the primary tumor. He remained without disease and had good function 5 years out from treatment.

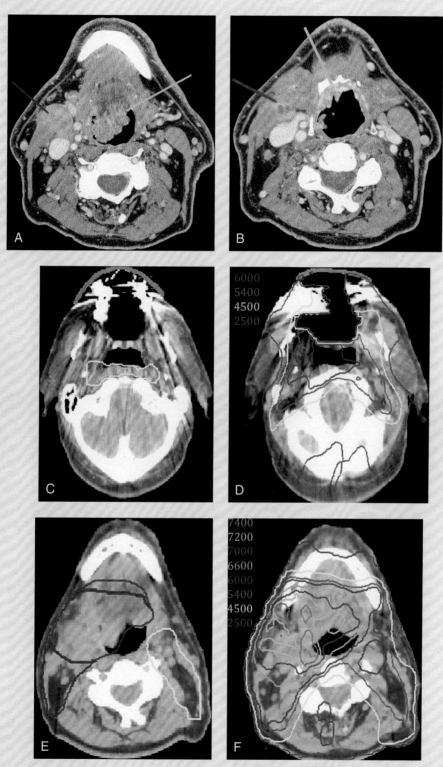

Case Figure 9.16 A–F

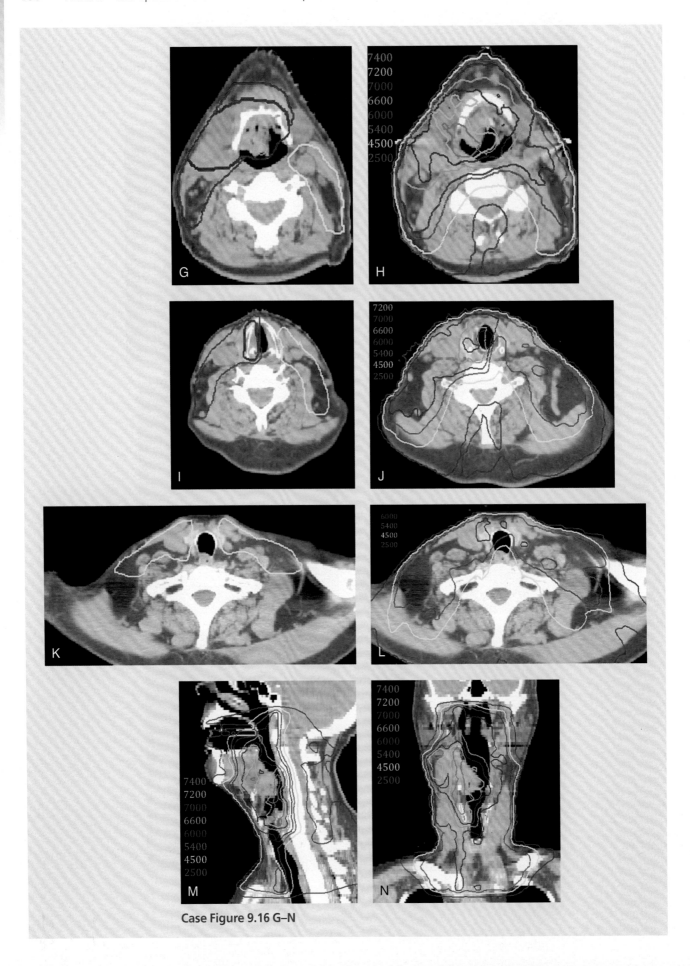

Case Figure 9.16 G–N

16 Gy in eight fractions to the boost volume or IMRT administering 66 Gy to CTV_{HD} given in 30 fractions over 6 weeks.

For patients with larger tumors who do not receive systemic therapy: options are (1) 70 Gy to CTV_{HD}, 63 Gy to CTV_{ID}, and 56 Gy to CTV_{ED} given in 35 fractions over 6 weeks (1 day a week of twice-a-day irradiation), (2) 70 Gy to CTV_{HD}, 60 Gy to CTV_{ID}, and 57 Gy to CTV_{ED} given in 33 fractions over 6.5 weeks, or (3) a concomitant boost-type regimen, which requires two IMRT plans (see IMRT Section of Chapter 1).

For patients with T3 to T4 or N2 to N3 tumors who receive systemic therapy: 70 Gy in 35 fractions over 7 weeks (when combined with three cycles of concurrent cisplatin) or either 70 Gy given in 35 fractions over 6 weeks (1 day a week of twice-a-day irradiation) or 70 Gy to CTV_{HD} given in 33 fractions over 6.5 weeks when combined with two cycles of high-dose cisplatin or weekly cetuximab.

Postoperative Radiotherapy

Adjuvant radiotherapy is indicated in occasional patients treated with upfront surgery. The principles are similar to those described in the section "Tonsillar Fossa."

Target Volume

The initial target volume encompasses the surgical bed and the entire neck. In patients who have had laryngectomy, the initial target volume includes the tracheal stoma if there is tumor extension into the soft tissues of the neck (including nodes with extracapsular extension), or the patient underwent an emergency tracheostomy prior to resection.

The boost volume encompasses areas of known disease locations with 1- to 2-cm margins.

For patients who are operated with intraoral techniques for smaller tumors, a vGTV is recreated from the surgical, radiographic, and pathologic findings. A 0.5- to 1.5-cm margin is placed around this primary vGTV to define a CTVHD.

An addition 5 mm is taken for subclinical targets at the primary site. Neck targets are similar to that described in the section "Tonsillar Fossa."

Setup and Field Arrangement

The general technique is the same as that described under "Primary Radiotherapy." Marking of the external surgical scar facilitates portal design. The *anterior* and *superior field borders* or CTVs are mainly determined by the local spread of the primary tumor and the extent of surgery (scar/flap).

Dose

- 60 Gy in 30 fractions to areas with high-risk features, that is, close or microscopically positive margins, perineural extension, vascular invasion, positive nodes, or extranodal extension. An additional boost dose of 6 Gy may be given when indicated, for example, when multiple adverse features are present or when the interval between surgery and radiotherapy is much longer than 6 weeks.
- 56 Gy in 28 fractions to the surgical bed.
- 50 Gy in 25 fractions to undissected regions to receive elective irradiation.

Similar dosing is applied if IMRT is used with treatment typically delivered in 30 fractions. CTV_{HD}, CTV_{ID}, and CTV_{ED} are prescribed 60 Gy, 57 Gy, and 54 Gy, respectively. The ECOG-ACRIN Cancer Research Group is currently randomizing patients who are deemed to require postoperative radiation following transoral robotic surgery for HPV- associated oropharyngeal cancers and do not have high-risk features (positive margins or extracapsular extension) to 50 Gy versus 60 Gy. Patients with high-risk features are treated to 60 Gy with concurrent chemotherapy. Whether patients with high-risk features require chemotherapy is subject to debate, and many now quantify ECE; nodes with ECE < 1 mm from the capsule are not considered high risk **(Case Study 9.17)**.

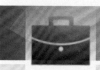

CASE STUDY 9.17

A 56-year-old male presented an with asymptomatic right neck mass. A fine needle aspiration was performed on a right neck node in level II and revealed metastatic squamous cell carcinoma, p16 positive. On physical examination, in addition to the node, a suspicious abnormality was seen in the inferior right base of tongue. The subtle abnormality can be appreciated on the contrast CT scan (Fig. 9.17A, *red* arrow), though it is better appreciated with hindsight. The staging PET/CT revealed the small lesion with SUV 6.9 (Fig. 9.17B). Two nodes were appreciated in level II, with maximum SUV 12.3.

He was dispositioned for treatment with transoral robotic surgery (TORS) with a right neck dissection (levels II to IV). Pathology revealed the primary tumor to be 3 mm, with negative margins, and the neck dissection recovered 38 lymph nodes, 2 of which were positive. There was no extracapsular extension (ECE).

Per ECOG definitions, he was determined to be at intermediate risk due to the two nodes. vGTVs of the nodes and primary were determined based on all the clinical, surgical, and pathologic findings. Only two CTVs were defined; CTV_{HD} and CTV_{ED}. Per the ECOG trial, patients are treated with sequential plans, so all targets are treated at 2 Gy to 50 Gy and then CTV_{HD} is boosted 10 Gy to a total dose of 60 Gy. CTV_{HD} is the vGTV with an approximately 5 mm margin, and CTV_{ED} covers the uninvolved bilateral cervical lymphatics (levels II to IV) and the ipsilateral retropharyngeal nodes. Figure 9.17C–E demonstrates the contours and isodose distributions in the axial, coronal, and sagittal planes, respectively. The targets are shown in colorwash: vGTV primary *light green*, vGTV nodes, *dark green*, CTV_{HD} *red* and CTV_{ED} *yellow*.

The patient remains well over 1 year from therapy with minimal toxicity.

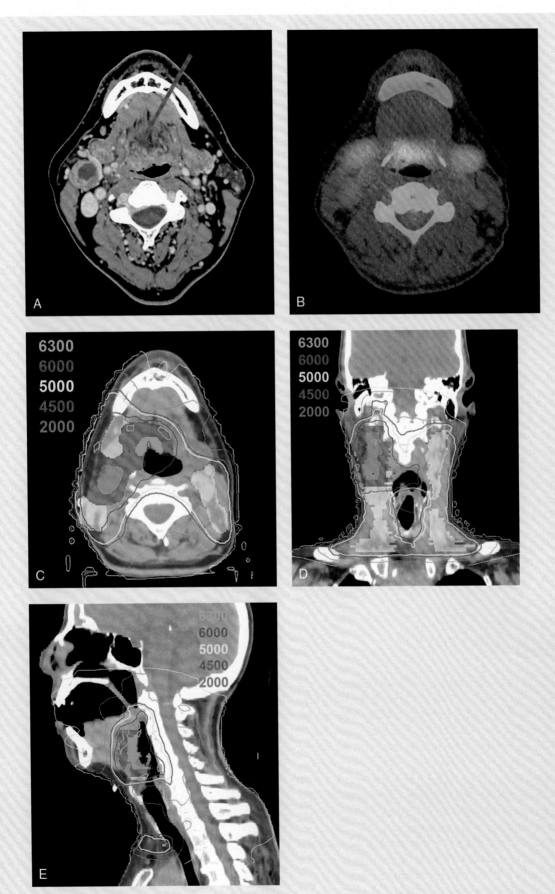

Case Figure 9.17 A–E

Timing of Postoperative Radiotherapy

It is desirable to commence postoperative radiotherapy as soon as possible after healing of surgical wounds. With good communication between surgical, radiation, and dental oncologists, simulation can usually take place 3 to 4 weeks after surgery, and radiotherapy can start within a week in most patients. When delayed wound healing postpones commencement of postoperative radiation to beyond 5 to 6 weeks, we administer accelerated fractionation, such as concomitant boost, by delivering twice-a-day irradiations for 5 treatment days, either once a week or daily toward the end of the radiation course, to reduce the potential hazard of prolonged cumulative treatment time.

However, commencing treatment too soon after tonsillectomy or intraoral surgery prior to the wound healing can lead to soft tissue necrosis. Wound healing may require 4 to 6 weeks, but as the majority of these patients have favorable prognoses, and many get concurrent chemotherapy, the need to accelerate radiation in the event of delay is moot.

Background Data

See Tables 9.9 and 9.10.

TABLE 9.9 Local Control ("Local Nonfailure") and Complications Following Curative Irradiation for Base of Tongue Carcinoma: Literature Review

Author, Year, Institution	Boost Technique	Local Control[a] by T Stage				Incidence of Soft Tissue ± Bone Necrosis[b]
		T1	T2	T3	T4	
Housset et al., 1987, Hopital Necker, Paris, France	Implant	6/6	17/23 (74%)	—	—	3/29 (10%)
Puthawala et al., 1988, Memorial Med. Center, Long Beach, California	Implant	2/2	14/16 (88%)	30/40 (75%)	8/12 (67%)	10/70 (14%)
Crook et al., 1988, Hopital Henri Mondor, Creteil, France	Implant	11/13 (85%)	25/35 (71%)	—	—	12/48 (25%)
Lusinchi et al., 1988, Inst. Gustave Roussy, Paris, France	Implant	15/18 (83%)	20/39 (51%)	35/51 (69%)	—	29/108 (27%)
Sessions et al., 1988, Memorial-Sloan Kettering, New York	Implant	4/4	5/6	5/6	1/1	6/17 (35%)
Goffinet et al., 1988, Stanford Univ., Stanford, California	Implant	4/5	7/7	9/10	5/7	8/29 (28%)[c]
Spanos et al., 1976, M.D. Anderson, Houston, Texas	External beam	29/32 (91%)	35/49 (71%)	50/64 (78%)	15/29 (52%)	15/91 (16%)[d]
Jaulerry et al., 1991, Curie Institute, Paris, France	External beam	21/22 (95%)	25/45 (56%)	26/64	4/31	ND
Mendenhall et al., 2000, Univ. of Florida, Gainesville, Florida	External beam	29[e] (96%)	76 (91%)	70 (81%)	42 (38%)	8/217 (4%)[f]

[a]No. continuously free of disease at the primary site/total no. treated.
[b]All degrees of severity.
[c]Three patients with development of hemorrhage are included.
[d]Bone only.
[e]Total patients and 5-year actuarial control.
[f]Severe late complications.
ND, not described.
Data from Foote RL, Parsons JT, Mendenhall WM, et al. Is interstitial implantation essential for successful radiotherapeutic treatment of base of tongue carcinoma? *Int J Radiat Oncol Biol Phys* 1990;18:1293; Mendenhall WM, Amdur RJ, Stringer SP, et al. Radiation therapy for squamous cell carcinoma of the base of tongue: a preferred alternative to surgery? *J Clin Oncol* 2000;18:35.

TABLE 9.10 Patterns of Failure in Patients Irradiated for Base of Tongue Carcinoma 2003 to 2012

| | Total | HPV+ (n = 321) | | | | | | | |
| | | Pattern of failure | | | | | | | |
		None	L	R	D	LR	LD	RD	LRD
T1	107	96	1	3	6	0	0	1	0
T2	123	102	5	2	7	2	1	2	2
T3	60	51	2	3	3	1	0	0	0
T4A	22	17	0	1	3	1	0	0	0
T4B	9	7	0	1	1	0	0	0	0
	Total	All (n = 689)							
		None	L	R	D	LR	LD	RD	LRD
T1	198	178	1	5	10	3	0	1	0
T2	258	223	8	4	14	2	1	3	3
T3	150	119	10	3	11	3	0	2	2
T4A	58	40	3	3	8	2	0	2	0
T4B	25	18	1	1	4	0	0	1	0

HPV+, Human papillomavirus related; All, HPV status not tested; None, No evidence of recurrence; L, Local; R, Regional; D, Distant.
Adapted from raw data from Dahlstrom KR, Garden AS, William WN Jr, et al. Proposed staging system for patients with HPV-related oropharyngeal cancer based on nasopharyngeal cancer N categories. *J Clin Oncol* 2016;34(16):1848–1854.

POSTERIOR OROPHARYNGEAL WALL

Treatment Strategy

Primary radiotherapy is preferred for T1 to T2 N0 to N1 carcinomas. Combination of radiation with systemic therapy is the treatment of choice for T3 and selected T4 or N2 to N3 tumors. Radiation with concurrent cisplatin is the favored combination.

As with other oropharyngeal carcinomas, there is now a consensus that patients presenting with N2 to N3 nodal disease achieving a complete clinical and radiographic response do not require a planned neck dissection. The value of PET-CT scan obtained 12 weeks after the completion of therapy in determining the need for a neck dissection for those with small, indeterminate residual nodal mass has recently been investigated in an randomized clinical trial showing noninferior results of response-based neck dissection versus planned neck dissection.

T4a tumors causing swallowing or laryngeal dysfunction are best treated with surgery followed by adjuvant radiotherapy and, in the presence of extracapsular extension or positive margin, combined with concurrent chemotherapy.

Primary Radiotherapy

Target Volume

The initial target volume encompasses the primary tumor with 2- to 3-cm margins (as submucosal spread can be extensive for this disease site) and retropharyngeal and levels II to IV nodes. The target volume also includes ipsilateral level IB in the presence of level II node. Level V is typically included in the node positive hemineck.

The boost volume encompasses the primary tumor and involved nodes with 1- to 2-cm margins.

Setup and Field Arrangement for Conventional Technique

The patient is immobilized in a supine position with a thermoplastic mask. Lateral parallel–opposed photon fields are used for treatment of the primary tumor and upper neck nodes (**Case Study 9.18**).

CASE STUDY 9.18

A 55-year-old man presented with a globus sensation on swallowing. A tumor was detected on the posterior oropharyngeal wall, and biopsy was positive for SCC. The tumor was approximately 5 mm in thickness and extended from the level of the soft palate superiorly to the level of mid tongue base inferiorly. There was no clinical adenopathy. Stage T2 N0 M0. He was treated with primary radiotherapy with concomitant boost regimen to a total dose of 72 Gy in 42 fractions.

Figure 9.18A shows the lateral portals on a sagittal digital reconstruction. Initial fields received 41.4 Gy in 23 fractions with 6 MV photons. A lower neck and supraclavicular field with a larynx block was matched on isocenter above the arytenoid. This anterior field received 50 Gy in 25 fractions prescribed at D_{max}. The lateral fields were reduced off the spinal cord and continued to 54 Gy. The posterior cervical strips excluded from the off–spinal cord photon fields were supplemented with 9 MeV electrons, 12.6 Gy at D_{max} in seven fractions. The boost was delivered as second daily fractions, 18 Gy in 12 fractions, with 18 MV photons. Figure 9.18B,C shows axial and sagittal isodose distributions through the middle of the tumor (T), respectively.

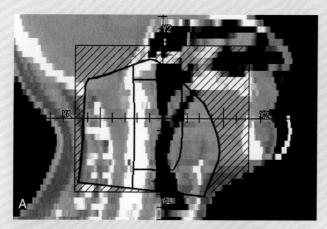

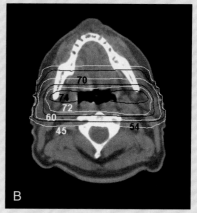

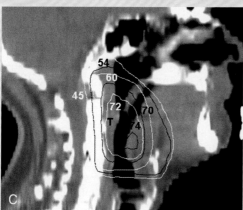

Case Figure 9.18 A–C

- *Anterior border:* at least 2 cm anterior to the known extent of the tumor, but when feasible, short of falloff anteriorly.
- *Superior border:* at the base of skull to cover parapharyngeal lymphatics and level II nodes.
- *Posterior border:* just behind the spinous processes or more posteriorly in the presence of large nodal masses. After off-cord reduction, the posterior portal margin is at the posterior one third of vertebral bodies to include the retropharyngeal nodes and provide the margin for the posterior pharyngeal wall.
- *Inferior border:* because the caudal extent of these tumors is often poorly defined, and submucosal extension beyond gross disease is frequent, a generous inferior margin (3 cm or more) is used to include the whole pharynx in the initial target volume.

An anterior appositional portal is used for treating lower neck nodes.

For the boost volume, the lateral fields are reduced to include the primary tumor with 1.5- to 2-cm margins; involved lymph nodes are either encompassed by lateral fields or, when overlying the spinal cord or low in the neck, by an appositional electron field or glancing photon portals.

Intensity-Modulated Radiation Therapy

IMRT is best suited for treating posterior pharyngeal wall tumors as it can produce a horseshoe-shaped isodose distribution to cover the paravertebral region without overdosing the spinal cord **(Case Study 9.19)**. The patient is immobilized in a supine position with an extended head and shoulder thermoplastic mask. Thin-cut CT scans are obtained in treatment position. The GTV, CTVs, and PTVs are outlined for dosimetric planning. The CTV_{HD} encompasses the GTV with 1- to 1.5-cm cranial and caudal margins, and CTV_{ID}

provides additional 1 to 2 cm of mucosal coverage. Tighter margins are used posteriorly due to the spinal cord, but more generous margins are used in the cranial–caudal dimension due to potential of submucosal spread. The role of image-guided therapy and PET scanning to identify tumor borders is under investigation. These studies are particularly pertinent in posterior pharyngeal tumors where the borders are frequently ill defined.

Dose

The dose is the same as that for tonsillar fossa primary lesion.

Postoperative Radiotherapy

Target Volume

The initial target volume encompasses the entire surgical bed and retropharyngeal and level II to IV nodes. The target volume also includes ipsilateral level IB in the presence of level II node. Level V is typically included in the node positive hemineck. When a laryngectomy is performed, indications for treatment of the tracheal stoma are as outlined for a base of tongue tumor.

The boost volume encompasses areas of known disease locations with 1- to 2-cm margins.

Setup and Field Arrangement

The general technique is the same as that described under "Primary Radiotherapy." Marking of the external surgical scar facilitates portal design. The *anterior* and *superior field borders* or CTVs are mainly determined by the local spread of the primary tumor and the extent of surgery (scar/flap). It is prudent to include 1- to 2-cm margins beyond the mucosal scar.

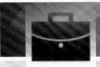

CASE STUDY 9.19

A 49-year-old woman, heavy smoker and alcohol user, presented with an otalgia, odynophagia, and dyphagia. Examination revealed a large tumor of the posterior pharyngeal wall extending from the inferior aspect of the nasopharynx to the inferior oropharynx. It did not extend into the pyriform sinuses or postcricoid region. There was no clinical or radiographic evidence of adenopathy. A biopsy was positive for papillary SCC.

She was treated with IMRT and three cycles of concurrent high-dose cisplatin. Two dose levels were used. CTV_{HD} (70 Gy) encompassed GTV with margin and

CTV_{ED} (57 Gy) covered the nodal levels II to V and the remaining pharyngeal walls, including hypopharynx. Therefore, it was decided to treat all the target volumes with IMRT, rather than match above the thyroid notch.

Figure 9.19 shows representative axial CT slices displaying the isodose distributions along the pharyngeal axis (Fig. 9.19A–E) with CTV_{HD} contoured in khaki and CTV_{ED} in blue. Figure 9.19F shows a sagittal isodose distribution through midplane with the tumor identified with *arrows*. The patient did well for 1 year posttreatment and was subsequently lost to follow-up.

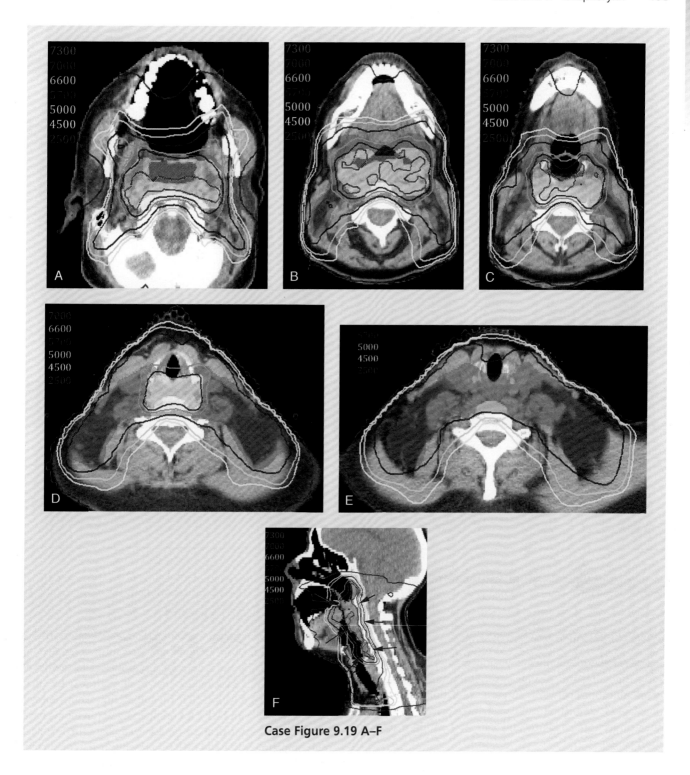

Case Figure 9.19 A–F

Dose

- 60 Gy in 30 fractions to areas with high-risk features, that is, close or microscopically positive margins, perineural extension, vascular invasion, positive nodes, or extranodal extension. An additional boost dose of 6 Gy may be given when indicated, for example, when multiple adverse features are present or when the interval between surgery and radiation is much longer than 6 weeks.
- 56 Gy in 28 fractions to the surgical bed.
- 50 Gy in 25 fractions to undissected regions to receive elective irradiation.

TABLE 9.11 SCCs of the Pharyngeal Walls Treated with Irradiation Alone: Failure Rates for Treatment of Primary Tumor in Patients Treated at the M.D. Anderson Cancer Center Between 1954 and 1974 (Analysis in October 1976)

Stage	Primary Tumor Control (%)	No. Salvaged by Surgery	Ultimate Primary Control (%)	No. of Complications[a] (%)
T1	10/11 (91)	1	11/11 (100)	0 (0)
T2	33/45 (73)	2	35/45 (78)	3 (7)
T3	38/62 (61)	6	44/62 (71)	9 (15)
T4	17/46 (37)	2	19/46 (41)	8 (17)

[a]Pharyngeal wall necrosis, 3, carotid rupture, 8 (5 associated with salvage surgery); osteonecrosis, 3; radiation myelitis, 2; severe larynx edema, 2; and severe neck fibrosis, 2.
Modified from Meoz-Mendez RT, Fletcher GH, Guillamondegui OM, et al. Analysis of the results of irradiation in the treatment of squamous cell carcinomas of the pharyngeal walls. *Int J Radiat Oncol Biol Phys* 1978;4:579–585.

TABLE 9.12 SCC of the Pharyngeal Walls Treated with Combination of Surgery and Preoperative or Postoperative Irradiation: Primary Control by Stage

Stage	No. of Patients	Primary Control (%)	Alive and NED at 1 yr	Died of Intercurrent Diseases <1 yr
T2	5	5/5 (100)	4	1
T3 + T4	20	15/20 (75)	10	5

NED, no evidence of disease.
Modified from Meoz-Mendez RT, Fletcher GH, Guillamondegui OM, et al. Analysis of the results of irradiation in the treatment of squamous cell carcinomas of the pharyngeal walls. *Int J Radiat Oncol Biol Phys* 1978;4:579–585, with permission.

Timing of Postoperative Radiotherapy

It is desirable to commence postoperative radiotherapy as soon as possible after healing of surgical wounds. With good communication between surgical, radiation, and dental oncologists, simulation can usually take place 3 to 4 weeks after surgery, and radiotherapy can start within a week in most patients.

Background Data

See Tables 9.11 and 9.12.

INTENSITY-MODULATED PROTON THERAPY

Advances in active scanning planning and delivery and IMPT techniques have provided the ability to treat geometrically complex oropharyngeal carcinoma target volumes. IMPT reduces integral dose to nontarget structures compared to IMRT, particularly those anterior and posterior to the target volumes, and this may reduce the "beam path toxicity" that has been observed with IMRT. The initial clinical outcomes of patients treated with IMPT for oropharyngeal carcinoma have recently been reported, and a randomized phase II/III clinical trial comparing IMRT and IMPT is presently being conducted. Examples of IMPT used for ipsilateral and bilateral neck treatment for tonsillar cancer are **Case Study 9.20 and Case Study 9.21**. An example of IMPT used for a patient with base of tongue cancer is shown in **Case Study 9.22**. Representative IMPT beam arrangements and dose distributions for two oropharyngeal carcinoma cases are shown in Figure 9.23.

Background Data

See Table 9.13.

A 69-year-old female presented with an asymptomatic neck mass. A fine needle aspiration was performed and was positive for metastatic squamous cell carcinoma, HPV 16 positive. An obvious 3-cm tumor was noted in the left tonsil, and the tumor was felt to be isolated to the tonsillar region, with no palate or tongue involvement. CT scan of the head and neck was performed and revealed the primary tumor (Fig. 9.20A, *red arrow*) and two nodes in level II of the left neck (the larger node seen in Fig. 9.20B, *green arrow*). Her clinical stage was T2N2b.

She was dispositioned to radiation with concurrent cetuximab. Because the primary disease was confined to the tonsil, she was treated with ipsilateral radiation, and protons were the chosen radiation modality.

An IMPT plan using single-field optimization (SFO) with three beams was designed. Three targets were defined: CTV_{HD} covered gross disease with margin, CTV_{ID} added additional margin to CTV_{HD} and also covered level II, while CTV_{ED} covered the left retropharyngeal nodes and the remaining uninvolved left sided nodal levels. Representative contours on two axial images where gross disease of both the tonsil and involved lymph nodes are shown in Figure 9.20C,D (CTV_{HD}, *purple*, CTV_{ID}, *blue*, and CTV_{ED}, *yellow*). Doses prescribed to CTV_{HD}, CTV_{ID}, and CTV_{ED} were 70 Gy, 62 Gy, and 56 Gy, respectively, and treatment delivered in 33 fractions. Representative views of the isodose distribution are shown in Figure 9.20E–H. Figure 9.20E–G are three axial views through the primary tumor, nodal disease, and uninvolved lower neck, respectively, and Figure 9.20H is a coronal view of the distribution through the primary tumor.

She remains without disease over 1 year out from therapy.

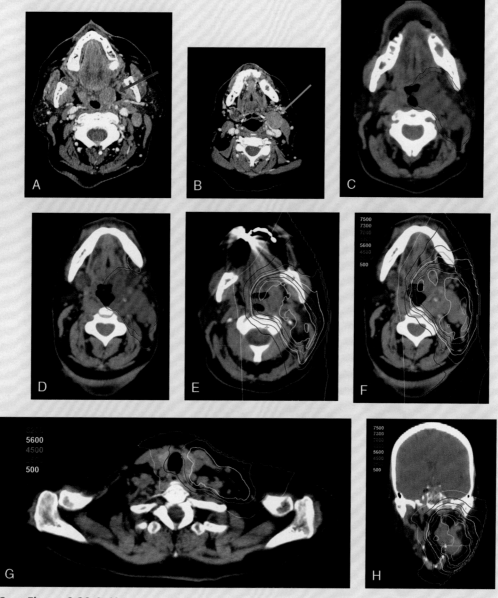

Case Figure 9.20 A–H

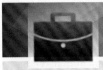

CASE STUDY 9.21

A 74-year-old male with a previous history of prostate cancer treated with radiation self-palpated a mass in his left tonsil. A biopsy was performed of the tonsillar mass and revealed poorly differentiated squamous cell carcinoma, p16 positive.

A staging workup ensued, and included a contrast CT scan and PET/CT scan. The primary tumor is seen on the CT scan (Fig. 9.21A, *red arrow*), and 2 level II nodes are evident on the PET/CT (Fig. 9.21B).

He was dispositioned for induction chemotherapy, and treated with 3 cycles of carboplatin and taxol, and achieved a partial response. He then proceeded to receive single-modality IMPT. As the primary tumor extended to the glossopharyngeal sulcus and base of tongue, it was elected to treat both sides of the neck, including right levels II to IV in CTV$_{ED}$.

Three targets were delineated. A vGTV of the primary tonsil tumor and left neck disease was defined from the prechemotherapy images and exam findings. CTV$_{HD}$ was then defined as vGTV with margin. Additional margin was added to CTV$_{HD}$ to create CTV$_{ID}$, and the remaining subclinical sites at risk (levels IB to V on the left, II to IV on the right, and the retropharyngeal nodes) were included in CTV$_{ED}$. Doses prescribed to CTV$_{HD}$, CTV$_{ID}$, and CTV$_{ED}$ were 66 Gy, 60 Gy, and 54 Gy, respectively, and delivered in 30 fractions. The IMPT was planned with multi-field optimization (MFO) using a posterior beam and two additional noncoplanar beams that entered anteriorly and cranially. Figure 9.21C shows the beam arrangement on an axial image through the primary tumor, and a colorwash presentation of the dose distribution. Additional views of the isodose distribution are seen in Figure 9.21D, a more inferior axial view through the tumor, and Figure 9.21E, a coronal view through the primary tumor.

The patient is doing well 3 years out from therapy.

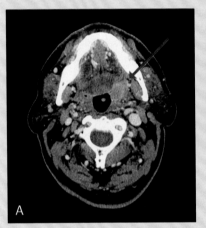
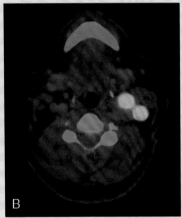
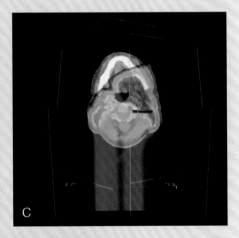
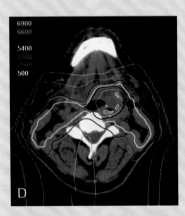
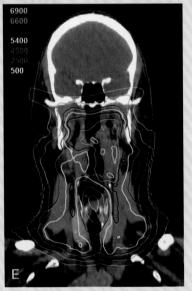

Case Figure 9.21 A–E

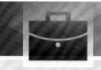

CASE STUDY 9.22

A 62-year-old male presented with left neck adenopathy, and was found to have a base of tongue mass. He was imaged with PET/CT, and a representative axial view (Fig. 9.22A) demonstrates the primary tumor and left neck adenopathy in level II. An additional node was detected in level III. The mass was biopsied, and pathology revealed a p16 positive squamous cell carcinoma. His primary tumor was >4 cm, so his clinical stage was T3N2b. He was treated with IMPT and weekly cisplatin. IMPT was planned with MFO using three beams.

Three targets were defined: CTV_{HD} covered gross disease with margin, CTV_{ID} added additional margin to CTV_{HD} and also covered left level II, and CTV_{ED} covered the retropharyngeal (RP) nodes, the remaining uninvolved left-sided nodal levels (IB to V), and the contralateral level II to IV nodes. Representative contours (CTV_{HD}, *purple*, CTV_{ID}, *blue*, and CTV_{ED}, *yellow*) are shown in an axial slice (Fig. 9.22B) and a sagittal view through midline (Fig. 9.22C). On the sagittal view, the use of a mouth opening tongue depressing stent for positioning can be appreciated. Doses prescribed to CTV_{HD}, CTV_{ID}, and CTV_{ED} were 70 Gy, 62 Gy, and 56 Gy, respectively, and treatment delivered in 33 fractions. A matching isodose distribution through midline in the sagittal plane is shown in Figure 9.22D. Additional isodose distributions are demonstrated in Figure 9.22E–G at the level of the RP nodes, through the tumor in the base of tongue, and at level IV of the neck, respectively.

One year following therapy, he developed lung metastases.

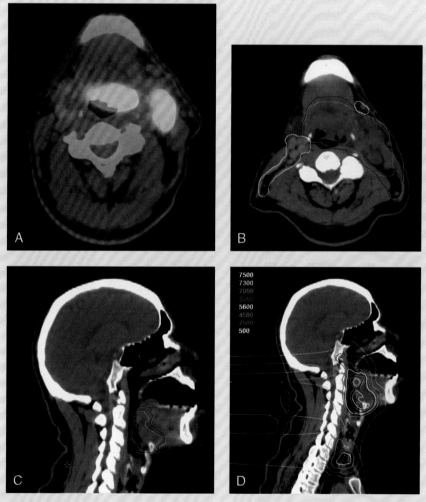

Case Figure 9.22 A–D

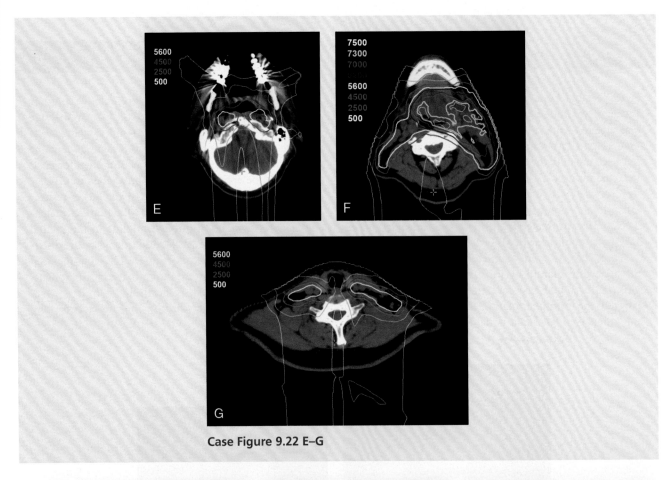

Case Figure 9.22 E–G

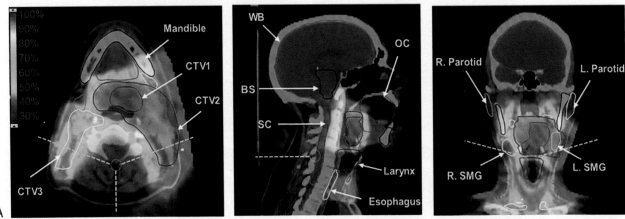

Figure 9.23 Representative dose distributions in the axial, sagittal, and coronal plane are shown for two cases of oropharyngeal squamous carcinoma treated with intensity-modulated proton therapy (IMPT) using active scanning beam and multi-field optimization (see Chapter 2). *Dashed white lines* show the beam arrangement (two anterior oblique and one posterior field). Case A: 50-year-old male, left base of tongue, T1 Nx(2b). Mean doses (in Gy radiobiologic equivalent): ipsi parotid 23.4, contra parotid 16.8, ipsi SMG 63.6, contra SMG 34.6, OC 9, larynx 28.3, esophagus 29.5, man 27.4, SPC 54, MPC 59.9, IPC 34.9. Prescription dose to CTV1, 2, and 3 were 66, 60, and 54 Gy, respectively, delivered in 30 fractions. Case B: 75-year-old male, left tonsil, T2 N2b. Mean doses (in Gy radiobiologic equivalent): ipsi parotid 35.1, contra parotid 14.6, ipsi SMG 68.6, contra SMG 27.3, OC 13.4, larynx 29.9, esophagus 11.7, man 18.5, SPC 59.7, MPC 44.8, IPC 27.9. Prescription dose to CTV1, 2, and 3 were 70, 63, and 57 Gy, respectively, delivered in 33 fractions. BS, brainstem; contra, contralateral; CTV, clinical target volume; IPC, inferior pharyngeal constrictor; ipsi, ipsilateral; L, left; man, mandible; MPC, middle pharyngeal constrictor; OC, oral cavity; R, right; SC, spinal cord; SMG, submandibular gland; SPC, superior pharyngeal constrictor; Thyroid G, thyroid gland; WB, whole brain. (Reproduced from Gunn GB, Blanchard P, Garden AS, et al. Clinical outcomes and patterns of disease recurrence following intensity modulated proton therapy for oropharyngeal squamous carcinoma. *Int J Radiat Oncol Biol Phys* 2016;95:360–367, with permission.)

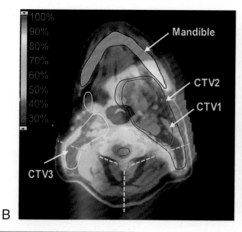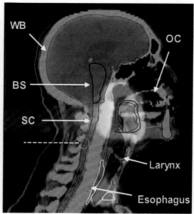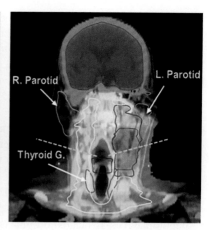

Figure 9-23 *(Continued)*

TABLE 9.13 Outcomes of Patients with Squamous Carcinoma of the Oropharynx Treated with Intensity-Modulated Proton Therapy at the M.D. Anderson Cancer Center

No. of Patients	% With Smoking History	% p16 Positive	% Stage III/IV	Median Follow-Up (mo)	No. with Gastrostomy Placed During Therapy	No. with Local-Regional Recurrence	% OS (2-yr)
50	50	98	98	29	11[a]	4	95

[a]No patient had a feeding tube at last follow-up.

Data from Gunn GB, Blanchard P, Garden AS, et al. Clinical outcomes and patterns of disease recurrence following intensity modulated proton therapy for oropharyngeal squamous carcinoma. *Int J Radiat Oncol Biol Phys* 2016;95:360–367.

SUGGESTED READINGS

Ang KK, Harris J, Wheeler R, et al. Human papillomavirus and survival of patients with oropharyngeal cancer. *N Engl J Med* 2010;363:24.

Ang KK, Peters LJ, Weber RS, et al. Concomitant boost radiotherapy schedules in the treatment of carcinoma of the oropharynx and nasopharynx. *Int J Radiat Oncol Biol Phys* 1990;19:1339.

Bataini JP, Asselain B, Jaulerry C, et al. A multivariate primary tumor control analysis in 465 patients treated by radical radiotherapy for cancer of the tonsillar region: clinical and treatment parameters as prognostic factors. *Radiother Oncol* 1989;14:265.

Blanchard P, Garden AS, Gunn GB, et al. Intensity-modulated proton beam therapy (IMPT) versus intensity-modulated photon therapy (IMRT) for patients with oropharynx cancer—A case matched analysis. *Radiother Oncol* 2016;120:48.

Chera BS, Amdur RJ, Hinerman RW, et al. Definitive radiation therapy for squamous cell carcinoma of the soft palate. *Head Neck* 2008;30:1114.

Chronowski GM, Garden AS, Morrison WH, et al. Unilateral radiotherapy for the treatment of tonsil cancer. *Int J Radiat Oncol Biol Phys* 2012;83:204.

Cooper RA, Slevin NJ, Carrington BM, et al. Radiotherapy for carcinoma of the posterior pharyngeal wall. *Int J Radiat Oncol Biol Phys* 2000;16:611.

Dahlstrom KR, Garden AS, William WN Jr, et al. Proposed staging system for patients with HPV-related oropharyngeal cancer based on nasopharyngeal cancer N categories. *J Clin Oncol* 2016;34:1848.

Daly ME, Le QT, Maxim PG, et al. Intensity-modulated radiotherapy in the treatment of oropharyngeal cancer: clinical outcomes and patterns of failure. *Int J Radiat Oncol Biol Phys* 2010;76:1339.

Denis F, Garaud P, Bardet E, et al. Final results of the 94-01 French Head and Neck Oncology and Radiotherapy Group randomized trial comparing radiotherapy alone with concomitant radiochemotherapy in advanced-stage oropharynx carcinoma. *J Clin Oncol* 2004;22:69.

Eisbruch A, Harris J, Garden AS, et al. Multi-institutional trial of accelerated hypofractionated intensity-modulated radiation therapy for early-stage oropharyngeal cancer (RTOG 00-22). *Int J Radiat Oncol Biol Phys* 2010;76:1333.

Fein DA, Mendenhall WM, Parsons JT, et al. Pharyngeal wall carcinoma treated with radiotherapy: impact of treatment technique and fractionation. *Int J Radiat Oncol Biol Phys* 1993;26:751.

Fletcher GH. Oral cavity and oropharynx. In: Fletcher GH, ed. *Textbook of radiotherapy*, 3rd ed. Philadelphia, PA: Lea & Febiger, 1980.

Garden AS, Dong L, Morrison WH, et al. Patterns of disease recurrence following treatment of oropharyngeal cancer with intensity modulated radiation therapy. *Int J Radiat Oncol Biol Phys* 2013;85:941.

Garden AS, Gunn GB, Hessel A, et al. Management of the lymph node-positive neck in the patient with human papillomavirus-associated oropharyngeal cancer. *Cancer* 2014;120:3082.

Garden AS, Kies MS, Morrison WH, et al. Outcomes and patterns of care of patients with locally advanced oropharyngeal carcinoma treated in the early 21st century. *Radiat Oncol* 2013;8:21.

Gunn GB, Blanchard P, Garden AS, et al. Clinical outcomes and patterns of disease recurrence following intensity modulated proton therapy for oropharyngeal squamous carcinoma. *Int J Radiat Oncol Biol Phys* 2016;95:360.

Gunn GB, Debnam JM, Fuller CD, et al. The impact of radiographic retropharyngeal adenopathy in oropharyngeal cancer. *Cancer* 2013;119:3162.

Hansen E, Panwala K, Holland J. Post-operative radiation therapy for advanced-stage oropharyngeal cancer. *J Laryngol Otol* 2002;116:920.

Housset M, Baillet F, Dessard-Diana B, et al. A retrospective study of three treatment techniques for T1–T2 base of tongue lesions: surgery plus postoperative radiation, external radiation plus interstitial implantation and external radiation alone. *Int J Radiat Oncol Biol Phys* 1987;13:511.

Keus RB, Pontvert D, Brunin F, et al. Results of irradiation in squamous cell carcinoma of the soft palate and uvula. *Radiother Oncol* 1988;11:311.

Lusinchi A, Eskandari J, Son Y, et al. External irradiation plus curietherapy boost in 108 base of tongue carcinomas. *Int J Radiat Oncol Biol Phys* 1989;17:1191.

Lusinchi A, Wibault P, Marandas P, et al. Exclusive radiation therapy: the treatment of early tonsillar tumors. *Int J Radiat Oncol Biol Phys* 1989;17:273.

Mendenhall WM, Amdur RJ, Stringer SP, et al. Radiation therapy for squamous cell carcinoma of the tonsillar region: a preferred alternative to surgery? *J Clin Oncol* 2000;18:2219.

Mendenhall WM, Stringer SP, Amdur RJ, et al. Is radiation therapy a preferred alternative to surgery for squamous cell carcinoma of the base of tongue? *J Clin Oncol* 2000;18:35.

Meoz-Mendez RT, Fletcher GH, Guillamondegui OM, et al. Analysis of the results of irradiation in the treatment of squamous cell carcinomas of the pharyngeal walls. *Int J Radiat Oncol Biol Phys* 1978;4:579.

Nien HH, Sturgis EM, Kies MS, et al. Comparison of systemic therapies used concurrently with radiation for the treatment of human papillomavirus-associated oropharyngeal cancer. *Head Neck* 2016;38(Suppl 1):E1554.

O'Sullivan B, Huang SH, Su J, et al. Development and validation of a staging system for HPV-related oropharyngeal cancer by the International Collaboration on Oropharyngeal cancer Network for Staging (ICON-S): a multicentre cohort study. *Lancet Oncol* 2016;17:440.

O'Sullivan B, Warde P, Grice B, et al. The benefits and pitfalls of ipsilateral radiotherapy in carcinoma of the tonsillar region. *Int J Radiat Oncol Biol Phys* 2001;51:332.

Parsons JT, Mendenhall WM, Stringer SP, et al. Squamous cell carcinoma of the oropharynx: surgery, radiation therapy or both. *Cancer* 2002;94:2967.

Rosenthal DI, Harari PM, Giralt J, et al. Association of Human Papillomavirus and p16 Status With Outcomes in the IMCL-9815 Phase III Registration Trial for Patients With Locoregionally Advanced Oropharyngeal Squamous Cell Carcinoma of the Head and Neck Treated With Radiotherapy With or Without Cetuximab. *J Clin Oncol* 2016;34:1300.

Selek U, Garden AS, Morrison WH, et al. Radiation therapy for early-stage carcinoma of the oropharynx. *Int J Radiat Oncol Biol Phys* 2004;59:743.

Setton J, Caria N, Romanyshyn J, et al. Intensity-modulated radiotherapy in the treatment of oropharyngeal cancer: an update of the Memorial Sloan-Kettering Cancer Center experience. *Int J Radiat Oncol Biol Phys* 2012;82:291.

Setton J, Lee NY, Riaz N, et al. A multi-institution pooled analysis of gastrostomy tube dependence in patients with oropharyngeal cancer treated with definitive intensity-modulated radiotherapy. *Cancer* 2015;121:294.

Tiwari RM, et al. Advanced squamous cell carcinoma of the base of the tongue treated with surgery and post-operative radiotherapy. *Eur J Surg Oncol* 2000;26:556.

Weber RS, Peters LJ, Wolf P, et al. Squamous cell carcinoma of the soft palate, uvula, and anterior faucial pillar. *Otolaryngol Head Neck Surg* 1988;99:16,23.

Withers HR, Peters LJ, Taylor JM, et al. Late normal tissue sequelae from radiation therapy for carcinoma of the tonsil: patterns of fractionation study of radiobiology. *Int J Radiat Oncol Biol Phys* 1995a;33(3):563.

Withers HR, Peters LJ, Taylor JM, et al. Local control of carcinoma of the tonsil by radiation therapy: an analysis of patterns of fractionation in nine institutions. *Int J Radiat Oncol Biol Phys* 1995b;33(3):549.

Yildirim G, Morrison WH, Rosenthal DI, et al. Outcomes of patients with tonsillar carcinoma treated with post-tonsillectomy radiation therapy. *Head Neck* 2010;32:473.

Zelefsky MJ, Harrison LB, Armstrong JG. Long-term treatment results of postoperative radiation therapy for advanced stage oropharyngeal carcinoma. *Cancer* 1992;70:2388.

10

Larynx

Key Points

- The larynx is divided into three anatomic sites: supraglottis, glottis, and subglottis.

- The majority of tumors present in the glottis, often at an early stage. Subglottic carcinoma is very rare.

- The glottis does not have a rich lymphatic supply, so nodal involvement is rare, and thus, elective treatment of the nodes is not required for stage I and II disease.

- The supraglottic larynx has greater access to the lymphatics, and thus, elective nodal irradiation is recommended.

- Radiation alone and transoral laser microsurgery are effective therapies for early laryngeal cancer. The choice of treatment is generally based on the anticipated voice quality, expertise, and personal preference.

- Concurrent radiation and cisplatin are often recommended for patients with intermediate-stage disease (bulky T2, T3, or node-positive disease) aiming at preserving the larynx. Some centers prefer induction chemotherapy (docetaxel, cisplatin, and fluorouracil) followed by radiotherapy in patients having at least a partial response.

- Patients at risk for aspiration or with advanced disease extending through the cartilage are generally not suited for larynx preservation. These patients are treated with laryngectomy followed by adjuvant radiotherapy and, in the presence of extracapsular nodal extension or positive surgical margins, the postoperative radiation is combined with concurrent cisplatin.

- When treated properly, few patients with early- or intermediate-stage laryngeal carcinoma die of their index cancer. Therefore, in addition to tumor eradication, preservation of natural speech, swallowing function, and avoidance of permanent tracheostomy are major therapy objectives.

SUPRAGLOTTIS CARCINOMA: EARLY STAGE

Treatment Strategy

Primary radiotherapy is preferred for most T1 tumors. The preferred larynx-preserving therapy for T2 depends on the disease and patient characteristics. For lesions that are non-bulky and exophytic, therapy consists of hyperfractionated or concomitant boost radiotherapy.

For T2 lesions, bulky or infiltrating:

- Good pulmonary function and general condition: supraglottic laryngectomy or transoral laser microsurgery (TLM) with or without postoperative radiotherapy
- Medically unfit or technically not suitable for supraglottic laryngectomy: if medically fit for chemotherapy, radiation with concurrent cisplatin or induction chemotherapy (docetaxel, cisplatin, and fluorouracil) followed by radiation; alternatively, hyperfractionated or concomitant boost radiotherapy

Primary Radiotherapy

Target Volume

Initial Target Volume

- T1 and T2 N0: larynx and nodes at levels II to IV (**Case Study 10.1 and Case Study 10.2**). Within level II, only the subdigastric nodes need be included.
- T1 and T2 N1: larynx and nodes at levels II to IV. Level II nodes are covered to the jugular fossa. Posterior level 1B nodes are also included.

For boost volume: primary tumor and, when present, involved nodes with 1- to 2-cm margins.

Setup and Field Arrangement for Conventional Radiotherapy Technique

The patient is immobilized in a supine position with a thermoplastic mask. Marking of shoulders and, when present, involved nodes facilitates portal design. Lateral parallel–opposed photon fields are used to treat the primary tumor and upper neck nodes.

- *Superior border:* approximately 2 cm above the angle of mandible when N0 or approximately 1 cm above the tip of mastoid process when N+.
- *Anterior border:* fall-off anteriorly; when there is extension into the oropharynx, a generous part of the base of tongue is encompassed in the field.
- *Posterior border:* behind the spinous processes or more posteriorly in the presence of large nodal mass.
- *Inferior border:* depends on the disease extent—middle or bottom of cricoid cartilage for tumors of the epiglottis or false cord; upper trachea when there is subglottic extension (at least 2 cm below inferior tumor extent).

An anterior portal is used to treat the lower neck. It may be necessary to use anterior and inferior tilts for patients with a short neck. In this case, the supraclavicular fossa is included in the primary portal.

For boost volume, the lateral fields are reduced to 1- to 2-cm margins around the primary tumor and involved nodes. Nodes overlying the spinal cord can usually receive boost dose through oblique-lateral primary boost portals and those in the lower neck through an appositional electron portal or glancing photon fields.

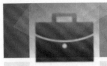

CASE STUDY 10.1

A 57-year-old woman presented with hoarseness, right otalgia, and odynophagia. A biopsy of a 1-cm tumor confined to the right false vocal cord was positive for squamous cell carcinoma. The vocal cord mobility was normal, and there was no palpable adenopathy. The final stage was T1 N0 M0. She was treated with primary radiation. Treatment started with parallel–opposed fields covering the levels II and III nodes and the primary tumor. An off–spinal cord reduction was made at 42 Gy and treatment continued to 50 Gy. A boost of 16 Gy was delivered to the primary tumor. Figure 10.1 shows the three pairs of lateral–opposed portals (Fig. 10.1A) and an isodose distribution through the isocenter (Fig. 10.1B). The beams were modified by the use of 30- and 45-degree wedges.

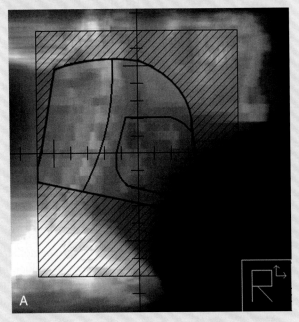

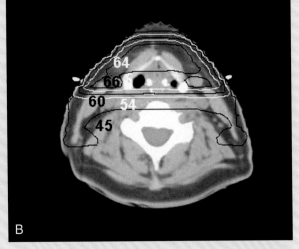

Case Figure 10.1 A,B

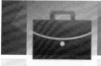

CASE STUDY 10.2

A 39-year-old man presented with intermittent hoarseness for 6 months. Examination showed a tumor on the left false cord, extending upward to the left aryepiglottic fold and downward to obliterate the left ventricle. There was no evidence of glottic or pyriform sinus involvement. The mobility of both true vocal cords was normal. There was no palpable neck adenopathy. Biopsy showed moderately differentiated squamous cell carcinoma. The final stage was T2 N0 M0. This patient was treated with primary radiotherapy using a hyperfractionation schedule. The primary tumor and upper and middle neck nodes were treated with lateral parallel–opposed fields (Fig. 10.2). Because the tumor was mainly located in the posterior part of the larynx, it was thought that the anterior skin could be excluded from the boost volume. Lower neck nodes were irradiated through an anterior appositional portal. The primary tumor received 76.6 Gy over 7 weeks (55.2 Gy in 46 fractions for 4.6 weeks + 21.6 Gy in 18 fractions for 2 weeks), uninvolved upper neck nodes 55.2 Gy in 46 fractions over 4.6 weeks, and lower neck nodes 50 Gy in 25 fractions for 5 weeks. He had no evidence of disease and worked full time 3 years after therapy.

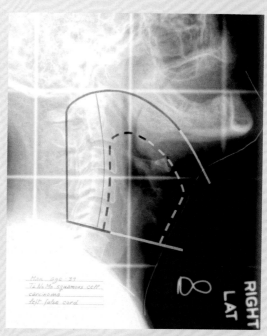

Case Figure 10.2

Dose

For T1 N0 tumors: 50 Gy in 25 fractions to the initial target volume followed by 16 Gy in eight fractions to the primary tumor. For T1 N1 tumors, an additional 4 Gy in 2 fractions can be delivered to the neck node with either an appositional electron beam or glancing photon beams.

For T2 N0 or T2 N1 tumors: hyperfractionated or concomitant boost regimen. Hyperfractionation delivers 55.2 Gy in 46 fractions to the initial target volume and then 21.6 Gy in 18 fractions (1.2-Gy fractions, twice daily, 6-hour interval); the spinal cord dose is limited to 44.4 to 45.6 Gy or less, and uninvolved posterior cervical nodes are supplemented with 2 Gy daily to approximately 55 Gy. Concomitant boost delivers 1.8-Gy fractions to 54 Gy in 30 fractions to the initial target volume and 1.5-Gy fractions to 15 to 18 Gy given as second daily fractions during the last 2 to 2.5 weeks; the spinal cord dose is limited to 45 Gy or less.

Positive nodes receive doses appropriate for the size. The fractionation schedules used, and include 66 to 70 Gy in 2-Gy fractions, 69 to 72 Gy with concomitant boost, or 74.4 to 79.2 Gy with hyperfractionation. The dose to uninvolved lower neck nodes is 50 Gy in 25 fractions (treated once a day).

Intensity-Modulated Radiation Therapy Planning

Most patients are now treated with IMRT with a goal of sparing normal tissues, most importantly the parotid glands (**Case Study 10.3**). The primary tumor is treated with a minimum of 8- to 10-mm margin; though due to laryngeal motion, it is prudent to encompass the majority of the larynx in the high–dose-target volume (CTV_{HD}), particularly in the cranial–caudal dimension. Involved node(s) with 8- to 10-mm margin are also encompassed in CTV_{HD}. The neck compartments outside CTV_{HD} with a 2-cm (cranial–caudal) margin are delineated as CTV_{ID}. The remaining nodal levels (II, III, IV, and V) are contoured as CTV_{ED}. Level Ib is included in CTV_{ED} on the side(s) of lymphadenopathy.

For patients with T2 tumors treated with IMRT, we have escalated treatment through the use of a modified DAHANCA fractionation or a concomitant boost schedule. In the modified DAHANCA fractionation, we use a single IMRT plan with a prescription dose of 70 Gy to CTV_{HD}, 60 to 63 Gy to CTV_{ID}, and 56 to 57 Gy to CTV_{ED}; this is delivered in 35 fractions over 6 weeks, by administering 6 fractions a week for 5 weeks with a 6-hour interfraction interval on the day when 2 fractions are delivered. Alternatively, we have used concomitant boost fractionation, which requires two separate IMRT plans. The first plan delivers 57 Gy in 30 fractions to CTV_{HD} and CTV_{ID} and 54 Gy to CTV_{ED}, and the second plan is for 18 Gy in 10 fractions to CTV_{HD}. The fractionation regimen is similar to non-IMRT radiotherapy.

Background Data

See Tables 10.1 and 10.2.

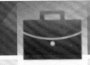

CASE STUDY 10.3

A 65-year-old male with a 100-pack-year cigarette smoking history presented to his local physician with a feeling of fullness and soreness in his throat. On evaluation, he was found to have a left supraglottic mass involving the arytenoid, aryepiglottic fold, and laryngeal surface of the epiglottis (Fig. 10.3A). A CT scan revealed lymph node in the left neck (Fig. 10.3B). Biopsy was positive with a final stage of T2 N1 M0 supraglottic larynx squamous carcinoma.

The patient was treated with concurrent chemoradiation using IMRT. The treatment was delivered using VMAT, with two arcs. Figure 10.3C–E shows CTV$_{HD}$ (*red*) encompassing the primary tumor (GTV, *green*) and the positive lymph node with generous margin, CTV$_{ID}$ (*blue*) the nodal region immediately adjacent to the involved node, and CTV$_{ED}$ (*yellow*) the remaining uninvolved neck nodes. The spinal cord and brainstem contours are seen in Figure 10.3C and D, and additionally, the PRV (5mm expansion) of the spinal cord used for planning purposes is seen (Fig. 10.3C). The bilateral parotids are contoured in Figure 10.3E.

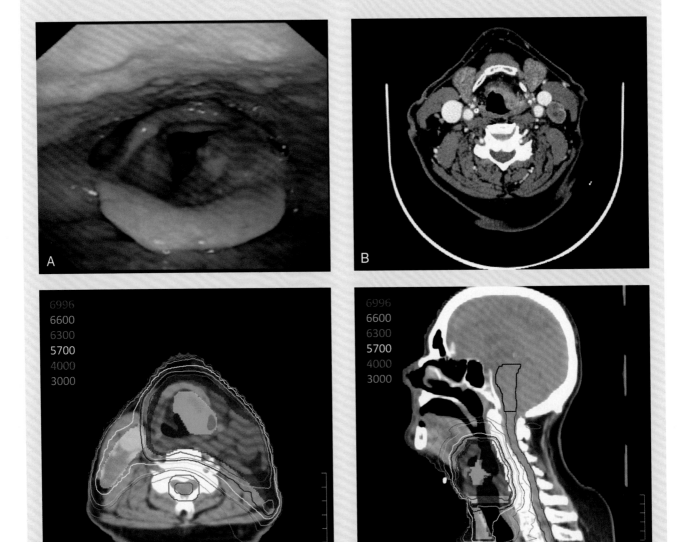

Case Figure 10.3 A–D

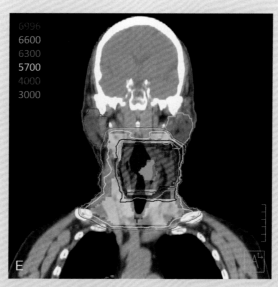

Case Figure 10.3 E

TABLE 10.1 Local Control and Complication Rates Following Radical Radiation of T2 to T3, N0 to N3 Carcinoma of the Supraglottic Larynx

Radiation Schedules	Local Control			Severe Complication[a] (%)
	No. of Patients	2 Years	5 Years	
Hyperfractionation[b] (1984–1991)	77	87%	80%	2.7
Standard fractionation[b] (1970–1981)	98	78%	70%	3.0

Note: Patients treated in 1982 and 1983 were excluded because some received treatment with conventional fractionation and others with hyperfractionation.
[a]Requiring tracheotomy or laryngectomy.
[b]$P = 0.04$.
Data from the M.D. Anderson Cancer Center. Analysis, July 1992.

TABLE 10.2 T2 to T3 Carcinoma of Supraglottic Larynx: Local Control Following Radiotherapy According to Medical and Anatomic Suitability for Surgery in 83 Patients Treated at the University of Florida[a]

Stage	Anatomically Suitable for Supraglottic Laryngectomy			Anatomically Unsuitable
	Medically Suitable	Medically Unsuitable	Total	
T2	35/41 (85%)	14/16 (88%)	49/57 (86%)	44/52 (85%)
T3	9/13 (69%)	8/13 (62%)	17/26 (66%)	17/26 (65%)
Total	44/54 (81%)	22/29 (76%)	66/83 (80%)	61/78 (78%)

[a]Excludes patients who died within 2 years of radiotherapy with primary site continuously disease free.
Modified from Hinerman RW, Mendenhall WM, Amdur RJ, et al. Carcinoma of the supraglottic larynx: treatment results with radiotherapy alone or with planned neck dissection. *Head Neck* 2002;24:456–467.

GLOTTIS CARCINOMA: EARLY STAGE

Treatment Strategy

Primary radiotherapy is preferred for most T1 to T2 tumors.

Primary Radiotherapy

Target Volume

The target volume encompasses the larynx proper (sparing the suprahyoid epiglottis) **(Case Study 10.4 and Case Study 10.5)**.

Setup and Field Arrangement for Conventional Radiotherapy Technique

The patient is immobilized in a supine position with a thermoplastic mask. Lateral parallel–opposed photon fields are used. In patients with a short neck, a 5- to 10-degree inferior tilt may be necessary to avoid irradiation through the wider part of the shoulder:

- *Superior border:* top of thyroid cartilage for T1 or higher for T2 tumor with supraglottic extension
- *Anterior border:* approximately 1-cm falloff
- *Posterior border:* anterior margin of the vertebral bodies
- *Inferior border:* lower edge of the cricoid cartilage for T1 or lower for T2 tumor with subglottic extension

Dose

For microscopic disease (e.g., after "stripping" or excisional biopsy of T1 tumors): 60 Gy in 30 fractions.

Other T1 tumors: Several dose fractionation schedules have been described. The key element is that the dose per fraction should be ≥2 Gy. Options are 66 Gy in 33 daily fractions or 63 Gy in 28 daily fractions.

T2 tumors: Altered fractionation schedules are preferred. Hyperfractionation to a dose of 76.6 to 79.2 Gy at 1.2 Gy per fraction delivered twice daily (with at least 6 hours between fractions) is an option. An alternative is 70 Gy in 35 fractions over 6 weeks by treating twice daily once per week (6 fractions per week) for 5 weeks.

Bulky T2 tumors: 70 Gy in 35 fractions over 7 weeks with concurrent cisplatin (see T3 tumors below).

The radiation dose is specified at an isodose line. For patients treated with conventional techniques, treatment is

CASE STUDY 10.4

A 66-year-old man presented with a 6-month history of progressive hoarseness. Examination showed mild edema and leukoplakia of the anterior commissure and the anterior one third of both true vocal cords. There was no supraglottic or subglottic spread and vocal cord mobility was normal. No lymph nodes were palpated in the neck. Biopsies showed microinvasive squamous cell carcinoma on both true vocal cords. The final stage was T1 N0 M0. The patient was treated with lateral parallel–opposed fields (Fig. 10.4). A dose of 64 Gy specified in the isocenter was delivered in 2-Gy fractions. After a dose of 50 Gy, the posterior border was moved 1 cm anteriorly to reduce the dose to the arytenoids. This field reduction is no longer recommended. A 15-degree wedge was used to produce a slight dose gradient delivering a higher dose to the thickest part of the lesion at the anterior third of the cords. He had no evidence of disease and had good voice quality 4 years after therapy.

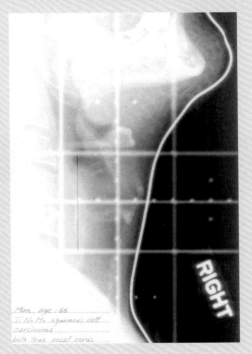

Case Figure 10.4

CASE STUDY 10.5

A 52-year-old woman who smoked cigarettes presented with hoarseness. Examination revealed a tumor involving the entire length of the right true vocal cord. The vocal cord mobility was normal, and the tumor did not extend into the supraglottic or subglottic larynx. A biopsy was positive for invasive squamous cell carcinoma. Final stage was T1 N0 M0. She was treated with primary radiation to the larynx only. Parallel-opposed fields were used to deliver a dose of 66 Gy in 33 fractions. Figure 10.5 shows the digitally reconstructed portal radiograph (Fig. 10.5A) and the isodose distribution through the larynx (Fig. 10.5B). A combination of 30- and 45-degree wedges was used to modify the beam, and the dose was delivered preferentially from the right side.

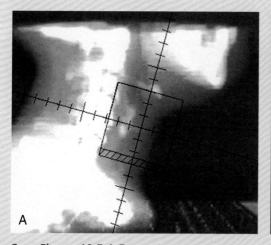
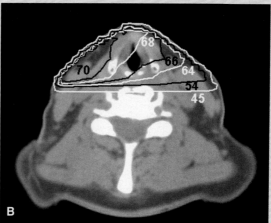

Case Figure 10.5 A,B

usually given with 15- or 30-degree wedges, with the heels oriented anteriorly. Differential loading (2:1 or 3:2) may be used for unilateral lesions.

Intensity-Modulated Radiation Therapy Planning

IMRT is an option for treatment of early-stage larynx cancer with a goal of improved carotid artery sparing **(Case Study 10.6)**. The CTV is the entire larynx excluding the suprahyoid epiglottis. The superior and inferior borders are similar to those used for conventional therapy. Volumetric modulated arc therapy (VMAT) has been adopted, when available, due to the ability to create a homogeneous plan with quick delivery time.

Background Data

See Tables 10.3 to 10.6.

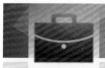

CASE STUDY 10.6

This 59-year-old patient was diagnosed with squamous cell carcinoma of the right true glottis larynx, stage T1a N0 M0 (stage I). He was treated with IMRT, delivered as VMAT using two arcs. Figure 10.6 shows an endoscopic image of his pretreatment disease extent (Fig. 10.6A), the diagnostic CT scan demonstrating right vocal cord thickening (Fig. 10.6B), and the treatment plan (Fig. 10.6C,D). The red color wash delineates the CTV$_{HD}$; the dose prescribed to the CTV$_{HD}$ was 63 Gy (in 28 fractions). Note the carotid vessels are spared from full dose through the use of this technique.

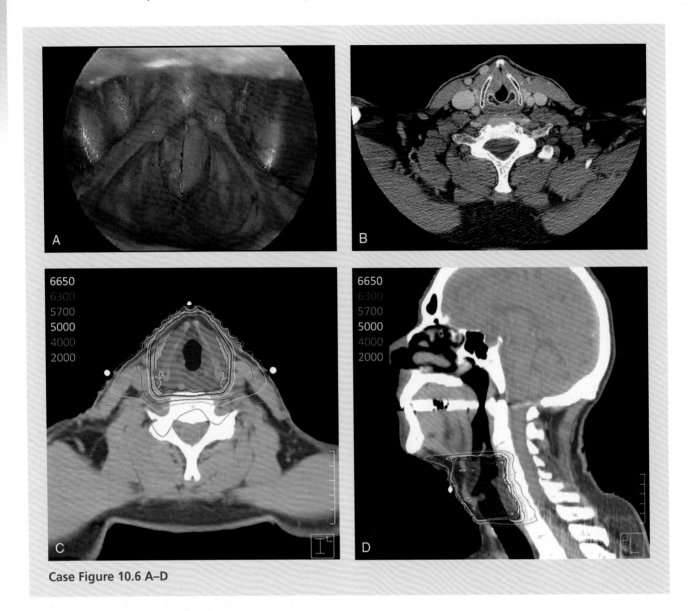

Case Figure 10.6 A–D

TABLE 10.3 Results of Radiation for T1 Carcinomas of the True Vocal Cords (Review)		
Series	No. of Patients	Local Control
Harwood et al. (1979)	333	86% (5-yr A)
Fletcher and Goepfert (1980)	332	89% (C)
Lustig et al. (1984)	342	90% (3-yr A)
Hendrickson (1985)	364	90% (C)

TABLE 10.3 Results of Radiation for T1 Carcinomas of the True Vocal Cords (Review) *(Continued)*

Series	No. of Patients	Local Control
Wang (1997)	665	93% (5-yr A)
Le et al. (1997)	315	84% (C)
Warde et al. (1998)	449	91% (T1a, 5-yr A) 82% (T1b, 5-yr A)
Cellai et al. (2005)	831	84% (5-yr A)
Chera et al. (2010)	325	94% (T1a, 5-yr A) 83% (T1b, 5-yr A)

A, actuarial; C, crude.

TABLE 10.4 Results of Radiation for T2 Carcinomas of the True Vocal Cords (Review)

Series	No. of Patients	Local Control
Lustig et al. (1984)	109	78% (3-yr A)
Karim et al. (1987)	156	78% (5-yr A)
Barton et al. (1992)	327	69% (5-yr A)
Wang (1996)	237	77% (T2a, 5-yr A) 71% (T2b, 5-yr A)
Warde et al. (1998)	230	69% (C)
Garden et al. (2003)	230	72% (5-yr A)
Frata et al. (2005)	256	73% (5-yr A)
Chera et al. (2010)	260	80% (T2a, 5-yr A) 70% (T2b, 5-yr A)

A, actuarial; C, crude.

TABLE 10.5 Five-Year Local Control Rates in 230 Patients with T2 N0 Glottic Carcinoma: Prognostic Variables

	No. of Patients	5-yr Control Rate (%)	*P*-value
No subglottic extension	111	81	
Subglottic extension	119	63	0.004
T2A	114	74	
T2B	116	70	0.37
Daily dose >2 Gy[a]	138	80	
Daily dose ≤2 Gy	90	59	<0.001
Once-daily fractionation[a]	147	67	0.06
Twice-daily fractionation	81	79	
Total	230	72	

[a]Two patients with compliance difficulties had fractionation schedule changes during their treatments and are excluded.
Data from M.D. Anderson Cancer Center.
Modified from Garden AS, Forster K, Wong PF, et al. Results of radiotherapy for T2 N0 glottic carcinoma: does the "2" stand for twice-daily treatment? *Int J Radiat Oncol Biol Phys* 2003;55:322–328.

TABLE 10.6 Causes of Death After Treatment of T2 Glottic Carcinoma in 230 Patients Treated at the MD Anderson Cancer Center

Causes	No. of Patients
Index cancer	
Recurrence above clavicles	15[a]
Distant metastases	15
Surgical complications	3
Second cancers	32
Other intercurrent disease (or unknown)	55
Total	119

[a]One patient died with both local recurrence and distant disease.
Adapted from Garden AS, Forster K, Wong PF, et al. Results of radiotherapy for T2 N0 glottic carcinoma: does the "2" stand for twice-daily treatment? *Int J Radiat Oncol Biol Phys* 2003;55:322–328.

LOCALLY ADVANCED CARCINOMA OF THE LARYNX

Treatment Strategy

For patients with T2 N2-3 and T3 larynx cancer who are good candidates for larynx preservation, concurrent chemoradiation with concurrent cisplatin is the preferred approach; the majority of data supports the use of a high-dose regimen (cisplatin 100 mg/m² every 3 weeks) although weekly regimens (cisplatin 40 mg/m² weekly) are increasing employed. An alternative option is three cycles of induction chemotherapy, consisting of docetaxel, cisplatin, and fluorouracil, followed by radiation therapy in responders or total laryngectomy in nonresponders.

The standard treatment for resectable T4 tumors is total laryngectomy; adjuvant radiation therapy is typically prescribed with adjuvant chemoradiation with cisplatin when the pathology reveals positive margins or extracapsular extension. Selected patients may be enrolled in ongoing trials to assess the optimal concurrent chemotherapy regimens.

Primary Radiotherapy for T3 or N+ Tumors

Target Volume

For patients without nodal involvement, the initial target volume encompasses larynx and levels II, III, and IV (subdigastric, midjugular, and lower neck) nodes **(Case Study 10.7)**. For patients with involved node(s), the initial target volume includes ipsilateral levels IB and/or V nodes. The boost volume encompasses primary tumor and involved nodes with 1- to 2-cm margins.

Setup and Field Arrangement for Conventional Radiotherapy Technique

The patient is immobilized in a supine position with a thermoplastic mask. Marking of shoulders and palpable lymph nodes, when present, facilitates portal design. Lateral parallel–opposed photon fields are used to treat the primary tumor and level II to III nodes. Field borders are similar to those used for supraglottic carcinoma. A matching anterior portal is used for treatment of the level IV nodes.

CASE STUDY 10.7

A 55-year-old man presented with a long history of persistent hoarseness and recent onset of left ear pain. Mirror examination showed a whitish exophytic lesion over the entire length of the left true vocal cord, which was fixed. The tumor extended into the left ventricle, and there was minimal edema of the left false cord. The right true vocal cord showed an area of leukoplakia, but the mobility was normal. There was no palpable neck lymphadenopathy. Computed tomography (CT) scan of the larynx confirmed the physical findings. Biopsy showed a well-differentiated squamous cell carcinoma of the left true vocal cord. The final stage was T3 N0 M0. He was treated with a standard fractionation (70 Gy in 35 fractions over 7 weeks with concurrent cisplatin.

The lateral portals (Fig. 10.7) were designed to encompass the primary tumor, level II and III lymph nodes. The level IV neck nodes were treated with a matching anterior appositional field. The boost dose was delivered through small lateral fields as used for T1 to T2 vocal cord tumors. The primary tumor received 70 Gy over 7 weeks, and the uninvolved neck nodes 50 Gy in 25 fractions over 5 weeks. This patient continued to smoke during and after treatment. Follow-up examination 2.5 years later revealed no evidence of disease, but the arytenoids were edematous.

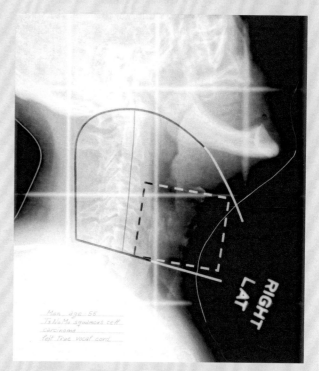

Case Figure 10.7

It may be necessary to use anterior and inferior tilts for patients with a short neck. In this case, the supraclavicular fossae are included in the primary portal **(Case Study 10.8)**.

For boost volume, lateral portals are reduced to encompass gross disease. Nodes overlying the spinal cord can usually receive boost dose through oblique-lateral primary boost portals and those in the lower neck through an appositional electron portal or glancing photon fields.

Intensity-Modulated Radiation Therapy Planning

Most patients are now treated with IMRT to spare parotid function **(Case Study 10.9 and Case Study 10.10)**. The primary disease is treated with a minimum of 8- to 10-mm margin, though due to laryngeal motion, it is prudent to encompass the majority of the larynx in the high-dose target (CTV_{HD}). Involved node(s) with 8- to 10-mm margin is also encompassed in CTV_{HD}. The neck compartments outside CTV_{HD} with a 2-cm (cranial-caudal) margin are delineated as CTV_{ID}. The remaining nodal levels (II, III, IV, V and VI) are contoured as CTV_{ED} (CTV3). Level Ib is included in CTV_{ED} on the side(s) of lymphadenopathy.

Dose

In combination with concurrent cisplatin, radiation is given in the conventional 2-Gy fractions to a dose of 50 Gy to the initial target volume and 70 Gy to the boost volume. Positive nodes receive 66 to 70 Gy depending on the size. The spinal cord dose is limited to 45 Gy or less. If treating with IMRT,

dose prescription is 70 Gy to CTV_{HD}, 60 to 63 Gy to CTV_{ID}, and 56 Gy to CTV_{ED}. Treatment is delivered in 33-35 fractions.

Postoperative Radiotherapy

Target Volume

The initial target volume encompasses the entire surgical bed, levels II–IV nodes and, when indicated, levels IB and V nodes and the tracheal stoma (see indications list in the following text) **(Case Study 10.8 and Case Study 10.11)**. The boost volume encompasses areas of known disease locations with 1- to 2-cm margins. Indications for postoperative radiotherapy to the tracheal stoma are subglottic extension, emergency tracheostomy, tumor invasion into the soft tissues of the neck (including ECE), close or positive tracheal margin, or surgical scar crosses the stoma.

Setup and Field Arrangement for Conventional Radiotherapy Technique

The patient is immobilized in a supine position with a thermoplastic mask. Marking of surgical scar, tracheal stoma, and shoulders facilitates portal design. Lateral parallel–opposed fields are used to treat the tumor bed and upper neck nodes:

- *Anterior, superior, and posterior borders:* similar to those of primary radiotherapy (ensure an adequate coverage of the entire surgical bed).
- *Inferior border:* just above the tracheal stoma.

CASE STUDY 10.8

A 52-year-old man presented with a transglottic tumor of the larynx and bilateral adenopathy. CT scan revealed a large primary laryngeal tumor invading the thyroid cartilage. He underwent a total laryngectomy and bilateral neck dissection. Histologic examination revealed basaloid squamous cell carcinoma of the right hemilarynx and pyriform sinus. The tumor invaded the thyroid cartilage, hyoid bone, and skeletal muscle of the neck. The margins were negative. Two of 32 right neck nodes were involved but without extracapsular extension. Left neck nodes were free of carcinoma. Final stage was T4 N2 M0. Radiation commenced 4 weeks after surgery. It was thought that the initial tumor volume extended inferiorly, and parallel-opposed fields would inadequately cover the volume at risk. It was elected instead to use oblique portals angled caudally and posteriorly (Fig. 10.8A). These two fields

encompassed the primary tumor volume at risk as well as the retropharyngeal nodes and nodal levels II through V. The stoma was covered in these fields, as well. At 42 Gy, the fields were reduced off the spinal cord. The caudal angulation was continued, but the fields were placed in true lateral position (Fig. 10.8B) to facilitate matching the electron fields for delivering supplemental dose to the posterior cervical strips. The final dose was 60 Gy. A reduction was not made off the superior border because the larger tissue diameter in this region resulted in a lower dose per fraction to the retropharyngeal and highest jugular nodes. Thus, the higher-risk volume received 60 Gy, while the lower-risk subclinical volume received 54 Gy (all in 30 fractions). Figure 10.8C, D shows representative isodose distributions through axial cuts of the mid- and low neck.

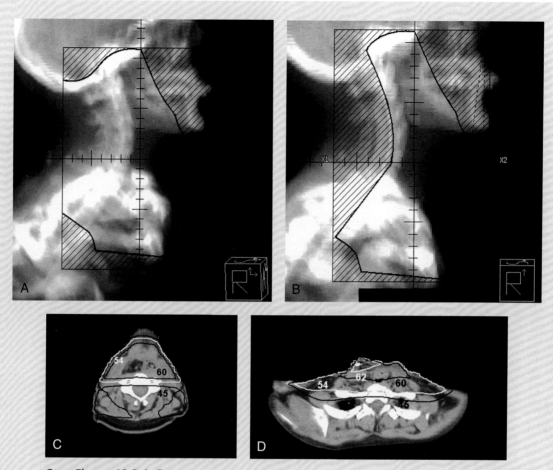

Case Figure 10.8 A–D

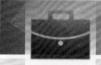

CASE STUDY 10.9

A 61-year-old male with a 60-pack-year smoking history presented with progressive hoarseness. Further evaluation revealed a bulky mass in the left hemilarynx with supraglottic and subglottic extension; the left hemilarynx was fixed. Biopsy was positive for squamous carcinoma. Final stage was T3 N0 M0. Figure 10.9A shows the

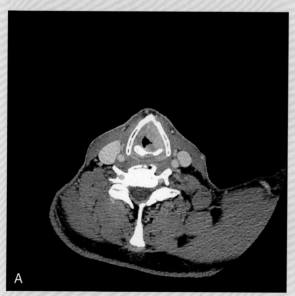

Case Figure 10.9 A,B

extent of the primary tumor on an axial CT image. He was treated with concurrent chemoradiation to a dose of 70 Gy in 33 fractions to CTV$_{HD}$, encompassing the pri-

mary tumor with margin, 63 Gy to CTV$_{ID}$ (approximately 1-cm additional margin around CTV$_{HD}$), and 57 Gy to CTV$_{ED}$ (Fig. 10.9B–D).

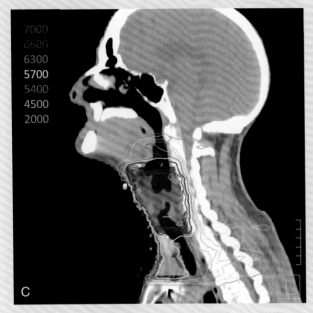

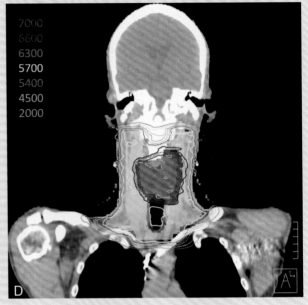

Case Figure 10.9 C,D

CASE STUDY 10.10

A 67-year-old male with a 44-year pipe-smoking history presented with hoarseness after intubation for a colon surgery. He then developed a right neck mass. Further evaluation revealed a bulky mass in the right supraglottis involving the right AE fold, arytenoid, false cord, true cord, and pyriform sinus. He also had right neck adenopathy. Biopsy was positive for squamous carcinoma; his stage was T3 N2b M0. Figure 10.10A shows the extent of the primary tumor and adenopathy on an axial CT image. He was treated with induction chemotherapy with a dramatic response at the

primary site (Fig. 10.10B). He was then treated with concurrent chemoradiation to a dose of 70 Gy in 33 fractions to CTV$_{HD}$, which encompassed the prechemotherapy primary tumor and nodal disease with margin (vGTV contours shown in light and dark green), 63 Gy to CTV$_{ID}$ (approximately 1-cm additional margin around CTV$_{HD}$), and 57 Gy to CTV$_{ED}$ (Fig. 10.10C–E). Figure 10.10D and Figure 10.10E show CTVED included the pre- and paratracheal nodes. Additionally, due to the extensive pyriform sinus involvement, the retropharyngeal nodes were treated.

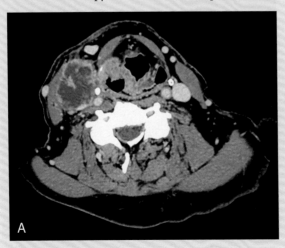

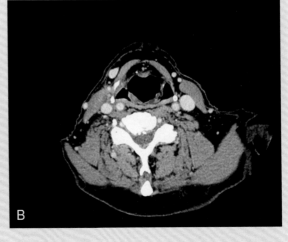

Case Figure 10.10 A,B

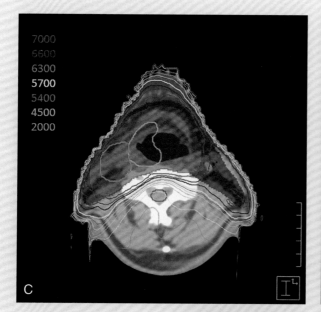
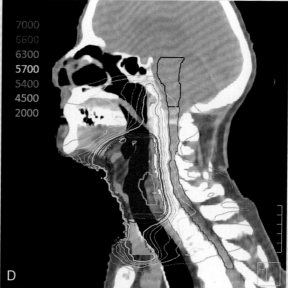
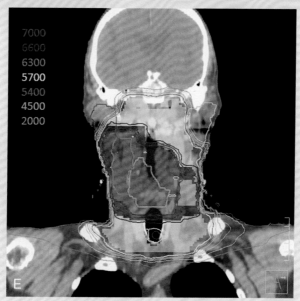

Case Figure 10.10 C–E

CASE STUDY 10.11

A 56-year-old man presented with a 3-month history of hoarseness and dysphagia. Examination showed a tumor of the infrahyoid epiglottis and both false cords. The true cords could not be visualized because of the swelling of the false cords. The pyriform sinuses appeared free of disease. There were no palpable neck nodes. A computed tomography (CT) scan showed a large tumor of the larynx involving both true cords with upward extension to the false cords and infrahyoid epiglottis and downward extension to the right lateral subglottic area. There was significant destruction of the thyroid cartilage and extension of the tumor into the anterior soft tissues of the neck. A biopsy showed squamous cell carcinoma. Stage: cT4 N0 M0. This patient underwent a wide-field laryngectomy. Pathologic examination showed a moderately differentiated squamous cell carcinoma involving both true vocal cords, right false cord, and infrahyoid epiglottis. There was 1.9-cm subglottic extension at the right side. The tumor penetrated through the thyroid cartilage into the anterior soft tissues of the neck. One of 14 recovered lymph nodes contained tumor. This node was located in the left paratracheal area and measured 1 cm in its largest diameter without extracapsular extension. Stage: pT4 N1 M0.

The surgical scar, tracheal stoma, and anterior skin of the neck and shoulders were wired at simulation. The tumor bed and level II to III nodes were irradiated through lateral–opposed fields (Fig. 10.11). The level IV nodal bed and tracheal stoma were treated with an anterior field. Primary tumor bed received a total dose of 60 Gy in 30 fractions, and dissected nodal areas along with tracheal stoma received a dose of 56 Gy in 28 fractions. He had no evidence of disease 3 years later.

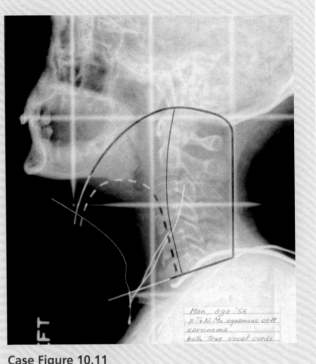

Case Figure 10.11

A matching anterior portal is used for the lower neck nodes and, when indicated, the tracheal stoma.

For the boost volume, lateral portals are reduced to encompass the areas of known tumor bed with 1- to 2-cm margins. Nodal areas overlying the spinal cord can usually receive boost dose through oblique-lateral primary boost portals and those in the lower neck through an appositional electron portal or glancing photon fields.

Dose

General guidelines after total laryngectomy are:

- 60 Gy in 30 fractions to areas with adverse features, that is, close or microscopically positive margins, perineural extension, vascular invasion, positive nodes, or extranodal extension. An additional boost dose of 6 Gy in three fractions may be given when indicated, for example, when multiple adverse features are present or when the interval between surgery and radiation is much longer than 6 weeks.
- 56 Gy in 28 fractions to the surgical bed.
- 50 Gy in 25 fractions to undissected regions to receive elective irradiation.
- When delayed wound healing postpones commencement of postoperative radiation to beyond 5 to 6 weeks, we prescribe accelerated fractionation, such as concomitant boost, by delivering twice-a-day irradiations for 1 week, usually at the end of the radiation

course, to reduce the potential hazard of prolonged cumulative treatment time.

After supraglottic laryngectomy, the dose is decreased to 55 Gy in 30 fractions over 6 weeks to minimize potential exacerbation of postsurgical edema by irradiation and facilitate rehabilitation of swallowing. Nodal beds at increased risk (ECE) are boosted an additional 6 to 10 Gy in 3 to 5 fractions with electrons or glancing photon fields.

The dose to the tracheal stoma is usually 50 Gy in 25 fractions.

Intensity-Modulated Radiation Therapy Planning

Most patients are now treated with IMRT to spare parotid function (**Case Study 10.12**). CTV_{HD} covers the preoperative tumor volume with 1- to 2-cm margins, CTV_{ID} defines the remaining operative bed, and CTV_{ED} encompasses the undissected, clinically uninvolved nodal levels along with the stoma. If there is substantial subglottic extension or paratracheal disease, the stoma can be delineated as CTV_{ID}.

Prescribed doses are 60 Gy to CTV_{HD}, 57 Gy to CTV_{ID}, and 54 Gy to CTV_{ED}. Regions containing positive margins or extensive ECE can be delineated separately to deliver doses of up to 63 to 66 Gy.

Background Data

See Tables 10.7 to 10.9.

CASE STUDY 10.12

A 59-year-old male with a 66-pack-year smoking history presented with sore throat, voice changes, and orthopnea. Physical examination revealed a large tumor of the entire larynx with extension anteriorly into the soft tissues in the neck (Fig. 10.12A) as well as left-sided nodal disease. Biopsy was positive for squamous carcinoma. Final stage was T4 N2b M0 larynx carcinoma.

He underwent a total laryngectomy and bilateral neck dissections. Pathology revealed a 4.2-cm primary tumor involving the transglottic larynx and extending into the soft tissue of the neck. There were two lymph nodes positive in the left neck with ECE. He was dis-

positioned to adjuvant chemoradiation. The primary tumor bed (neopharynx) and involved nodal areas (left neck) were identified as CTV$_{HD}$ (*red*) and prescribed 60 Gy. The uninvolved, but dissected, neck areas were treated as CTV$_{ID}$ and prescribed 57 Gy (*blue*). The uninvolved and undissected nodal areas were contoured as CTV$_{ED}$ and prescribed 54 Gy (*yellow*); CTV$_{ED}$ included the stoma, deemed at risk, but given the lowest dose level to balance the risk of recurrence versus the toxicity of microstomia. Figure 10.12B–D shows the dose distribution in axial, sagittal, and coronal views as well as the 3 CTVs in colorwash. The patient was alive 2 years later without evidence of disease.

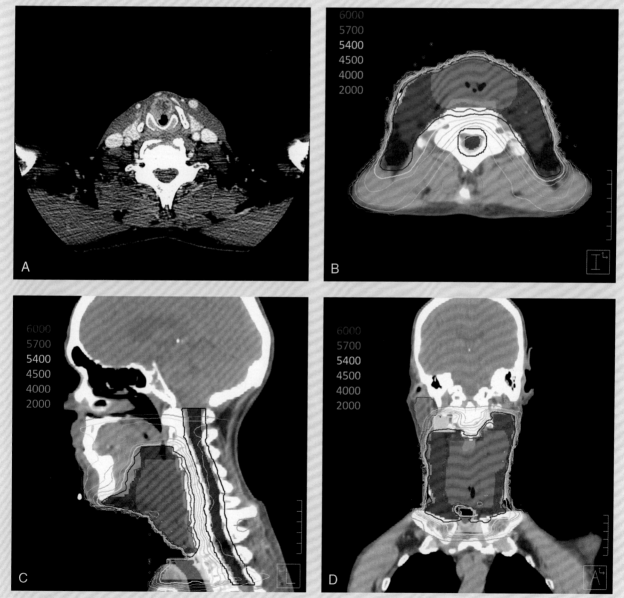

Case Figure 10.12 A–D

TABLE 10.7 Results of Radiation and Chemotherapy for Organ Preservation in Larynx Cancer: RTOG 91-11

	Radiotherapy Alone	Cisplatin+5-FU followed by Radiotherapy	Radiation+ Concurrent Cisplatin
Patient number	173	173	172
Supraglottic/glottic (%)	72/28	68/32	66/34
T2/T3/T4 (%)	12/79/9	12/78/10	11/78/10
Node positive (%)	50	50	50
2-yr local control (%)	58	64	80
2-yr laryngeal preservation (%)	70	75	88
2-yr distant failure (%)	16	9	8
2-yr overall survival (%)	75	74	75
2-yr difficulty swallowing (%)	14	16	15

Adapted from Forastiere AA, Goepfert H, Maor M, et al. Concurrent chemotherapy and radiotherapy for organ preservation in advanced laryngeal cancer. *N Engl J Med* 2003;349:2091–2098.

TABLE 10.8 Summary of Phase III Laryngeal Preservation Trials

Study Group (Year)	Eligibility	Sample Size	Study Arms	Overall Survival	Larynx Preservation
VA Laryngeal Cancer Study Group (1991)	Stage III–IV larynx cancer	332	A. Surgery B. Induction chemotherapy (CF)	68% 68% (NS, 2-yr A)	64%
GETTEC (1998)	T3 larynx cancer	68	A. surgery B. induction chemotherapy (CF)	84% 69% (P < 0.006, 2-yr A)	ND
EORTC (2009)	Stage III–IV larynx or hypopharynx cancer requiring total laryngectomy	450	A. induction chemotherapy (CF) B. alternating chemotherapy (CF) and radiation	62% 65% (NS, 3-yr A)	40%[a] 45% (NS)

TABLE 10.8 Summary of Phase III Laryngeal Preservation Trials *(Continued)*

Study Group (Year)	Eligibility	Sample Size	Study Arms	Overall Survival	Larynx Preservation
Intergroup -RTOG, SWOG, and ECOG (2013)	Stage III–IV larynx cancer requiring total laryngectomy	547	A. radiation B. radiation + cisplatin C. induction chemotherapy (CF)	32% 28% 39% (NS, 10-yr A)	64% 82% (*P* < 0.001) 68%
GORTEC 2000–2001 (2016)	Stage III–IV larynx or hypopharynx cancer requiring total laryngectomy	213	A. induction chemotherapy (CF) B. induction chemotherapy (TPF)	30% 24% (NS, 10-yr A)	46% 70% (*P* < 0.03)

[a]A 3-year actuarial laryngectomy-free survival.
CF, cisplatin and 5-FU; TPF, docetaxel, cisplatin, and 5-FU; NS, not significant; y A, year, actuarial; ND, not described.
Adapted from The Department of Veterans Affairs Laryngeal Study Group. Induction chemotherapy plus radiation compared with surgery plus radiation in patients with advanced laryngeal cancer. *N Engl J Med* 1991;324:1685; Richard J, et al. Randomized trial of induction chemotherapy in larynx carcinoma. *Oral Oncol* 1998;34:224; Lefebvre JL, et al. Phase 3 randomized trial on larynx preservation comparing sequential vs alternating chemotherapy and radiotherapy. *J Natl Cancer Inst* 2009;101:142; Forastiere AA, et al. Long-Term Results of RTOG 91-11: A Comparison of Three Nonsurgical Treatment Strategies to Preserve the Larynx in Patients With Locally Advanced Larynx Cancer. *J Clin Oncol* 2013;31:845; Pointreau et al. Randomized trial of induction chemotherapy with cisplatin and 5-fluorouracil with or without docetaxel for larynx preservation. *J Natl Cancer Inst* 2009;101:498.

TABLE 10.9 Failures Above the Clavicles by Primary and Nodal Staging in Patients with Advanced Glottic Carcinomas[a] Treated with Surgery (With or Without Postoperative Radiotherapy)

Stage	T3 (*n* = 185)		T4 (*n* = 57)	
	Surgery Alone	Combined Treatment	Surgery Alone	Combined Treatment
N0	22/135 (16)	2/22 (9)	10/32 (31)	1/16 (6)
N1	4/17 (24)	1/4 (25)	0/1 (0)	—
N2a	—	0/1 (0)	1/1 (100)	—
N2b	1/2 (50)	0/2 (0)	1/1 (100)	0/2 (0)
N3a	—	—	—	0/2 (0)
N3b	1/1 (100)	0/1 (0)	0/2 (0)	—
Total	28/155 (18)	3/30 (10)	12/37 (32.4)	1/20 (5)

[a]Values in parentheses are percentages.
Data from the M.D. Anderson Cancer Center.
Modified from Yuen A, Medina JE, Goepfert H, et al. Management of stage T3 and T4 glottic carcinomas. *Am J Surg* 1984;148:467–472.

SUGGESTED READINGS

Al-Mamgani A, Kwa SL, Tans L, et al. Single vocal cord irradiation: image guided intensity modulated hypofractionated radiation therapy for T1a glottic cancer: early clinical results. *Int J Radiat Oncol Biol Phys* 2015;93:337.

Barton MB, Keane TJ, Gadalla T, et al. The effect of treatment time and treatment interruption on tumour control following radical radiotherapy of laryngeal cancer. *Radiother Oncol* 1992;23:137.

Bron LP, Soldati D, Zouhair A, et al. Treatment of early stage squamous-cell carcinoma of the glottic larynx: endoscopic surgery or cricohyoidoepiglottopexy versus radiotherapy. *Head Neck* 2001;23:823.

Bryant GP, Poulsen MG, Tripcony L, et al. Treatment decision in T3N0M0 glottic carcinoma. *Int J Radiat Oncol Biol Phys* 1995;31:285.

Cellai E, Frata P, Magrini S, et al. Radical radiotherapy for early glottic cancer: results in a series of 1087 patients from two Italian radiation oncology centers. I. The case of T1N0 disease. *Int J Radiat Oncol Biol Phys* 2005;63:1378.

Chera BS, Amdur RJ, Morris CG, et al. T1N0 to T2N0 squamous cell carcinoma of the glottic larynx treated with definitive radiotherapy. *Int J Radiat Oncol Biol Phys* 2010;78(2):461.

Chera BS, Amdur RJ, Morris CG, et al. Carotid-sparing intensity-modulated radiotherapy for early-stage squamous cell carcinoma of the true vocal cord. *Int J Radiat Oncol Biol Phys* 2010;77:1380.

Fields JN, Marks JE. A technique for treatment of advanced carcinomas of the larynx and hypopharynx using low-megavoltage X-rays. *Radiother Oncol* 1986;7:281.

Fletcher GH. History of irradiation in squamous cell carcinomas of the larynx and hypopharynx. *Int J Radiat Oncol Biol Phys* 1986;12:2019.

Fletcher GH, Goepfert H. Larynx and pyriform sinus. In: Fletcher GH, ed. *Textbook of radiotherapy*, 3rd ed. Philadelphia, PA: Lea & Febiger, 1980.

Fletcher GH, Goepfert H. Irradiation in management of squamous cell carcinoma of the larynx. In: English GM, ed. *Otolaryngology*. Philadelphia, PA: Harper & Row, 1984.

Forastiere AA, Goepfert H, Maor M, et al. Long-term results of RTOG 91-11: a comparison of three nonsurgical treatment strategies to preserve the larynx in patients with locally advanced larynx cancer. *J Clin Oncol* 2013;31:845.

Frata P, Cellai E, Magrini S, et al. Radical radiotherapy for early glottic cancer: results in a series of 1087 patients from two Italian radiation oncology centers. II. The case of T2N0 disease. *Int J Radiat Oncol Biol Phys* 2005;63:1387.

Fuller CD, Mohamed AS, Garden AS, et al. Long-term outcomes after multidisciplinary management of T3 laryngeal squamous cell carcinomas: Improved functional outcomes and survival with modern therapeutic approaches. *Head Neck* 2017;38:1739.

Garden AS, Forster K, Wong PF, et al. Results of radiotherapy for T2 N0 glottic carcinoma: does the "2" stand for twice-daily treatment? *Int J Radiat Oncol Biol Phys* 2003;55:322.

Goepfert H, Jesse RH, Fletcher GH, et al. Optimal treatment for the technically resectable squamous cell carcinoma of the supraglottic larynx. *Laryngoscope* 1975;85:145.

Harwood AR, Beale FA, Cummings BJ, et al. Supraglottic laryngeal carcinoma: an analysis of dose-time-volume factors in 410 patients. *Int J Radiat Oncol Biol Phys* 1983;9:311.

Harwood AR, Hawkins NV, Beale FA, et al. Management of advanced glottic cancer. *Int J Radiat Oncol Biol Phys* 1979;5:899.

Harwood AR, Hawkins NV, Rider WD, et al. Radiotherapy of early glottic cancer—I. *Int J Radiat Oncol Biol Phys* 1979;5:473.

Hendrickson FR. Radiation therapy treatment of larynx cancers. *Cancer* 1985;55(suppl 9):2058.

Hinerman RW, Mendenhall WM, Amdur RJ, et al. Carcinoma of the supraglottic larynx: treatment results with radiotherapy alone or with planned neck dissection. *Head Neck* 2002;24:456.

Hinerman RW, Mendenhall WM, Morris CG, et al. T3 and T4 true vocal cord squamous carcinomas treated with external beam irradiation: a single institution's 35-year experience. *Am J Clin Oncol* 2007;30:181.

Janoray G, Pointreau Y, Garaud P, et al. Long-term results of a multicenter randomized phase III trial of induction chemotherapy with cisplatin, 5-fluorouracil, + docetaxel for larynx preservation. *J Natl Cancer Inst* 2016;108:pii.

Johansen LV, Grau C, Overgaard J. Supraglottic carcinoma: patterns of failure and salvage treatment after curatively intended radiotherapy in 410 consecutive patients. *Int J Radiat Oncol Biol Phys* 2002;53:948.

Johansen LV, Grau C, Overgaard J. Laryngeal carcinoma—multivariate analysis of prognostic factors in 1252 consecutive patients treated with primary radiotherapy. *Acta Oncol* 2003;42:771.

Johansen LV, Overgaard J, Hjelm-Hansen M, et al. Primary radiotherapy of T1 squamous cell carcinoma of the larynx: analysis of 478 patients treated from 1963 to 1985. *Int J Radiat Oncol Biol Phys* 1990;18:1307.

Karim AB, Kralendonk JH, Yap LY, et al. Heterogeneity of stage II glottic carcinoma and its therapeutic implications. *Int J Radiat Oncol Biol Phys* 1987;13:313.

Knab BR, Salama JK, Solanki A, et al. Functional organ preservation with definitive chemoradiotherapy for T4 laryngeal squamous cell carcinoma. *Ann Oncol* 2008;19:1650.

Le QX, Fu KK, Kroll S, et al. Influence of fraction size, total dose, and overall time on local control of T1-T2 glottic carcinoma. *Int J Radiat Oncol Biol Phys* 1997;39:115.

Lee NK, Goepfert H, Wendt CD, et al. Supraglottic laryngectomy for intermediate-stage cancer: U.T. M.D. Anderson Cancer Center experience with combined therapy. *Laryngoscope* 1990;100:831.

Lefebvre JL, Pointreau Y, Rolland F, et al. Induction chemotherapy followed by either chemoradiotherapy or bioradiotherapy for larynx preservation: the TREMPLIN randomized phase II study. *J Clin Oncol* 2013;31:853.

Lefebvre JL, Rolland F, Tesselaar M, et al. Phase 3 randomized trial on larynx preservation comparing sequential vs alternating chemotherapy and radiotherapy. *J Natl Cancer Inst* 2009;101:142.

Levendag P, Vikram B. The problem of neck relapse in early stage supraglottic cancer—results of different treatment modalities for the clinically negative neck. *Int J Radiat Oncol Biol Phys* 1987;13:1621.

Lundgren JA, Gilbert RW, van Nostrand AW, et al. T3N0M0 glottic carcinoma—a failure analysis. *Clin Otolaryngol Allied Sci* 1988;13:455.

Lustig RA, MacLean CJ, Hanks GE, et al. The patterns of care outcome studies: results of the national practice in carcinoma of the larynx. *Int J Radiat Oncol Biol Phys* 1984;10:2357.

Marks JE, Breaux S, Smith PG, et al. The need for elective irradiation of occult lymphatic metastases from cancers of the larynx and pyriform sinus. *Head Neck Surg* 1985;8:3.

Mendenhall WM, Parsons JT, Brant TA, et al. Is elective neck treatment indicated for T2N0 squamous cell carcinoma of the glottic larynx? *Radiother Oncol* 1989;14:199.

Nguyen-Tan PF, Le QT, Quivey JM, et al. Treatment results and prognostic factors of advanced T3-T4 laryngeal carcinoma: the University of California, San Francisco (UCSF) and Stanford University Hospital experience. *Int J Radiat Oncol Biol Phys* 2001;50:1172.

Parsons JT, Mendenhall WM, Mancuso AA, et al. Twice-a-day radiotherapy for T3 squamous cell carcinoma of the glottic larynx. *Head Neck* 1989;11:123.

Parsons JT, Mendenhall WM, Stringer SP, et al. T4 laryngeal carcinoma: radiotherapy alone with surgery reserved for salvage. *Int J Radiat Oncol Biol Phys* 1998;40:54.

Peters LJ, Thames HD Jr. Dose-response relationship for supraglottic laryngeal carcinoma. *Int J Radiat Oncol Biol Phys* 1983;9:421.

Richard J, Sancho-Garnier H, Pessey JJ, et al. Randomized trial of induction chemotherapy in larynx carcinoma. *Oral Oncol* 1998;34:224.

Robbins KT, Davidson W, Peters LJ, et al. Conservation surgery for T2 and T3 carcinomas of the supraglottic larynx. *Arch Otolaryngol Head Neck Surg* 1988;114:421.

Rosenthal DI, Fuller CD, Barker JL Jr, et al. Simple carotid-sparing intensity-modulated radiotherapy technique and preliminary experience for T1-2 glottic cancer. *Int J Radiat Oncol Biol Phys* 2010;77:455.

Rosenthal DI, Mohamed ASR, Weber RS, et al. Long-term outcomes after surgical or nonsurgical initial therapy for patients with T4 squamous cell carcinoma of the larynx: a 3-decade survey. *Cancer* 2015;121:1608.

Sailer SL, Sherouse GW, Chaney EL, et al. A comparison of postoperative techniques for carcinomas of the larynx and hypopharynx using 3-D dose distributions. *Int J Radiat Oncol Biol Phys* 1991;21:767.

Stalpers LJ, Verbeek AL, van Daal WA. Radiotherapy or surgery for T2N0M0 glottic carcinoma? A decision-analytic approach. *Radiother Oncol* 1989;14:209.

Terhaard CH, Karim AB, Hoogenraad WJ, et al. Local control in T3 laryngeal cancer treated with radical radiotherapy, time dose relationship: the concept of nominal standard dose and linear quadratic model. *Int J Radiat Oncol Biol Phys* 1991;20:1207.

The Department of Veterans Affairs Laryngeal Cancer Study Group. Induction chemotherapy plus radiation compared with surgery plus radiation in patients with advanced laryngeal cancer. *N Engl J Med* 1991;324:1685.

Trotti A, Zhang Q, Bentzen SM, et al. Randomized trial of hyperfractionation versus conventional fractionation in T2 squamous cell carcinoma of the vocal cord (RTOG 9512). *Int J Radiat Oncol Biol Phys* 2014;89:958.

Wang CC. Carcinoma of the larynx. *Radiation therapy for head and neck neoplasms.* New York: Wiley-Liss, 1997.

Wang CC, Nakfoor BM, Spiro IJ, et al. Role of accelerated fractionated irradiation for supraglottic carcinoma: assessment of results. *Cancer J Sci Am* 1997;3:88.

Warde P, Harwood A, Keane T. Carcinoma of the subglottis. Results of initial radical radiation. *Arch Otolaryngol Head Neck Surg* 1987;113:1228.

Wendt CD, Peters LJ, Ang KK, et al. Hyperfractionated radiotherapy in the treatment of squamous cell carcinomas of the supraglottic larynx. *Int J Radiat Oncol Biol Phys* 1989;17:1057.

Yamazaki H, Nishiyama K, Tanaka E, et al. Radiotherapy for early glottic carcinoma (T1N0M0): results of prospective randomized study of radiation fraction size and overall treatment time. *Int J Radiat Oncol Biol Phys* 2006;64:77.

Yom SS, Morrison WH, Ang KK, et al. Two-field versus three-field irradiation technique in the postoperative treatment of head-and-neck cancer. *Int J Radiat Oncol Biol Phys* 2006;66:469.

Yuen A, Medina JE, Goepfert H, et al. Management of stage T3 and T4 glottic carcinomas. *Am J Surg* 1984;148:467.

11

Hypopharynx

Key Points

- The hypopharynx is comprised of the pyriform sinuses and posterior pharyngeal wall. The pyriform sinus is conical in shape. Its medial wall is the lateral component of the supraglottic larynx, and the lateral wall is the lateral aspect of the pharynx. The majority of the posterior wall resides posterior to the larynx. Neoplasms in this location are referred to as postcricoid tumors.

- As the larynx essentially "resides in" the hypopharynx, strategies for management are similar for carcinomas originating from these two sites. The major objectives are tumor eradication, preservation of the natural speech, swallowing function, and avoidance of permanent tracheostomy.

- Hypopharyngeal carcinoma is usually diagnosed at more advanced T-category with higher incidence of nodal involvement than cancer of the larynx.

- Early tumors can be effectively controlled with definitive radiotherapy.

- Locally advanced tumors intermediate stage tumors (bulky T2 or T3) are effectively treated with concurrent chemoradiation with cisplatin; there are some data supporting use of induction chemotherapy (docetaxel, cisplatin, and 5-fluorouracil) for these patients, followed by either surgery or chemoradiation, depending on response.

- More advanced, resectable tumors are often managed with pharyngolaryngectomy followed by adjuvant radiation alone or radiation plus concurrent cisplatin, based on pathologic risk factors.

- The overall prognosis of patients with hypopharyngeal carcinoma is worse than those with laryngeal cancer.

PYRIFORM SINUS

Treatment Strategy

Primary radiotherapy is preferred for stage I and II tumors. Extrapolating from trials on laryngeal cancer (some European studies also enrolled hypopharyngeal carcinomas), radiation with three cycles of concurrent cisplatin (100 mg/m^2, q 3 weeks) is the preferred organ-preserving treatment for bulky T2 and T3 tumors. Posttreatment neck dissection can be used in patients with persistent neck adenopathy approximately 6 to 12 weeks after the completion of radiotherapy.

The standard treatment for resectable T4 tumors is total pharyngolaryngectomy. This is typically followed by postoperative radiation, with the use of concurrent chemotherapy if pathology reveals ECE or positive margins. Selected patients may be enrolled into ongoing trials; for example, testing various adjuvant concurrent chemotherapeutic agents and integrating molecularly targeted agents.

Indications for postoperative radiotherapy and irradiation of the tracheal stoma are similar to those for carcinoma of the larynx.

Primary Radiotherapy

Target Volume

The initial target volume encompasses the primary tumor with good margins and bilateral neck nodes, including the retropharyngeal, and levels II, III, IV, and V nodes. The target volume also includes ipsilateral level IB in the presence of level II node (**Case Study 11.1 and Case Study 11.2**).

The boost volume encompasses primary tumor and involved nodes with 1- to 2-cm margins.

Setup and Field Arrangement for Conventional Radiotherapy Technique

Marking of shoulders and palpable nodes facilitates portal design. The patient is immobilized in a supine position with the shoulders pulled down to the maximal extent. Lateral parallel–opposed photon fields are used to treat the primary tumor and upper and mid neck nodes:

- *Superior border:* at the level of the skull base to include the upper jugular and parapharyngeal lymphatics
- *Anterior border:* 1-cm fall-off
- *Posterior border:* behind the spinous processes or more posteriorly in the presence of large nodal mass
- *Inferior border:* encompasses primary lesion with margin (as low as possible while avoiding the shoulders)

A matching anterior portal is used to treat the lower neck nodes. It may be necessary to use anterior and inferior tilts for patients with a short neck or because of the inferior extent of the primary tumor or nodal mass. In this case, the supraclavicular fossae are included in the primary portal.

For the boost volume, reduced lateral fields are used as follows:

- *Superior and inferior borders:* depends on the extent of the disease, at least include aryepiglottic folds superiorly and cricoid cartilage inferiorly

CASE STUDY 11.1

A 54-year-old man had a routine checkup and was found to have a right neck mass. Physical examination showed discrete redness and mucosal irregularity in the medial and lateral walls of the right pyriform sinus without changes at the apex. There was a 5-cm firm node, fixed to the sternocleidomastoid muscle, palpated in the right lower jugular area. A biopsy from the right pyriform sinus showed moderately to well-differentiated squamous cell carcinoma. The final stage was T1 N2a M0. The primary tumor; bilateral levels II, III, IV; and retropharyngeal nodes were treated with lateral parallel–opposed photon fields (Fig. 11.1). The inferior border was placed just above the shoulders to encompass the involved lower jugular node (wired). Since all disease was located on the right side, the fields were weighted 3:2 in favor of the right side. A total dose of 66.6 Gy was delivered to the isocenter, which resulted in a dose of 68 Gy to the primary and 72 Gy to the involved node in 7 weeks. Off-cord reduction was made at 45 Gy. The posterior cervical nodes were supplemented with electrons to 54 Gy. The supraclavicular nodes were treated with an anterior appositional photon field to 54 Gy. Tissues directly posterior and inferior to the palpable node received additional irradiation to a cumulative dose of 63 Gy. Physical examination 6 weeks after completion of radiotherapy revealed a complete response at the primary site. In the neck, however, a 3-cm residual node was noted. Therefore, patient subsequently underwent a right neck dissection. He was alive and functioning well 2.5 years after therapy.

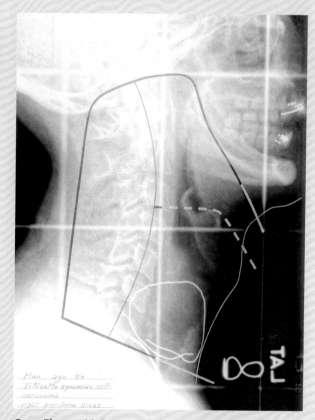

Case Figure 11.1

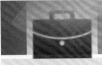

CASE STUDY 11.2

A 76-year-old man presented with a 10-month history of left-sided sore throat and otalgia. A 1.5-cm tumor was detected on the medial wall of the left pyriform sinus without extension to the apex. The larynx mobility was normal. A 1-cm lymph node was detected in level III in the left neck. Biopsy of the primary tumor revealed moderately differentiated squamous cell carcinoma. Final stage was T1 N1 M0. He was treated with 6 MV photons, with the primary tumor and upper and mid neck lymphatics as well as the retropharyngeal nodes encompassed in parallel–opposed fields (Fig. 11.2A). These portals received 42 Gy. An anterior supraclavicular and low neck field was matched on the skin and treated to 50 Gy. The upper fields were reduced off the spinal cord and continued to 54 Gy. An additional 12 Gy was delivered to coned down portals to a final dose of 66 Gy. The off spinal cord and boost fields were treated with parallel right anterior and left posterior oblique fields (Fig. 11.2B) to encompass the gross disease in the photon fields. The boost was preferentially weighted to the left. An isodose distribution through the central axis and primary tumor (*T*) and gross lymph node (*N*) is shown in (Fig. 11.2C). Both posterior cervical strips received 12-Gy supplement in six fractions with 9 MeV electrons, and then the left posterior strip received an additional boost of 12 Gy. The patient is without evidence of disease 2 years later.

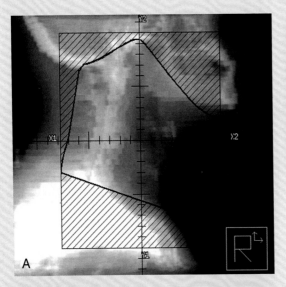

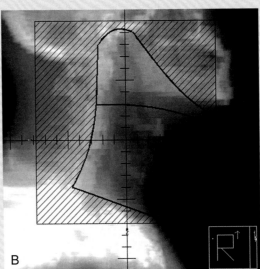

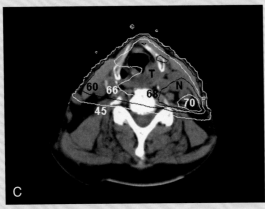

Case Figure 11.2A–C

- *Anterior border:* 1-cm fall-off, except when primary lesion is confined to the posterior structures where a small strip of anterior skin may be spared.
- *Posterior border:* mid-vertebral bodies, or posterior one third of vertebral bodies when the primary involves posterior pharyngeal wall.

Involved upper and midjugular nodes receive boost dose through lateral fields along with the primary tumor and lower neck nodes through a reduced anterior portal.

Nodes overlying the spinal cord can receive boost dose with electron beam(s) or, alternatively, the primary tumor and ipsilateral node can receive boost dose with oblique photon fields depending on the location of the node(s).

Intensity-Modulated Radiation Therapy Planning

Most patients are now treated with IMRT to spare parotid function (**Case Study 11.3 through Case Study 11.5**). The primary tumor and involved node(s) with a minimum of 8- to 10-mm margin constitute CTV_{HD}. However, because of laryngeal motion, it is prudent to encompass the majority of the larynx in the high-dose target volume. CTV_{ID} defines the neck compartments outside CTV_{HD} with a 2 cm

CASE STUDY 11.3

A 61-year-old male presented with sore throat, mild odynophagia, and weight loss. Examination revealed an extensive tumor of the oropharyngeal walls extending into the right pyriform sinus and postcricoid region; biopsy was positive for squamous cell carcinoma. There was no clinical evidence of lymphadenopathy. He received concurrent chemoradiation. While bulky disease was seen filling the right pyriform sinus, the disease had significant superficial spread. A PET–CT simulation was performed to assist in defining the targets, particularly the inferior extent of disease that could not be visualized clinically. An axial CT slice with adjacent fused PET image is shown (Fig. 11.3A). The high-dose clinical target volume (*red*) and subclinical target (*yellow*) are shown on the CT scan. A more inferior slice through the postcricoid region (Fig. 11.3B) did not demonstrate increase in FDG uptake. A high-dose clinical volume was outlined for boost volume definition, as this slice was approximately 1 cm below the identified gross target volume.

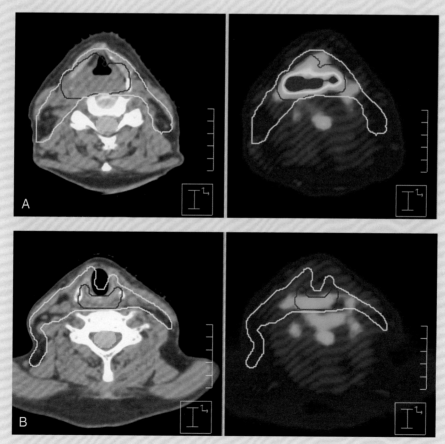

Case Figure 11.3A,B

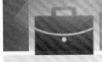

CASE STUDY 11.4

A 53-year-old male presented with a right upper neck mass and mild sore throat. Examination revealed a 2.5-cm upper jugular node and a lesion on the medial wall of the pyriform sinus (Fig. 11.4A). Axial CT images (Fig. 11.4B,C) show the right level II node and the superior aspect of the primary tumor at the vestibule of the right pyriform sinus and the bulk of the primary lesion at the level of the midpyriform sinus (T, tumor; N, node). The inferior aspect of the node can be seen abutting the anterior aspect of the sternocleidomastoid muscle. Biopsy of the primary tumor revealed squamous cell carcinoma. The final stage was T2 N1 M0.

He was treated with concurrent chemoradiation using IMRT.

CTV$_{HD}$ (70 Gy) encompassed the primary tumor and involved node with margins (Fig. 11.4D), CTV$_{ID}$ (60 Gy) the right posterior neck, and CTV$_{ED}$ (56 Gy) the left neck. The ipsilateral hypopharyngeal wall down to the cricoid level was included in CTV$_{HD}$ (Fig. 11.4E), right level III nodal region in CTV$_{ID}$ and left level III, and bilateral levels IV and IV nodes in CTV$_{ED}$ (Fig. 11.4F). Figure 11.4G shows the sagittal isodose distribution through the primary tumor. The patient had good function without evidence of disease 3 years after completing treatment.

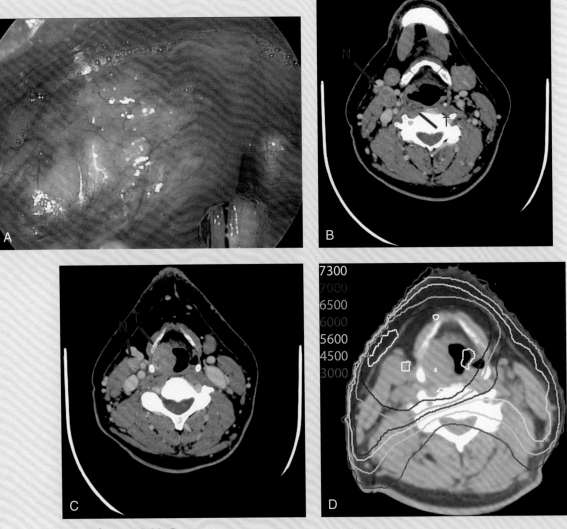

Case Figure 11.4A–D

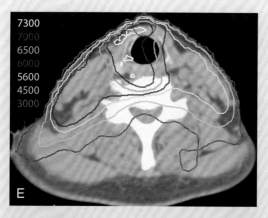

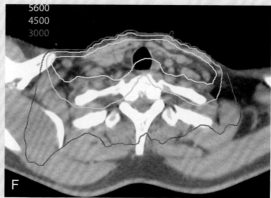

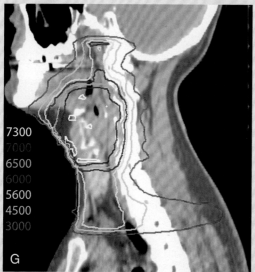

Case Figure 11.4E–G

CASE STUDY 11.5

A 76-year-old male with a history of cigarette and cigar smoking presented with a 6-month history of a globus sensation. Examination showed a large primary tumor of the left pyriform sinus that extended to the supraglottic larynx. There was no suspicious adenopathy. Biopsy of the primary tumor showed squamous cell carcinoma. Final stage was T4 N0 M0. Videostroboscopy and swallowing evaluation revealed excellent function.

Given his excellent function, he was dispositioned to induction chemotherapy followed by reevaluation for locoregional therapy based on response. He received weekly carboplatin, paclitaxel, and cetuximab (×6 cycles). Fig. 11.5A and Fig. 11.5B are axial CT views at the tumor

epicenter before and after chemotherapy). Due to the very good response and continued good function, he was dispositioned to definitive chemoradiation. He was treated with IMRT and concurrent weekly carboplatin (due to preexisting hearing loss). Figure 11.5C–E show axial, sagittal and coronal views. CTV$_{HD}$ (70 Gy—*red*) encompasses the prechemotherapy tumor with 8- to 10-mm margin, CTV$_{ID}$ (63 Gy—*blue*) covers the adjacent areas, and CTV$_{ED}$ (57 Gy—*yellow*) covers the uninvolved neck, including the bilateral retropharyngeal lymph nodes. Three years after completion of therapy, he remained free of disease, ate a near normal diet, and had normal speech.

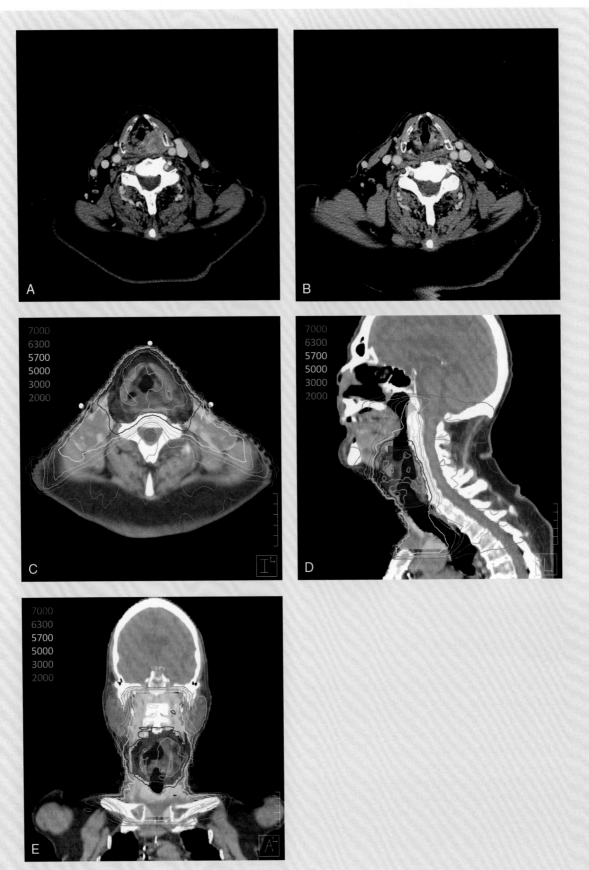

Case Figure 11.5A–E

(cranial–caudal). The remaining nodal levels (II, III, IV, and V) are contoured as CTV$_{ED}$. Level Ib on the side of involved node is included in CTV$_{ED}$.

Dose

Stage I (T1 N0) tumors: 50 Gy in 25 fractions to the initial target volume and then 16 Gy in 8 fractions to the primary tumor. For patients treated with IMRT, a dose of 66 Gy is prescribed to CTV$_{HD}$ and 54 Gy to CTV$_{ED}$. An alternative option is to treat with two sequential plans. The first delivers 50 Gy in 25 fractions to CTV$_{HD}$ and CTV$_{ED}$ followed by a plan that delivers 16 Gy in 8 fractions to CTV$_{HD}$.

Stage II (T2 N0) tumors: hyperfractionated or concomitant boost regimen. Hyperfractionation delivers 55.2 Gy in 46 fractions to the initial target volume and then 21.6 Gy in 18 fractions (1.2-Gy fractions, twice daily, 6-hour interval); the spinal cord dose is limited to 44.4 to 45.6 Gy or less and uninvolved posterior cervical nodes are supplemented with 2 Gy daily to approximately 55 Gy. Concomitant boost delivers 1.8-Gy fractions to 54 Gy in 30 fractions to the initial target volume and 1.5-Gy fractions to 15 to 18 Gy given as second daily fractions during the last 2 to 2.5 weeks; the spinal cord dose is limited to 45 Gy or less. For patients treated with IMRT, one option is to use the concomitant boost schedule, which requires two separate plans. The first plan delivers 54 Gy in 30 fractions to CTV$_{HD \, and}$ CTV$_{ED}$, and the second plan is for 18 Gy in 10 to 12 fractions to CTV$_{HD}$ (given as second daily fractions). An alternative choice is to use one plan that delivers 70 Gy to CTV$_{HD}$ and 56 Gy to CTV$_{ED}$. Treatment is given in 35 fractions over 30 treatment days, by delivering 6 fractions a week for 5 weeks with a 6-hour interfraction interval on the day 2 fractions.

Stage III and IV tumors: In combination with concurrent cisplatin, radiation is given in the conventional 2-Gy fractions to a dose of 50 Gy to the initial target volume and 70 Gy to the boost volume. Differential loading may be preferred for lateralized lesions with ipsilateral nodal disease only. In this situation, the dose is specified at an isodose line with maximal allowable dose heterogeneity of ±2.5%. The spinal cord dose is limited to 45 Gy or less. For patients treated with IMRT, the commonly prescribed doses are 70 Gy to CTV$_{HD}$, 60 to 63 Gy to CTV$_{ID}$, and 56 to 57 Gy to CTV$_{ED}$, given once daily in 33 to 35 fractions.

Postoperative Radiotherapy

The indications, technique, and dose prescriptions are similar to those for supraglottic carcinoma, except that the target volume also encompasses the retropharyngeal nodes. The superior border of the lateral fields is placed at the level of the base of skull (**Case Study 11.6**). For IMRT treatment planning, CTV$_{HD}$ encompasses the preoperative tumor bed and involved nodal regions with margin, CTV$_{ID}$ the operative bed, and CTV$_{ED}$ the undissected nodal volumes at risk including the retropharyngeal nodes. The stoma can be delineated as CTV$_{ID}$ or CTV$_{ED}$ depending on the risk features. Areas of very high risk (positive margin or extranodal extension) can be delineated separately, to a prescribed higher dose (e.g., 64 to 66 Gy).

Background Data

See Tables 11.1 and 11.2 for data regarding radiation for hypopharyngeal carcinoma and Table 11.3 for background data of radiation for early pyriform sinus cancer.

CASE STUDY 11.6

A 61-year-old man presented with several months of left otalgia and weight loss. Examination showed a large mass filling the left pyriform sinus, invading medially into the larynx. Biopsy of the primary tumor revealed moderately differentiated squamous cell carcinoma. Because of the weight loss and near obstruction of the larynx, a gastrostomy tube was placed and tracheostomy performed. He subsequently underwent total laryngectomy, partial pharyngectomy, and bilateral neck dissections. The defect was repaired with a radial forearm graft. Histologic examination revealed a carcinoma of the left pyriform sinus invading the left aryepiglottic fold and thyroid cartilage. There was perineural and lymph-vascular space invasion. Two of 25 nodes recovered from the left neck dissection contained metastatic disease without extracapsular extension. Stage: pT4 N2b M0. He received postoperative radiation. Figure 11.6A shows treatment began with large parallel–opposed fields that were progressively reduced after 42 Gy and 56 Gy to administer a total of 60 Gy to the high-risk regions. Figure 11.6B shows an isodose distribution through the central axis. The posterior cervical strips were supplemented with 12 MeV electrons to 56 Gy. A matching anterior field was used to treat the low neck and stoma to 50 Gy.

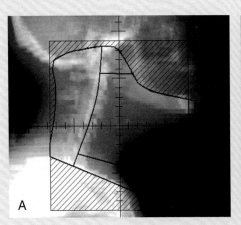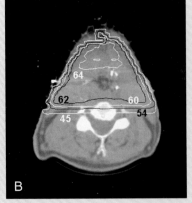

Case Figure 11.6A,B

TABLE 11.1 Distribution of Initial Failures in Patients with Early Stage (T1–T2) Carcinoma of the Hypopharynx Treated with Radiation Therapy

	T1	T2	Total
Type of Recurrence	(n = 58)	(n = 139)	(n = 197)
Primary relapse (P)	8	32	40
Nodal recurrence (N)	3	11	16
P + N	0	7	7
P + D	1	0	1
N + D	0	5	5
P + N + D	0	1	1
Distant metastasis (D)	3	8	10
Failure above clavicles without D	12 (21%)	50 (36%)	62 (31%)
Total failures	15 (26%)	58 (42%)	73 (37%)

Modified from Garden AS, et al. *Head Neck* 1996;18:317; Nakamura K. et al. *Int J Radiat Oncol Biol Phys* 2006;65:1045.

TABLE 11.2 Outcomes of Organ-preserving IMRT for Hypopharyngeal Carcinoma

	Patient Number	2-Yr OS	2-Yr LRC	2-Yr DMR
T1	14	85%	86%	14%
T2	39	70%	70%	16%
T3	28	76%	84%	20%
T4	17	70%	73%	13%
N0	18	88%	77%	6%
N1	19	88%	68%	6%
N2	49	72%	88%	11%
N3	12	42%	45%	72%
Total	98	74%	77%	17%

OS, overall survival; LRC, local regional control; DMR, distant metastasis rate.
Adapted from Edson MA, Garden AS, Takiar V, et al. Outcomes for hypopharyngeal carcinoma treated with organ-preservation therapy. *Head Neck* 2016;38(suppl 1):E2091–E2099.

TABLE 11.3 Local Control of Radiation for Early (T1–T2) Squamous Cell Carcinoma of the Pyriform Sinus (Literature Review)

Institution	Stage (No. of Patients)	5-Yr Actuarial Control
University of Florida	T1 (23)	85%
	T2 (100)	85%
University of Texas MD Anderson Cancer Center[a]	T1 (19)	89%
	T2 (63)	70%
Massachusetts General Hospital	T1 (24)	74%
	T2 (51)	76%
Japan (10 institutions)[b]	T1 (39)	85%[c]
	T2 (76)	68%[c]

[a]Includes all hypopharyngeal sites (69% of patients had pyriform sinus tumors).
[b]Includes all hypopharyngeal sites (70% of patients had pyriform sinus tumors)
[c]Crude local control rate.
Adapted from Rabbani A, et al. *Int J Radiat Oncol Biol Phys* 2008;72:351; Garden AS, et al. *Head Neck* 1996;18:317; Wang CC. In *Radiation therapy for head and neck neoplasms* 1997;212; Nakamura K. et al. *Int J Radiat Oncol Biol Phys* 2006;65:1045.

POSTERIOR HYPOPHARYNGEAL WALL

Treatment Strategy

Primary radiotherapy is preferred for T1 to T2 tumors. A combination of chemotherapy and radiation is the treatment of choice for T3 or N2 to N3 tumors. If the patient is not enrolled on a protocol, the combination of conventional radiation fractionation (70 Gy in 35 fractions over 7 weeks) with cisplatin (100 mg/m² given on days, 1, 22, and 43 of radiotherapy) is recommended. Consideration of a neck dissection is indicated for patients who have residual neck disease 6 to 10 weeks after completion of therapy.

Occasionally, advanced tumors (T4) are treated with surgery and postoperative radiotherapy. Carcinoma of the postcricoid region is very rare and is usually treated with surgery with or without postoperative radiotherapy.

Primary Radiotherapy

Target Volume

The initial target volume encompasses the primary with at least 2- to 3-cm margins (submucosal spread can be extensive) and levels II to V and retropharyngeal nodes (**Case Study 11.7**). The boost volume encompasses primary tumor and involved nodes with 1- to 2-cm margins.

IMRT target volumes are similar to those described for pyriform sinus cancers. CTV_{HD} should, however, include 3 to 5 mm of the anterior vertebral bodies even without demonstrable bone invasion. CTV_{ID} is often more generous, 2 to 3 cm in the cranial and caudal dimensions, because of the risk of submucosal lymphatic spread through the retropharyngeal space.

Setup and Field Arrangement for Conventional Radiotherapy Technique

Marking of palpable nodes and shoulders facilitates portal design. The patient is immobilized in a supine position with a thermoplastic mask with the shoulders pulled down as far as possible. Lateral parallel–opposed photon fields are used for treatment of the primary tumor and upper neck nodes:

- *Superior border:* at the base of skull to cover parapharyngeal lymphatics and upper jugular nodes.
- *Anterior border:* at least 2 cm anterior to the known extent of the tumor but when feasible short of fall-off anteriorly.
- *Posterior border:* just behind the spinous processes or more posteriorly in the presence of large nodal masses. After off-cord reduction, the posterior portal margin is at the posterior one third of vertebral bodies to include the retropharyngeal nodes and provide margin for the posterior pharyngeal wall.
- *Inferior border:* encompasses primary lesion with 3 cm or greater margin when possible.

CASE STUDY 11.7

A 68-year-old man had a 1-year history of dysphagia. Mirror examination revealed a mass in the left lateral and posterior hypopharyngeal walls. The medial wall and apex of the pyriform sinus were free. There were no palpable neck nodes. A CT scan confirmed the physical findings and in addition showed some thickening of the left aryepiglottic fold. Biopsy showed moderately differentiated squamous cell carcinoma. Final stage is

T2 N0 M0. This patient received radiotherapy with a hyperfractionation schedule. Figure 11.7 shows lateral fields designed to encompass the primary tumor and the majority of neck nodes while sparing a strip of anterior skin. The posterior border of the off-cord and boost portals at the level of the primary tumor was close to the posterior edge of the vertebral bodies to cover the lesion adequately. Supraclavicular nodes were treated with an anterior appositional photon field. The primary tumor received 76.6 Gy in 7 weeks (55.2 Gy in 46 fractions for 4.6 weeks + 21.6 Gy in 18 fractions for 2 weeks); uninvolved upper and midjugular nodes received 55.2 Gy in 4.6 weeks and uninvolved posterior cervical nodes 54 Gy in 5 weeks. Supraclavicular nodes received 50 Gy in five fractions for 5 weeks. Physical examination 6 months after radiotherapy revealed fullness of the left pyriform sinus. Biopsy of this area showed squamous cell carcinoma. He underwent total laryngopharyngectomy with left modified neck dissection and pharyngeal reconstruction with jejunal free flap. Second local recurrence occurred 5 months after surgery and he died of uncontrolled local disease.

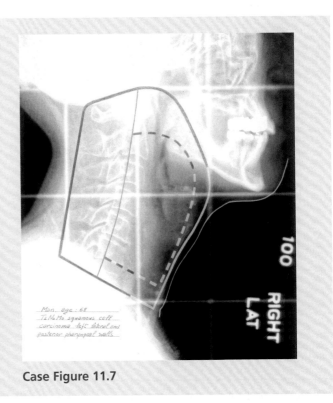

Case Figure 11.7

An anterior appositional portal is used for treating lower neck nodes. It may be necessary to use anterior and inferior tilts for patients with a short neck or because of the inferior extent of the primary tumor or nodal mass. In this case, the supraclavicular fossae are included in the primary portal.

For boost volume, the lateral fields are reduced:

- *Superior and inferior borders:* depends on extent of the primary tumor
- *Anterior border:* short of fall-off
- *Posterior border:* posterior one third of vertebral bodies

Involved levels II and III nodes are encompassed in lateral fields and lower neck nodes in a reduced anterior portal.

Nodes overlying the spinal cord can be boosted with electron beam(s) or, alternatively, the primary tumor and ipsilateral node can be boosted with oblique photon fields.

Intensity-Modulated Radiation Therapy Planning

IMRT is best suited for treating tumors extending to the paravertebral region without overdosing the spinal cord because this technique can produce a horseshoe-shape isodose distribution. The patient is immobilized in a supine position with an extended thermoplastic mask (**Case Study 11.8**) Thin-cut computed tomography scans are obtained in treatment position. Clinical target volumes, as described for

CASE STUDY 11.8

A 60-year-old man presented with dysphagia and was found to have biopsy proven squamous cell carcinoma of the posterior hypopharynx (Fig. 11.8A). Axial CT slices show disease in the posterior hypopharyngeal wall invading the preverterbral muscles (Fig. 11.8B) with left retropharyngeal adenopathy (Fig. 11.8C). He underwent total pharyngolaryngectomy and bilateral neck dissections including resection of the retropharyngeal space followed by a tubed shape anterolateral thigh free flap

reconstruction. Histologic examination revealed a 7-cm primary tumor, five positive nodes in the right neck and eight positive nodes in the left neck, as well as disease in the retropharyngeal space. He was treated with concurrent cisplatin and IMRT delivering 60 Gy in 30 fractions to CTV$_{HD}$. Figure 11.8D–F shows representative isodose distribution on axial, sagittal, and coronal views through isocenter. He developed lung metastasis without locoregional relapse <1 year from diagnosis.

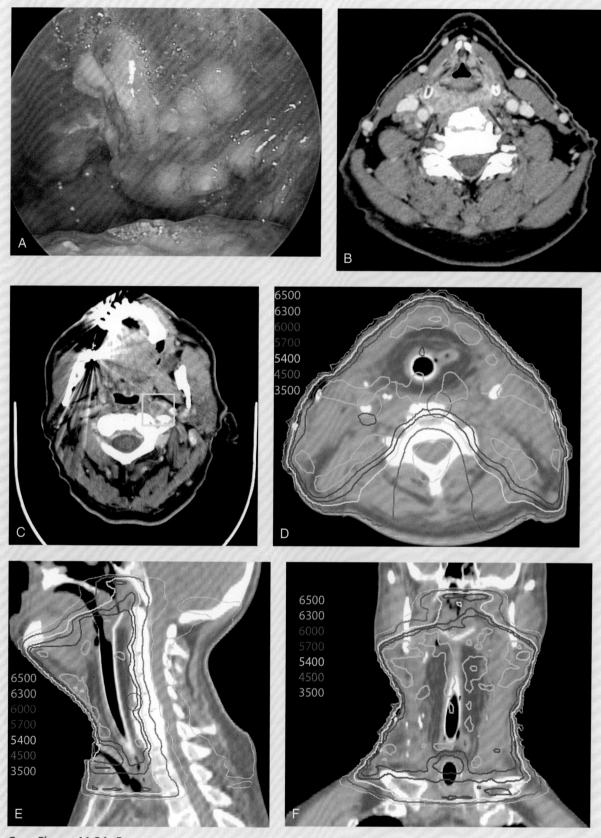

Case Figure 11.8A–F

pyriform sinus carcinomas above, are outlined for dosimetric planning.

Dose

T1 tumors: 50 Gy in 25 fractions to the initial target volume and then 16 Gy in 8 fractions to the primary tumor.

T2 tumors: hyperfractionated or concomitant boost regimen. Hyperfractionation delivers 55.2 Gy in 46 fractions to the initial target volume then 21.6 Gy in 18 fractions (1.2-Gy fractions, twice daily, 6-hour interval); the spinal cord dose is limited to 44.4 to 45.6 Gy or less and uninvolved posterior cervical nodes are supplemented with 2 Gy daily to approximately 55 Gy. Concomitant boost delivers 1.8-Gy fractions to 54 Gy in 30 fractions to the initial target volume and 1.5 Gy-fractions to 15 to 18 Gy given as second daily fractions during the last 2 to 2.5 weeks; the spinal cord dose is limited to 45 Gy or less.

Positive nodes, frequently present, receive doses appropriate for the size and the fractionation schedule used, for example, includes 66 to 70 Gy in 2-Gy fractions, 69 to 72 Gy with concomitant boost, or 74.4 to 79.2 Gy with hyperfractionation.

T3 tumors: In combination with three cycles of concurrent cisplatin, radiation is given in the conventional 2-Gy fractions to a dose of 50 Gy to the initial target volume and 70 Gy to the boost volume. The spinal cord dose is limited to 45 Gy or less.

Regimens for IMRT are similar to that described for pyriform sinus tumors.

Postoperative Radiotherapy

Indications and technique for postoperative radiotherapy are similar to those for pyriform sinus cancer, with the exception that the posterior border of the off-cord and boost fields are brought closer to the posterior edge of the vertebral bodies to ensure good coverage of the prevertebral and paravertebral

tissues. CTV_{HD} should, however, include 3 to 5 mm of the anterior vertebral bodies even without demonstrable bone invasion.

Background Data

See Table 11.4

SUGGESTED READINGS

Bataini P, et al. Results of radical radiotherapy treatment of carcinoma of the pyriform sinus: experience of the Institute Curie. *Int J Radiat Oncol Biol Phys* 1982;9:1277.

Edson MA, Garden AS, Takiar V, et al. Outcomes for hypopharyngeal carcinoma treated with organ-preservation therapy. *Head Neck* 2016;38(suppl 1):E2091–E2099.

El Badawi SA, et al. Squamous cell carcinoma of the pyriform sinus. *Laryngoscope* 1982;92:357.

Fein DA, et al. Pharyngeal wall carcinoma treated with radiotherapy: impact of treatment technique and fractionation. *Int J Radiat Oncol Biol Phys* 1993;26:751.

Fletcher GH, Goepfert H. Larynx and pyriform sinus. In: Fletcher GH, ed. *Textbook of radiotherapy*, 3rd ed. Philadelphia, PA: Lea & Febiger, 1980.

Frank JL, et al. Postoperative radiotherapy improves survival in squamous cell carcinoma of the hypopharynx. *Am J Surg* 1994;168:476.

Garden AS, et al. Early squamous cell carcinoma of the hypopharynx: outcomes of treatment with radiation alone to the primary disease. *Head Neck* 1996;18:317.

Hall SF, et al. Radiotherapy or surgery for head and neck squamous cell cancer: establishing the baseline for hypopharyngeal carcinoma. *Cancer* 2009;115:5711.

Hinerman RW, et al. Hypopharyngeal carcinoma. *Curr Treat Options Oncol* 2002;3:41.

Janoray G, et al. Long-term results of a multicenter randomized phase III trial of induction chemotherapy with cisplatin, 5-fluorouracil, +/− docetaxel for larynx preservation. *J Natl Cancer Inst* 2015;108(4). pii: djv368. doi: 10.1093/jnci/djv368.

Johansen LV, Grau C, Overgaard J. Hypopharyngeal squamous cell carcinoma—treatment results in 138 consecutively admitted patients. *Acta Oncol* 2000;39:529.

Kuo P, et al. Hypopharyngeal cancer incidence, treatment and survival temporal trends in the United States. *Laryngoscope* 2014;124:2064.

Lefebvre JL, et al. Larynx preservation with induction chemotherapy for hypopharyngeal squamous cell carcinoma: 10-year results of EORTC trial 24891. *Ann Oncol* 2012;23:2708.

Lefebvre JL, et al. Induction chemotherapy followed by either chemoradiotherapy or bioradiotherapy for larynx preservation: the TREMPLIN randomized phase II study. *J Clin Oncol* 2013;31:853–859.

TABLE 11.4 Local Control of Radiation Alone for Squamous Cell Carcinoma of the Hypopharyngeal Wall

Institution	Stage (No. of Patients)	Actuarial Local Control
University of Florida[a]	T1 (5)	100%
	T2 (24)	76%
	T3 (36)	51%
	T4 (10)	25%
Massachusetts General Hospital[b]	T1 (18)	88%
	T2 (46)	55%
	T3-4 (41)	49%

[a]2-Yr actuarial control.
[b]5-Yr actuarial control.
Modified from Fein DA, et al. *Int J Radiat Oncol Biol Phys* 1996;26:751–757; Wang CC. In *Radiation therapy for head and neck neoplasms* 1997:216.

Marks JE, et al. Pharyngeal wall cancer: an analysis of treatment results complications and patterns of failure. *Int J Radiat Oncol Biol Phys* 1978;4:587.

Nakamura K, et al. Multi-institutional analysis of early squamous cell carcinoma of the hypopharynx. *Int J Radiat Oncol Biol Phys* 2006;65:1045.

Pene F, et al. A retrospective study of 131 cases of carcinoma of the posterior pharyngeal wall. *Cancer* 1978;42:2490.

Pingree TF, et al. Treatment of hypopharyngeal carcinoma: a 10-year review of 1,362 cases. *Laryngoscope* 1987;97:901.

Posner MR, et al. Sequential therapy for locally advanced larynx and hypopharynx cancer subgroup in TAX 324: survival, surgery, and organ preservation. *Ann Oncol* 2009;20:921–927.

Prades JM, et al. Concomitant chemoradiotherapy in pyriform sinus carcinoma. *Arch Otolaryngol Head Neck Surg* 2002;128:384.

Pradhan SA. Post-cricoid cancer: an overview. *Semin Surg Oncol* 1989;5:331.

Rabbani A, et al. Definitive radiotherapy for T1-T2 squamous cell carcinoma of the pyriform sinus. *Int J Radiat Oncol Biol Phys* 2008;72:351.

Samant S, et al. Concomitant radiation therapy and targeted cisplatin chemotherapy for the treatment of advanced pyriform sinus carcinoma: disease control and preservation of organ function. *Head Neck* 1999;21:595.

Stell PM, et al. Management of post-cricoid carcinoma. *Clin Otolaryngol* 1982;7:145.

Vandenbrouck C, et al. Squamous cell carcinoma of the pyriform sinus: retrospective study of 351 cases treated at the Institut Gustave-Roussy. *Head Neck Surg* 1987;10:4.

Wang CC. Carcinoma of the hypopharynx. In: *Radiotherapy of head and neck neoplasms*. New York, NY: Wiley-Liss, 1997.

12

Nasal Cavity

Key Points

- The nasal cavity comprises the nasal vestibule and nasal fossa (posterior nasal cavity).

- The nasal vestibule is lined with squamous epithelium, and carcinomas originating in this location behave like common skin cancers.

- Nasal vestibule carcinomas can spread to the buccal, facial, and cervical lymph nodes.

- Radiation, often with brachytherapy alone or combined with external beam, is a primary treatment option for early carcinoma of the vestibule. Postoperative radiation is often recommended for advanced lesions.

- The nasal fossa proper is lined with respiratory mucosa inferiorly and olfactory epithelium superiorly. Neoplasms arising in this location include squamous cell carcinomas, adenocarcinomas, and neuroendocrine cancers that occasionally spread to level IB and/or IIA nodes at presentation.

- Management of nasal fossa cancers depend on histology and stage but often involve multimodality therapy including radiation.

- The superior aspect of the nasal fossa lies between the eyes and below the anterior cranial fossa and is, therefore, quite challenging for planning radiotherapy. Intensity-modulated radiation therapy is now commonly used to treat cancers in this location.

- Proton therapy, including intensity-modulated proton therapy, can be advantageous for targets at the anterior skull base.

NASAL VESTIBULE

Treatment Strategy

Primary radiotherapy is preferred for smaller tumors for better cosmetic outcome. Combination of surgery and radiotherapy may be necessary for large, locally destructive tumors.

Primary Radiotherapy

Target Volume

Initial Target Volume

The initial target volume for well-differentiated tumors with diameters of 1.5 cm or less without extension into adjacent structures is the primary tumor with approximately 2-cm margins. Radiation can be administered by brachytherapy, external beam, or a combination of both, depending on the location.

For poorly differentiated tumors or well-differentiated tumors >1.5 cm in diameter without palpable nodes (N0), the volume encompasses primary tumor with approximately 2-cm margins and bilateral facial lymphatics ("Manchu moustache area") and level IB (submandibular) and level IIA (subdigastric) nodes (**Case Study 12.1**). Patients with involved node(s) also receive irradiation to the level III and IV nodes.

CASE STUDY 12.1

A 41-year-old man presented with a "pimple" at the junction of right nasal vestibule and upper lip. A generous biopsy was taken, which showed squamous cell carcinoma with perineural and lymphatic invasion. The patient was referred for treatment.

Physical examination revealed a 2.5 × 1.5 ulcerative area in the nasal vestibule, extending halfway down the upper lip as shown in Figure 12.1A,B. There was no palpable adenopathy. The diagram (Fig. 12.1C) illustrates the primary and moustache fields. The lower half of the nose and upper lip were treated with an anterior appositional field using 20-MeV electrons and 6-MV photons weighted in the ratio 4:1. The facial lymphatics were treated with anterior appositional (15-degree gantry rotation) 6-MeV electron fields. The upper neck nodes received irradiations with parallel–opposed lateral photon fields (Fig. 12.1D). The primary tumor received 60 Gy (at 90%) in 30 fractions and facial lymphatics and upper neck nodes 50 Gy in 25 fractions. Dry skin reactions outline the portals at completion of treatment (Fig. 12.1E,F), but skin reactions subsided 3 weeks after completion of radiation. This patient had no evidence of disease 5 years after therapy.

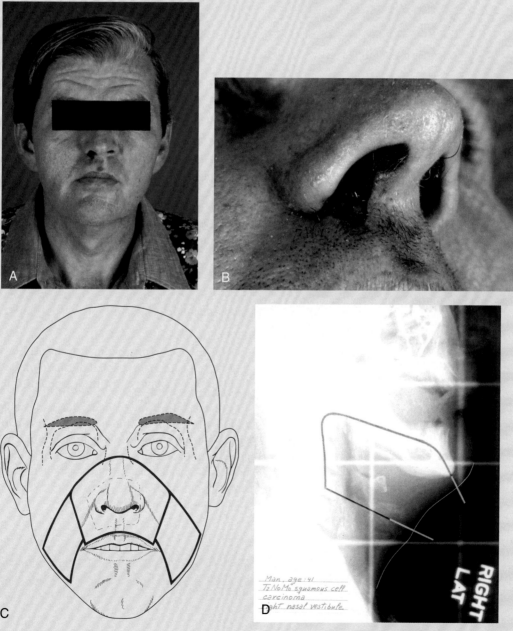

Case Figure 12.1A–D

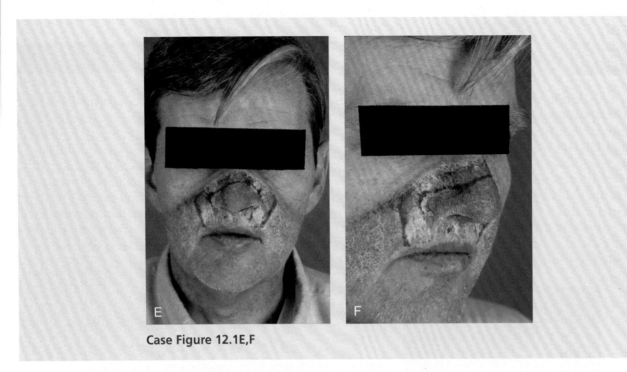

Case Figure 12.1E,F

The boost volume encompasses primary tumor and, when present, involved nodes with 1- to 2-cm margins.

Setup and Field Arrangement

An intraoral stent containing cerrobend is used to displace the tongue posteriorly and to partially shield the upper alveolar ridge (see Fig. 3.7). The patient is immobilized in a supine position.

With external beam irradiation, an anterior appositional field (combination of electrons and photons usually in a ratio of 4:1) is used to treat the nasal vestibule.

- *Superior border*: bridge of the nose or higher in large tumors.
- *Lateral borders*: approximately 1 cm lateral to the alae nasi.
- *Inferior border*: depends on the extent of upper lip invasion (e.g., from mid upper lip to the vermilion border).
- *Boost irradiation*: the anterior portal encompasses the primary tumor with 1- to 2-cm margins.

Technical details to improve the dose distribution are as follows:

- Nasal cavities are filled with bolus to reduce dose heterogeneity.
- Skin collimation is used and wax bolus is applied to smooth the contour for electron beam irradiations.
- If the overlying skin is involved, bolus is placed over the infiltrated area to eliminate the skin-sparing effect of photon irradiation.

For the moustache field, anterior right and left appositional electron fields (usually set up with an approximately 15- to 20-degree gantry angle) are used to treat the facial lymphatics. This field is set up clinically after approving the primary tumor and upper neck portals.

- *Medial border*: matches the lateral border of the anterior field (primary tumor).
- *Anterior border*: extends down from oral commissure to the middle of the horizontal ramus of the mandible.
- *Posterior border*: from the upper edge of the anterior field to just above the angle of the mandible.
- *Inferior border*: splits the horizontal ramus of the mandible and adjoins the upper neck field.

The upper neck nodes are treated with lateral parallel–opposed photon fields:

- *Anterior border*: 1-cm falloff
- *Superior border*: matches moustache fields
- *Posterior border*: just behind the mastoid processes
- *Inferior border*: just above the arytenoids

Patients with involved nodes receive irradiation to mid and lower neck nodes through an anterior portal. Involved nodes receive a boost dose with appositional electrons or glancing photon fields. Brachytherapy alone or a combination of external irradiation and brachytherapy is used to treat small lesions of the vestibule or lower septum (**Case Study 12.2 through Case Study 12.4**).

Dose

Small lesions (1.5 cm or less): 50 Gy in 25 fractions followed by 10 to 16 Gy in 5 to 8 fractions boost by external irradiation (usually prescribed at 90% isodose line) or 60 to 65 Gy over 5 to 7 days by implants.

CASE STUDY 12.2

A 71-year-old man underwent a single-plane iridium implant of the nasal septum for a 1.5-cm squamous cell carcinoma. Five-centimeter stainless steel needles were loaded with 5-cm active-length iridium 192 wires (0.65-mg Ra equivalent per cm) to deliver a dose of 70 Gy at 5 mm in 127 hours.

Figure 12.2 shows the primary lesion at the nasal septum (Fig. 12.2A) and the geometry of the iridium implant in anterior (Fig. 12.2B) and lateral (Fig. 12.2C) views.

On follow-up, the patient had occasional nasal bleeding caused by changes in weather. He was diagnosed with prostate cancer 12 years later and died of pneumonia and cardiac failure following surgery for an aneurysm of the aorta 13 years later without evidence of disease at the nasal septum. (From Delclos L. A second look at interstitial irradiation. In: Deeley TJ, ed. *Topical reviews in radiotherapy and oncology*, vol. II. Bristol, VA: John Wright & Sons Ltd., 1982:190–191, with permission.)

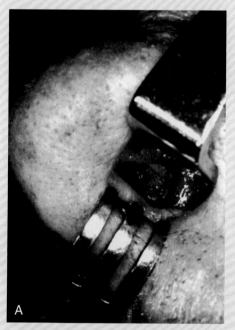

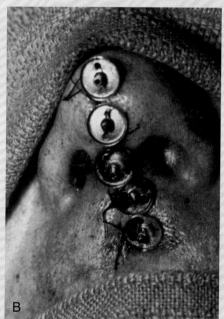

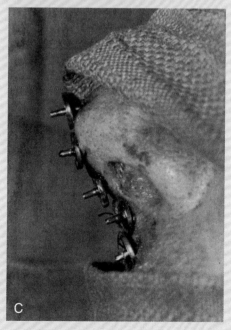

Case Figure 12.2A–C

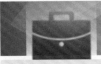

CASE STUDY 12.3

A 67-year-old man presented with T1 N0 squamous cell carcinoma of the right anterior nasal septum and received treatment with brachytherapy.

Figure 12.3 shows the implant with five needles with approximately 1-cm spacing (Fig. 12.3A) and an isodose distribution through the midplane (Fig. 12.3B). The cav-ity was packed with Vaseline gauze and the needles were afterloaded with iridium 192. The active lengths varied between 3 and 3.5 cm, providing approximately 1-cm margin beyond the tumor. The total dose was 60 Gy spec-ified to the 40 cGy per hour line. The patient was alive without disease 6 years later.

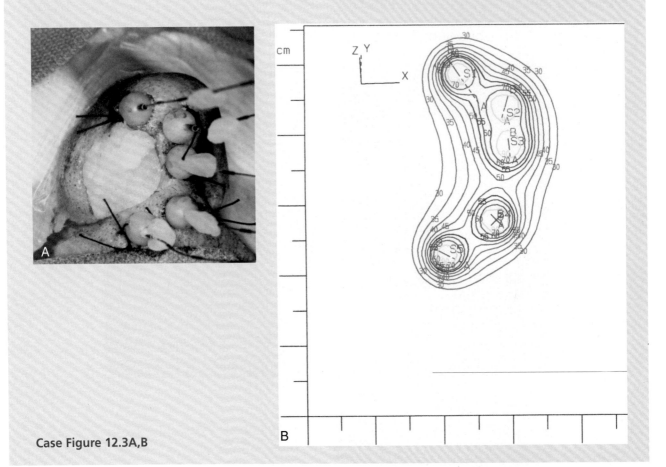

Case Figure 12.3A,B

Larger lesions: 50 Gy in 25 fractions followed by 16 to 20 Gy in 8 to 10 fractions boost. Elective treatment of facial (moustache area) and upper neck nodes: 50 Gy in 25 frac-tions. Palpable nodes receive a total dose of 66 to 70 Gy depending on the size.

Dose Specification: See "General Principles"

The electron beam to the nose should be of a sufficiently high energy (15 to 20 MeV) to provide an adequate deep mar-gin. The dose is specified at an isodose line (usually 90%). Moustache fields are irradiated with 6-MeV electrons pre-scribed at D_{max}.

NASAL FOSSA PROPER

Treatment Strategy

Our current treatment strategy is as follows:

- T1 to T2 N0 to N1: radiotherapy or surgery depending on the location and size. Postoperative radiation (with or without chemotherapy) may be indicated in patients treated with surgery, if margins are inadequate, if there is perineural invasion, or if a neck dissection is per-formed and reveals multiple nodes or nodal extracap-sular extension (ECE).

CASE STUDY 12.4

An 87-year-old man presented with epistaxis. A biopsy of a 1-cm lesion at the anterior left nasal septum was positive for well-differentiated squamous cell carcinoma.

Figure 12.4 shows a CT slide of the head and neck, which reveals the lesion (Fig. 12.4A). He was treated with brachytherapy. Ten stainless steel needles were placed in the left nasal ala, nasal tip, and left nasal septum

(Fig. 12.4B) and were afterloaded with ^{192}Ir wires. A total dose of 60 Gy was delivered over 3½ days. CT dosimetry was obtained, and isodose distributions are shown on an axial plane through the tumor (Fig. 12.4C) and on a lateral view (Fig. 12.4D). He had no evidence of disease and had no symptoms 3 years after treatment.

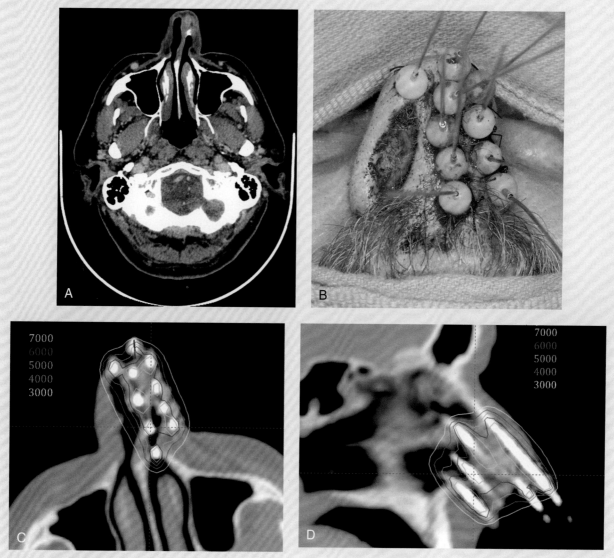

Case Figure 12.4A–D

- T3 to T4 or N2 to N3: surgery + postoperative radiotherapy. Patients are occasionally selected for treatment with systemic therapy. Patients with good partial or complete responses are treated with concurrent chemoradiation, and those with lesser responses are treated with surgery followed by radiation.

Primary Radiotherapy

The target volume encompasses primary tumor with 2- to 3-cm margins. Lesions of 1.5 cm or less in diameter that are located in the inferior nasal septum are generally treated with interstitial brachytherapy as described above for tumors of the nasal vestibule. Other lesions selected for radiotherapy receive external irradiation.

Setup and Field Arrangement for Conventional External Irradiation

Marking of lateral canthi, oral commissures, and limbus (particularly medial and inferior borders) facilitates portal design. An intraoral stent is used to open the mouth and to depress the tongue out of the radiation fields (see Chapter 3). The patient is immobilized in a supine position with the head positioned in such a way that the hard palate is perpendicular to the treatment couch.

The location and size of the tumor determine the appropriate portal borders and arrangement. Tumors in the anterior nasal cavity not suited for brachytherapy (see subsequent text) may be treated with an appositional mixed beam arrangement (**Case Study 12.5**). This requires careful CT scan–based treatment planning because it is very easy to underestimate the appropriate depth. Additionally, the isodose distribution can be heterogeneous in this location with irregular contours and significant bone and air interfaces, especially when using electron beam.

Three-field technique (see Chapter 13) is required for irradiation of primaries of the upper or posterior nasal cavity. This setup allows coverage of ethmoids without delivering high doses to the optic apparatus. CT scan–based treatment planning is necessary to determine the appropriate beam weighting and wedge sizes.

Intensity-Modulated Radiation Therapy

The complexity of the anatomy and the proximity to the optic structures and brain make tumors located in these areas well-suited for intensity-modulated radiation therapy (IMRT), which has become a preferred technique. The patient is immobilized in a supine position, with an extended head and shoulder thermoplastic mask. Thin-cut CT scans are obtained in treatment position. The target volumes are outlined for dosimetric planning (**Case Study 12.6 and Case Study 12.7**).

Gross Target Volume

Gross target volume (GTV) represents all areas determined from clinical examination and imaging studies to contain macroscopic disease.

Clinical Target Volumes

Three clinical target volumes (CTVs) are generally delineated.

- CTV_{HD} delineates volumes to receive the highest dose, which includes the primary tumor and nodal GTVs with 0.5- to 1-cm margins.
- CTV_{ID} outlines volumes to receive an intermediate dose, which encompasses an additional 0.5- to 1-cm margin around CTV_{HD} and, in the presence of

CASE STUDY 12.5

A 57-year-old woman presented with nasal fullness and epistaxis. Examination showed a tumor of the nasal septum, the biopsy of which revealed squamous cell carcinoma. Although the tumor was primarily at the anterior septum, the posterior and superior extent made it unfavorable for brachytherapy. Therefore, she was treated with external beam radiation.

Figure 12.5 shows lead skin collimation with additional thickness over the eyes (Fig. 12.5A) and customized beeswax bolus (Fig. 12.5B) used (also see Fig. 3.12). Axial isodose distribution with simulated skin collimation (because the lead cannot be scanned) and the beeswax bolus are shown at the levels of the midnose through the tumor (Fig. 12.5C) and through the inferior orbits (Fig. 12.5D). A total dose of 66 Gy was delivered to a 90% isodose line (actual doses shown). Beams were a mix of 20-MeV electrons and 6-MV photons, in approximately 4.5:1 ratio. Small reductions were made inferiorly and superiorly to minimize hot spots in the palate and ethmoids. The patient remains without disease 3.5 years from treatment. However, she developed epiphora 2 years following therapy, which was resolved with dacryocystorhinostomy and silicone tube placement.

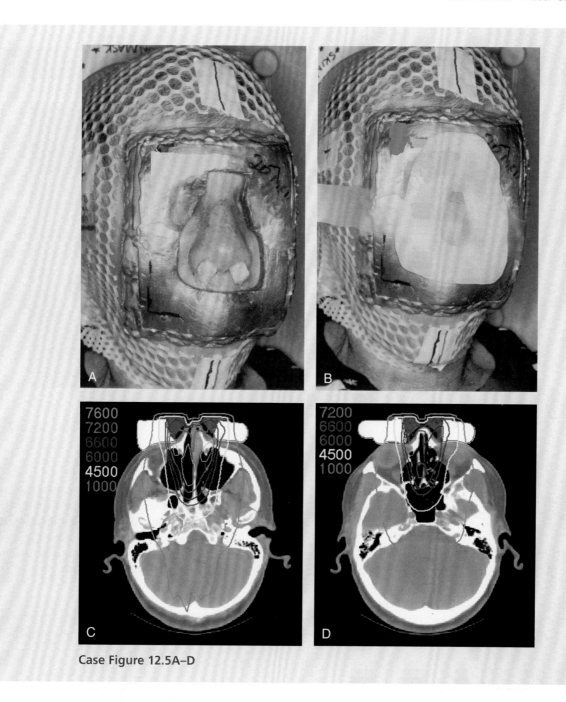

Case Figure 12.5A–D

positive node(s), the involved and adjoining nodal compartment(s).

- CTV$_{ED}$ delineates volumes to receive an elective dose for subclinical disease. If the tumor invades an adjacent sinus, CTV$_{ED}$ encompasses the entire sinus beyond CTV$_{ID}$. In the N0 neck, CTV$_{ED}$ may include retropharyngeal, levels IB and II nodes depending on the tumor type and stage. When level IB or II node is involved, CTV$_{ED}$ also includes clinically uninvolved ipsilateral levels III and IV nodes. Note that ipsilateral levels III and IV nodes can also be treated with a matching anterior oblique photon

portal with an isocenter placed above the thyroid cartilage.

Dose

- *External irradiation*: conventional technique delivering 50 Gy in 25 fractions to the initial target volume plus 16 to 20 Gy in 8 to 10 fractions to the boost volume depending on the size. IMRT regimen for T1 and small T2 tumors is 66, 60, and 54 Gy to CTV$_{HD}$, CTV$_{ID}$, and CTV$_{ED}$, respectively, given in 30 fractions. Regimens for larger tumors, or when combined with concurrent chemotherapy, are

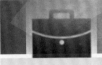

CASE STUDY 12.6

A 55-year-old male initially presented with T2 N0 squamous cell carcinoma of the oropharynx. He was treated with concomitant boost fractionation. Approximately 1 year later, a routine follow-up endoscopy discovered a mass in the posterior right nasal septum, biopsy positive for squamous cell carcinoma. The tumor was too deep for either brachytherapy or electron therapy. Given the previous radiotherapy, which encompassed the entire posterior pharynx, he was treated with IMRT to a total dose of 66 Gy delivered in 30 fractions.

Figure 12.6 shows a representative axial isodose through the tumor. He was without evidence of disease for both primary tumors.

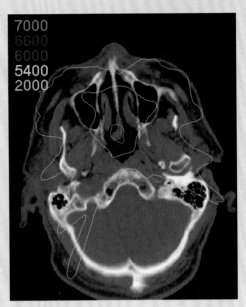

Case Figure 12.6

70, 60 to 63, and 56 to 57 Gy to CTV$_{HD}$, CTV$_{ID}$, and CTV$_{ED}$, respectively, in 33 or 35 fractions.
- *Brachytherapy*: approximately 60 to 65 Gy in 5 to 7 days specified at the margins of the lesion.

Postoperative Radiotherapy

Target Volume

The initial target volume encompasses the entire surgical bed. The boost volume encompasses areas of macroscopic disease with 1- to 2-cm margins.

Intensity-Modulated Radiation Therapy

The technique used is similar to primary radiotherapy presented above. The patient is immobilized in a supine position, with an extended head and shoulder thermoplastic mask. Thin-cut CT scans are obtained in treatment position. The target volumes are outlined for dosimetric planning (**Case Study 12.8 through Case Study 12.10**).

Virtual Gross Target Volume

There is no actual GTV after complete surgical tumor resection. However, it can be useful to formulate a virtual GTV

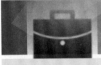

CASE STUDY 12.7

A 30-year-old man presented with nasal obstruction. Examination showed a right nasal mass, the biopsy of which revealed sinonasal undifferentiated carcinoma.

Figure 12.7A shows a T2-weighted axial magnetic resonance imaging revealing the lesion in the nasal cavity with secretions in the adjacent maxillary and sphenoid sinuses. He was treated with neoadjuvant VP-16 and cisplatin for three cycles with a good response, with only questionable residual disease in the posterior nasal cavity. He subsequently received IMRT with two additional cycles

of single-agent cisplatin. Figure 12.7B,C shows axial dose distributions through the nasal cavity and sagittal view through midline, respectively. The areas of residual abnormality (*yellow*) received 66 Gy, the pretreatment tumor volume received 63 Gy, and areas of potential microscopic spread including right level I and II nodes received 54 Gy, all given in 30 fractions. Brainstem (*magenta*), optic chiasm (*blue*), and an oral avoidance volume (*orange*) are shown. He was free of recurrence at the last follow-up, more than 3 years after completion of therapy.

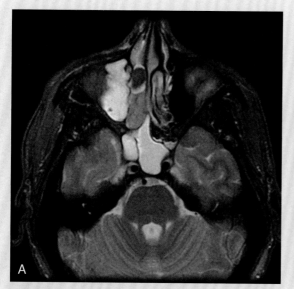

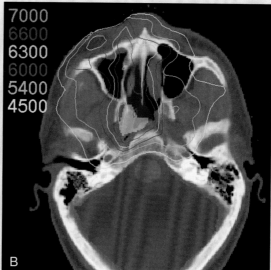

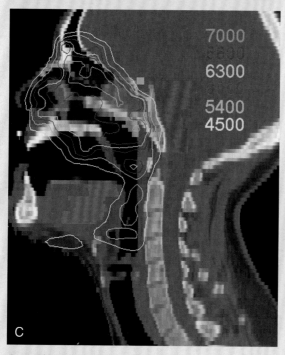

Case Figure 12.7A–C

CASE STUDY 12.8

A 60-year-old woman presented with nasal obstruction and epistaxis. She was found to have a lesion in the posterior right nasal septum. Biopsy was positive for squamous cell carcinoma.

Figure 12.8A shows the tumor (*green arrow*) in an axial slice of diagnostic CT scan. She underwent an endoscopic resection of the tumor. Margins were negative but contained high-grade dysplasia.

She was treated with postoperative IMRT. A mouth-opening, tongue-depressing stent was used to minimize dose to the oral structures. As the vGTV was relatively small, it was elected to omit CTV_{ID} but define CTV_{HD}

fairly generously to include the septum and right nasal cavity. The remaining left nasal cavity, medial aspect of the right maxillary sinus, hard palate (floor of the nasal cavity), anterior sphenoid sinus, and ethmoid sinuses were defined as CTV$_{ED}$. CTV$_{HD}$ and CTV$_{ED}$ were prescribed 60 and 54 Gy, respectively, and treatment was delivered in 30 fractions. An axial view of the isodose distribution is shown through the mid-nose (Fig. 12.8B) along with CTV$_{HD}$ (*red*) and CTV$_{ED}$ (*yellow*). A second axial view (Fig. 12.8C) through the

ethmoids and orbits shows only CTV$_{ED}$ at this level. The doses to the optic nerves and lenses were <45 and <10 Gy, respectively. Isodose distributions in sagittal (Fig. 12.8D) and coronal views through midplane of the head (Fig. 12.8E) are also shown. The contour color wash inside the 60-Gy line is removed so the underlying resected tissues can be appreciated. The mouth-opening stent can also be seen on these views. The patient has done well and is without disease 3 years later.

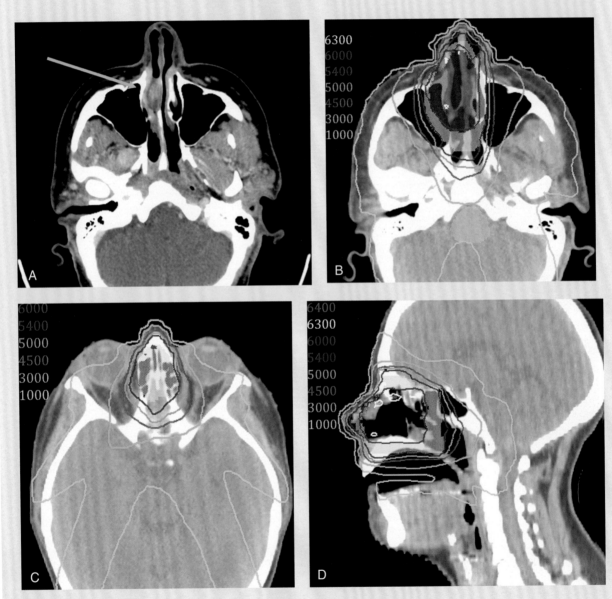

Case Figure 12.8A–D

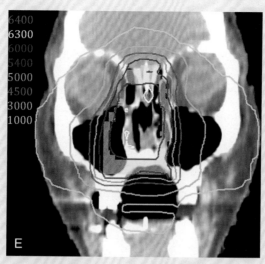

Case Figure 12.8E

CASE STUDY 12.9

A 74-year-old woman had a squamous cell carcinoma of the right nasal ala treated with Mohs surgery.

One year later, the tumor (*green arrow*) recurred locally as demonstrated on Figure 12.9A showing an axial view of the diagnostic head and neck CT scan. She was treated with surgery and postoperative IMRT.

Surgery consisted of a radical resection of the soft tissue of the face, right medial maxillectomy, partial ethmoidectomy, and lacrimal sac marsupialization. The defect was reconstructed with an anterolateral thigh-free flap. Histologic examination revealed a poorly differentiated squamous carcinoma that invaded the connective tissue and periosteum of the lateral nasal wall and medial maxilla. There was also perineural invasion.

Postoperative IMRT was delivered in 30 fractions starting 1 month later. Figure 12.9B shows an axial isodose distribution with contours of CTV_{HD} (tumor bed—

red), CTV_{ID} (surgical bed—*blue*), and CTV_{ED} (perineural route and upper neck nodes at risk—*yellow*). The surgical bed and reconstructed tissues can be better appreciated without CTV contours (Fig. 12.9C). The main nerve at risk was the infraorbital nerve to the maxillary nerve as it exits foramen rotundum. Since poorly differentiated carcinoma has a higher propensity for nodal spread, CTV_{ED} included the right buccal, facial, and upper cervical nodes. Also shown are axial isodose distributions at the level of the ethmoids and orbits (Fig. 12.9D), maxilla (Fig. 12.9E), buccal region (Fig. 12.9F), facial and upper neck nodes (Fig. 12.9G), and a coronal view through the orbits and anterior maxillary sinuses (Fig. 12.9H). The patient developed posttherapy ectropion and epiphora that was helped by removal of scar tissue and tarsorrhaphy to repair the ectropion 1 year later. She remains without disease 2 years later.

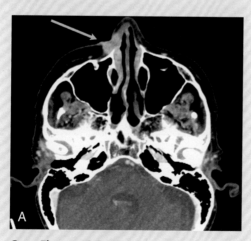
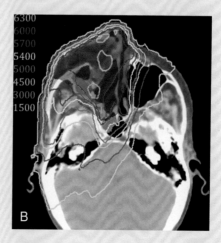

Case Figure 12.9A,B

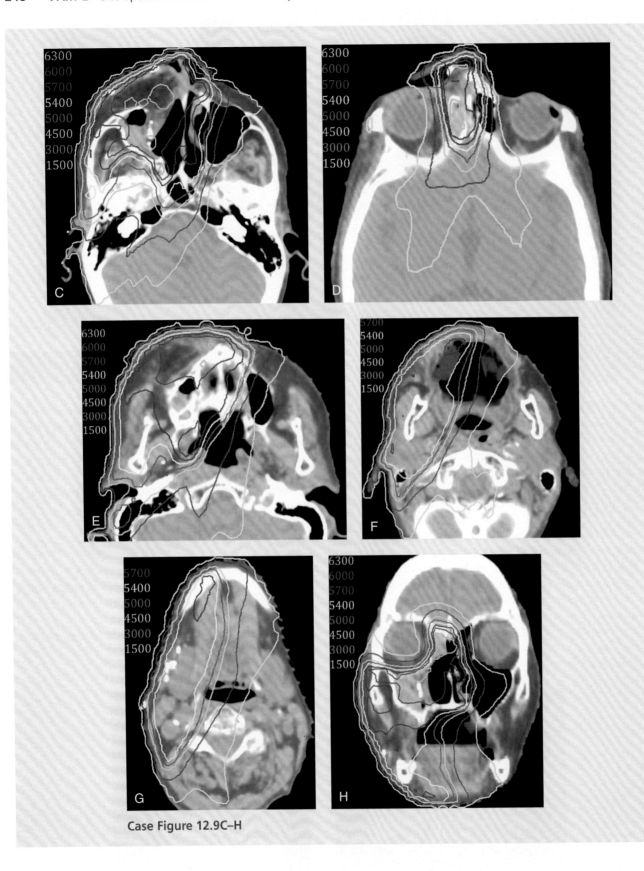

Case Figure 12.9C–H

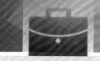

CASE STUDY 12.10

A 57-year-old man presented with chronic epistaxis and was found to have a tumor of the nasal septum. A biopsy revealed poorly differentiated squamous cell carcinoma.

Figure 12.10 shows representative images of staging CT scan revealing a bulky tumor (*green arrow*) primarily in the floor of the nasal cavity abutting the anterior maxilla (Fig. 12.10A) and more superiorly the septal defect with surrounding irregular tissue (Fig. 12.10B).

He underwent a partial rhinectomy, ethmoidectomy, partial resection of the upper lip, and sphenoidotomy, followed by plastic surgical reconstruction. The tumor was 3.5 cm in size and invaded the cartilage. Due to the

size and poor differentiation, postoperative IMRT was recommended to treat the nose, the remaining upper lip, and draining lymphatics. Tissue equivalent material was placed in the surgical defect to improve the dose distribution. Figure 12.10C–H shows axial isodose distributions at the level of the ethmoids (Fig. 12.10C), midmaxillary sinuses and the center of the rhinectomy defect (Fig. 12.10D), maxilla and residual upper lip (Fig. 12.10E), mandible and buccal region (Fig. 12.10F), upper neck (Fig. 12.10G), and a sagittal view through midplane (Fig. 12.10H). The patient was without disease but did have grade 2 xerostomia, 1 year after treatment.

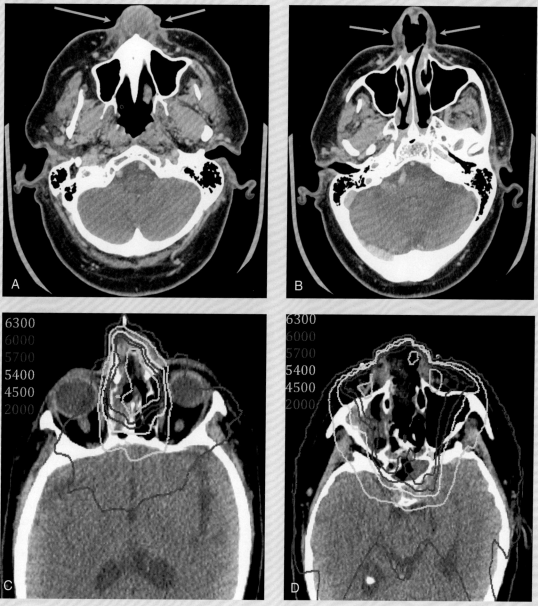

Case Figure 12.10A–D

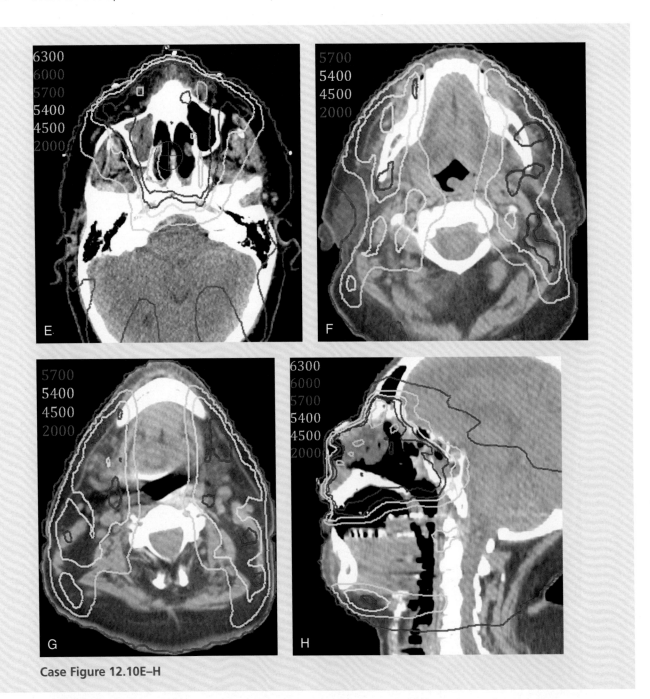

Case Figure 12.10E–H

(vGTV) to guide target volume contouring. The vGTV represents all areas determined from clinical examination, preoperative imaging studies, and the surgical–pathologic findings to likely contain high density of microscopic disease.

Clinical Target Volume

Three CTVs are generally delineated:

- CTV_HD delineates volumes to receive the highest dose, which includes the primary and nodal vGTVs with 0.5- to 1-cm margins.

- CTV_ID outlines volumes to receive an intermediate dose, which includes the operative bed outside of CTV_HD.

- CTV_ED delineates volumes to receive an elective dose for subclinical disease. When the tumor invades the adjacent sinus, then CTV_ED encompasses the entire sinus. In the N0 neck, CTV_ED may include retropharyngeal and levels IB and II nodes. When level IB or II node is involved, CTV_ED also includes clinically uninvolved ipsilateral level III and IV nodes. Note that ipsilateral level III and IV nodes can also be treated with a matching anterior oblique photon portal with an isocenter placed above the thyroid cartilage.

Setup and Field Arrangement

This setup is similar to that for the maxillary sinus (see Chapter 13); the field borders are adjusted to the location and extent of the tumor.

Dose

With conventional technique, 50 Gy in 25 fractions is delivered to the initial target volume, and 10 Gy in 5 fractions (negative margins) to 16 Gy in 8 fractions (positive margins) is delivered to the boost volume.

IMRT is delivered in 30 fractions. The doses prescribed are 60, 57, and 54 Gy to CTV$_{HD}$, CTV$_{ID}$, and CTV$_{ED}$, respectively. In the case of positive margins or extracapsular nodal extension, an additional 6 Gy can be given, as an integrated boost or in an additional three fractions, to the high-risk volume.

Proton Therapy and Intensity-Modulated Radiation Therapy

When the target is situated at the anterior skull base, proton therapy can deliver optimal dose distributions, conforming dose to the target volumes and reducing unnecessary dose outside. Combination plans using passive and active scanning proton beam can further optimize dose distributions, particularly when the boost target volumes are adjacent to critical structures (**Case Study 12.11**).

Background Data

See Tables 12.1 to 12.4.

CASE STUDY 12.11

A 55-year-old man developed epistaxis and tenderness at tip of the nose. There was expansion of the columella and friable mucosa of the left side of the nasal septum. Biopsy from nasal septum lesion showed poorly differentiated squamous carcinoma. CT sinuses and neck (Fig. 12.11A) showed enhancing tumor/mucosal irregularity tracking superiorly and posteriorly along the left side of the nasal septum (*white arrow*) with tumor involving tip of nose and columella. There were no regional or distant metastases detected. As an alternative to surgery, which would have included a total rhinectomy, an organ preservation strategy was pursued with definitive concurrent chemoradiation therapy.

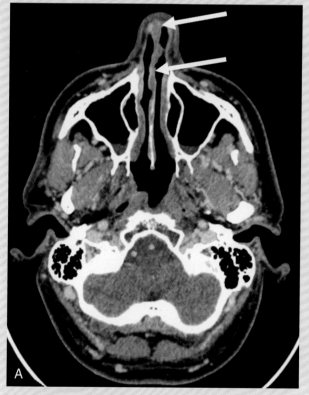
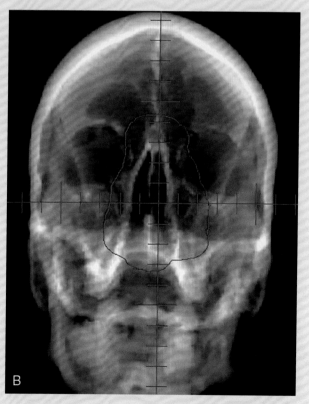

Case Figure 12.11A,B

Given the superior and posterior extent, the tumor was not amenable to brachytherapy. He was treated with proton therapy. The primary site, adjacent nasal septum and cavity, and bilateral facial and upper neck lymphatics (levels Ib and IIA) were treated to 50 Gy (radiobiologic equivalent [RBE]) in 25 fractions using active scanning IMPT multifield optimization technique (see Chapter 2). A 20 Gy(RBE) boost in 10 fractions was then given to

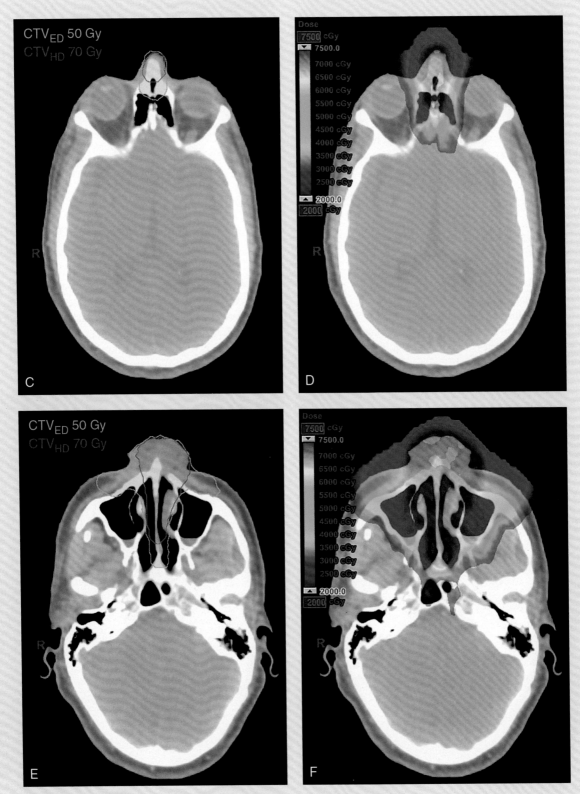

Case Figure 12.11C–F

the primary site with 1.5 cm margin using passive scatter proton beam. The total dose to CTV$_{HD}$ was 70 Gy(RBE) in 35 fractions. The boost fields were mostly anterior and employed apertures to reduce dose to the eyes. Digitally reconstructed radiograph of a boost field aperture is shown in Figure 12.11B.

CTVs and composite proton therapy dose distributions are shown (Fig. 12.11C–L). The clinical photographs show the sharply demarcated acute dermatitis in the last week of therapy (Fig. 12.11M) and subsequent resolution at 2 months after therapy (Fig. 12.11N). He remains in surveillance but has been free of tumor for 10 months.

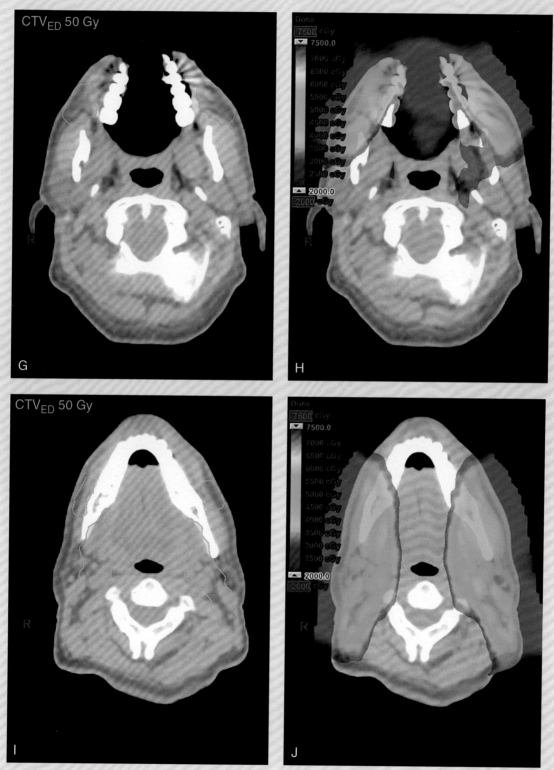

Case Figure 12.11G–J

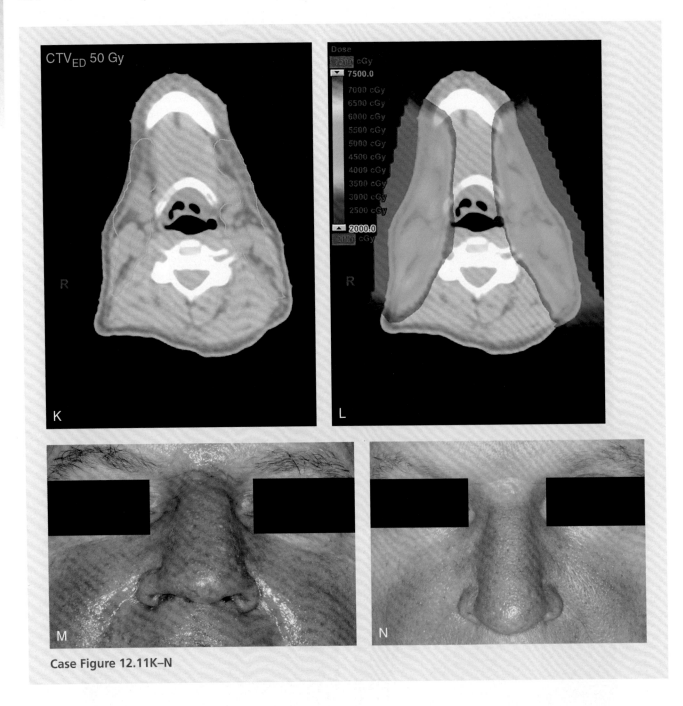

CTV$_{ED}$ 50 Gy

Case Figure 12.11K–N

TABLE 12.1 Locoregional Failures of Radiotherapy of Nasal Vestibule, 1983 to 1984 (Analysis, February 1986)

Treatment Category	No. of Patients	P	P + N	N	M ± N
Primary only interstitial	11	—	—	—	—
External beam	7	—	1	1	1
Primary + moustache[a]	2	—	—	1	—
Primary + neck	2	—	—	—	—
Primary + moustache + neck	10	—	—	—	—

[a]Intervening tissues between the nasal vestibule and the neck.
P, primary; N, neck; M, metastasis.
From Chobe R, McNeese M, Weber R, et al. Radiation therapy for carcinoma of the nasal vestibule. *Otolaryngol Head Neck Surg* 1988;98:67–71, with permission.

TABLE 12.2 Local Control and Regional Relapse for Carcinoma of the Nasal Vestibule Treated with Radiation Therapy (Literature Review)

Authors	Year of Publication	No. of Patients	Local Control (%)	Neck Failure[a] (%)
Wong and Cummings	1986	56	80 (C)	4
Chobe et al.	1988	32	97 (C)	17
Mazeron et al.	1988	64	75 (C)	13
Levendag and Pomp	1990	63	86 (C)	6
Wang	2000	54	81—T1 79—T2 53—T3 (5 yr)	NS
Langendijk et al.	2004	56	80 (2 yr)	12
Agger et al.	2009	120	61 (5 yr LRC)	11
Wray et al.	2016	58	89 (10 yr)	15
Vennette et al.	2016	81	86 (C)	10

[a]Neck failure in patients who did not receive elective nodal irradiation.
C, crude; NS, not stated; LRC, local–regional control.

TABLE 12.3 Pattern of Failure

Primary Site	No. of Patients	LR	RR	LR + DM	DM
After initial treatment					
Nasal septum	14	2	2	0	0
Lateral wall and floor	31	9	0	1	2
After salvage treatment					
Nasal septum	14	0	0	0	0
Lateral wall and floor	31	5	0	2	2

LR, local recurrence; RR, regional relapse; DM, distant metastases.
Modified from Ang KK, Jiang GL, Frankenthaler RA, et al. Carcinomas of the nasal cavity. *Radiother Oncol* 1992;24:163.

TABLE 12.4 Survival Rates by Site of Primary Disease

Actuarial Rates	Patient Number	5 Years (%)	*P* value
Overall survival			
Septum	31	90	0.04
Cavity	37	78	
Disease-specific survival			
Septum	31	90	0.13
Cavity	37	83	
Local–regional control			
Septum	31	79	0.49
Cavity	37	71	

Modified from Allen MW, Schwartz DL, Rana V et al. Long-term radiotherapy outcomes for nasal cavity and septal cancers. *Int J Radiat Oncol Biol Phys* 2008;71:401–406.

SUGGESTED READINGS

Agger A, von Buchwald C, Madsen AR, et al. Squamous cell carcinoma of the nasal vestibule 1993–2002: a nationwide retrospective study from DAHANCA. *Head Neck* 2009;31:1593.

Allen MW, Schwartz DL, Rana V, et al. Long-term radiotherapy outcomes for nasal cavity and septal cancers. *Int J Radiat Oncol Biol Phys* 2008;71:401.

Ang KK, Jiang GL, Frankenthaler RA, et al. Carcinomas of the nasal cavity. *Radiother Oncol* 1992;24:163.

Bhattacharyya N. Cancer of the nasal cavity: survival and factors influencing prognosis. *Arch Otolaryngol Head Neck Surg* 2002;128:1079.

Chobe R, McNeese M, Weber R, et al. Radiation therapy for carcinoma of the nasal vestibule. *Otolaryngol Head Neck Surg* 1988;98:67.

Diaz EM Jr, Johnigan RH 3rd, Pero C, et al. Olfactory neuroblastoma: the 22-year experience at one comprehensive cancer center. *Head Neck* 2005;27:138.

Jeannon JP, Riddle PJ, Irish J, et al. Prognostic indicators in carcinoma of the nasal vestibule. *Clin Otolaryngol* 2007;32:19.

Langendijk JA, Poorter R, Leemans CR, et al. Radiotherapy of squamous cell carcinoma of the nasal vestibule. *Int J Radiat Oncol Biol Phys* 2004;59:1319.

Levendag PC, Nijdam WM, van Moolenburgh SE, et al. Interstitial radiation therapy for early-stage nasal vestibule cancer: a continuing quest for optimal control and cosmesis. *Int J Radiat Oncol Biol Phys* 2006;66:160.

Levendag PC, Pomp J. Radiation therapy of squamous cell carcinoma of the nasal vestibule. *Int J Radiat Oncol Biol Phys* 1990;19:1363.

Mazeron JJ, Chassagne D, Crook J, et al. Radiation therapy of carcinomas of the skin of nose and nasal vestibule: a report of 1676 cases by the Groupe Europeen de Curietherapie. *Radiother Oncol* 1988;13:165.

Mendenhall WM, Amdur RJ, Morris CG, et al. Carcinoma of the nasal cavity and paranasal sinuses. *Laryngoscope* 2009;119:899.

Rosenthal DI, Barker JL Jr, El-Naggar AK, et al. Sinonasal malignancies with neuroendocrine differentiation: patterns of failure according to histologic phenotype. *Cancer* 2004;101:2567.

Schalekamp W, Hordijk GJ. Carcinoma of the nasal vestibule: prognostic factors in relation to lymph node metastasis. *Clin Otolaryngol* 1985;10:201.

Vanneste BG, Lopez-Yurda M, Tan IB, et al. Irradiation of localized squamous cell carcinoma of the nasal vestibule. *Head Neck* 2016;38(suppl 1):E1870.

Wallace A, Morris CG, Kirwan J, et al. Radiotherapy for squamous cell carcinoma of the nasal vestibule. *Am J Clin Oncol* 2007;30:612.

Wong CS, Cummings BJ. The place of radiation therapy in the treatment of squamous cell carcinoma of the nasal vestibule. A review. *Acta Oncol* 1988;27:203.

Wray J, Morris CG, Kirwan JM, et al. Radiation therapy for nasal vestibule squamous cell carcinoma: a 40-year experience. *Eur Arch Otorhinolaryngol* 2016;273:661.

13

Paranasal Sinuses

Key Points

- The paranasal sinuses include the maxillary, ethmoid, sphenoid, and frontal sinuses.

- Cancers of the paranasal sinuses are uncommon with the majority originating in the maxillary sinus.

- Carcinomas arising from the sinuses have a wide range of histologic types. Squamous cell cancer is most common, but neoplasms arising from minor salivary glands and respiratory and olfactory cells can also develop in sinuses.

- Most paranasal sinus cancers are treated with surgery. Radiation with or without chemotherapy is often recommended postoperatively.

- Rare neoplasms, including undifferentiated carcinomas, can be addressed with definitive radiation in combination with chemotherapy.

- The proximity of the eyes, optic pathways, and brain makes treatment of these cancers quite challenging because of the complexity of target volumes. Intensity-modulated radiation therapy (IMRT) can circumvent some of these challenges.

- Proton therapy and intensity-modulated proton therapy for paranasal sinus and skull base tumors may further improve patient outcomes by reducing integral dose to nontarget avoidance structures for the subsites discussed in this chapter.

MAXILLARY SINUS

Treatment Strategy

Surgery alone is the preferred treatment of T1 tumors (uncommon). Postoperative radiotherapy is only indicated when the margin is close or positive. Surgery plus postoperative radiotherapy is the standard therapy for T2 to T4 tumors.

Patients with larger T3 and T4 tumors are occasionally selected for treatment with systemic therapy in an attempt to reduce the need for orbital exenteration. The response to chemotherapy determines the type of local regional treatment. For complete or near-complete response, the treatment is radiotherapy with concurrent chemotherapy (uncommon), and for less than near-complete response, the treatment is surgery plus postoperative radiotherapy, with concurrent chemotherapy in case of the presence of positive margins or nodal disease with extracapsular extension.

Postoperative Radiotherapy

Target Volume

The initial target volume encompasses the entire surgical bed (**Case Study 13.1 and Case Study 13.2**), ipsilateral levels IB and II (submandibular and subdigastric) and retropharyngeal regions for patients with squamous cell or undifferentiated carcinomas with no clinical evidence of nodal involvement at diagnosis, or whole ipsilateral or bilateral neck for patients with N+ at diagnosis.

The boost volume encompasses areas of known disease with 1- to 2-cm margins.

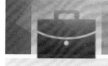

CASE STUDY 13.1

A 77-year-old woman presented with tingling of the left anterior maxillary gingiva. Physical examination showed a mass in the gingiva extending to the hard palate. Imaging studies revealed that the epicenter of the mass was in the inferior maxillary sinus, with extension to both the posterior wall and the premaxillary soft tissue. She underwent an infrastructure maxillectomy. Histologic examination revealed grade 2 mucoepidermoid carcinoma.

Figure 13.1 illustrated postoperative radiation delivered using anterior (Fig. 13.1A) and left lateral (Fig. 13.1B), wedged-pair, portals with 45-degree wedges. The total dose was 60 Gy, with a serial reduction made at 54 Gy. An isodose distribution through the resected sinus is shown in Figure 13.1C.

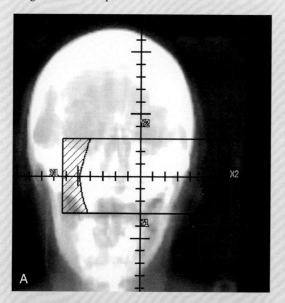

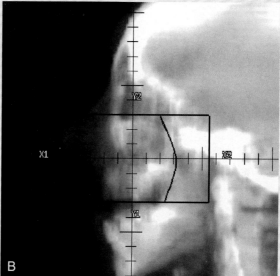

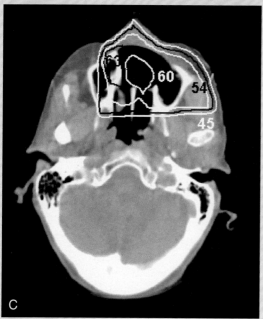

Case Figure 13.1A–C

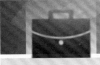

CASE STUDY 13.2

A 46-year-old woman was found to have a right nasal polyp, biopsy of which revealed neuroblastoma. Imaging revealed the bulk of tumor in the medial wall of the right maxillary sinus. She underwent a medial maxillectomy and postoperative radiation.

Figure 13.2 shows details of radiation treatment delivered through an anterior (Fig. 13.2A) and two lateral–

opposed portals (Fig. 13.2B) with 6 MV photons, with 60-degree wedges being used on the lateral fields with the heels oriented anterior. The loading of anterior to lateral was 1:0.07:0.07. The lateral fields were reduced after 40 Gy, and the total dose was 56 Gy specified at the 95% line. Representative isodose distributions through the maxillary sinus and between the orbits are shown in Figure 13.2C,D.

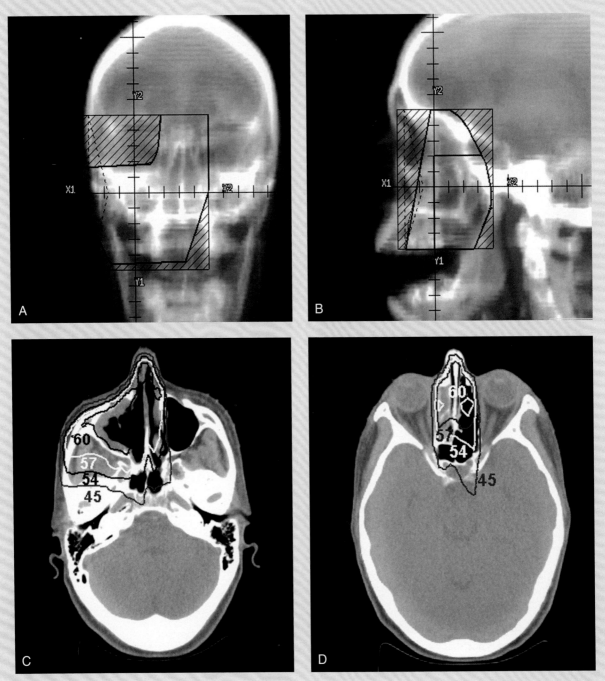

Case Figure 13.2A–D

Setup and Field Arrangement for Conventional Technique

An intraoral stent is used to open the mouth and depress the tongue. When surgical resection includes removal of the hard palate, the stent can be designed to hold a water-filled balloon to occlude the surgical defect (see Chapter 3). Orbital exenteration defect, if present, is filled directly with a water-containing balloon (**Case Study 13.3**) or other types of bolus material.

The patient is immobilized in a supine position with a slight hyperextension of the head to bring the floor of the orbit parallel to the axis of the anterior beam. This position allows delivery of the desired dose to the orbital floor without irradiating through a large volume of the ipsilateral eye.

Marking of lateral canthi, oral commissures, and external scar facilitates portal design. When there is no external scar (e.g., after craniofacial resection), a wire is placed on the premaxillary skin to indicate the slope of this structure. In addition, it is helpful to mark the position of the medial and inferior limbus with the eyes gazing forward for the purpose of corneal shielding. The location and size of the tumor determine the appropriate portal borders and arrangement.

For tumors of the **infrastructure with no extension into the orbit or ethmoids** (uncommon), anterior and ipsilateral wedge-pair (usually 45-degree wedges) photon fields are used. The use of the "half-beam" technique (i.e., placing the isocenter at the level of the orbital floor and shielding of the upper half of the fields) prevents exposure of the contralateral eye by beam divergence.

Anterior portal borders:

- *Superior:* just above the floor of the orbit but below the cornea
- *Lateral:* 1 cm beyond the lateral wall of the maxillary sinus (or falling off when there is tumor extension into the facial soft tissues)
- *Medial:* 1 to 2 cm across midline
- *Inferior:* 1 cm below the floor of the maxillary sinus or below the surgical bed

Lateral portal borders:

- *Superior and inferior:* same as the anterior portal
- *Anterior:* in front of the anterior wall
- *Posterior:* behind the pterygoid plates or more posteriorly depending on the extent of the contiguous tumor spread

For tumors of the **infrastructure spreading across midline** through the hard palate, lateral–opposed photon fields are preferred. The use of the "half-beam" technique (i.e., placing the isocenter at the level of the orbital floor and shielding of the upper half of the fields) prevents exposure of the contralateral eye by beam divergence. The portal borders are similar to the lateral field described previously.

For tumors involving the **suprastructure or ethmoids,** a three-field technique is used (**Case Study 13.2 and Case Study 13.3**). An anterior portal is combined with right and left lateral fields. Loading varies from 1:0.15:0.15 to 1:0.07:0.07 depending on the tumor location and photon energy. The lateral fields have 60-degree wedges and can have a slight posterior tilt.

Anterior portal borders:

- *Superior:* above the crista galli to cover the ethmoids and, in the absence of orbital invasion, at the lower edge of the cornea to cover the orbital floor. When the orbit is involved, an attempt is made to shield the lacrimal gland whenever possible to avoid occurrence of dry, painful eye. Tumor extension into the frontal sinus or cranial fossa calls for a more generous superior coverage.
- *Inferior:* 1 cm below the floor of the maxillary sinus or below the surgical bed.
- *Medial:* 1 to 2 cm, or farther, across midline to cover the contralateral ethmoidal extension.
- *Lateral:* depends on the tumor extent (1 cm beyond lateral orbital wall when this structure is intact or falling off when there is tumor extension into facial soft tissues or infratemporal fossa).

Lateral portal borders:

- *Superior:* follows the contour of the floor of the anterior cranial fossa.
- *Inferior:* corresponds to that of anterior portal.
- *Anterior:* behind the lateral bony canthus parallel to the slope of the face as marked by the wire.
- *Posterior:* behind the pterygoid plates or more posteriorly, depending on the extent of the contiguous tumor spread and the surgery.

For boost volume, the portal size is reduced to encompass the tumor bed and to exclude as much optic pathway as possible. The contralateral optic nerve and chiasm are excluded from the field after a dose of 54 Gy in 27 fractions. Sometimes, this requires two field reductions (i.e., after 50 and 54 Gy, respectively). When the lesion abuts these structures, the benefits and risks of delivering a maximum dose of 60 Gy in 30 fractions, which carries a 5% to 10% risk of blindness resulting from nerve injury, are discussed with the patient.

For treatment of the **neck nodes,** ipsilateral upper neck irradiation is given to patients with squamous cell or undifferentiated carcinomas, stages T2 to T4 N0. This is accomplished through a lateral appositional electron field.

- *Superior border:* sloping up from the horizontal ramus of the mandible anteriorly to match the inferior border of the primary portal posteriorly. This portal matching creates a small triangle over the cheek, which is irradiated with an abutting triangular, appositional electron field (6 MeV) when there is tumor extension into facial soft tissues.
- *Anterior border:* just behind the oral commissures.
- *Posterior border:* at the mastoid process.
- *Inferior border:* at the thyroid notch (above the arytenoids).

CASE STUDY 13.3

A 67-year-old man underwent a removal of a polyp of the right nasal cavity. Histologic examination showed an inverted papilloma. Three years later, he underwent a second polypectomy for recurrence. Histologic examination revealed a small focus of carcinoma within inverted papilloma. Eight months after the second surgery, this patient was referred to the M.D. Anderson Cancer Center for treatment of a large recurrence located in the right maxillary sinus, orbit, and infratemporal fossa. He underwent resection of this tumor with orbital exenteration. Histologic examination revealed inverted papilloma with multiple foci of squamous cell carcinoma.

The margins of resection contained papilloma but were free of invasive carcinoma. He received postoperative radiotherapy as shown in Figure 13.3. The surgical bed was treated with an anterior (Fig. 13.3A) and right lateral fields loaded 1:0.15:0.15, respectively. A stent was used to depress the tongue. A water-filled balloon was placed in the surgical defect. The surgical scar, lateral orbital canthi, and oral commissures are marked. The initial target volume received a dose of 50 Gy in 25 fractions, specified at the isocenter. Subsequently, the fields were reduced to administer a boost dose of 10 Gy in 5 fractions to the tumor bed. A CT scan was obtained for treatment planning, which showed good filling of the surgical defect with the water-filled balloon (Fig. 13.3C,D). This patient did well until 22 months later when a pedunculated lesion was noted in the right ethmoid remnant along with a firm area in the floor of the maxillary defect. Biopsy of both lesions revealed diffusely infiltrating inverting papilloma with focal squamous cell carcinomas.

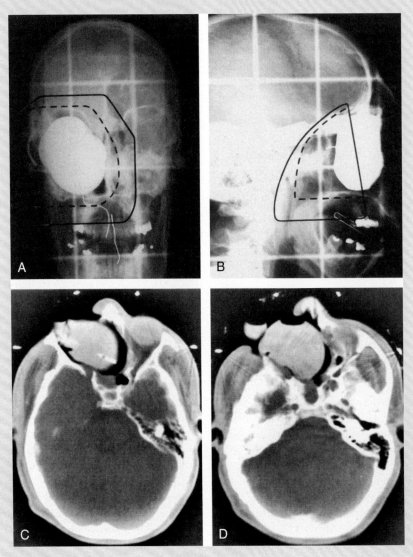

Case Figure 13.3A–D

Bilateral neck treatment is indicated in patients presenting with clinically positive nodes. Proper field-matching technique should be selected in this setting to minimize dose heterogeneity, particularly to prevent overdosing in the depth by beam divergence. This can be accomplished by treating both the primary tumor bed and the upper neck with half-beam technique (shielding the caudal half of maxillary fields and the cephalad half of neck fields) to eliminate divergence and thereby prevent beam overlap. The central axis of the primary tumor portals and that of the opposed–lateral upper neck fields are placed at the axial plane of the inferior portal border of the maxillary fields (i.e., usually 1 cm below the floor of the maxillary sinus). It is prudent to move the junction line between the primary and neck fields during the course of treatment. The mid and lower neck is irradiated with an anterior appositional photon field matched to the inferior border of opposed–lateral upper neck fields (see "General Principles").

The portal borders of the maxillary fields are as defined previously. The borders of the upper neck fields are determined by the extent of the nodal disease. If the initial lateral fields are on the spinal cord, portal reduction is made after approximately 45 Gy. The posterior cervical areas are then irradiated to the desired dose with abutting electron fields.

Intensity-Modulated Radiation Therapy Planning

The complex anatomy of the paranasal sinuses makes it appealing to use high-precision conformal radiotherapy for the treatment of sinonasal tumors to reduce normal tissue toxicity without compromising the dose to the tumor bed. IMRT generally yields better dose distribution for these tumors (**Case Study 13.4 and Case Study 13.5**).

The patient is immobilized in a supine position with an extended head and shoulder thermoplastic mask.

CASE STUDY 13.4

A 60-year-old woman presented with a loose right maxillary tooth. A biopsy taken from the tissue adjacent to the tooth was positive for squamous cell cancer (SCC).

A CT scan was obtained and demonstrated a mass in the inferior aspect of the right maxillary sinus. The mass (*green arrows*) can be seen on axial (Fig. 13.4A) and coronal views (Fig. 13.4B). She underwent an infrastructure maxillectomy. Histologic examination revealed SCC with bone invasion (stage pT4 cN0).

Postoperative IMRT was administered in 30 fractions. CTV_{HD} (*red* color wash), CTV_{ID} (*blue*), and CTV_{ED} (*yellow*) were prescribed 60 Gy, 57 Gy, and 54 Gy,

respectively. CTV_{HD} encompassed the right maxillary sinus and medial aspect of the resected palate, CTV_{ID} an additional margin on the operative bed, and CTV_{ED} the undissected, ipsilateral lymphatics considered at risk including the right facial nodes and right level I and II nodes. Figure 13.4 displays contours and isodose distribution on axial views at the level of the midsinus (Fig. 13.4C), inferior sinus (Fig. 13.4D), facial and superior level II nodes (Fig. 13.4E), and midlevel I and II nodes (Fig. 13.4F). The patient was in an excellent general condition and had no evidence of disease at the last follow-up.

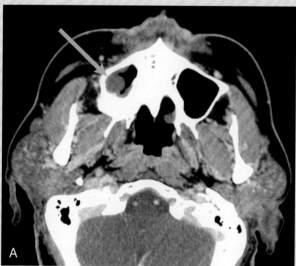
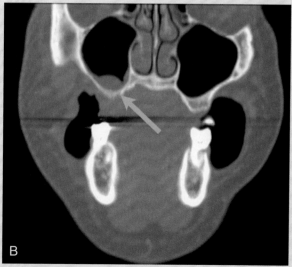

Case Figure 13.4A,B

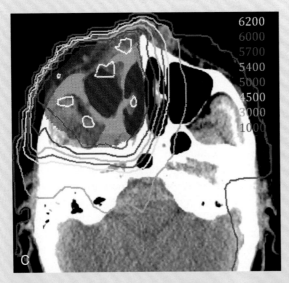

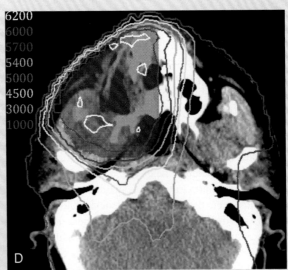

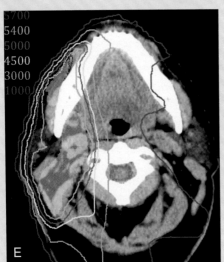

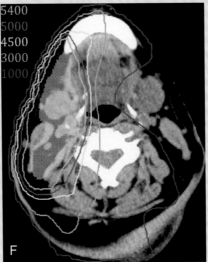

Case Figure 13.4C–F

CASE STUDY 13.5

A 58-year-old man presented with a right facial mass and oral pain.

A CT scan showed a large mass in the right maxillary sinus invading the right buccal space and soft tissues of the cheek (Fig. 13.5A,B). He underwent a total maxillectomy. Histologic examination revealed a 5-cm squamous cell carcinoma of the sinus invading the hard palate. He was treated with postoperative IMRT, delivered in 30 fractions.

A vGTV (*green* color wash) was defined based on the clinical, surgical, and pathologic findings. CTV$_{HD}$ (*orange*), CTV$_{ID}$ (*aqua*), and CTV$_{ED}$ (*yellow*) were prescribed 60 Gy,

57 Gy, and 54 Gy, respectively. Axial views at the level of the ethmoids (Fig. 13.5C), superior sinus and floor of the orbit (Fig. 13.5D), midmaxillary sinus (Fig. 13.5E), and upper neck (Fig. 13.5F) are shown with target contours in color wash and isodose distribution. Matched coronal slice through the sinus with and without contours are shown in Figure 13.5G,H. Figure 13.5I,J shows a coronal isodose distribution (Fig. 13.5I) posterior to the sinus and a sagittal isodose distribution (Fig. 13.5J) through the mid right orbit and resected sinus. The patient had no evidence of disease 2 years posttreatment.

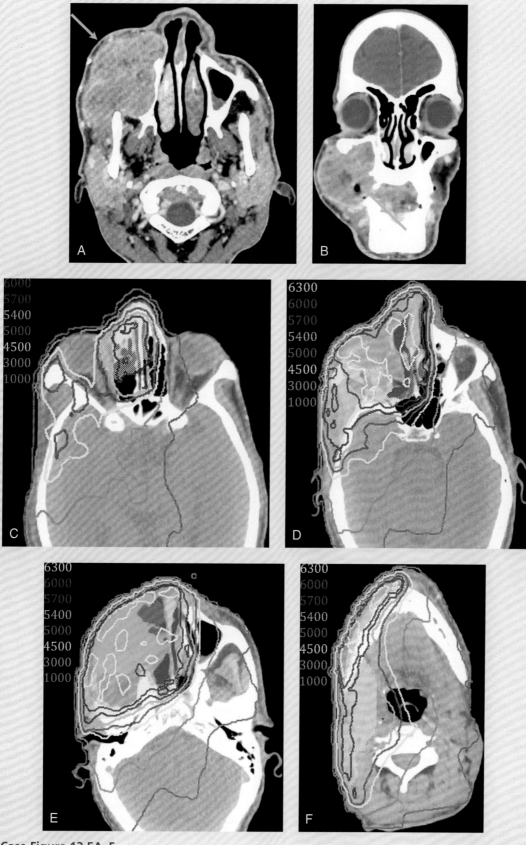

Case Figure 13.5A–F

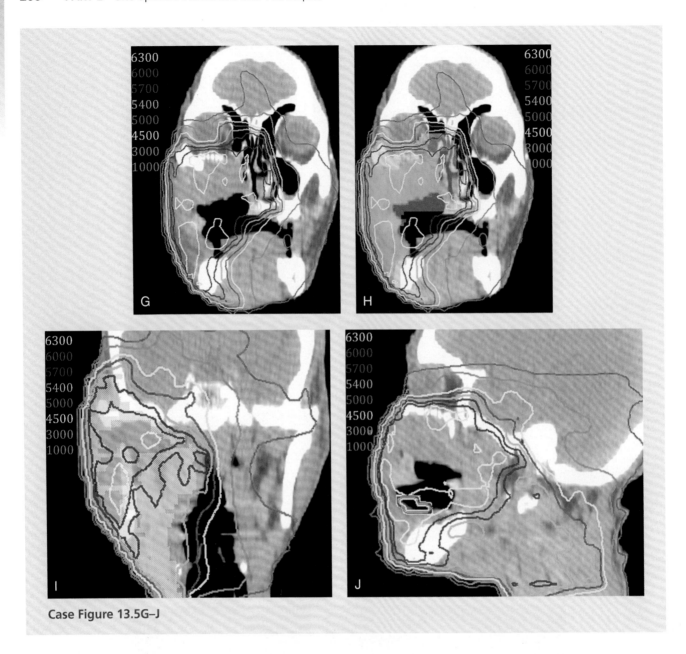

Case Figure 13.5G–J

Thin-cut computed tomography (CT) scans are obtained in treatment position. The clinical target volume (CTV) and planning target volume are outlined for dosimetric planning.

Virtual Gross Target Volume

There is no actual gross target volume (GTV) after a complete surgical tumor resection. However, it can be useful to formulate a virtual GTV (vGTV) to facilitate target volume definition. The vGTV is the best approximation of the tissues having high likelihood of harboring microscopic tumor reconstructed based on findings of preoperative clinical examination, imaging studies, and surgical pathologic assessment. Bulky flaps can cause substantial distortions in the tumor bed and should, therefore, be taken into account in reconstructing the vGTV.

Clinical Target Volumes

Three CTVs are generally delineated.

- CTV$_{HD}$ delineates volumes to receive the highest dose. This includes the primary and nodal vGTVs with 1-cm margins. The entire sinus is included in this volume. Medially, the ipsilateral nasal cavity to the septum is included. Generous coverage is given posteriorly into the residual masticator space and pterygomaxillary tissues as this is a frequent site of recurrence. The lateral edge includes the masticator space. In patients with partial palate resection, CTV$_{HD}$ includes at least 1 cm of the remaining palate. If the floor of the orbit was involved, CTV$_{HD}$ needs to cover the inferior orbital tissues as a minimum. For disease extension beyond the sinus, CTV$_{HD}$ should cover these tissues with a 0.5- to 1-cm margin.

- CTV$_{ID}$ delineates volumes to receive an intermediate dose. For the primary tumor bed, CTV$_{ID}$ encompasses a 0.5- to 1-cm additional margin beyond CTV$_{HD}$. For anterior tumors in particular, the skin, if not covered by CTV$_{HD}$, will need to be included, and bolus may be required. For the neck, CTV$_{ID}$ covers the dissected nodal region not harboring involved nodes.

- CTV$_{ED}$ delineates volumes to receive an elective dose for subclinical disease. When microscopic perineural invasion is present, the maxillary nerve up to foramen rotundum, if not covered in higher-dose CTVs, should be encompassed in CTV$_{ED}$. For extensive perineural extension (involvement of large nerve or presence of clinical signs), CTV$_{ED}$ includes the proximal V2 up to the trigeminal ganglion. In squamous cell or undifferentiated carcinomas without clinical nodal involvement, CTV$_{ED}$ encompasses the ipsilateral nodal levels I and II, retropharyngeal, and buccal and facial nodes. For tumors crossing midline, CTV$_{ED}$ covers bilateral nodes.

The isocenter is generally placed in the center of the treated volume. In the node-positive patient, the isocenter can be placed at a level just above the arytenoids. Nodal levels III and IV are preferentially treated with a matching anterior beam similar to convention techniques. The dissected uninvolved nodal levels are boosted to 56 Gy, and an additional 4 Gy is added if these lower neck nodes harbored disease.

Dose

Primary tumor bed: 50 Gy in 25 fractions to the initial target volume plus 10 Gy in 5 fractions (negative margins) to 16 Gy in 8 fractions (positive margins) to the boost volume.

Elective nodal irradiation: 50 Gy in 25 fractions.

Involved nodal regions (particularly in the presence of extracapsular nodal disease): 60 to 66 Gy in 30 to 33 fractions.

IMRT: 60 Gy to the primary tumor bed and 57 Gy to the surgical bed in 30 fractions. In case of close or positive margins, a small volume within CTV$_{HD}$ receives 66 Gy in 30 fractions (2.2 Gy per fraction). CTV$_{ED}$ is prescribed 54 Gy (in 30 fractions) Therefore, the fraction size varies from 2.0 to 2.2 Gy to the tumor bed and from 1.8 to 1.9 Gy to the surgical bed and subclinical target volumes.

Instructing the patients to open the eye during irradiation to take advantage of the photon-dose buildup characteristics can minimize the dose to the cornea. The dose to the macula, optic nerve, and chiasm is limited to 54 Gy or less whenever possible to minimize the risk of blindness.

Dose Specification

For the primary tumor bed, specification is at an isodose line with dose heterogeneity of no more than ±5%. A planning CT scan is obtained, and loading, wedges, and field margins are adjusted when necessary or for conformal radiation planning.

Primary Radiotherapy

The radiation techniques are the same as those in the postoperative radiotherapy setting. Portal borders are determined by radiologically demonstrable tumor extent. With conventional technique, the prescribed dose is 50 Gy in 25 fractions to the initial target volume plus 16 to 20 Gy in 8 to 10 fractions to the boost volume.

Intensity-Modulated Radiation Therapy Planning

The complexity of the anatomy and the proximity to the brain and optic structures makes tumors located in these areas well suited for IMRT, which has become our preferred technique. The patient is immobilized in a supine position, with an extended head and shoulder thermoplastic mask. Thin-cut CT scans are obtained in treatment position. The target volumes are outlined for dosimetric planning (**Case Study 13.6**).

CASE STUDY 13.6

A 46-year-old man presented with maxillary tooth pain and numbness of the left palate and cheek. A left maxillary sinus mass was found, and a Caldwell-Luc procedure was performed. Histologic examination of the tissue revealed sarcomatoid carcinoma. Magnetic resonance imaging (MRI) revealed the maxillary sinus mass with perineural invasion through foramen rotundum extending to the cavernous sinus. He was treated with concurrent cisplatin (100 mg/m² given every 3 weeks) and radiation. IMRT was used given the tumor shape. A dose of 70 Gy in 35 fractions was prescribed to CTV$_{HD}$. The 66 Gy isodose line encompassed the entire volume at risk.

Figure 13.6 shows axial (Fig. 13.6A), coronal (Fig. 13.6B), and sagittal isodose (Fig. 13.6C) distributions through the sinus. The left upper neck received 50 Gy in 25 fractions through a matching 12-MeV electron field. Postradiation imaging revealed residual abnormality in the maxillary sinus. A maxillectomy was performed revealing squamous cell carcinoma with extensive degenerative changes. The nerve specimens did not contain tumor. Three months after surgery, osteoradionecrosis of the anterior maxilla and palate developed. He was treated with hyperbaric oxygen and sequestrectomy. The patient remains without evidence of disease 2 years after treatment.

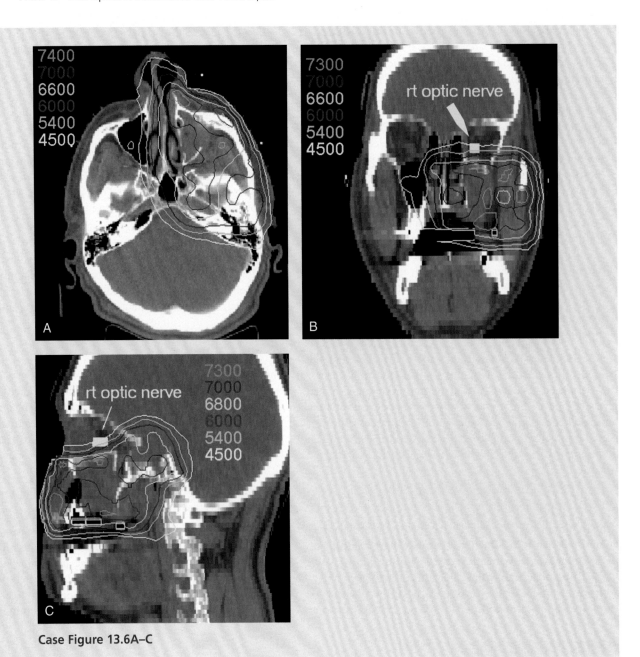

Case Figure 13.6A–C

Gross Target Volume

GTV represents all areas determined from clinical examination and imaging studies to contain gross disease.

Clinical Target Volume

Three CTVs are generally delineated.

- CTV_{HD} delineates volumes to receive the highest dose. This includes the primary and nodal GTVs with 0.5- to 1-cm margins.
- CTV_{ID} delineates volumes to receive an intermediate dose, which includes a 0.5- to 1-cm margin around CTV_{HD}. In the node-positive neck, CTV_{ID} covers the involved nodal bed outside CTV_{HD} and an additional 1 to 2 cm in cranial caudal directions.

- CTV_{ED} delineates volumes to receive an elective dose for subclinical disease. If not already included in higher-dose targets (rare), CTV_{ED} should cover the entire sinus and the floor of the orbit, ethmoid sinuses, masticator space, and pterygomaxillary tissues. If perineural invasion is present, CTV_{ED} includes V2 as per the guidelines described in the postoperative setting. In squamous cell or undifferentiated carcinoma without clinical nodal involvement, CTV_{ED} encompasses ipsilateral facial, buccal, retropharyngeal, and levels I and II nodes. If the tumor crosses midline, bilateral nodal irradiation is recommended. If level I or II node is involved, CTV_{ED} covers levels III and IV regions. Alternatively, levels III and IV regions can be irradiated with a separate matched anterior beam with an isocenter placed above the thyroid cartilage.

CASE STUDY 13.7

A 43-year-old woman presented with right periorbital pain and nasal obstruction. She underwent bilateral endoscopic surgery removing a mass from the right nasal cavity and ethmoids, which was positive for sinonasal undifferentiated carcinoma. MRI revealed residual disease in the right nasoethmoidal region with extension to the nasopharynx. She was treated with three cycles of cisplatin and etoposide yielding a partial response. This was followed by IMRT using nine fields and dynamic multileaf collimation. The gross residual tumor received 70 Gy, the prechemotherapy volume received 60 Gy, and bilateral upper neck nodes received 56 Gy.

Figure 13.7 shows axial (Fig. 13.7A) and sagittal (Fig. 13.7B) isodose distributions. The residual tumor and prechemotherapy tumor (*bright red* and *pale red*) and optic pathways (*yellow* for chiasm) are shown. Concurrent cisplatin was administered every 3 weeks. Posttreatment imaging revealed a residual mass. Therefore, a resection was performed. Histologic examination revealed fibrotic tissue only. She developed a solitary larynx metastasis 2 years later and received radiation and chemotherapy to the larynx only. She is without disease 4 years from her initial diagnosis.

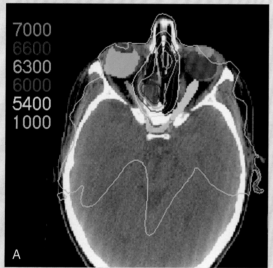
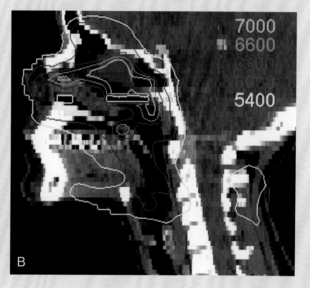

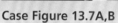
Case Figure 13.7A,B

A dose of 70 Gy is prescribed to CTV$_{HD}$, 60 to 63 Gy to CTV$_{ID}$, and 56 to 57 Gy to CTV$_{ED}$. The nodal volumes are the same as in the postoperative setting. The fraction number ranges from 33 to 35 and is usually determined by the volume of central nervous system (CNS) adjacent to the target encompassed in the high-dose regions. It is desirable to keep the fraction size to the CNS below 2 Gy.

ETHMOID SINUSES

Treatment Strategy

Till recently, most patients have been treated with surgery and postoperative radiotherapy. A combination of chemotherapy

and radiation has been used in select cases for organ preservation (**Case Study 13.7**).

Postoperative Radiotherapy

The radiation techniques are the same as those for carcinoma of the suprastructure of the maxillary sinus (**Case Study 13.8**). In the event of a craniofacial resection, no attempt is made to cover the incision site along the scalp.

The total dose usually does not exceed 54 Gy without a detailed consent from the patient because it is extremely difficult to exclude optic nerves from the target volume due to the proximity. IMRT often provides better dose distribution in this setting and is the preferred technique (**Case Study 13.9**). The dose to the chiasm may exceed 54 Gy if necessary for target coverage, again, provided a detailed consent is obtained from the patient. The fundamentals for target definition are similar to those applied for tumors of the suprastructure.

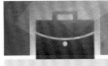

CASE STUDY 13.8

A 56-year-old man sought medical attention because of nasal stuffiness and pressure discomfort below the right eye. A polypoid mass was removed from the right nasal cavity, which was diagnosed as adenocarcinoma. CT scan revealed a tumor in the right ethmoid sinuses and upper part of the right nasal cavity involving the floor of the right orbit. The tumor was resected through a craniofacial approach. The right antrum and sphenoid sinus were inspected and found free of gross disease, but the mucosal lining was removed. Histologic examination revealed an adenocarcinoma at the ethmoid sinuses spreading to the mucosa of the nasal septum.

The patient received postoperative radiotherapy.

Figure 13.8 shows anterior field (Fig. 13.8A) and right (Fig. 13.8B) and left lateral fields used to treat the surgical bed with 6 MV photons. The lateral orbital canthi, external auditory canals, oral commissures, and position of the cornea of the right eye were marked at simulation. The thick, straight wire indicated the slope of the face. A dose of 56 Gy was delivered to the isocenter in 28 fractions.

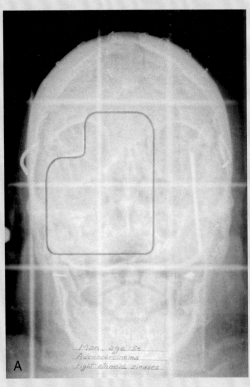
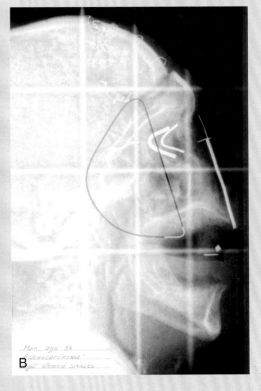

Case Figure 13.8A,B

Intensity-Modulated Radiation Therapy Planning

The patient is immobilized in a supine position, with an extended head and shoulder thermoplastic mask. Thin-cut CT scans are obtained in treatment position. The target volumes are outlined for dosimetric planning.

Gross Target Volume

GTV represents all areas determined from clinical examination and imaging studies to contain gross disease. There is no actual GTV after complete surgical tumor resection. However, it can be useful to formulate a vGTV to facilitate target volume definition in the postoperative setting. The vGTV is the best approximation of the tissues having high likelihood of harboring microscopic tumor reconstructed based on findings of preoperative clinical examination, imaging studies, and surgical pathologic assessment.

Clinical Target Volume

Three CTVs are generally delineated.

- CTV$_{HD}$ delineates volumes to receive the highest dose. This includes the primary and nodal GTVs (or vGTV in the postoperative setting) with 0.5- to 1-cm margins.

CASE STUDY 13.9

This 47-year-old woman presented with anosmia and nasal obstruction.

As shown in Figure 13.9, CT scan demonstrates a tumor epicentered in the ethmoid sinuses (Fig. 13.9A, *green arrows*) broken through the floor of the anterior cranial fossa in coronal view (Fig. 13.9A, *blue arrow*). She underwent resection of the mass with an endoscopic approach inferiorly and a bifrontal craniotomy to address the superior aspect of the tumor. Histologic examination revealed an esthesioneuroblastoma extended through the cribriform plate to involve the dura mater. Margins were positive.

She was treated with postoperative IMRT delivered in 30 fractions. CTV$_{HD}$ (60 Gy) covered the vGTV as reconstructed from the imaging and operative and pathology reports. A small higher-risk volume, at the right anterior cranial fossa floor where the margin was not cleared, was defined and given 63 Gy. CTV$_{ID}$ (57 Gy) covered the additional margin on the cranial fossa floor, as well as the remaining sinuses that were uninvolved but were in the surgical bed. Figure 13.9B shows a coronal view through the posterior orbits with an isodose distribution. Note the 63-Gy line at the superior aspect of the surgical cavity and the 60-Gy line encompassing the resected ethmoids between the orbits. The 57-Gy line in this view covers the bilateral maxillary sinuses and nasal cavity. Figure 13.9C shows a sagittal view through midline. Again, the 63-Gy line and 60-Gy line are appreciated covering a small portion of the inferior aspect of the anterior cranium and the resected tumor bed,

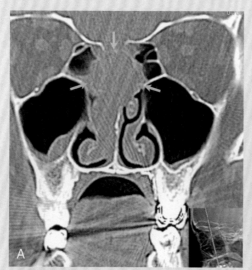

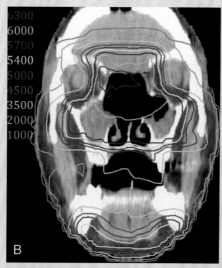

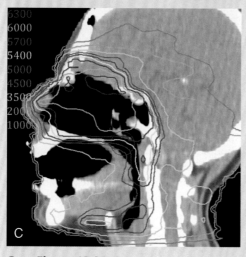

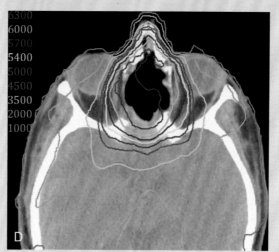

Case Figure 13.9A–D

respectively. The 57-Gy line covers the sphenoid sinus. Also note the isodose gradient achieved to keep the optic chiasm within tolerance. Axial isodose distributions are shown at the level of the orbits and optic pathways (Fig. 13.9D), the epicenter of the surgical cavity (Fig 13.9E), and midmaxillary sinuses (Fig. 13.9F). CTV_{ED} (54 Gy) encompassed the retropharyngeal (Fig. 13.9G) and the upper neck (Fig. 13.9H) nodes. She remains without disease 3 years later.

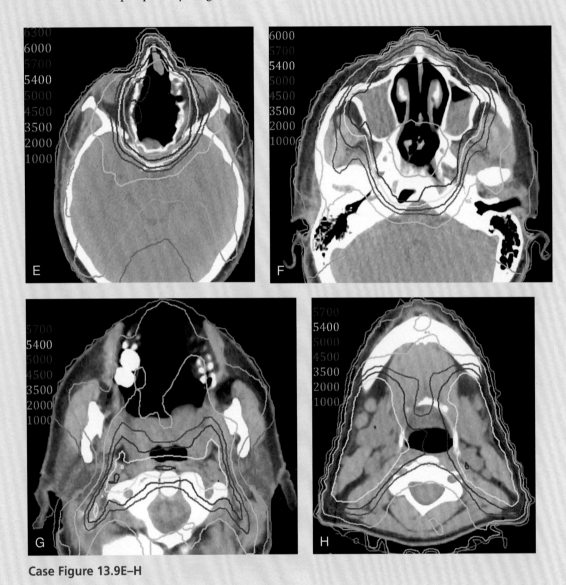

Case Figure 13.9E–H

- CTV_{ID} delineates volumes to receive an intermediate dose, which includes a 0.5- to 1-cm margin around CTV_{HD}. In the node-positive neck, CTV_{ID} covers the involved nodal bed outside CTV_{HD} and additional 1 to 2 cm in cranial caudal directions.
- CTV_{ED} delineates volumes to receive an elective dose for subclinical disease. If not already included in higher-dose targets (rare), CTV_{ED} should cover the entire sinus, the medial orbital wall, sphenoid sinus, nasal cavity, medial aspect of the maxillary sinus (or sinuses for bilateral disease), and floor of the anterior

cranial fossa. In clinically N0 neck (except for low-grade tumors), CTV_{ED} encompasses levels I and II nodes. If level I or II node is involved, CTV_{ED} covers levels III and IV regions. Alternatively, levels III and IV regions can be irradiated with a separate matched anterior beam with an isocenter placed above the thyroid cartilage.

Background Data

See Tables 13.1 to 13.5.

TABLE 13.1 Influence of Disease and Therapy Variables on the Treatment Outcome

Variables	No. of Patients	Local 5-yr Control (%)	Regional 5-yr Control (%)	5-Yr Overall Survival (%)
Pathologic T stage[a]				
T1 + T2	22	73	76	66
T3	47	84	82	57
T4	77	68	84	50
N stage				
N0	126	73	83	56
N1–N2	20	79	75	44
Histologic findings				
SCC	89	68	80	49
Undifferentiated	11	91	73	40
Adenocarcinoma	6	80	75	37
Adenoid cystic carcinoma	33	85	96	69
Other	7	64	80	71
Nerve invasion[a]				
No	82	81	83	61
Yes	60	66	82	45
Margin of resection[a]				
Negative/close	107	74	84	59
Positive	37	73	77	41
Elective nodal treatment	51	69	93	47

[a]Patients with unknown status excluded.

Bristol IJ, Ahamad A, Garden AS, et al. Postoperative radiotherapy for maxillary sinus cancer: long-term outcomes and toxicities of treatment. *Int J Radiat Oncol Biol Phys* 2007;68:719, with permission.

TABLE 13.2 Influence of Disease and Therapy Variables on the Treatment Outcome of 34 Patients Irradiated for Carcinoma of the Ethmoid Sinuses

Variables	No. of Patients	5-Yr Actuarial Local Control (%)	5-Yr Actuarial Disease-Specific Survival (%)
T stage			
T1	6	100	100
T2	13	79	62
T3	15	53	51
Dura invasion[a]			
No	13	100	83
Yes	5	30	40
Histologic findings[b]	12	82	72
Undifferentiated carcinoma	8	53	70
Squamous cell carcinoma and adenoid cystic and adenocarcinoma	13	73	50
Local treatment			
Surgery + radiation	21	74	68
Radiation alone	13	64	56
Chemotherapy			
No	25	80	62
Yes	9	50	67

[a]Patients treated with postoperative irradiation only.
[b]Excludes one patient with transitional cell carcinoma.
Modified from Jiang GL, Morrison WH, Garden AS, et al. Ethmoid sinus carcinomas: natural history and treatment results. *Radiother Oncol* 1998;49:21–27, with permission.

TABLE 13.3 Patterns of Failure in Patients with Sinonasal Carcinomas with Neuroendocrine Differentiation

Histology	Patient No.	Local Failure[a] (%)	Regional Failure[a] (%)	Distant Failure[a] (%)
Esthesioneuroblastoma	31	4	9	0
Neuroendocrine carcinoma	18	27	13	12
Sinonasal undifferentiated carcinoma	16	21	16	25
Small cell carcinoma	7	33	44	75

Data from the M.D. Anderson Cancer Center.
[a]5-Yr actuarial rates.
Modified from Rosenthal DI, Barker JL Jr, El-Naggar AK, et al. Sinonasal malignancies with neuroendocrine differentiation: patterns of failure according to histologic phenotype. *Cancer* 2004;101:2567, with permission.

TABLE 13.4 Control of Paranasal Sinus Malignancies Treated with IMRT

First Author (Year)	Patient Number	% of Patients Treated Postoperatively	Local Control (%)
Combs (2006)	46	ND	81 (2 yr)
Daly (2007)	36	89	62 (2 yr)
Hoppe (2008)	37	100	75 (2 yr)
Madani (2009)	84	89	71 (2 yr)
Dirix (2010)	40	100	76 (2 yr)
Al-Mamgani (2012)	82	78	74 (5 yr)
Wiegner (2012)	52	90	64[a] (5 yr)

[a]Local–regional control.
ND, not described.
Data from Combs SE, et al. *Radiat Oncol* 2006;1:23; Daly ME, et al. *Int J Radiat Oncol Biol Phys* 2007;67:151; Hoppe BS, et al. *Head Neck* 2008;30:925; Madani I, Bonte K, Vakaet L, et al. Intensity-modulated radiotherapy for sinonasal tumors: Ghent University Hospital update. *Int J Radiat Oncol Biol Phys* 2009;73:424; Dirix P, et al. *Int J Radiat Oncol Biol Phys* 2010;78:998; Al-Mamgani A, Monserez D, Rooij PV, et al. *Oral Oncol* 2012;48:905; Wiegner EA, Daly ME, Murphy JD, et al. *IJROBP* 2012;83:243.

TABLE 13.5 Disease Control and Survival for Patients Receiving Radiation Therapy for Clinically Node-Negative Esthesioneuroblastoma

Patient No.	No. Kadish C	No. with Local Failure	No. with Regional Failure		No. with Distant Failure	Median Time to Recurrence (Months)	10-Yr Overall Survival (%)
			No ENI (n = 49)	With ENI (n = 22)			
71[a]	52	3	13[b]	0	7[b]	60	73

[a]65 were treated postoperatively.
[b]Two had simultaneous regional and distant failure.
No., number; ENI, elective nodal irradiation.
Data from the M.D. Anderson Cancer Center 1970–2013; Jiang W, Mohamed AS, Fuller CD, et al. The role of elective nodal irradiation for esthesioneuroblastoma patients with clinically negative neck. *Pract Radiat Oncol* 2016;6:241.

SPHENOID AND FRONTAL SINUSES

Treatment Strategy

Cancers of the sphenoid sinus and frontal sinuses are very rare. Treatment is individualized and modalities are chosen based on the extent of disease and the histologic type. Radiation is often recommended either as an adjunct to surgery or as a frontline therapy in patients with inoper-able tumor or with tumor type that is thought to be (chemo) radiosensitive.

Nodal disease is uncommon. Radiation targets are the primary site with margin. IMRT is preferred due to the proximity to the optic structures and brain. Examples of treatment of a patient with sphenoid sinus cancer with frontline radiotherapy (**Case Study 13.10**) and a case with frontal sinus cancer treated with postoperative radiation (**Case Study 13.11**) are shown.

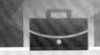

CASE STUDY 13.10

A 66-year-old man presented with headache. An MRI showed a mass (*green arrow*) in the sphenoid sinus (Fig. 13.10A). An endoscopic biopsy revealed squamous cell carcinoma. He was treated with induction chemotherapy yielding a partial response.

He was then treated with IMRT with concurrent chemotherapy. Target delineation was done by fusing the prechemotherapy MRI onto the postchemotherapy planning CT set. CTV$_{HD}$ encompassed the prechemotherapy gross disease. Margin was only added anteriorly into the ethmoids where it was deemed safe. Figure 13.10 shows a sagittal view of isodose distribution through midline (Fig. 13.10B) with the optic chiasm highlighted by *yellow* color wash and *arrow*.

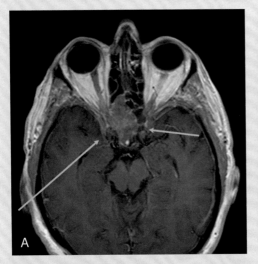
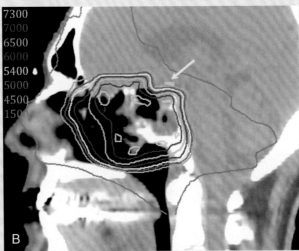
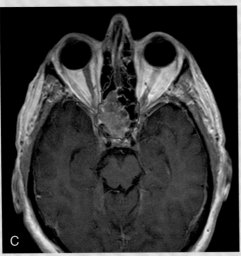
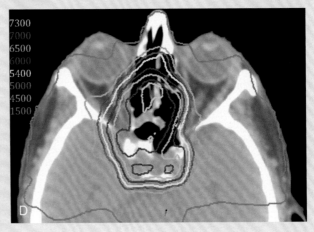

Case Figure 13.10A–D

Figure 13.10C–F shows two matched pairs of contours as shown on the prechemotherapy MRI and isodose distributions on the planning CT. CTV$_{HD}$ (*red* contour) was prescribed 70 Gy. A third matched pair (Fig. 13.10G,H) shows axial views below the optic pathways. CTV$_{ED}$ (*blue*) provided an additional 0.5-cm margin on the ethmoids and was prescribed 60 Gy. The patient remains well over 2 years from treatment without disease, and there was no vision impairment.

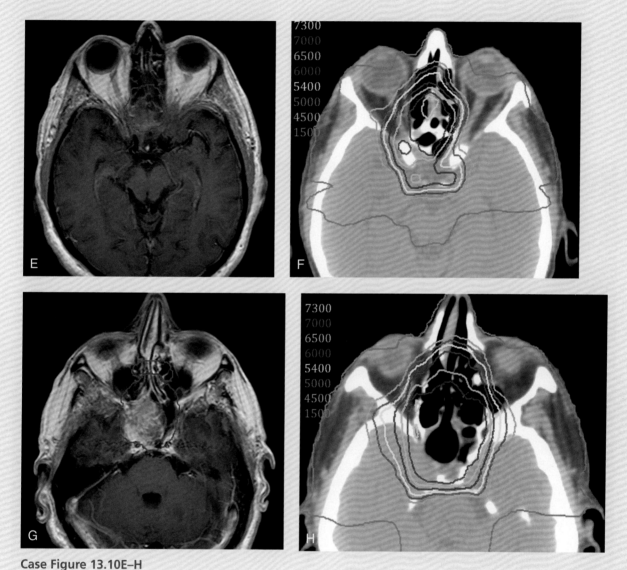

Case Figure 13.10E–H

PROTON THERAPY AND INTENSITY-MODULATED PROTON THERAPY

Proton therapy, and specifically intensity-modulated proton therapy, can deliver conformal dose distributions for tumors of the paranasal sinuses and skull base while minimizing integral dose to critical structures and nontarget regions (**Case Study 13.12 through Case Study 13.14**). Combination plans using passive and active scanning proton beam can further optimize dose distributions, particularly when the boost target volumes are adjacent to critical structures. General principles, site-specific target volume delineation, and dose specification for proton therapy are similar to that described in the previous sections.

CASE STUDY 13.11

A 71-year-old man presented with headache. An MRI showed changes that were thought to be consistent with a mucocele of the left frontal sinus. He underwent resection, and histologic examination revealed poorly differentiated squamous cell carcinoma. Restaging revealed no gross residual disease, so it was elected to treat him with postoperative IMRT as the multidisciplinary team did not believe further surgery would be of benefit.

IMRT was designed to address the primary tumor bed only with two target volumes. Because he had a debulk-

ing rather than an oncologic surgical approach, CTV$_{HD}$ encompassing the left frontal sinus was prescribed 66 Gy. CTV$_{ED}$ added additional 0.5- to 1-cm margins, more generous margin into the right frontal sinus, and was prescribed 60 Gy.

Figure 13.11 shows contours (*orange* color wash for CTV$_{HD}$ and *aqua* for CTV$_{ED}$) and isodose distributions on a coronal view (Fig. 13.11A) and three axial views through the sinus (Fig. 13.11B–D). The patient is without disease at the last follow-up.

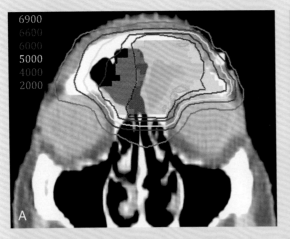
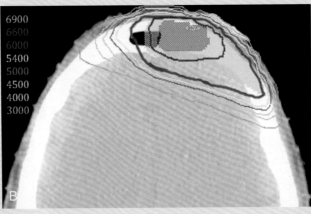
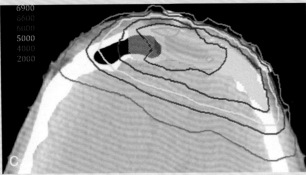
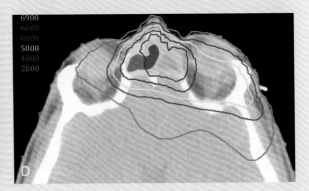

Case Figure 13.11A–D

CASE STUDY 13.12

A 61-year-old female presented with right-sided epiphora and nasal congestion. Imaging revealed a destructive maxillary sinus mass and biopsy showed sarcomatoid squamous cell carcinoma. Coronal projection of staging PET–CT in Figure 13.12A demonstrates the hypermetabolic tumor extending through all walls of the maxillary sinus and the floor of the orbit. The axial T1 MRI with gadolinium in Figure 13.12B shows the enhancing tumor filling the maxillary sinus with central necrosis and tumor extending anteriorly into soft tissues of face (*white arrows*) and posterolaterally into the masticator space. There was no sign of regional or distant disease on imaging.

She was treated with total maxillectomy and ethmoidectomy with sphenoidotomy and removal of sphenoid sinus contents, masticator and pterygopalatine space dissection, and resection of involved hard palate. The floor of the orbit was resected but the globe preserved. Final pathology confirmed poorly differentiated sarcomatoid squamous carcinoma. There was bone and soft tissue involvement. Final surgical margins were free of tumor. The ethmoid sinus specimen contained tumor, while the sphenoid sinus contents did not. There was no perineural or lymphovascular

invasion. Reconstruction of the defect was accomplished using a free fibula osseocutaneous flap, and the floor or orbit was also reconstructed with a titanium plate.

She was then treated with postoperative radiation therapy using active scanning intensity-modulated proton therapy. She was simulated and treated with a mouth-opening and tongue-depressing stent with bite block. The tumor bed, including the reconstruction flap with margin (CTV_{HD}), was treated to 60 Gy(radiobiologic equivalent [RBE]), the operative bed (CTV_{ID}) to 57 Gy(RBE), and the right upper neck levels Ib to II (CTV_{ED}) to 54 Gy(RBE) all in 30 daily fractions. The CTVs and proton therapy dose distributions are shown in paired images in Figures 13.12C–J, highlighting the conformality of the high-dose regions with limited integral dose to brain, brainstem, and nontarget oral cavity. The maximum dose to the right optic nerve (*white arrow* in Fig. 13.12G) was limited to 60 Gy(RBE). One year after completing therapy, she has retained functional vision in both eyes and is free of disease, but she is dealing with low-grade keratopathy and an emerging cataract on the right, being managed conservatively with ocular hydration.

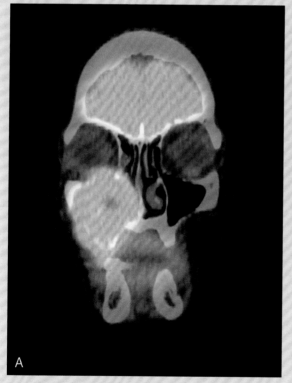
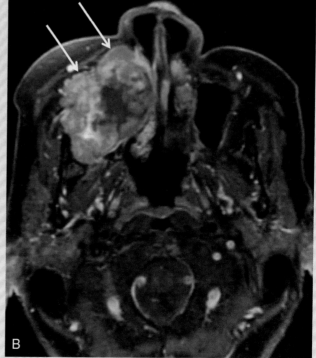

Case Figure 13.12A,B

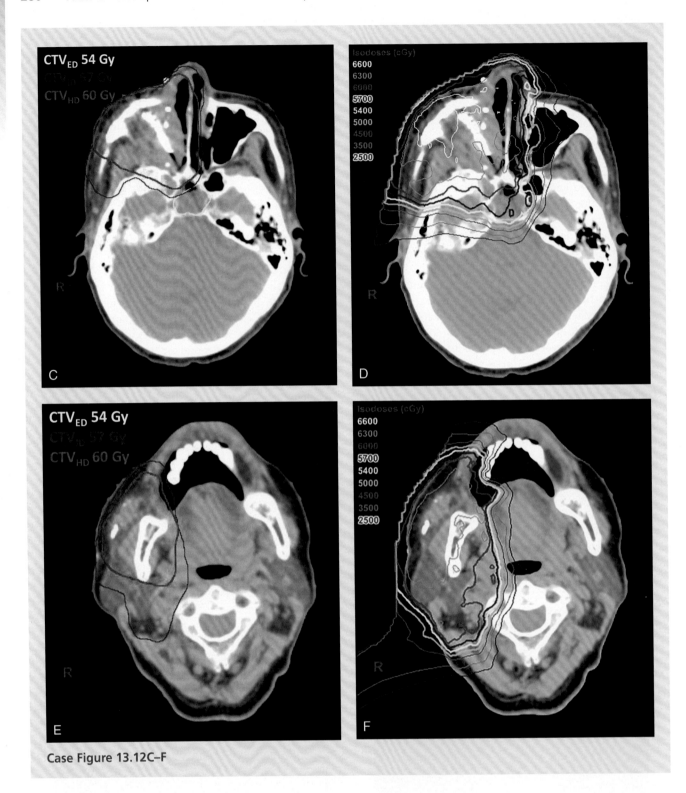

Case Figure 13.12C–F

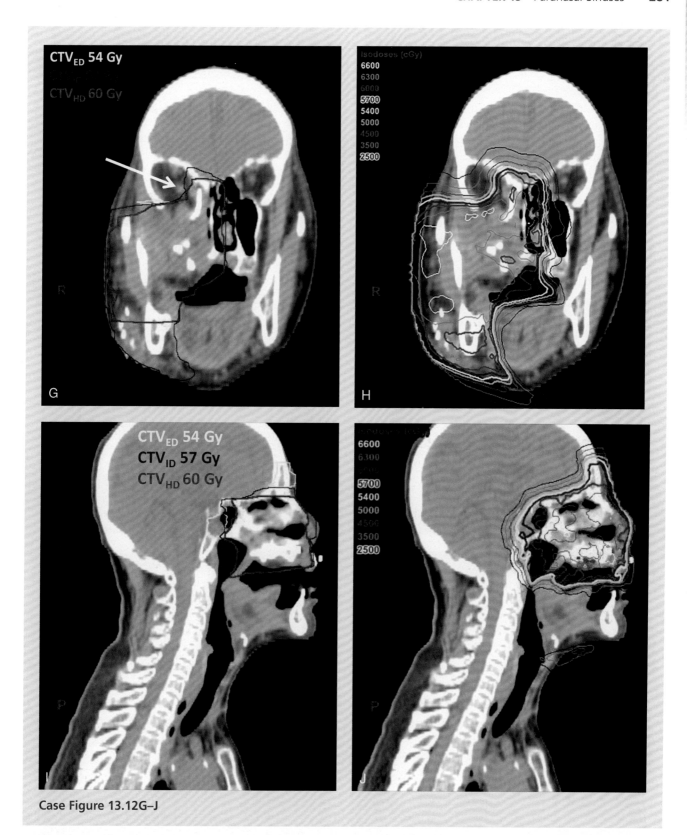

Case Figure 13.12G–J

CASE STUDY 13.13

A 39-year-old man presented to his physician after 4 months of persistent nasal congestion. Initial imaging showed an infiltrative and destructive process of the anterior and central skull base and regional adenopathy. Biopsy of the primary mass revealed sinonasal undifferentiated carcinoma. Representative images from his initial T1-weighted MRI with gadolinium are shown in the coronal and sagittal plane in Figure 13.13A,B. The mass was centered in the left nasoethmoid region, filled the nasopharynx, and destroyed the clivus. T2 images of the neck show the left lateral retropharyngeal adenopathy (*white arrow* in Fig. 13.13C) and bilateral level II adenopathy (*white arrows* in Fig. 13.13D).

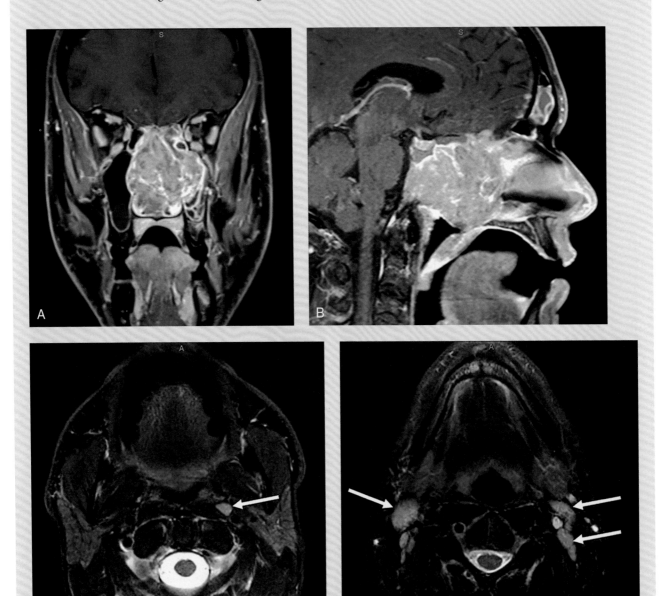

Case Figure 13.13A–D

He then came to our center for additional evaluation and treatment. PET scan showed no additional sites of disease or distant metastases. He received induction chemotherapy consisting of cisplatin and etoposide. Restaging MRI after two cycles of chemotherapy showed excellent response. Axial images at the epicenter of the primary tumor before and after induction chemotherapy are shown in Figure 13.13E,F, respectively. The *white arrows* in Figure 13.13F point to the postchemotherapy residual tumor. He then went on to receive two additional cycles of chemotherapy concurrent with definitive radiation therapy.

He was treated using active scanning intensity-modulated proton therapy. The prechemotherapy extent of primary and nodal disease with margin (CTV$_{HD}$) were treated to 66 Gy(radiobiologic equivalent [RBE]), the adjacent sinuses and involved nodal levels (CTV$_{ID}$) to 57 Gy(RBE), and the remainder of the at-risk bilateral neck (levels Ib through V and bilateral lateral retropharyngeal lymph nodes) (CTV$_{ED}$) to 54 Gy(RBE) all in 33 daily fractions. The CTVs and proton therapy dose distributions are shown in paired images in Figures 13.13G–T. Dose distributions on the coregistered prechemotherapy MRI are shown in Figure 13.13U. He recently completed therapy without interruption. There was grade 3 dermatitis but minimal oral reactions.

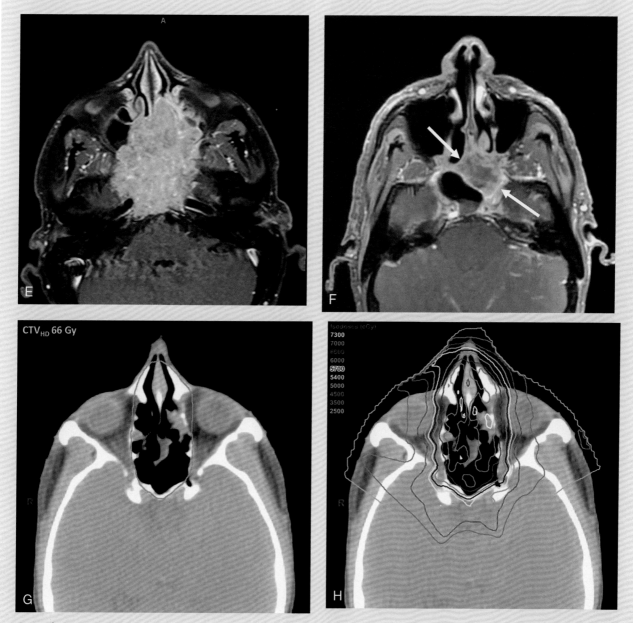

Case Figure 13.13E–H

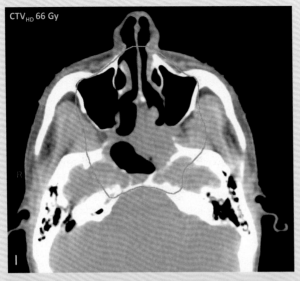

CTV_{HD} 66 Gy

I

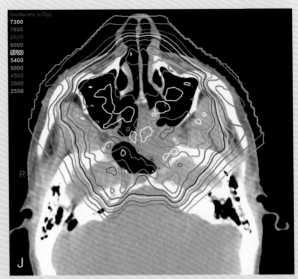

J

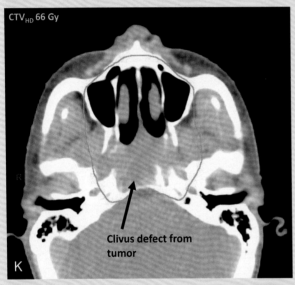

CTV_{HD} 66 Gy

Clivus defect from
tumor

K

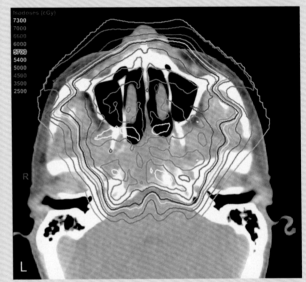

L

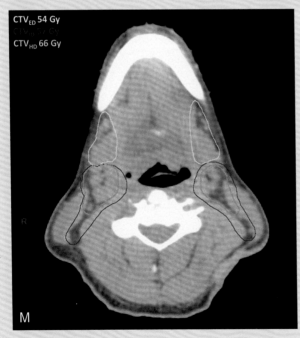

CTV_{ED} 54 Gy
CTV_{ID} 57 Gy
CTV_{HD} 66 Gy

M

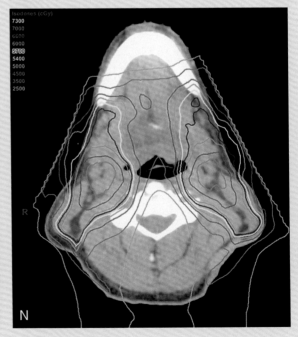

N

Case Figure 13.13I–N

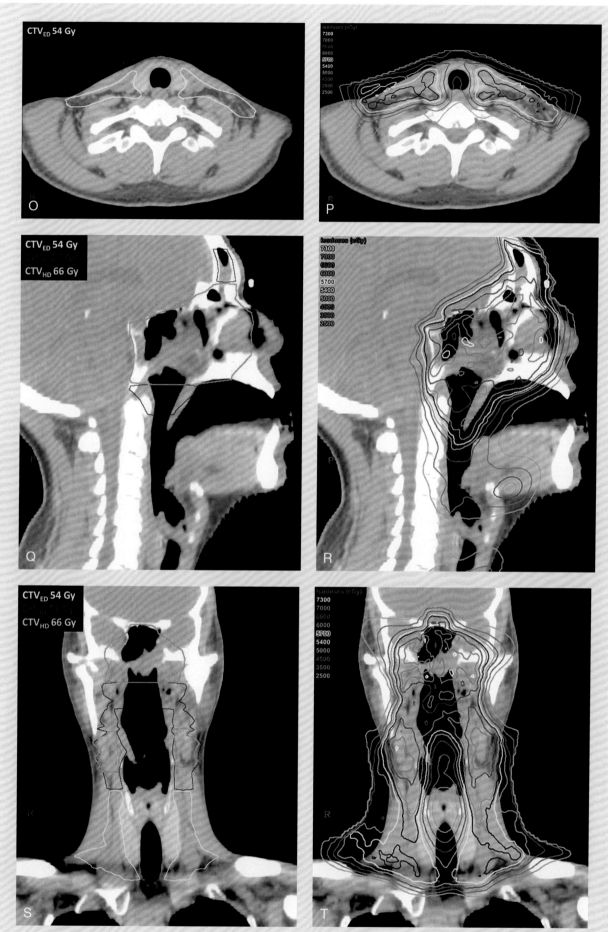

Case Figure 13.13O–T

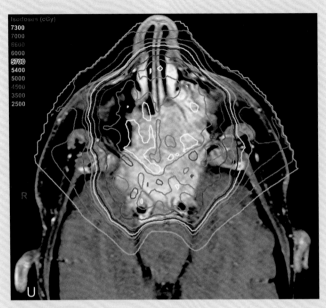

Case Figure 13.13U

CASE STUDY 13.14

A 48-year-old man presented to his physician initially with left-sided nasal obstructive symptoms. These symptoms further progressed to anosmia, dysgeusia, headache, double vision, and blurry vision in the left eye. Initial imaging included an MRI, which showed a left-sided nasoethmoid mass with extension into the left orbit and sphenoid and maxillary sinuses. Biopsy revealed sinonasal undifferentiated carcinoma. His initial T1-weighted MRI with gadolinium is shown in the axial and coronal plane in Figure 13.14A,B, respectively. The *white arrows* point to the extension into the left orbit. He underwent endoscopic resection of his tumor at an outside facility.

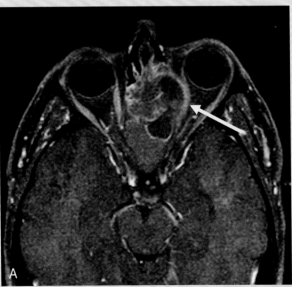
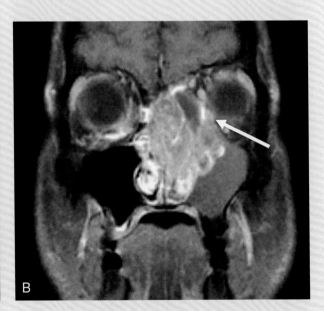

Case Figure 13.14A,B

Pathology confirmed sinonasal undifferentiated carcinoma, and multiple specimens were taken, many with positive margins. The surgeon communicated the most concerning area of disease to be at the left orbital region, adjacent to the left orbital apex.

He then came to our center for additional evaluation and treatment. Repeat MRI showed only postoperative changes with no clear imaging evidence of residual gross tumor. PET scan showed no regional or distant metastases. Postoperative chemotherapy and radiation therapy using proton therapy were recommended. He received his first cycle of cisplatin and etoposide prior to, the second cycle concurrent with, and the third and fourth cycles after radiation therapy.

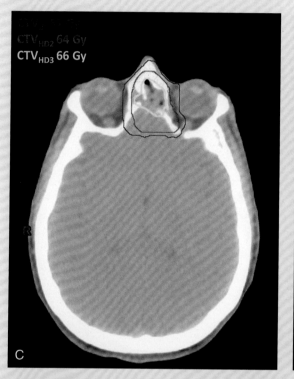

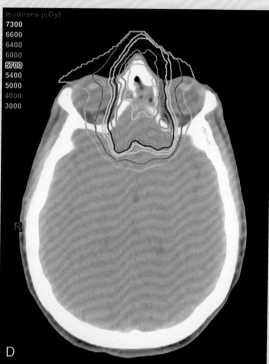

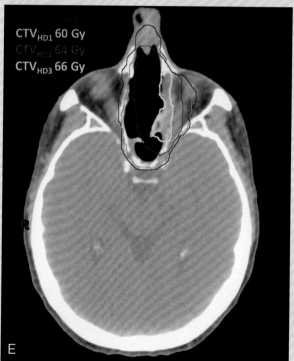

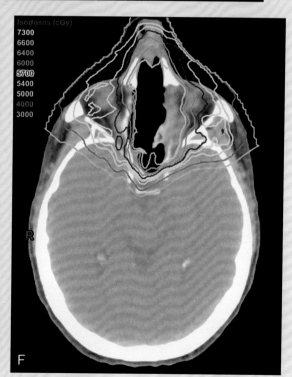

Case Figure 13.14C–F

He was treated using active scanning intensity-modulated proton therapy. He was simulated and treated with a mouth-opening and tongue-depressing stent with bite block. The highest risk tumor bed at the medial aspect of the left orbit (CTV_{HD3}) was treated to 66 Gy(radiobiologic equivalent [RBE]), the remainder of the tumor bed (CTV_{HD1} and CTV_{HD2}) to 60 to 64 Gy(RBE), operative bed (CTV_{ID}) to 57 Gy(RBE), and the bilateral level II and bilateral lateral retropharyngeal lymph nodes (CTV_{ED}) to 54 Gy(RBE) all in 33 daily fractions. The CTVs and proton therapy dose distributions are shown in paired images in Figures 13.14C–L. He remains disease free now 6 months since treatment completion.

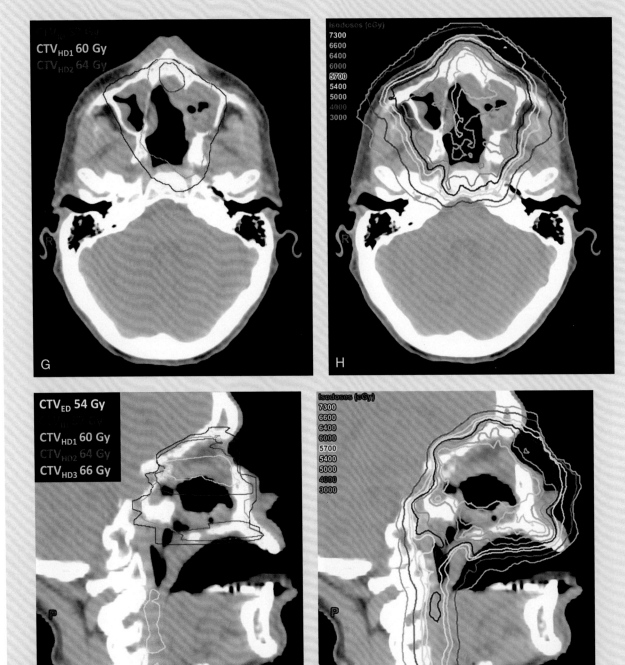

Case Figure 13.14G–J

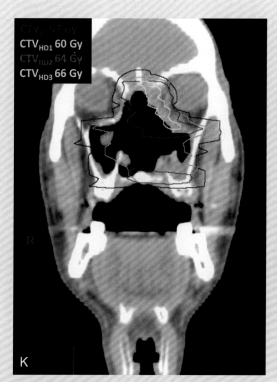
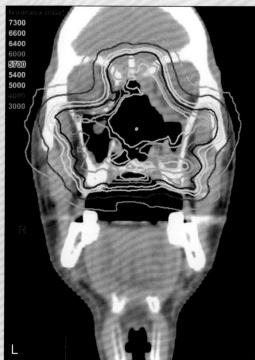

Case Figure 13.14K,L

SUGGESTED READINGS

Al-Mamgani A, Monserez D, Rooij PV, et al. Highly-conformal intensity-modulated radiotherapy reduced toxicity without jeopardizing outcome in patients with paranasal sinus cancer treated by surgery and radiotherapy or (chemo)radiation. *Oral Oncol* 2012;48:905.

Bristol IJ, Ahamad A, Garden AS, et al. Postoperative radiotherapy for maxillary sinus cancer: long-term outcomes and toxicities of treatment. *Int J Radiat Oncol Biol Phys* 2007;68:719.

Christopherson K, Werning JW, Malyapa RS, et al. Radiotherapy for sinonasal undifferentiated carcinoma. *Am J Otolaryngol* 2014;35:141.

Claus F, De Gersem W, De Wagter C, et al. An implementation strategy for IMRT of ethmoid sinus cancer with bilateral sparing of the optic pathways. *Int J Radiat Oncol Biol Phys* 2001;51:318.

Dagan R, Bryant C, Li Z, et al. Outcomes of sinonasal cancer treated with proton therapy. *Int J Radiat Oncol Biol Phys* 2016;95:377.

Demonte F, Ginsberg LE, Clayman GL. Primary malignant tumors of the sphenoidal sinus. *Neurosurgery* 2000;46:1084.

Duprez F, Madani I, Morbee L, et al. IMRT for sinonasal tumors minimizes severe late ocular toxicity and preserves disease control and survival. *Int J Radiat Oncol Biol Phys* 2012;83:252.

Fletcher GH, Goepfert H, Jesse RH. Nasal and paranasal sinus carcinoma. In: Fletcher GH, ed. *Textbook of radiotherapy*, 3rd ed. Philadelphia, PA: Lea & Febiger, 1980.

Jiang W, Mohamed AS, Fuller CD, et al. The role of elective nodal irradiation for esthesioneuroblastoma patients with clinically negative neck. *Pract Radiat Oncol* 2016;6(4):241–247.

Jiang GL, Morrison WH, Garden AS, et al. Ethmoid sinus carcinomas: natural history and treatment results. *Radiother Oncol* 1998;49:21.

Le QT, Fu KK, Kaplan MJ, et al. Lymph node metastasis in maxillary sinus carcinoma. *Int J Radiat Oncol Biol Phys* 2000;46:541.

Madani I, Bonte K, Vakaet L, et al. Intensity-modulated radiotherapy for sinonasal tumors: Ghent University Hospital update. *Int J Radiat Oncol Biol Phys* 2009;73:424.

Mendenhall WM, Amdur RJ, Morris CG, et al. Carcinoma of the nasal cavity and paranasal sinuses. *Laryngoscope* 2009;119:899.

Mock U, Georg D, Bogner J, et al. Treatment planning comparison of conventional, 3D conformal and intensity-modulated photon (IMRT) and proton therapy for paranasal sinus carcinoma. *Int J Radiat Oncol Biol Phys* 2004;58:147.

Patel SH, Wang Z, Wong WW, et al. Charged particle therapy versus photon therapy for paranasal sinus and nasal cavity malignant diseases: a systematic review and meta-analysis. *Lancet Oncol* 2014;15:1027.

Paulino AC, Marks JE, Bricker P, et al. Results of treatment of patients with maxillary sinus carcinoma. *Cancer* 1998;83:457.

Pommier P, Ginestet C, Sunyach M, et al. Conformal radiotherapy for paranasal sinus and nasal cavity tumors: three-dimensional treatment planning and preliminary results in 40 patients. *Int J Radiat Oncol Biol Phys* 2000;48:485.

Rosenthal DI, Barker JL Jr, El-Naggar AK, et al. Sinonasal malignancies with neuroendocrine differentiation: patterns of failure according to histologic phenotype. *Cancer* 2004;101:2567.

Takes RP, Ferlito A, Silver CE, et al. The controversy in the management of the N0 neck for squamous cell carcinoma of the maxillary sinus. *Eur Arch Otorhinolaryngol* 2014;271:899.

Tsien C, Eisbruch A, McShan D, et al. Intensity-modulated radiation therapy (IMRT) for locally advanced paranasal sinus tumors: incorporating clinical decisions in the optimization process. *Int J Radiat Oncol Biol Phys* 2003;55:776.

Waldron JN, O'Sullivan B, Gullane P, et al. Carcinoma of the maxillary antrum: a retrospective analysis of 110 cases. *Radiother Oncol* 2000;57:167.

Waldron JN, O'Sullivan B, Warde P, et al. Ethmoid sinus cancer: twenty-nine cases managed with primary radiation therapy. *Int J Radiat Oncol Biol Phys* 1998;41:361.

Wiegner EA, Daly ME, Murphy JD, et al. Intensity-modulated radiotherapy for tumors of the nasal cavity and paranasal sinuses: clinical outcomes and patterns of failure. *Int J Radiat Oncol Biol Phys* 2012;83:243.

14

Salivary Glands

Key Points

- Salivary gland neoplasms originate both from the major salivary glands (parotid, submandibular, and sublingual glands) and from thousands of minor salivary glands spread throughout the mucosa of the head and neck.

- The most common neoplasm is a benign pleomorphic adenoma. Malignant tumors comprise a wide variety of histologic types, including mucoepidermoid carcinoma, adenoid cystic carcinoma, salivary duct carcinoma, and acinic cell carcinoma.

- Histologic grade of differentiation is a strong prognostic factor. Distant metastases are more common in patients with high-grade tumors.

- Surgery is the recommended frontline treatment for resectable salivary gland cancers. Many of these tumors are locally infiltrative with ill-defined borders, which make obtaining resections with negative margins challenging.

- Adjuvant radiation is often recommended based on pathologic risk factors and histology. Indications for radiation include extraglandular extension, close or positive surgical margins, nodal involvement, high-grade histology, and perineural invasion. The combination of chemotherapy delivered concurrent with radiation for the treatment of high-risk salivary cancers is being investigated.

- In order to account for perineural spread, particularly with adenoid cystic carcinoma, radiation volumes often include the nerve pathways from the primary tumor to the skull base.

- Primary radiation therapy is reserved for unresectable tumors. The role of concurrent chemotherapy in this setting is controversial. Historically, neutron therapy had been utilized for these cases, particularly for adenoid cystic carcinoma, but this has largely fallen out of favor due to concerns for toxicity and lack of availability of neutron treatment facilities. The use of high LET particle therapy remains of interest with reports suggesting benefit from both proton therapy and carbon ion therapy.

- In both adjuvant and definitive settings, the standard of care in modern practice is the use of IMRT, when available. This allows optimal coverage of the tumor bed, any at-risk lymph nodes (depending on histology and stage), and perineural tracts; the potential benefit is largely based on data extrapolated from other head and neck sites. If IMRT is not available, traditional conventional photon or electron fields may be employed.

INTRODUCTION

Despite the realization of the diverse natural history and variation of radiation technique by specific site of origin, the rarity of salivary cancers led many investigators to report treatment outcomes in aggregate. Therefore, this chapter begins by summarizing the general background outcome data before addressing individual subsites.

Background Data

See Tables 14.1 to 14.4.

TABLE 14.1 Histologic Distribution of Salivary Neoplasms by Site

Site	Benign	Mucoepidermoid	Adenoid Cystic	Adenocarcinoma	MMT	Acinic	Epidermoid	Anaplastic
Parotid	1,342	272	54	62	107	75	45	8
Submandibular	106	37	45	9	24	2	8	—
Palate	60	37	67	41	18	1	—	4
Lip/cheek	13	23	12	20	2	3	—	—
Antrum	—	13	31	23	3	1	—	1
Tongue	2	14	30	12	2	—	—	3
Nasal cavity	4	12	17	23	—	1	—	3
Gingiva	—	13	10	6	3	1	—	1
Floor of the mouth	1	6	7	8	—	—	—	—
Larynx	—	3	3	7	—	—	—	8[a]
Tonsil	—	4	3	3	1	—	—	2
Ethmoid	—	1	1	6	—	—	—	1
Nasopharynx	—	2	1	5	1	—	—	—
Pharyngeal wall	1	2	—	—	—	—	—	—

[a]All neuroendocrine carcinomas.
MMT, malignant mixed tumor.
From Spiro RH. Salivary neoplasms: overview of a 35-year experience with 2,807 patients. *Head Neck Surg* 1986;8:177–184, with permission.

TABLE 14.2 Local Failure of Adenoid Cystic Carcinomas Treated with Surgery and Postoperative Irradiation Stratified by Positive Margins and Named Nerve Involvement

Site	No. of Failures/No. of Patients (%)	No. of Failures/No. of Patients with Positive Margins (%)	No. of Failures/No. of Patients with Named Nerve Involvement (%)
Minor salivary gland	16/122 (13)	10/54 (19)	5/31 (16)
Submandibular/sublingual gland	1/41 (2)	1/11 (9)	1/14 (7)

TABLE 14.2 Local Failure of Adenoid Cystic Carcinomas Treated with Surgery and Postoperative Irradiation Stratified by Positive Margins and Named Nerve Involvement *(Continued)*

Site	No. of Failures/No. of Patients (%)	No. of Failures/No. of Patients with Positive Margins (%)	No. of Failures/No. of Patients with Named Nerve Involvement (%)
Parotid gland	4/30 (13)	3/15 (20)	4/10 (40)
All patients	21/193 (11)	14/80 (18)	10/55 (18)

Data from M.D. Anderson Cancer Center.
Modified from Garden AS, Weber RS, Morrison WH, et al. The influence of positive margins and nerve invasion in adenoid cystic carcinoma of the head and neck treated with surgery and radiation. *Int J Radiat Oncol Biol Phys* 1995;32:619.

TABLE 14.3 Outcomes of 146 Patients with Adenoid Cystic Carcinomas Treated with Postoperative IMRT

Outcome	5 Years	7 Years	10 Years
Overall survival	84.0%	79.2%	73.7%
Local recurrence	8.6%	8.6%	13.7%
Regional recurrence	3.3%	3.3%	3.3%
Distant metastases	28.4%	36.6%	43.7%
Any recurrence	33.9%	41.9%	50.3%

Median follow-up of 71 mo. Unpublished data from M.D. Anderson Cancer Center; manuscript in preparation, 2016.

TABLE 14.4 Overall Survival Rates of Patients with Adenoid Cystic Treated with Particle Therapy

First Author	Modality	Patient Number	Median Follow-Up (Months)	Overall Survival
Douglas	Neutrons	151	32	72% (5-yr)
Pommier	Protons	23	ND	77% (5-yr)
Linton	Protons	26	25	93% (2-yr)
Takagi	Protons/carbon ion	40—protons 40—carbon ion	38	82% (3-yr)
Mizoe	Carbon ion	69	ND	68% (5-yr)
Jensen	IMRT + carbon ion boost	309	34	75% (5-yr)

ND, not described.
From Douglas JG, et al. *Int J Radiat Oncol Biol Phys* 2000;46:551; Pommier P, et al. *Arch Otolaryngol Head Neck Surg* 2006;132:1242; Linton OR, et al. *JAMA Otolaryngol Head Neck Surg* 2013;139:1306; Takagi M, et al. *Radiother Oncol* 2013;113:364; Mizoe, et al. *Radiother Oncol* 2012;103:32; Jensen AD, et al. *Radiother Oncol* 2016;118:272.

PAROTID

Treatment Strategy

Surgery is the preferred treatment for operable cases. Postoperative radiotherapy is indicated in the following clinical settings: high-grade tumors, close or positive surgical margins (including incompletely resected recurrent pleomorphic adenoma), tumor adherence to or invasion of the facial nerve or presence of perineural invasion on microscopic evaluation, bone and/or connective tissue involvement, lymph node metastases (particularly with extracapsular extension), or after resection of recurrent disease, even with negative margins.

Postoperative Radiotherapy

Target Volume

Initial Target Volume

The target volume for benign and low-grade tumors without lymph node involvement is the operative bed only. For high-grade tumors and tumors with lymph node involvement, the volume encompasses the parotid bed and ipsilateral lymph nodes of the neck.

For tumors with perineural invasion, the course of the facial nerve should be included to the stylomastoid foramen; if there is macroscopic invasion of the facial nerve, the volumes should be even more generous and extend to the facial canal and geniculate ganglion.

Setup, Field Arrangement, and Dose for Conventional Technique

A conventional technique should be utilized if IMRT is not available.

If the target volume is 5 cm or less deep (superficial lobe and deep lobe in thin patients) **(Case Study 14.1 and Case Study 14.2)**.

A lateral appositional field is used to cover the parotid bed and upper neck nodes. Radiation is delivered with a combination of electrons (16 to 20 MeV depending on the depth) and photons (6 MV) usually in the ratio of 4:1.

An intraoral stent containing cerrobend is used to shield the posterior oral tongue (see Chapter 3).

Marking of the surgical scar and lateral canthus of the ipsilateral orbit facilitates portal design.

Patient is immobilized in an open neck position with a thermoplastic mask. Flattening of the ipsilateral ear against the mastoid process minimizes dose heterogeneity resulting

CASE STUDY 14.1

A 39-year-old woman presented with a 4-month history of a right parotid swelling. She underwent a surgical exploration, which revealed a large mass extending from the base of skull to the subdigastric muscle inferiorly. This lesion was dissected off the facial nerve and removed in two major pieces. Histologic examination showed a pleomorphic adenoma. Five months later, she presented with a recurrent nodule in the upper posterior cervical region. This was excised and was also found to contain pleomorphic adenoma. Four months after the second intervention, a small mass developed at the posterior auricular region. Fine-needle aspiration showed carcinoma. She was then referred to MD Anderson Cancer Center. Review of the slides revealed carcinoma ex-pleomorphic adenoma (considered a high grade malignancy) in the specimens of the first and second surgical procedures. Physical examination upon referral revealed no palpable residual disease and an intact facial nerve. It was decided to deliver postoperative radiotherapy to the parotid bed and upper neck with a lateral appositional field (Fig. 14.1) using a combination of electrons and photons (20 MeV and 6 MV, respectively). An intraoral stent was used to protect the mucosa of the oral tongue and contralateral oral cavity. The mid and lower neck nodes on the ipsilateral side were treated with a separate electron field. The tumor bed received a dose of 60 Gy in 30 fractions prescribed to the 90% isodose line and the mid and lower neck prescribed a dose of 50 Gy in 25 fractions.

Off-cord reduction is made after reaching a dose of approximately 44 Gy and the posterior strip is supplemented with lower-energy electrons (usually 9 MeV).

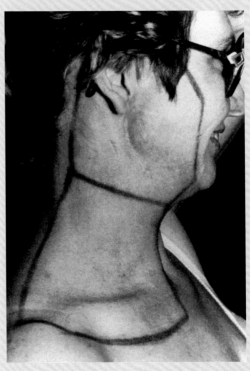

Case Figure 14.1

CASE STUDY 14.2

A 66-year-old man presented with a 2-cm left preauricular mass. Radiographic imaging revealed a mass in the superficial lobe of the left parotid gland. He underwent a superficial parotidectomy and upper neck dissection. Histologic examination revealed an adenoid cystic carcinoma with positive anterior and deep margins but none of five lymph nodes harbored metastases. The patient received postoperative radiotherapy in the open neck position. As shown in Figure 14.2B, a tongue-displacing stent (S) was used, and bolus material (B) applied to modulate the depth of the electron range. An initial 50 Gy was delivered to the parotid bed and upper neck (Fig. 14.2A) with a 4:1 mix of 16 MeV electrons and 6 MV photons. A boost of 16 Gy to the high-risk area was delivered with 12 MeV electrons. A representative axial isodose distribution is shown in Figure 14.2B.

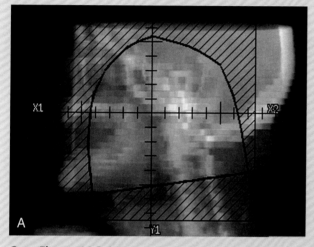

Case Figure 14.2 A,B

from electron perturbation. For the same reason, the external auditory canal is filled with Burow's solution prior to each electron treatment.

Bolus is used to cover the superior aspect of the portal when it extends above the zygomatic arch to minimize the dose to the temporal lobe of the brain.

Portal borders are as follows:

- *Superior:* zygomatic arch or higher as indicated by tumor extent or surgical scar
- *Anterior:* anterior edge of the masseter muscle
- *Inferior:* thyroid notch
- *Posterior:* just behind the mastoid process

A 1.5- to 2-cm beveled bolus or a computer-generated custom bolus is placed at the superior part of the portal (above the line connecting the orbital floor and the mastoid process) to reduce the dose to the temporal lobe. A lateral appositional electron field is used to treat the mid and lower neck nodes when indicated (for borders of neck field; see "General Principles"). Field reduction takes place after 50 to 54 Gy in 25 to 27 fractions to deliver the boost dose when indicated. If the anterior edge of the portal is close to the eye, skin collimation is applied and the beam may be angled 5 to 10 degrees posteriorly to minimize the dose to the orbital content.

For more deep-seated tumors or when facial canal is part of the target volume, a wedge-pair technique **(Case Study 14.3 and Case Study 14.4)** with photon beams is often preferable.

With these techniques, the patient is immobilized in a supine position with the head hyperextended with thermoplastic mask. The axial plane of the fields is chosen so that the posterolateral portal does not exit through the contralateral eye. A relatively simple wedge-pair technique uses anterolateral and posterolateral oblique photon fields (the anterolateral oblique field is on the spinal cord and the posterolateral oblique field is off cord). The simulation focuses on marking of the surgical scar and both inferior orbital rims and selection of a provisional isocenter. The provisional isocenter is generally placed at the center of the square defined by the zygomatic arch, anterior edge of the masseter, thyroid notch, and mastoid, and halfway between the skin and the oropharyngeal wall.

Thin-slice computed tomography (CT) scan is obtained in the treatment position for outlining the target volume and planning the portal sizes, hinge angle, and thickness of wedges using treatment planning system. No off–spinal cord reduction is required with a wedge-pair technique because the posterolateral field is off the cord from the beginning. Field reduction for boost dose, when indicated, occurs after 50 to 54 Gy.

CASE STUDY 14.3

A 46-year-old woman presented with a 1-year history of intermittent left facial swelling and left parietal headache. Physical examination of the parotid region and other head and neck areas was unremarkable. The facial nerve was intact. A computed tomography (CT) scan, however, showed a soft tissue mass in the deep lobe of the parotid. The patient underwent a total parotidectomy with sparing of the facial nerve. The tumor was removed from beneath the facial nerve with some difficulty. Histologic examination revealed a benign pleomorphic adenoma measuring

3.5 × 3 × 2.5 cm. The deep margin of resection was positive. Two intraparotid lymph nodes and 16 periparotid nodes, removed to gain access to the parotid, were all free of tumor. It was decided to treat this patient with postoperative radiotherapy because of the difficult and incomplete resection. The target volume extended to 6 cm from the surface, which was too deep for the highest available electron energy (20 MeV). Therefore, it was elected to treat with wedge-pair fields (Fig. 14.3A,B). A total dose of 50 Gy was delivered to the 95% isodose line in 25 fractions.

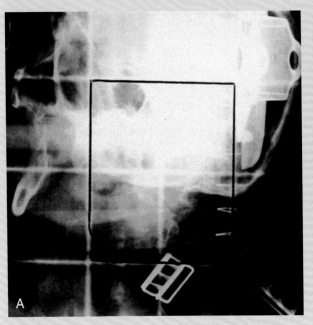 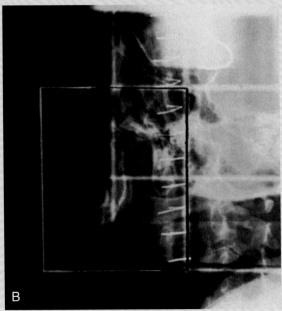

Case Figure 14.3 A,B

CASE STUDY 14.4

A 46-year-old man presented with a left parotid mass associated with facial pain and facial palsy. Magnetic resonance imaging (MRI) showed a mass occupying most of the superficial lobe and extending into the deep lobe, measuring 5 cm in greatest dimension. He underwent a resection of the mass consisting of left total parotidectomy, left parapharyngeal space dissection, left upper neck dissection, and left segmental mandibulectomy. Histopathologic evaluation of resected tumor showed cribriform, grade 2, adenoid cystic carcinoma, 5.5 × 4.0 × 3.0 cm, extending to

the surgical margin. None of 11 lymph nodes contained metastatic deposits. The patient received postoperative radiotherapy with a left anterior oblique and left posterior oblique pair of portals with 60-degree wedges. This was chosen because of the disease deep in the dissected parapharyngeal space. A field reduction was made at 50 Gy. The total dose was 66 Gy in 33 fractions. Figure 14.4 shows axial (Fig. 14.4A) and coronal (Fig. 14.4B) isodose distributions. The patient remains free of disease 30 months from diagnosis.

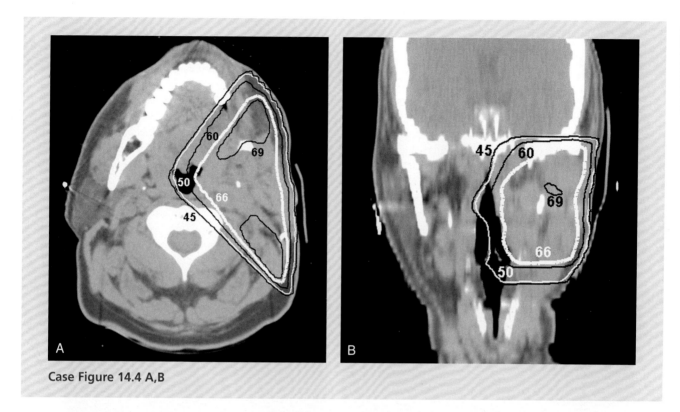

Case Figure 14.4 A,B

For patients treated with conventional radiation therapy (electrons or photons), conventional fractionation is typically used, with a series of field reductions to accomplish boosting to the resection bed. For benign and low-grade tumors with negative section margins, a dose of 50 to 54 Gy in 25 to 27 fractions is prescribed. For patients with close or positive margins, the prescribed dose is 60 to 66 Gy. Patients with multiple recurrence of benign disease or with multinodular disease are treated to 60 Gy.

For high-grade tumors and those with lymph node metastases, the commonly prescribed dose is 60 Gy in 30 fractions after complete resection or 64 to 66 Gy in 32 to 33 fractions in the presence of positive margin or extracapsular tumor extension (ECE). Off-spinal cord reduction, with ipsilateral electron–photon technique, takes place at approximately 44 Gy and field size is reduced after 50 to 54 Gy. For elective neck irradiation, a dose of 50 Gy in 25 fractions is prescribed.

For a lateral appositional field, the dose is prescribed at the 90% isodose line. The energy of electrons is chosen according to the depth of the tumor bed. For wedge-pair technique, the dose is prescribed at the isodose line encompassing the target volume.

Intensity-Modulated Therapy: Targets and Dose

IMRT is considered standard of care for adjuvant treatment of patients with parotid cancers in the modern era, when available. With IMRT, the patient is immobilized with an extended head and shoulder thermoplastic mask in a supine position. Extending the head aids in minimizing exposure to oral cavity. A tongue-lateralizing oral stent may be used to displace and immobilize the tongue away from the tumor bed. Thin-slice CT scan is obtained for delineation of target volumes (Case Study 14.5 through Case Study 14.7).

IMPT is an alternative for adjuvant treatment of patients with parotid cancer. It is unclear if the use of protons, a high LET particle, offers a biologic advantage for salivary gland cancers, particularly in the adjuvant setting. However, it does allow for greater lateralization of the dose, and so is attractive for treatment of patients with parotid cancers who are principally treated to the side of involvement (Case Study 14.8 and Case Study 14.9).

Virtual Gross Target Volume

There is no actual GTV after complete surgical tumor resection. However, it can be useful to formulate a virtual GTV (vGTV) to facilitate target volume definition. The vGTV is a best approximation of the tissues having high likelihood of harboring microscopic tumor reconstructed based on findings of preoperative clinical examination, imaging studies, and surgical–pathologic assessment.

Clinical Target Volumes

Three clinical target volumes (CTVs) are generally delineated.

- CTV$_{HD}$ delineates volumes to receive the highest dose. This includes the primary and nodal vGTVs with 8- to 10-mm margins.
- CTV$_{ID}$ delineates volumes to receive an intermediate dose, which typically encompasses the remaining operative bed not included in CTV$_{HD}$.

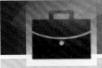

CASE STUDY 14.5

A 22-year-old woman man presented with a left parotid mass. The lesion was present for 6 years, but it had recently become larger and uncomfortable. A magnetic resonance imaging (MRI) revealed the left parotid mass, involving both the superficial and deep lobes (Fig. 14.5A, *white arrow*). An FNA was positive for carcinoma. She underwent a total parotidectomy with facial nerve sparing. Histologic examination revealed a 1.7-cm acinic cell carcinoma with a poorly differentiated component, extending to the periglandular soft tissue, with no perineural invasion and a positive margin; there was also one intraparotid lymph node positive for carcinoma. She received postoperative radiotherapy using IMRT to the tumor bed and ipsilateral neck (because of the poorly differentiated component). Figure 14.5B shows an axial isodose distribution at approximately the same level as the preoperative MRI image (Fig. 14.5A). A total dose of 66 Gy was delivered in 30 fractions due to the positive margin (prescribed to CTV in maroon colorwash). Additional CTV targets in red and blue colorwash were prescribed 60 Gy and 57 Gy, respectively. The IMRT field was matched to a conventional low-neck field with a half-beam block. The patient is now 2 years posttreatment with no evidence of disease and intact facial nerve function.

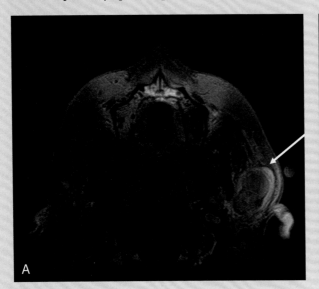
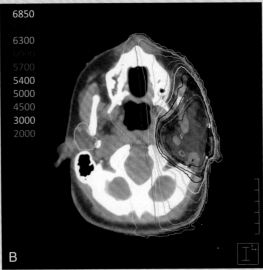

Case Figure 14.5 A,B

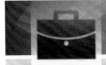

CASE STUDY 14.6

A 41-year-old woman presented with an enlarging right parotid mass for 6 years, with steady growth and increasing trismus over the last year. An MRI revealed a left-sided parotid mass with invasion of the parapharyngeal space and soft tissue extension to the stylomastoid foramen (Fig. 14.6A). An FNA was positive for adenoid cystic carcinoma. She underwent a left radical parotidectomy, mastoidectomy, and modified radical neck dissection; she underwent a flap reconstruction. Histologic examination revealed a 4.5-cm adenoid cystic carcinoma, cribriform pattern, with extensive perineural invasion. Soft tissue at the stylomastoid foramen and TMJ were positive for carcinoma, with a focally positive margin. All lymph nodes were negative. She was treated with postoperative IMRT delivered in 30 fractions. Given the concern for the margin and soft tissue findings at the stylomastoid foramen, a dose of 66 Gy was prescribed to that area, 60 Gy to the entire parotid bed, and 57 Gy to the remaining operative bed including the dissected upper neck. The left lower neck was not treated given the pathologically negative neck dissection and histology of the primary tumor (adenoid cystic carcinoma). Figure 14.6B shows an axial slice demonstrating the boost volume (red colorwash) at the level of the TMJ, where the concern for residual disease was centered. Figure 14.6C demonstrates a caudal axial slice, demonstrating coverage of the flap reconstruction and positioning of the tongue with a tongue-deviating stent. The 60 Gy target is in blue colorwash, and the 57 Gy target in yellow colorwash. Figure 14.6D,E shows the isodose lines and coverage of the resection bed and entirety of the flap in the coronal and sagittal planes. Five years after completing treatment, she has no evidence of locoregional recurrence; she did develop small volume lung metastases 2 years after treatment.

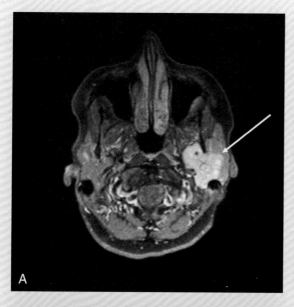

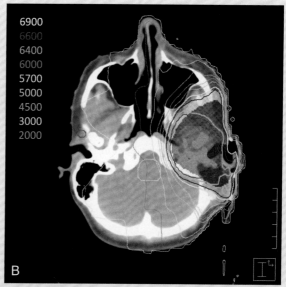

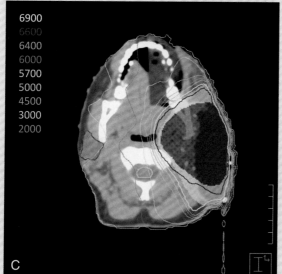

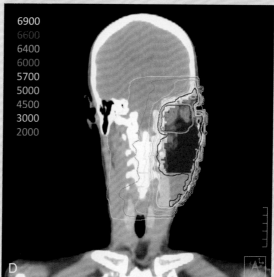

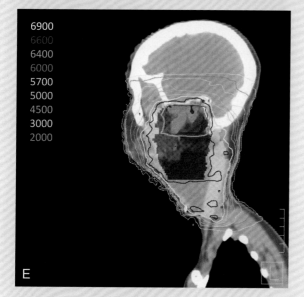

Case Figure 14.6 A–E

CASE STUDY 14.7

A 50-year-old woman presented with a painless left parotid mass. An MRI revealed a mass in the left parotid (Fig. 14.7A, *white arrow*) with a suspicious level II lymph node. She underwent a total parotidectomy with sacrifice of the lower division of the facial nerve and a left modified neck dissection. Pathology examination revealed salivary duct carcinoma measuring 3 cm with perineural invasion; margins were negative. Forty resected lymph nodes were negative for carcinoma. She was treated with postoperative IMRT delivered in 30 fractions. The region of the resected tumor was defined as CTV_{HD} (*red color wash*) and prescribed 60 Gy. The entire operative bed, including the parotid bed and dissected neck, was defined as CTV_{ID}

(*blue* color wash). The facial nerve was treated to the stylomastoid foramen to account for the perineural invasion. The left lower neck was treated with a matched oblique photon beam. Figure 14.7B shows an axial slice of the plan with coverage of the stylomastoid foramen (arrow) to account for perineural invasion. Additional axial views of the plan are shown in Figure 14.7C–E, including the conventional low-neck field match (Fig 14.7E), which preferentially spares the larynx, esophagus, and spinal cord. The tongue displacing stent can be seen in Figure 14.7C, moving the tongue out of the 30-45 Gy region. Figure 14.7F shows a coronal view and isodose distribution of the full plan. Two years later, she has no evidence of disease.

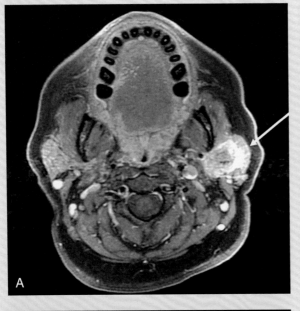

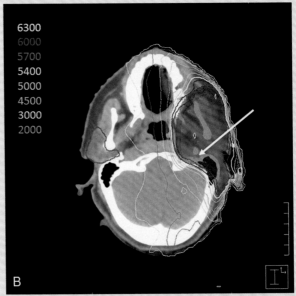

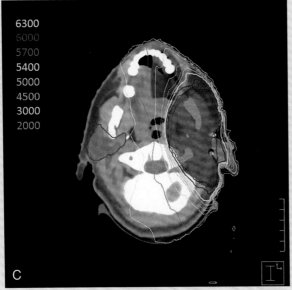

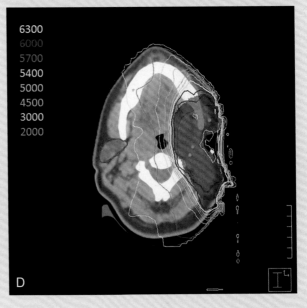

Case Figure 14.7 A–D

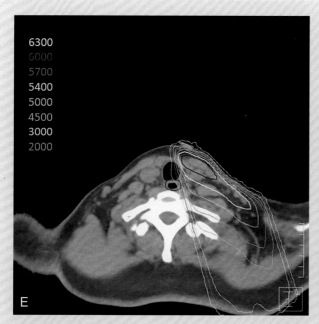 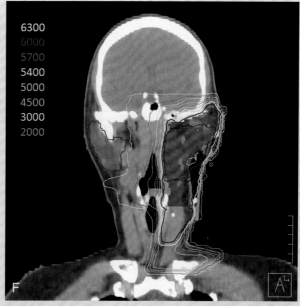

Case Figure 14.7 E,F

CASE STUDY 14.8

A 64-year-old man presented with an otherwise asymptomatic left preauricular lump. There was no facial weakness detected on clinical examination. CT scan of the head and neck with contrast showed an enhancing mass in the superficial lobe of the left parotid gland with central necrosis (Fig. 14.8A, *white arrow*) and multiple enlarged enhancing lymph nodes in left level IIa (Fig. 14.8B, *white arrows*). Fine-needle aspiration of the parotid mass showed high-grade carcinoma. PET–CT (Fig. 14.8C,D) showed these same lesions to be moderately FDG-avid, but there were no additional lesions or distant metastases.

He underwent left superficial parotidectomy with dissection and preservation of the facial nerve and left neck dissection levels II to IV. Operative findings describe a 2.5-cm firm mass in the left parotid with infiltration of the underlying masseter muscle that required resection of a cuff of muscle, the buccal branch of the facial nerve that was adherent to the mass, and resection of multiple enlarged periparotid and upper neck lymph nodes. The remainder of the facial nerve was preserved. Final pathology showed high-grade salivary duct carcinoma, arising as a carcinoma ex-pleomorphic adenoma, with periglandular extension, muscle invasion, perineural invasion, and lymphovascular invasion. Surgical margins were negative. Multiple lymph nodes in levels II and III contained metastatic carcinoma, all with extracapsular extension. Final stage was PT3N2b.

He was treated with postoperative chemoradiation using intensity-modulated proton therapy (IMPT), single-field optimization (SFO) technique, using active-scanning beam. He was simulated and treated using a posterior head, neck and shoulder mold, tongue-deviating stent with bite block, and a full-length custom mask. The parotid tumor bed and positive lymph node beds with margin (CTV_{HD}) were treated to 60 Gy (radiobiologic equivalent [RBE]), the operative bed (CTV_{ID}) to 56 Gy(RBE), and the remainder of the at-risk neck (CTV_{ED}) to 54 Gy(RBE) all in 30 fractions in a single integrated plan. Neck levels I to V were included in the treatment volume. He received weekly cisplatin 40 mg/m² for 5 of the 6 weeks of IMPT.

The CTVs and IMPT dose distributions are shown in paired images through the axial plane in Figure 14.8E through L. Care was taken to include the deep lobe of the parotid and parapharyngeal space in CTV_{ID} (*white arrow* of Fig. 14.8E) and generous coverage of the aspects of the masseter which were invaded, in CTV$_{HD}$ (*white arrow* Fig. 14.8G). Given multilevel lymph node involvement and extracapsular extension, broad coverage of the left neck and adequate surface dose along surgical scars were ensured at the

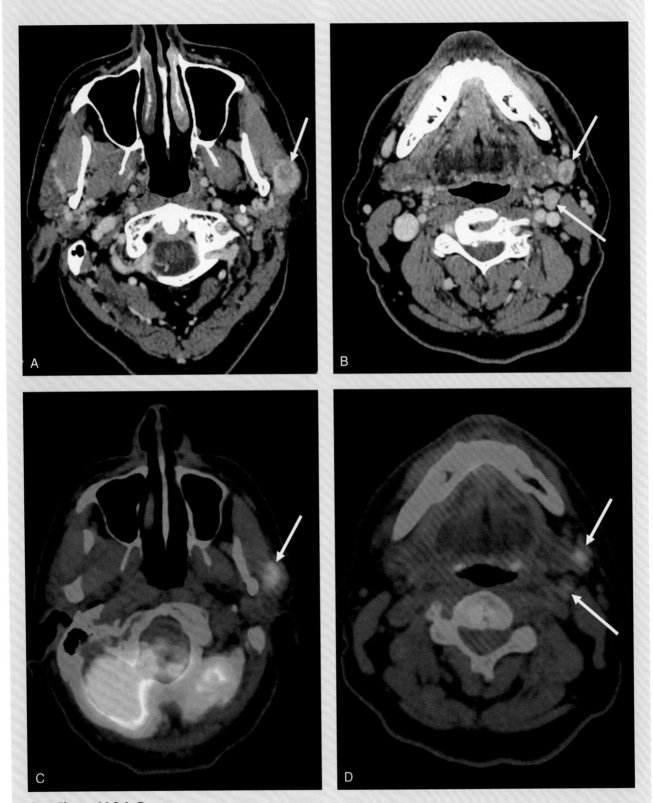

Case Figure 14.8 A–D

time of proton planning. Using the combination of a tongue-deviating stent and proton therapy, the dose of the oral tongue was exceedingly low. The medical photographs taken during week 6 of IMPT show no visible buccal or oral tongue acute mucosal reactions (Fig. 14.8M,N).

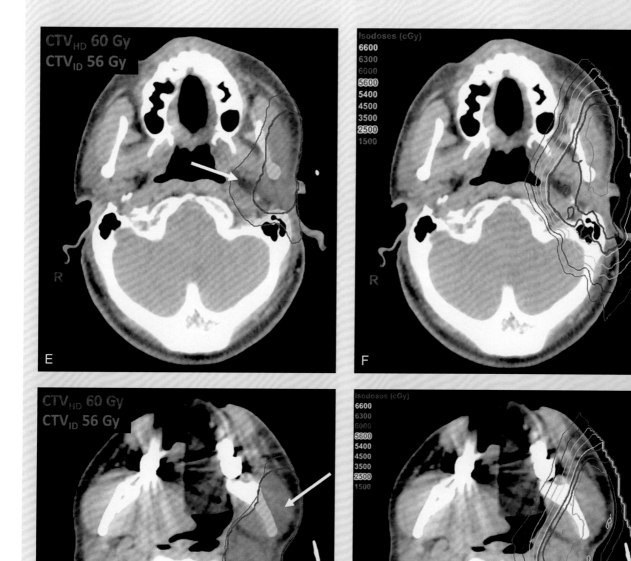

Case Figure 14.8 E–H

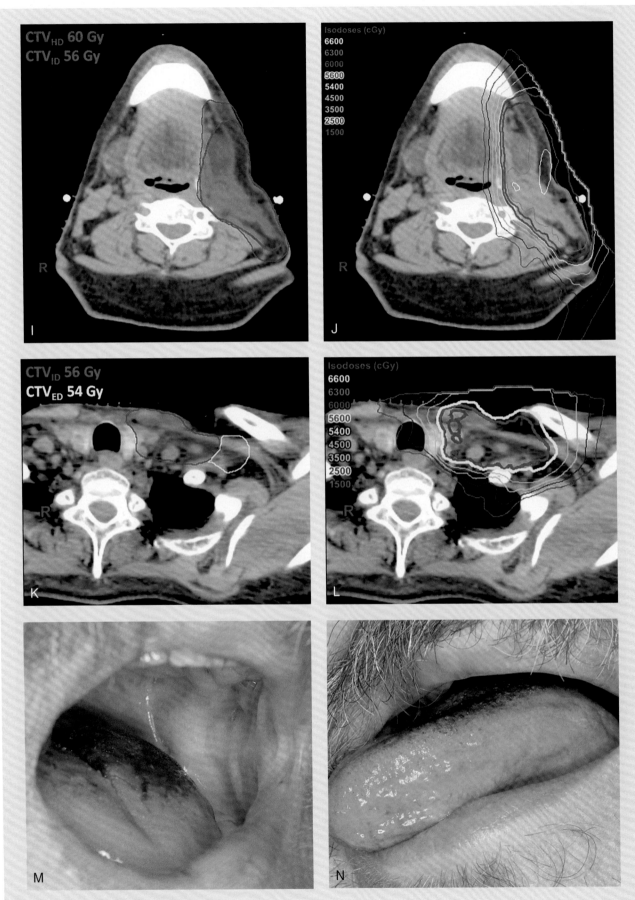

Case Figure 14.8 I–N

CASE STUDY 14.9

A 68-year-old male presented with a left parotid mass, and fine-needle aspiration confirmed malignancy. He underwent a total parotidectomy, radical neck dissection, and reconstruction with a fasciocutaneous flap. Pathology revealed high-grade salivary duct carcinoma in the parotid with extension to adjacent fibrous and soft tissue. The facial nerve was involved and there was perineural and intraneural involvement. In the dissected neck, levels I to V harbored 42 nodes positive for disease.

He was treated postoperatively with IMPT using single-field optimization (SFO) with active scanning. He was treated with concurrent paclitaxel and carboplatin. Figure 14.9A–F is axial images showing the contours of CTV$_{HD}$ (*red*) and CTV$_{ED}$ (*blue* superiorly and *turquoise*

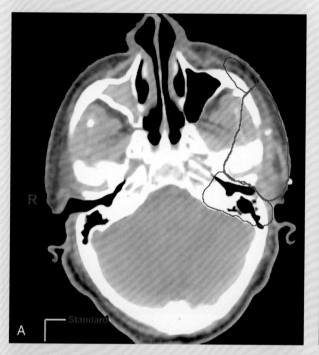

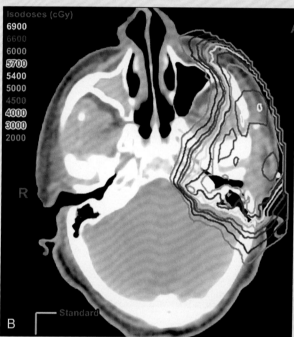

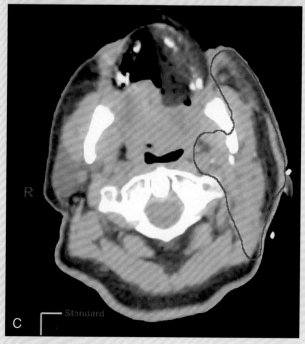

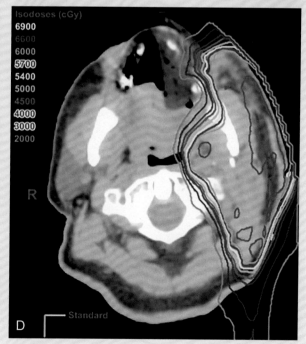

Case Figure 14.9 A–D

inferiorly), prescribed 60 and 54 Gy, respectively, in 30 fractions. These images are paired with the respective isodose distribution. Figure 14.9A,B is an axial representation through the superior parotid bed and temporal bone (covering the facial nerve going through the bone due to the extensive nerve involvement). Figure 14.9C,D is a representation through the midparotid bed (the contralateral normal parotid is well seen), and Figure 14.9E,F demonstrates the contours and isodose at the junction of

neck nodal levels II and III. Figure 14.9G through J shows similar views of paired contours and isodoses in coronal and sagittal orientations.

He developed expected radiation dermatitis and minimal lateral oral mucositis. His pain was controlled with ibuprofen. He remained without local–regional disease for 1 year but was found to have pulmonary and hepatic metastases that progressed on conventional therapies.

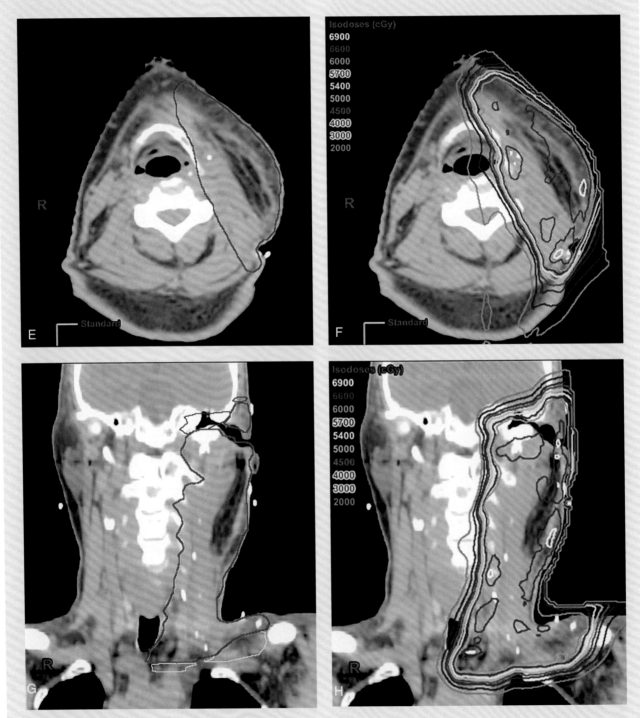

Case Figure 14.9 E–H

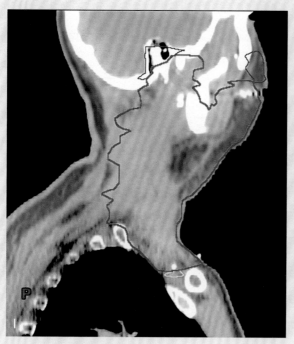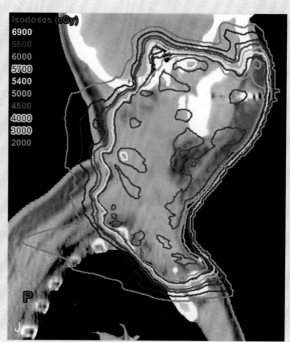

Case Figure 14.9 I,J

- CTV$_{ED}$ delineates volumes to receive an elective dose for subclinical disease including the stylomastoid foramen. If the facial nerve is involved, CTV$_{ED}$ extends into the facial canal to the geniculate ganglion. For patients treated with a superficial parotidectomy, CTV$_{ED}$ extends medial to CTV$_{HD}$ or CTV$_{ID}$ to the lateral pharyngeal wall to ensure coverage of the entire deep lobe. Anteriorly, CTV$_{ED}$ extends lateral to and along the masseter to encompass the accessory gland and Stensen's duct. In patients with high-grade cancers without clinical evidence of nodal involvement, CTV$_{ED}$ covers ipsilateral nodal levels II to IV. In patients with nodal involvement, CTV$_{ED}$ encompasses ipsilateral nodal levels not included in higher-dose CTVs.

The isocenter is placed in the center of the treatment volume when the parotid bed alone is treated. If the entire neck is to be treated, a half-beam matching technique might be preferable.

In this case, the isocenter is placed above the level of the arytenoids. Ipsilateral levels III and IV are included in a matching anterior (or parallel anterior and posterior) photon portal. Alternatively, VMAT may be used to treat the entirety of the parotid bed and ipsilateral neck in a comprehensive IMRT plan.

With IMRT, doses prescribed to CTV$_{HD}$, CTV$_{ID}$, and CTV$_{ED}$ are 60, 57, and 54 Gy, respectively, and treatment is given in 30 fractions. In the case of a high-risk area, such as a positive margin, the dose can be boosted to a total dose of 66 Gy in 30 fractions (2.2 Gy per fraction). For low-grade tumors treated to a lower total dose, CTV$_{HD}$ receives 2 Gy per fraction, and the fraction number adjusted accordingly. For IMRT, the dose is prescribed at the isodose line encompassing the target volume.

Background Data

See Table 14.5.

TABLE 14.5 Local Failures after Postoperative Radiotherapy for Parotid Gland Malignancies by Patient, Surgical, and Pathologic Features

Feature	No. of Patients	No. of Failures
Facial nerve sacrificed	42	9 (21%)
Positive margins	37	6 (16%)
Close or uncertain margins	66	5 (8%)
Low histologic grade	46	1 (2%)

(Continued)

TABLE 14.5 Local Failures after Postoperative Radiotherapy for Parotid Gland Malignancies by Patient, Surgical, and Pathologic Features *(Continued)*

Feature	No. of Patients	No. of Failures
Focal perineural invasion	36	4 (11%)
Named nerve involvement	20	5 (25%)
Extraglandular disease extension	78	11 (14%)
All patients	166	15 (9%)

Data from M.D. Anderson Cancer Center.
Modified from Garden AS, El-Naggar AK, Morrison WH, et al. Postoperative radiotherapy for malignant tumors of the parotid gland. *Int J Radiat Oncol Biol Phys* 1997;37:79–85.

SUBMANDIBULAR GLAND

Treatment Strategy

As in parotid gland tumors, surgery is the preferred treatment for submandibular gland neoplasms. Indications of postoperative radiotherapy are the same as those listed in the "Parotid" section; similar to parotid cancers, IMRT is considered the standard of care in the modern era, when available.

Postoperative Radiotherapy

Target Volume

The initial target volume for low-grade tumors without lymph node involvement encompasses the surgical bed; the target volume for high-grade tumors or tumors with positive lymph nodes encompasses the surgical bed and ipsilateral neck nodes (**Case Study 14.10**).

For cases in which there is perineural invasion from a submandibular gland primary cancer, the tracts of the lingual and hypoglossal nerves should be covered. For focal or small nerve

CASE STUDY 14.10

An 82-year-old man noted an asymptomatic mass in the left submandibular area and sought medical attention immediately. Examination revealed a 3-cm left submandibular mass. This tumor was resected along with a left modified neck dissection, and histologic examination revealed an adenoid cystic carcinoma in the submandibular gland measuring 2.5 × 2 × 2 with perineural invasion. One of the eight nodes (a subdigastric node) in the specimen contained metastatic disease. The lingual and hypoglossal nerves were free of gross tumor invasion. Postoperative radiotherapy was delivered through a left lateral appositional field (Fig. 14.10) encompassing the tumor bed, the proximal extension of the nerves at risk, and the upper neck. A combination of 20 MeV electrons and 6 MV photons was used weighted 4 to 1. A dose of 50 Gy in 25 fractions was delivered, after which the field was reduced to administer an additional 10 Gy in 5 fractions boost to the tumor bed. The mid and lower neck nodes were treated with a matching 9-MeV electron field to a dose of 50 Gy in 25 fractions.

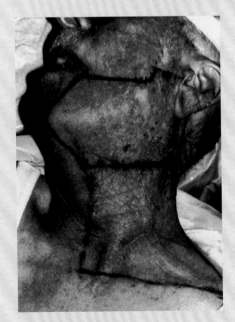

Case Figure 14.10

invasion, the primary tumor and neck coverage typically includes the distal branches. For more extensive invasion and involvement of the named nerves, both should be covered to the skull base (to foramen ovale and the hypoglossal canal, respectively).

Setup, Field Arrangement, and Dose for Conventional Technique

For patients with submandibular gland primaries, ipsilateral radiation with electron beam is typically sufficient (exceptions: medial extent of primary tumor or coverage of the skull base beyond the range of electrons). The patient is immobilized in the open neck position with a thermoplastic mask. Marking of the scar and oral commissure facilitates portal design.

A lateral appositional field encompasses the tumor bed and upper neck nodes. Radiation is delivered with a combination of electrons (12 to 20 MeV depending on the depth) and photons (6 MV) in a ratio of 4:1. Portal borders are as follows:

- *Superior:* from the oral commissure sloping up to cover the ascending ramus of the mandible just short of the temporomandibular joint. The field is extended up to the base of the skull when there is perineural invasion of a major nerve.
- *Anterior:* determined by the extent of surgery; the oral commissure and skin of the chin are shielded when possible.

- *Inferior:* thyroid notch.
- *Posterior:* just behind the mastoid process.

An off-cord reduction is made at approximately 44 Gy and the posterior strip is supplemented with lower-energy electrons. A lateral appositional electron field is used for irradiation of the mid and lower neck nodes when indicated (see "General Principles").

For high-grade tumors and those with lymph node metastases, the commonly prescribed dose is 60 Gy in 30 fractions after complete resection or 64 to 66 Gy in 32 to 33 fractions in the presence of positive margin or ECE. Field reduction is made after 50 to 54 Gy. For elective neck irradiation, a dose of 50 Gy in 25 fractions is prescribed.

Intensity-Modulated Radiation Therapy

In the modern era, IMRT is often the technique of choice to treat submandibular cancers, when available. For IMRT, the patient is immobilized in a supine position with extended thermoplastic head and shoulder mask. A thin-slice CT scan is obtained in the treatment position for outlining the target volumes **(Case Study 14.11 and Case Study 14.12)**. IMPT is an alternative for patients and, with lateralization of dose, may result in less toxicity **(Case Study 14.13)**.

CASE STUDY 14.11

A 46-year-old woman presented with fullness under her left jaw; an evaluation noted a left submandibular mass. A CT revealed a 4-cm left submandibular mass (Fig. 14.11A, *white arrow*). She underwent resection of the mass at an outside hospital, which revealed adenoid cystic carcinoma, cribriform and tubular type, with perineural invasion of large nerves and positive margins. She was treated with postoperative radiation therapy to the tumor bed and ipsilateral perineural tracts of the lingual and hypoglossal nerves. She was treated unilaterally, with a tongue-elevating stent, to separate the tongue from the tumor bed (Fig. 14.11B). Figure 14.11C and D

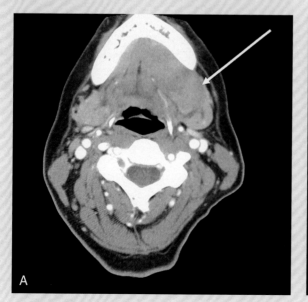
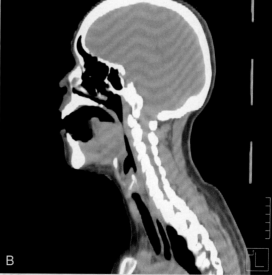

Case Figure 14.11 A,B

shows isodose distributions depicting the comprehensive IMRT plan. Figure 14.11E and F demonstrates coverage of the lingual (V3) nerve along the inner aspect of the mandible (*dashed arrow*) to foramen ovale (*solid arrow*). Two years following treatment, she has no evidence of disease.

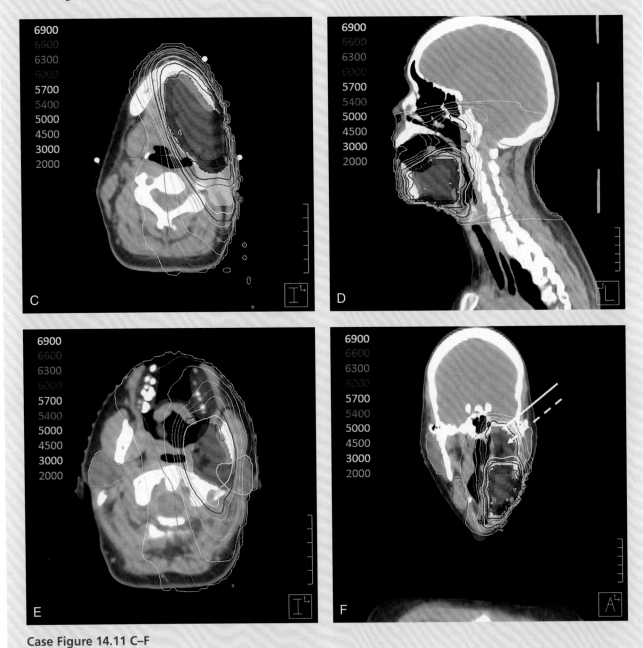

Case Figure 14.11 C–F

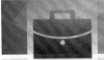

CASE STUDY 14.12

A 78-year-old man presented with an enlarging right submandibular mass. He noted that a lesion had been present in that location for almost 20 years; over the last 2 years, he noted growth. The lesion was excised for diagnosis at a local hospital; pathology revealed high-grade salivary duct carcinoma with soft tissue extension and positive margins. A postoperative PET–CT demonstrated post-treatment changes in the right submandibular area and multiple ipsilateral lymph nodes (Fig. 14.12A); the solid arrows indicate the postoperative changes, and the dashed arrow indicates an FDG-avid lymph node. He underwent oncologic resection of the submandibular tumor bed and a right selective neck dissection, which demonstrated no residual tumor at the primary site and two lymph nodes positive for salivary duct carcinoma with extracapsular extension. He was dispositioned to adjuvant radiation to the right submandibular region and right neck. Given the soft tissue extension in the primary tumor and extracapsular extension in the lymph nodes, the dose to CTV_{HD} was increased to 63 Gy (*red* color wash), covering the submandibular bed and area of positive neck lymph nodes. CTV_{ID} (57 Gy, *blue* color wash) encompassed an additional margin on CTV_{HD} and the remainder of the operative bed within the upper neck. The upper neck IMRT field was matched to oblique conventional low-neck fields. Figure 14.12B and C shows contours and isodose distributions in an axial and coronal view. The patient remains without disease 2 years later.

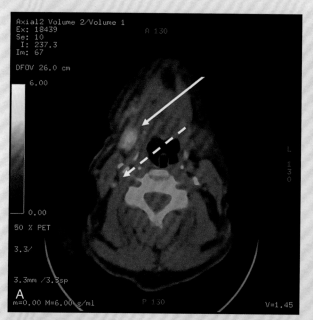

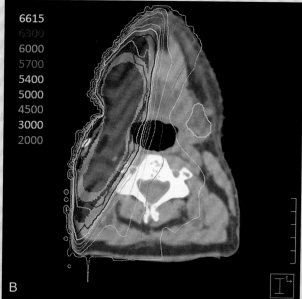

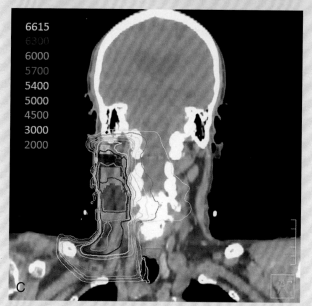

Case Figure 14.12 A–C

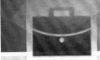

CASE STUDY 14.13

A 72-year-old female presented with a right submandibular mass (Fig. 14.13A). She underwent resection and right selective neck dissection. Pathology revealed a low-grade adenoid cystic carcinoma with a 2-mm margin. All nodes were negative.

She was treated with postoperative IMPT using single-field (SFO) optimization and active scanning.

Figure 14.13B through I shows paired axial images demonstrating the treatment contours and isodose distributions. The patient was prescribed 60 Gy to CTV$_{HD}$ (red), 56 Gy to CTV$_{ID}$ (blue), and 54 Gy to CTV$_{ED}$ (yellow). The latter is shown in Figure 14.13B, as coverage included the perineural pathway to just below foramen ovale. Figure 14.13D,E are at the same level as seen in

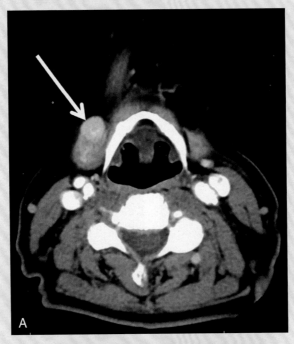

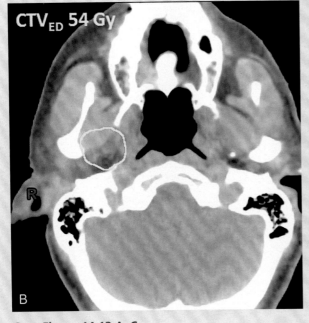

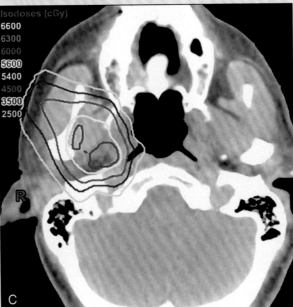

Case Figure 14.13 A–C

Figure 14.13A, the preoperative diagnostic CT scan. Figure 14.13F,G shows coronal views, as Figure 14.13F demonstrates levels II and III inferiorly (operative bed), and the perineural coverage superiorly to the inferior aspect of foramen ovale. Figure 14.13H,I is a more anterior coronal view with CTV$_{HD}$ covering the tumor bed, CTV$_{ID}$ covering the more inferior operative bed, and CTV$_{ED}$ covering the perineural path of the lingual nerve. She tolerated her treatment well, with minimal mucositis as seen in Figure 14.13J, an intraoral photograph taken at the end of treatment. She remains well and without disease 1 year posttreatment.

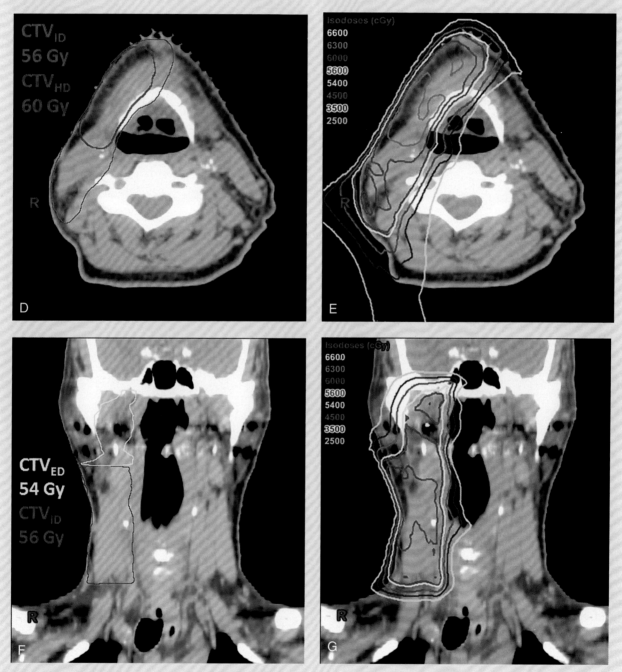

Case Figure 14.13 D–G

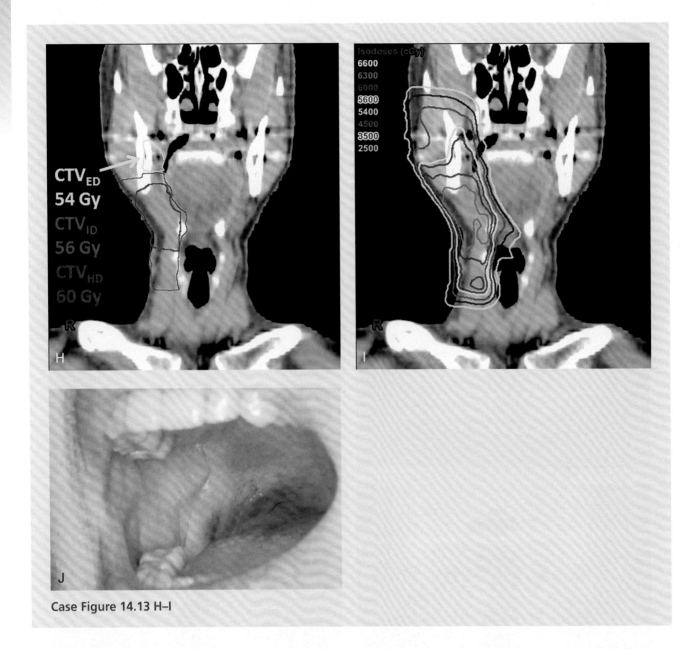

Case Figure 14.13 H–I

Virtual Gross Target Volume

There is no actual GTV after complete surgical tumor resection. However, it can be useful to formulate a virtual GTV (vGTV) to facilitate target volume definition. The vGTV is a best approximation of the tissues having high likelihood of harboring microscopic tumor reconstructed based on findings of preoperative clinical examination, imaging studies, and surgical–pathologic assessment.

Clinical Target Volumes

Three clinical target volumes (CTVs) are generally delineated.

- CTV_{HD} delineates volumes to receive the highest dose. This includes the primary and nodal vGTVs with 8- to 10-mm margins.

- CTV_{ID} delineates volumes to receive an intermediate dose, which typically encompasses the remaining operative bed not included in CTV_{HD}.

- CTV_{ED} delineates volumes to receive an elective dose for subclinical disease. Perineural spread from submandibular gland tumors affects branches of V3 (particularly the lingual nerve) and the hypoglossal nerve. The mandibular nerve exits foramen ovale. The lingual nerve branches off medial to the lateral pterygoid muscle and lies anterior to the inferior alveolar nerve (also a branch of V3). While the inferior alveolar nerve enters its canal in the mandible, the lingual nerve continues between the pterygoid muscle and the ramus of the mandible, crosses the submandibular duct (the usual origin point of perineural spread) before branching off in the tongue. In patients with high-grade cancers without clinical evidence of nodal involvement, CTV_{ED} covers ipsilateral nodal levels II to IV. In patients with nodal involvement, CTV_{ED} encompasses ipsilateral nodal levels not included in higher-dose CTVs.

The isocenter is placed in the center of the treatment volume when the submandibular bed alone is treated. If the entire neck is to be treated, a half-beam matching technique might be preferable. The isocenter is placed above the level of the arytenoids. Ipsilateral levels III and IV are included in a matching anterior (or parallel anterior and posterior) photon portal. Alternatively, the entirety of the targets can be covered with a single VMAT plan.

With IMRT, doses prescribed to CTV_{HD}, CTV_{ID}, and CTV_{ED} are 60, 57, and 54 Gy, respectively, and treatment

is given in 30 fractions. A high-risk volume (e.g., positive margin) can receive a total dose of 66 Gy in 30–33 fractions (2.0–2.2 Gy per fraction). If using more than 30 fractions, the lower dose CTVs should have their dose increased 1-2 Gy accordingly.

Background Data

See Table 14.6.

MINOR SALIVARY GLAND TUMORS

Treatment Strategy

Surgery is the preferred treatment for operable patients if the cosmetic and functional repercussions are not too severe. Indications for postoperative radiotherapy are listed in the "Parotid" section. For tumors of the minor salivary glands that are not resectable, or for which resection would be highly morbid, concurrent chemoradiation may be used, extrapolating from other head and neck sites and histologies; however, data for this are limited and outcomes are likely nonoptimal.

Postoperative Radiotherapy

Target Volume

Initial Target Volume

- Low-grade tumors without lymph node involvement: surgical bed.
- High-grade tumors or lymph node involvement: surgical bed and neck nodes. The extent of elective neck treatment varies with histology and the anatomical site of the primary lesion.
- Adenoid cystic carcinoma or presence of perineural invasion: more generous coverage of the perineural tracks **(Case Study 14.14 through Case Study 14.17)**.

The boost volume encompasses the tumor bed and involved nodal bed.

Setup and Field Arrangement

Varies with the site of the primary lesion (see respective sites). Knowledge of the nerves at risk and their specific proximal pathways to the respective foramina in the base of skull is essential for planning IMRT.

Dose

See "Parotid" section

Background Data

See Tables 14.7 and 14.8.

TABLE 14.6 Submandibular Gland Neoplasms: 5-Year Local–Regional Control Rates (Stratified by Risk Variables) of Surgery and Postoperative Irradiation

Variable	No. of Patients	Control (%)
Adenocarcinoma	10	41
Adenoid cystic carcinoma	50	98
High grade	23	69
Positive resection margin	19	79
Perineural invasion	54	94
Named nerve involvement	17	88
Positive nodes	21	78
Extraglandular extension	58	85
All patients	83	88

Data from the M.D. Anderson Cancer Center.
Modified from Storey MR, Garden AS, Morrison WH, et al. Postoperative radiotherapy for malignant tumors of the submandibular gland. *Int J Radiat Oncol Biol Phys* 2001;51:952.

CASE STUDY 14.14

A 59-year-old man presented with obstructive right ear symptoms. A mass was found in the posterior wall of the right nasopharynx. A transoral piecemeal excision was performed and histologic examination revealed adenoid cystic carcinoma with perineural invasion and positive margins. Examination was suspicious for a residual mass, so a wide reexcision using a transpalatal approach was performed. The pathologic studies on the reexcision were negative, but because of the original findings and tumor location, postoperative radiation was recommended. Radiation was delivered through a pair of parallel–opposed beams (Fig. 14.14). The initial fields encompassed the primary tumor and operative bed. The generous margin superiorly allowed for coverage of the perineural pathways. The fields were reduced off the spinal cord at 42 Gy and reduced further at 50 Gy to boost the tumor bed to 60 Gy. The patient remains free of disease 10 years from his therapy.

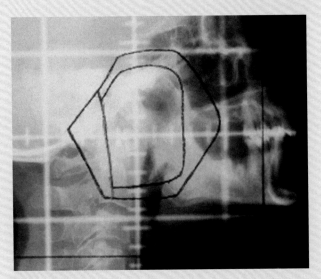

Case Figure 14.14

CASE STUDY 14.15

A 51-year-old man presented with an asymptomatic hard palate mass. Tumor biopsy revealed adenoid cystic carcinoma, cribriform and tubular type. He underwent resection, which included an infrastructure maxillectomy and drill-out of the maxillary nerve. Tumor was present at the proximal section margin of the nerve, where clips were placed. He received postoperative IMRT. The region of positive margin and V2 through foramen rotundum received 66 Gy and a more generous margin including the operative bed received 60 Gy in 30 fractions. Figure 14.15 shows isodose distributions through the clipped margin (*pink arrow*) on axial (Fig. 14.15A) and coronal (Fig. 14.15B) views.

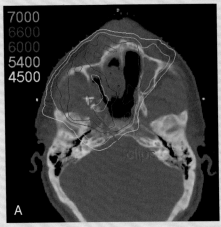
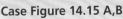
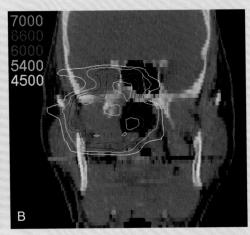

Case Figure 14.15 A,B

CASE STUDY 14.16

A 38-year-old man presented with epistaxis. Fiberoptic nasopharyngoscopy noted a large left sinonasal mass. He was taken for endoscopic sinus surgery, with a planning CT scan for the procedure (Fig. 14.16A). Pathology showed adenoid cystic carcinoma, cribriform type. An MRI revealed residual disease postbiopsy with suspected involvement of the left medial pterygopalatine fossa, foramen rotundum, and superior orbital fissure (Fig. 14.16B). He was taken to surgery. Pathology revealed a 3.5-cm adenoid cystic carcinoma, cribriform type, with bone invasion. There was a separate focus of carcinoma in the pterygopalatine fissure. He was dispositioned to postoperative IMRT which was delivered in 30 fractions. Figure 14.16C–E shows representative contours and isodose distributions. Given the focus of disease in soft tissue, a small volume was taken to 66 Gy (*red* color wash). The resected tumor bed was treated to CTV$_{HD}$ (*blue* color wash) and taken to a dose of 60 Gy. The CTV$_{ED}$ (*yellow* color wash) was prescribed 57 Gy. CTV$_{ED}$ was delineated to cover the cavernous sinus, given concern for potential perineural spread to the skull base. The maximal dose to the optic nerves and chiasm was kept below 54 Gy. The lymph nodes were not treated due to the histology (adenoid cystic). Four years after treatment, the patient has no evidence of recurrent disease.

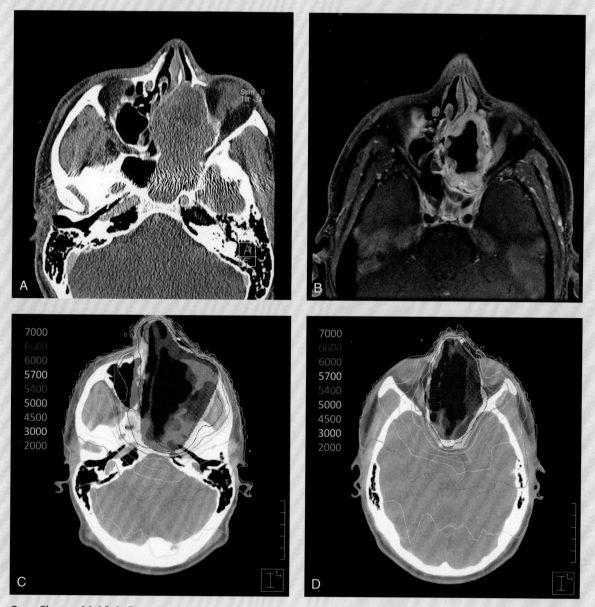

Case Figure 14.16 A–D

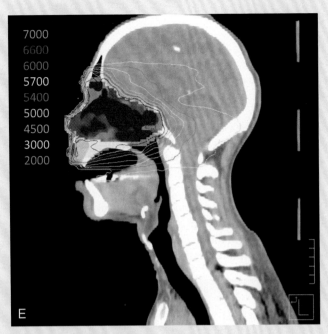

Case Figure 14.16 E

CASE STUDY 14.17

A 77-year-old man presented with a painless mass at the midline of his mucosa of his upper lip, near the frenulum. A biopsy revealed adenoid cystic carcinoma (ACC), cribriform and tubular type, with focal perineural inva- sion. A CT scan failed to note the primary tumor; how- ever, there was a suspicious right level IB lymph node (Fig. 14.17A—*arrow*). FNA was also positive for ACC. He was taken for oncologic resection of the lip lesion with

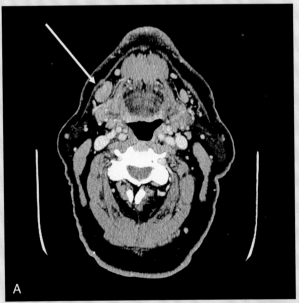

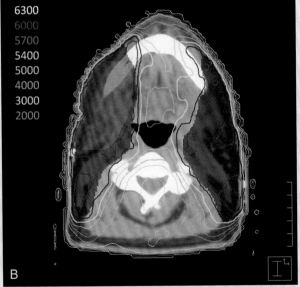

Case Figure 14.17 A,B

bilateral neck dissections, due to the midline nature of the primary. Pathology revealed adenoid cystic carcinoma in the primary specimen with negative margins. There was metastatic disease in two of seven right IB lymph nodes. The remainder of the bilateral neck dissections was negative for disease. He was dispositioned to postoperative radiation with IMRT matched to an appositional low-neck field. Since the lymph nodes were pathologically positive in level IB, the entire bilateral necks were treated. Dose volumes were as follows, as shown in Figure 14.17B through D: CTV$_{HD}$ (60 Gy, *red* color wash) covered the

vGTV (the site of resected disease in the lip and right level 1B) with 8- to 10-mm margins, CTV$_{ID}$ (57 Gy, *blue* color wash) encompassed the remaining operative bed, and CTV$_{ED}$ (54 Gy, *yellow* color wash) delineated the perineural tracts of V2 bilaterally. Isodose distributions are also shown. In Figure 14.17B, the coverage of the right IB and bilateral upper necks is shown. In Figure 14.17C, the coverage of the lip, bilateral facial nodes, and bilateral V2 distribution is shown. In Figure 14.17D, the coverage of the bilateral low necks with a matched appositional field is shown.

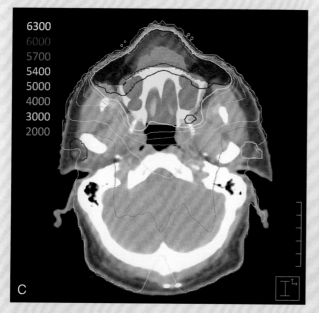

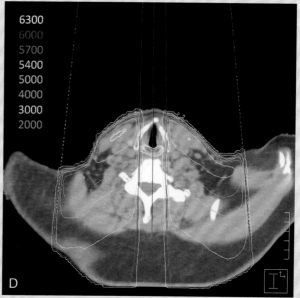

Case Figure 14.17 C,D

TABLE 14.7 Cervical Node Metastases in 434 Patients with Malignant Tumors of Minor Salivary Gland Origin

Distribution by	No. of Patients	Metastases Previously Excised	Present on Admission	Appeared Later	Total with Metastases
By histologic findings					
Adenoid cystic	174	1	13	10	24 (14%)
Mucoepidermoid	76	—	12	11	23 (30%)
Solid duct					
Adenocarcinoma	106	—	19	11	30 (28%)
Variants of duct					
Adenocarcinoma	37	1	4	4	9 (24%)

(Continued)

TABLE 14.7 Cervical Node Metastases in 434 Patients with Malignant Tumors of Minor Salivary Gland Origin *(Continued)*

Distribution by	No. of Patients	Metastases Previously Excised	Present on Admission	Appeared Later	Total with Metastases
Malignant mixed	13	1	3	1	5 (38%)
Acinic cell	2	—	—	—	—
Oat cell	14	—	5	2	7 (50%)
Colonic type	12	—	1	—	1 (8%)
Anatomic site					
Palate	140	—	10	12	22 (16%)
Sinuses or nasal	127	1	9	9	19 (15%)
Tongue	52	1	15	6	22 (42%)
Cheek or lips	40	—	4	2	6 (15%)
Gingivae	29	—	2	4	6 (21%)
Floor of the mouth	17	—	5	2	7 (41%)
Larynx	15	1	5	4	10 (67%)
Tonsil	11	—	7	—	7 (65%)
Pharynx	3	—	—	—	—
Total	434	3	57	39	99 (23%)

Modified from Spiro RH, Koss LG, Hajdu SI, et al. Tumors of minor salivary origin. A clinicopathologic study of 492 cases. *Cancer* 1973;31:117.

TABLE 14.8 Local Control of Minor Salivary Gland Carcinomas Treated with Postoperative Radiation

First Author, Year	Patient Number	Adenoid Cystic Carcinoma	10-yr Local Control Rate
Garden, 1994	160	71%	86%
Le, 1999	54	59%	88%
Cianchetti, 2009	76	58%	86%

DEFINITIVE RADIOTHERAPY

Target Volume

For patients with unresectable tumors of the salivary glands, the target is typically the GTV with 8- to 10-mm margins, encompassing CTV_{HD}. CTV_{ID} typically is an expansion around the high-dose area of approximately 1 cm. CTV_{ED} typically encompasses any at-risk nodal regions and perineural tracts.

Setup and Field Arrangement

Varies with the site of the primary lesion (see respective sites). Knowledge of the nerves at risk and their specific proximal pathways to the respective foramina in the base of skull is essential for planning IMRT/IMPT.

Dose

For patients with unresectable tumors, the doses are typically extrapolated from squamous histologies. Hence, CTV_{HD} is taken to 70 Gy, CTV_{ID} to 63 Gy, and CTV_{ED} to 57 Gy in 33 to 35 fractions. However, unresectabliity is often due to proximity to the brain, eyes or optic pathways, and the doses need to be balanced with the normal tissue tolerances (see Chapter 6). Chemotherapy is often used concurrently to escalate treatment in these cases **(Case Study 14.18)**; however, the data supporting the use of concurrent chemotherapy are sparse.

CASE STUDY 14.18

A 33-year-old female noticed anisocoria with associated headache and nasal congestion, which prompted evaluation with an otolaryngologist. A nasopharyngeal mass was evident with clival destruction and sphenoid sinus involvement. Biopsy revealed adenoid cystic carcinoma. Sagittal view of T1-weighted MRI is shown in Figure 14.18A (*white arrow* shows sphenoid sinus involvement), and the axial T2-weighted image in Figure 14.18B shows tumor filling the nasopharynx. There were no regional or distant metastases, and the tumor was judged to be unresectable.

She was treated with definitive concurrent chemoradiation using active-scanning proton therapy, IMPT-MFO technique. A mouth-opening tongue-depressing oral stent and bite block were used for simulation and treatment. Following CT simulation, she underwent volumetric MRI in the treatment position, which was fused with the treatment planning CT in order to accurately delineate targets and avoidance structures at the base of skull. She was treated to 70 Gy(RBE) in 33 fractions to the GTV with narrow margin. Aspects of the GTV adjacent to the brainstem, temporal lobes, and optic structures were targeted to 66 Gy(RBE) but were optimized to respect critical structure tolerance. Surrounding soft tissue regions at risk were treated to 56 Gy(RBE). She initially received weekly cisplatin (40 mg/m²) but was transitioned to carboplatin toward the end of treatment due to ototoxicity.

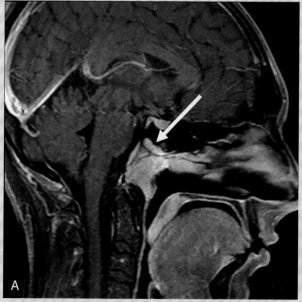

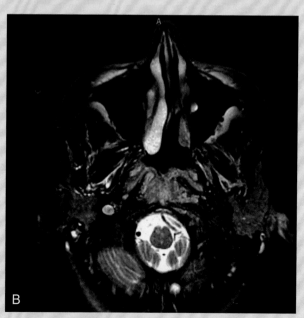

Case Figure 14.18 A–B

Two anterior oblique and a single vertex field were used. Paired images of the contoured CTVs and the respective IMPT dose distributions are displayed in all three planes in Figure 14.18C–L and highlight the sparing of brain and oral cavity and ability of IMPT to generate the concave conformal dose distributions around the brainstem. Figure 14.18G,H shows coverage of tumor extension into left occipital condyle (*green arrow*).

Figure 14.18M shows the pretherapy PET–CT with avid tumor of the nasopharynx with clival destruction. Figure 14.18N shows the posttherapy PET–CT (obtained 3 months after treatment completion) with resolution of all FDG-avid tumor. Figure 14.18O shows a medical photograph taken during the final week of IMPT with only grade 1 (erythematous) mucositis evident.

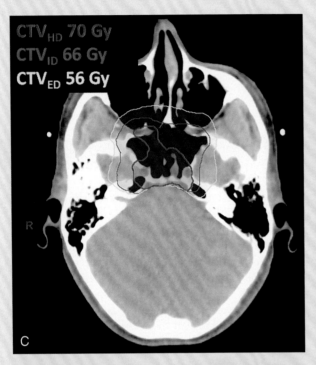

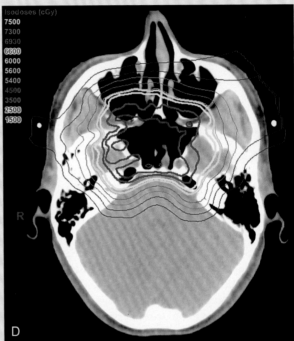

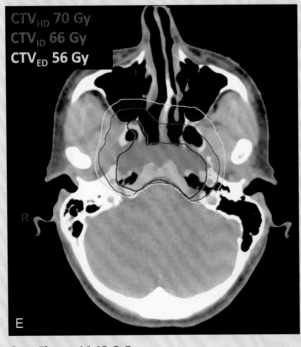

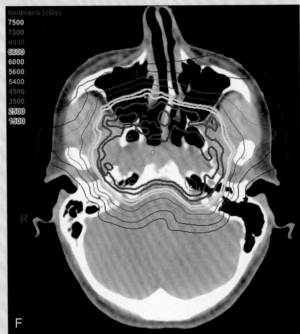

Case Figure 14.18 C–F

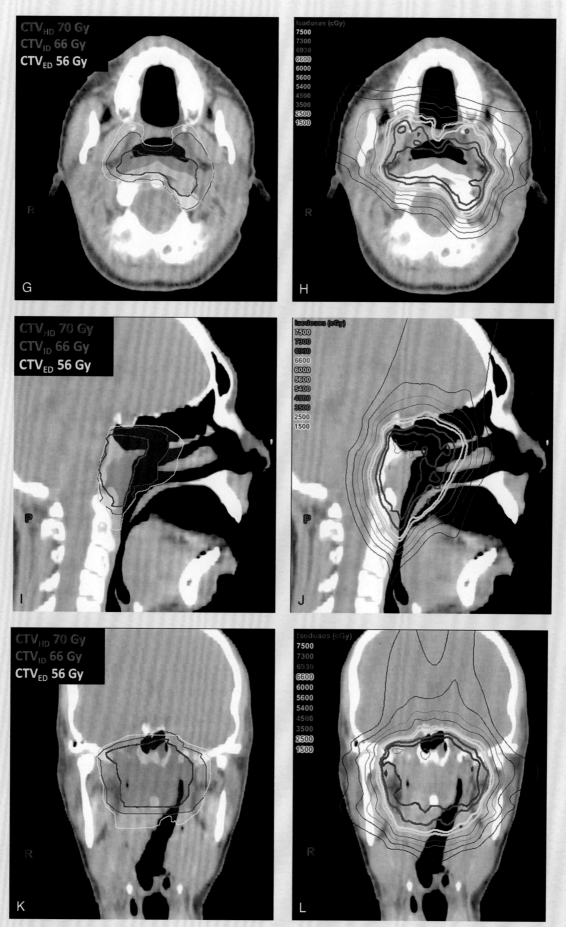

Case Figure 14.18 G–L

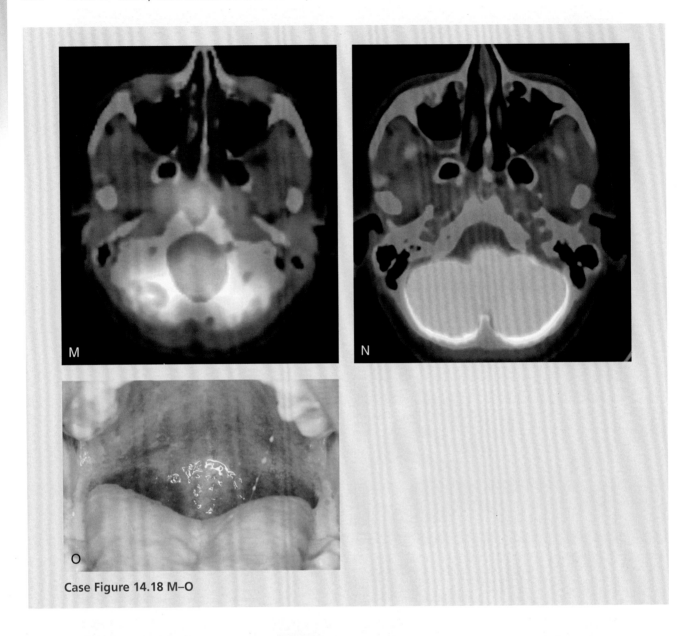

Case Figure 14.18 M–O

SUGGESTED READINGS

Armstrong JG, Harrison LB, Thaler HT, et al. The indications for elective treatment of the neck in cancer of the major salivary glands. *Cancer* 1992;69:615.

Barton J, Slevin NJ, Gleave EN. Radiotherapy for pleomorphic adenoma of the parotid gland. *Int J Radiat Oncol Biol Phys* 1992;22:925.

Bissett RJ, Fitzpatrick PJ. Malignant submandibular gland tumors. A review of 91 patients. *Am J Clin Oncol* 1988; 11:46.

Chen AM, Granchi PJ, Garcia J, et al. Local-regional recurrence after surgery without postoperative irradiation for carcinomas of the major salivary glands: implications for adjuvant therapy. *Int J Radiat Oncol Biol Phys* 2007; 67:982.

Cianchetti M, Sandow PS, Scarborough LD, et al. Radiation therapy for minor salivary gland carcinoma. *Laryngoscope* 2009;119:1334.

Douglas JG, Koh WJ, Austin-Seymour M, et al. Treatment of salivary gland neoplasms with fast neutron radiotherapy. *Arch Otolaryngol Head Neck Surg* 2003;129:944.

Douglas JG, Laramore GE, Austin-Seymour M, et al. Treatment of locally advanced adenoid cystic carcinoma of the head and neck with neutron radiotherapy. *Int J Radiat Oncol Biol Phys* 2000;46:551.

Fordice J, Kershaw C, El-Naggar A, et al. Adenoid cystic carcinoma of the head and neck: predictors of morbidity and mortality. *Arch Otolaryngol Head Neck Surg* 1999; 125:149.

Frankenthaler RA, Luna MA, Lee SS, et al. Prognostic variables in parotid gland cancer. *Arch Otolaryngol Head Neck Surg* 1991;117:1251.

Fu KK, Leibel SA, Levine ML, et al. Carcinoma of the major and minor salivary glands: analysis of treatment results and sites and causes of failures. *Cancer* 1977;40:2882.

Garden AS, El-Naggar AK, Morrison WH, et al. Postoperative radiotherapy for malignant tumors of the parotid gland. *Int J Radiat Oncol Biol Phys* 1997;37:79.

Garden AS, Weber RS, Ang KK, et al. Postoperative radiation therapy for malignant tumors of minor salivary glands. Outcome and patterns of failure. *Cancer* 1994;73:2563.

Garden AS, Weber RS, Morrison WH, et al. The influence of positive margins and nerve invasion in adenoid cystic carcinoma of the head and neck treated with surgery and radiation. *Int J Radiat Oncol Biol Phys* 1995;32:619.

Goepfert H, Luna MA, Lindberg RD, et al. Malignant salivary gland tumors of the paranasal sinuses and nasal cavity. *Arch Otolaryngol* 1983;109:662.

Guillamondegui OM, Byers RM, Luna MA, et al. Aggressive surgery in treatment for parotid cancer: the role of adjunctive postoperative radiotherapy. *AJR Am J Roentgenol* 1975;123:49.

Huber PE, Debus J, Latz D, et al. Radiotherapy for advanced adenoid cystic carcinoma: neutrons, photons or mixed beam? *Radiother Oncol* 2001;59:161.

Laramore GE, Krall JM, Griffin TW, et al. Neutron versus photon irradiation for unresectable salivary gland tumors: final report of an RTOG-MRC randomized clinical trial. *Int J Radiat Oncol Biol Phys* 1993;27:235.

Le QT, Birdwell S, Terris DJ, et al. Postoperative irradiation of minor salivary gland malignancies of the head and neck. *Radiother Oncol* 1999;52:165.

Liu F-F, Rotstein L, Davison AJ, et al. Benign parotid adenomas: a review of the Princess Margaret Hospital experience. *Head Neck* 1995;17:177.

Loh KS, Barker E, Bruch G, et al. Prognostic factors in malignancy of the minor salivary glands. *Head Neck* 2009;31:58.

Luna MA. Pathology of tumors of the salivary glands. In: Thawley SE, Panje WR, Batsakis JG et al., eds. *Comprehensive management of head and neck tumors*, 2nd ed. Philadelphia, PA: WB Saunders, 1999.

Lupinetti AD, Roberts DB, Williams MD, et al. Sinonasal adenoid cystic carcinoma: the M.D. Anderson Cancer Center experience. *Cancer* 2007;110:2726.

Mendenhall WM, Morris CG, Amdur RJ, et al. Radiotherapy alone or combined with surgery for salivary gland carcinoma. *Cancer* 2005;103:2544.

Mifsud MJ, Tanvetyanon T, Mccaffrey JC, et al. Adjuvant radiotherapy versus concurrent chemoradiotherapy for the management of high-risk salivary gland carcinomas. *Head Neck* 2016;38:1628–1633.

Orlandi E, Iacovelli NA, Bonora M, et al. Salivary gland. Photon beam and particle radiotherapy: present and future. *Oral Oncol* 2016;60:146–156.

Schoenfeld JD, Sher DJ, Norris CM, et al. Salivary gland tumors treated with adjuvant intensity-modulated radiotherapy with or without concurrent chemotherapy. *Int J Radiat Oncol Biol Phys* 2012;82:308.

Spiro RH. Salivary neoplasms: overview of a 35-year experience with 2,807 patients. *Head Neck Surg* 1986;8:177.

Spiro RH, Koss LG, Hajdu SI, et al. Tumors of minor salivary origin. A clinicopathologic study of 492 cases. *Cancer* 1973;31:117.

Storey MR, Garden AS, Morrison WH, et al. Postoperative radiotherapy for malignant tumors of the submandibular gland. *Int J Radiat Oncol Biol Phys* 2001;51:952.

Tanvetyanon T, Fisher K, Caudell J, et al. Adjuvant chemoradiotherapy versus radiotherapy alone for locally advanced salivary gland carcinoma among older patients. *Head Neck* 2016;38:863.

Terhaard CH, Lubsen H, Rasch CR, et al. The role of radiotherapy in the treatment of malignant salivary gland tumors. *Int J Radiat Oncol Biol Phys* 2005;61:103.

Waldron CA, El-Mofty SK, Gnepp DR. Tumors of the intraoral minor salivary glands: a demographic and histologic study of 426 cases. *Oral Surg Oral Med Oral Pathol* 1988; 66:323.

Wang CC, Goodman M. Photon irradiation of unresectable carcinomas of salivary glands. *Int J Radiat Oncol Biol Phys* 1991;21:569.

Weber RS, Byers RM, Petit B, et al. Submandibular gland tumors. Adverse histologic factors and therapeutic implications. *Arch Otolaryngol Head Neck Surg* 1990;116:1055.

Weber RS, Palmer JM, El-Naggar AE, et al. Minor salivary gland tumors of the lip and buccal mucosa. *Laryngoscope* 1989;99:6.

15

Thyroid

Key Points

- Thyroid carcinomas are classified into four histologic types. Papillary and follicular carcinomas are often grouped together as differentiated thyroid cancers. Medullary and particularly anaplastic carcinomas have more aggressive clinical behavior but, fortunately, are much less common.

- Surgery is the primary therapy for thyroid carcinomas.

- The objectives of radioactive iodine (RAI) after surgery for differentiated thyroid carcinomas (which take up iodine) are as follows: first, to ablate residual thyroid tissue to allow more effective detection of the presence of metastatic deposits that take up iodine, and, second, to ablate "functional" metastatic disease using higher doses (e.g., 100 to 150 mCi) of RAI.

- Adjuvant external beam radiation has a limited role in the treatment of differentiated carcinomas. At our center, we consider its use in patients judged to be at high risk for subsequent nonsalvageable (or overly morbid) local–regional recurrence, which is largely surgeon determined. This generally represents older patients, pT4 tumors (visceral invasion or adherence), extensive soft tissue infiltration, multiply recurrent disease, and/or aggressive histologic variants. Other than for purely palliative situations, we rarely irradiate gross disease in the neck.

- Because of a higher risk for local–regional recurrence, adjuvant external beam radiation is also considered in the treatment of medullary thyroid carcinoma with the same relative indications as differentiated thyroid cancers. As for differentiated thyroid carcinomas, due to lack of any randomized clinical trials, it is difficult to estimate the magnitude of effect of adjuvant radiotherapy in improving the local–regional tumor control and the impact of radiation on overall survival for patients with medullary carcinoma.

- Anaplastic carcinoma is one of the most aggressive human cancers. The median survival of patients presenting with this cancer is measured in months, and even for those with localized disease, long-term survival rates are <20%. Treatment is often multimodal, but RAI generally has no role. Surgery and adjuvant chemoradiation are recommended for those few cases where the disease is localized and resectable. When surgery is not feasible, urgent initiation of radiation, often with concurrent chemotherapy, is recommended for inducing local tumor regression as these patients can rapidly develop airway obstruction, severe dysphagia, and death due to overwhelming local tumor burden (often despite tracheostomy). Given lack of effective therapies for anaplastic carcinomas, priority should be given to treatment on clinical study. These often involve the use of targeted agents that are either approved or being tested for efficacy in these diseases.

- The horseshoe-shaped geometry of the target volumes, which often include the entirety of the central compartment, laryngeal inlet, bilateral tracheo-esophageal grooves, bilateral superior paratracheal nodal basins, and at-risk lateral neck nodes, coupled with significant changes in depth, width, and curvature from the neck to the mediastinum and proximity of the spinal cord makes treatment planning and delivery of traditional postoperative radiation doses with conventional radiation technique very complex. Therefore, intensity-modulated radiation therapy is the preferred technique.

TREATMENT STRATEGY

The primary treatment for thyroid cancers is surgery, and for differentiated cancers, followed by thyroid-stimulating hormone suppression. RAI is a generally accepted adjuvant therapy to surgery for most functioning papillary or follicular carcinomas.

The relative indications for postoperative external beam radiotherapy are influenced by tumor histology and disease extent.

For patients with differentiated (follicular/papillary) cancers, postoperative external beam radiotherapy is considered for those judged to be at high risk for subsequent nonsalvageable (or overly morbid) local–regional recurrence. Most frequently, this involves disease located in the central compartment and disease that involves the esophagus, trachea, and/or larynx (pT4), or there is extensive soft tissue infiltration (muscle and/or nerve), multiply recurrent disease, and/or aggressive histologic variants (e.g., poorly differentiated or tall cell). Other relative indications include positive microscopic surgical margin, extensive nodal extracapsular extension, and extensive mediastinal nodal involvement. The sequence of external beam radiation therapy and RAI (when

indicated) is individualized. This decision is often made based on the patient being staged with an iodinated contrast CT of the neck, forcing a delay in RAI staging and therapy. Treatment of gross differentiated thyroid cancer is limited to palliative situations.

Medullary carcinoma has the same relative indications as that of differentiated cancer plus persistent elevation of calcitonin levels after surgery, without demonstrable distant metastatic disease. With high competing risk of distant failure and emergence of FDA-approved targeted therapy for medullary carcinoma, the use of postoperative radiation at our center has declined in recent years.

For anaplastic carcinoma, rapid evaluation for surgery for those with localized disease is critical. Almost all patients receive radiation, if possible, after maximal surgical debulking. Given the potential for rapid recurrence, postoperative radiation therapy should be initiated as soon as possible. Patients with locally advanced anaplastic carcinoma should be prioritized for enrollment into ongoing protocols testing the combination of chemotherapy and, more recently, targeted agents (varies with protocol) with local–regional treatment. The presence of distant metastases should not necessarily preclude the use of upfront palliative local–regional therapy to treat or prevent impending symptoms of tracheal or esophageal compromise, and medically fit patients with smaller volume distant disease may still benefit from more aggressive upfront local–regional therapy. Iodine 131 imaging and RAI generally have no role.

POSTOPERATIVE RADIOTHERAPY

Target Volume

The initial target volume encompasses the surgical bed, bilateral upper paratracheal and lateral neck nodes at risk, upper mediastinum, and mid-mediastinum when the upper mediastinum is involved **(Case Study 15.1)**. Unless the tumor volume is well lateralized, both left and right tracheoesophageal grooves are included in the subclinical target volume. The high-dose volume encompasses the area of known disease locations with 1- to 2-cm margins.

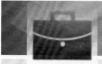

CASE STUDY 15.1

A 64-year-old woman was found to have a thyroid nodule on routine physical examination. She had no family history of thyroid cancer and had never received radiotherapy. CT scan showed a mass in the right lobe of the thyroid gland. There was no evidence of associated lymphadenopathy or disease in the mediastinum. Fine-needle

aspiration showed medullary thyroid carcinoma. Serum calcitonin levels were elevated. Carcinoembryonic antigen level was normal. Metastatic workup results were negative. The patient underwent a thyroidectomy and right neck dissection. Histologic examination showed a 2-cm medullary carcinoma of the right lobe. Eight right paratracheal nodes and four jugular nodes were positive, the largest measuring 1.2 cm. Postoperatively, serum calcitonin levels remained elevated. Because of extensive nodal involvement and persistent elevated serum calcitonin level, it was decided to deliver postoperative radiotherapy.

Figure 15.1 shows opposed AP–PA portals, with a compensating filter for the anterior field, used to treat the initial target volume (Fig. 15.1A,B). The wire indicates the surgical scar. A dose of 44 Gy was delivered in 22 fractions following which the left anterior oblique and right posterior oblique fields (Fig. 15.1C,D) were used to boost the tumor bed and right neck. After reaching a tumor dose of 50 Gy, the length of the oblique fields was reduced to encompass the areas of known tumor involvement for an additional 10 Gy. Therefore, the primary tumor bed and involved nodal areas received a total dose of 60 Gy, the right neck received a dose of 50 Gy, and the contralateral neck and mediastinum received a dose of 44 Gy, all delivered in 2 Gy per fraction. This patient was alive without evidence of disease and without complications 6 years after completion of therapy.

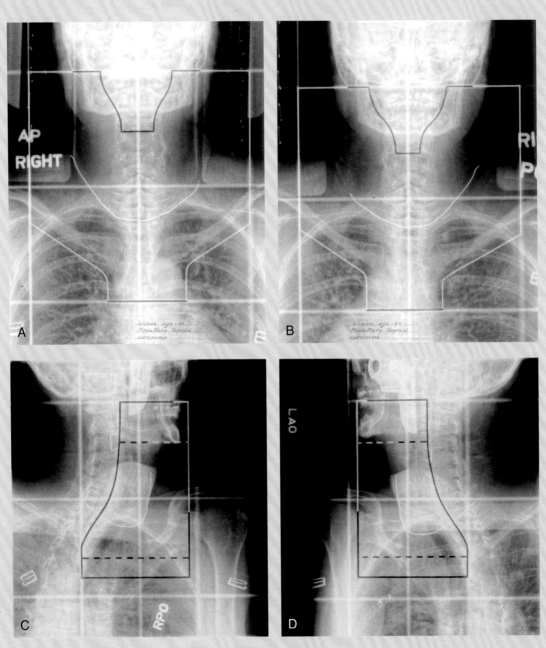

Case Figure 15.1 A–D

Setup and Field Arrangement for Conventional Technique

Marking of the surgical scar facilitates portal design. A 2-3-mm bolus is placed over the thyroidectomy scar. The patient is immobilized with a thermoplastic mask in a supine position, with the head hyperextended to minimize inclusion of the oral cavity in the portals. If the patient is unable to hyperextend the neck, a cephalad gantry tilt can be used to achieve the same goal. Opposed anterior and posterior (AP–PA) photon fields are used for the initial target volume:

- *Superior border*: at the level of the hyoid bone. If there is significant nodal disease warranting treatment of the upper neck, the superior extent should be at the level of the mastoid process on the side of the neck requiring this additional coverage. However, in most cases the goal is to control the central compartment, so extending above the hyoid is discouraged except when there is very extensive level 2 disease.
- *Lateral borders*: covering the medial two thirds of the clavicles.
- *Inferior border*: at the carina; (when the upper mediastinum is involved, it is 3 to 4 cm below the mediastinal component).

The use of missing tissue compensating filter or field-in-field technique (see Chapter 3) minimizes dose heterogeneity, and therefore potential overdose to a segment of the spinal cord, because of the large differences in the diameter of the patient at different anatomic levels.

For fields that extend superior to the hyoid, the oral cavity and oropharynx can be shielded to the extent possible without compromising on the coverage of the tumor bed and neck.

CASE STUDY 15.2

A 48-year-old woman underwent a total thyroidectomy for papillary carcinoma followed by postoperative RAI ablation. A year later, she represented with a 2-cm left neck mass. Fine-needle aspiration confirmed recurrence, and she underwent a left neck and central compartment dissection. Histologic examination revealed recurrent thyroid carcinoma in the connective tissues of the neck. A postoperative iodine scan was negative. She received postoperative external beam radiation.

The radiation treatment commenced with parallel-opposed anterior (6-MV photons) and posterior (18-MV photons) fields. The portals covered the neck and upper mediastinum. After a dose of 42 Gy, the fields were reduced off–spinal cord by using parallel-opposed right anterior oblique and left posterior oblique fields. At 50 Gy, a reduction was made off the superior and inferior borders, and the areas felt to be at the highest risk were irradiated to 60 Gy. The right neck was supplemented with 12-MeV electron beam to bring the dose to the mid and lower right neck to 50 Gy.

Figure 15.2 shows representative axial isodose distributions through the mid (Fig. 15.2A) and lower (Fig. 15.2B) neck.

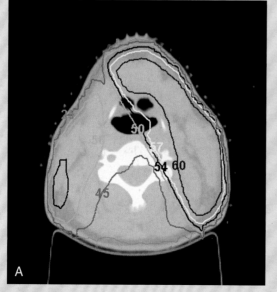
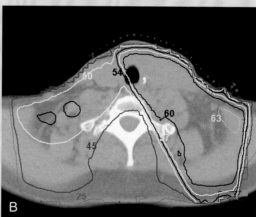

Case Figure 15.2 A,B

The boost dose is usually delivered through opposed anterior oblique and posterior oblique off-cord photon fields encompassing the tumor bed and the side of the neck with nodal involvement. A planning computed tomography (CT) scan is obtained to determine the angle and width of these fields.

If the contralateral neck or thyroid bed is also at high risk, it can receive boost dose through an appositional electron field with a gantry angle corresponding to that of the anterior oblique photon field to avoid overlap **(Case Study 15.2)**.

Intensity-Modulated Radiation Therapy

Intensity-modulated radiation therapy (IMRT) generally offers better coverage of the rather complex anatomy and geometry of the inferior neck.

With IMRT, the patient is immobilized with an extended head and shoulder thermoplastic mask in a supine position. If the targets extend superior to the hyoid bone, extending the head aids in minimizing exposure to the oral cavity. Thin-slice CT scan is obtained for delineation of target volumes **(Case Study 15.3 through Case Study 15.6)**.

CASE STUDY 15.3

A 57-year-old man presented with left neck swelling. A fine-needle aspiration revealed papillary thyroid carcinoma (PTC). He underwent a total thyroidectomy with selective dissection of the left levels II to IV and Vb and a left superior mediastinum nodal dissection. The primary tumor was 3.5 cm in size, multifocal, and extending into the extrathyroidal tissues. All nodal levels dissected were positive, including seven out of seven paratracheal nodes. Because a postoperative iodine scan revealed residual activity in the thyroid bed, he received 150 mCi ^{131}I to ablate the residual thyroid tissue. This was followed by external beam IMRT, recommended because of the extent of the disease.

Figure 15.3 shows CTV$_{HD}$ (60 Gy, *green*) and CTV$_{ED}$ (54 Gy, *blue*) contours and isodose curves on a coronal image (Fig. 15.3A), an axial slice at the level of the cricoid (Fig. 15.3B), and an axial image at the paratracheal level (Fig. 15.3C). Note that the involved nodal basins of the left neck was defined as CTV$_{HD}$, whereas right posterior level III and IV uninvolved nodes were outlined as CTV$_{ED}$. Right level II nodes were not irradiated to spare the right submandibular salivary gland. He had no evidence of disease 2 years posttherapy.

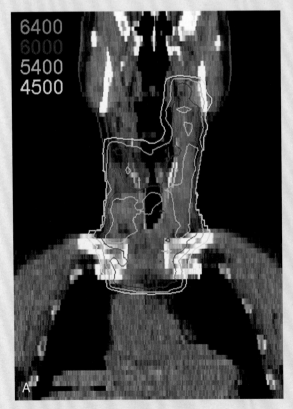

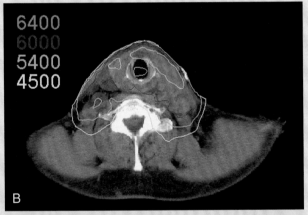

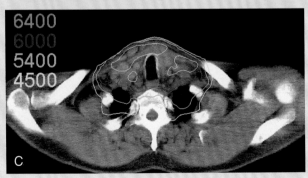

Case Figure 15.3 A–C

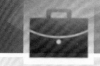

CASE STUDY 15.4

A 56-year-old man presented with cough and was found to have a thyroid mass. He underwent partial thyroidectomy, which revealed a 6.5-cm mass with positive margins and six of six positive nodes. Microscopic residual disease persisted even after a subsequent completion of thyroidectomy. On presentation to the M.D. Anderson Cancer Center, restaging with ultrasonography revealed bilateral adenopathy. He underwent bilateral neck and paratracheal dissections including exploration of level I nodes. Histologic examination revealed multiple positive nodes with extracapsular extension and soft tissue involvement. He received ^{131}I followed by IMRT.

Figure 15.4 shows CTV$_{HD}$ and CTV$_{ED}$ contours and isodose curves on a coronal image (Fig. 15.4A), an axial slice at level II in the neck (Fig. 15.4B), and an axial image at the paratracheal level (Fig. 15.4C). It is noted that because of the extent of the disease in level II and in the operative bed, the plan has generous anterior coverage including level Ib (Fig. 15.4B), and the TE groove, which is covered in CTV$_{HD}$ (Fig. 15.4C). He remains without evidence of disease 2 years since completing radiation.

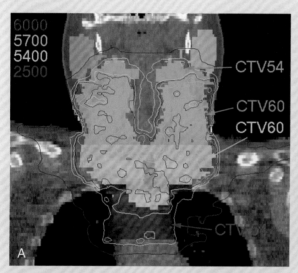

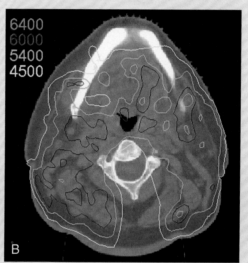

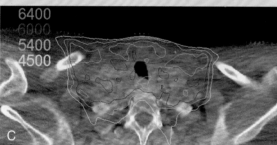

Case Figure 15.4 A–C

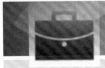

CASE STUDY 15.5

A 61-year-old female presented with a right neck mass. A CT scan of the head and neck demonstrated a mass of the right thyroid gland (Fig. 15.5A, *green arrow*) extending up to the level of the hyoid bone with involvement of the lateral pharyngeal wall (Fig. 15.5B, *green arrows*). A fine-needle aspiration revealed PTC. She underwent a total thyroidectomy with microdissection of the right recurrent laryngeal nerve. Histologic examination revealed a 5-cm mass with extension of PTC into the soft tissues. Two nodes were positive.

As she had extensive T4 tumor, external beam radiation followed by RAI was recommended. Note that Figure 15.5A and 15.5B are images of the CT scan with contrast. Thus, RAI was delayed till after the external therapy to allow for adequate time for clearance of the iodinated contrast material. CTV$_{HD}$ (60 Gy) covered the preoperative tumor volume, right levels II to IV, and paratracheal nodes. While the tumor was predominantly right sided, the left thyroid bed and adjacent nodal bed was also encompassed in CTV$_{HD}$ (Fig. 15.5C, *red*) as the precise location of the positive nodes was unclear. Figure 15.5D shows a matched image with the isodose distribution alone. Though the tumor was anterior, care was taken to encompass the bilateral TE grooves in CTV$_{ED}$ (56 Gy),

which also covered the left level III and IV, and upper mediastinal nodes along with an additional 1-cm margin around right level II nodes. Figure 15.5E shows both CTV$_{HD}$ (*red*) and CTV$_{ED}$ (*blue*) in a coronal view through the larynx. As the tumor was right sided, it was elected not to treat left level II nodes and, thereby, spare the left submandibular gland (*light green*) as well as further spare the parotids. Figure 15.5F shows an axial view at level II region. Note that the 60-Gy isodose line encompasses tumor bed and the 56-Gy isodose line covers the remainder of the right level II region. Also shown is the sparing of the left submandibular gland, which received a mean dose of <10 Gy. Figure 15.5G shows the isodose distribution at the level of the larynx. Because tumor was dissected off the right recurrent laryngeal nerve, the right hemilarynx (with intention to cover the laryngeal inlet where the nerve enters the larynx) is encompassed in CTV$_{HD}$. The remaining neck at this level is covered in CTV$_{ED}$. Figure 15.5H shows an axial view at the upper mediastinum. The nodes at this level were delineated as CTV$_{ED}$ and treated to 56 Gy. The patient retained local–regional control but ultimately developed distant disease.

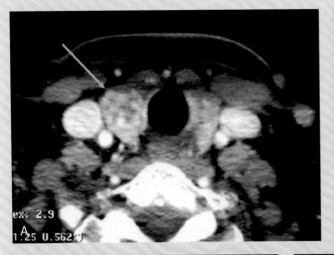

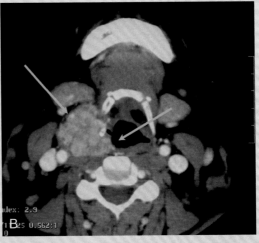

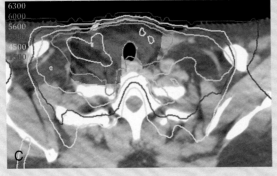

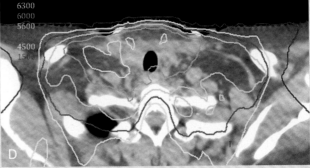

Case Figure 15.5 A–D

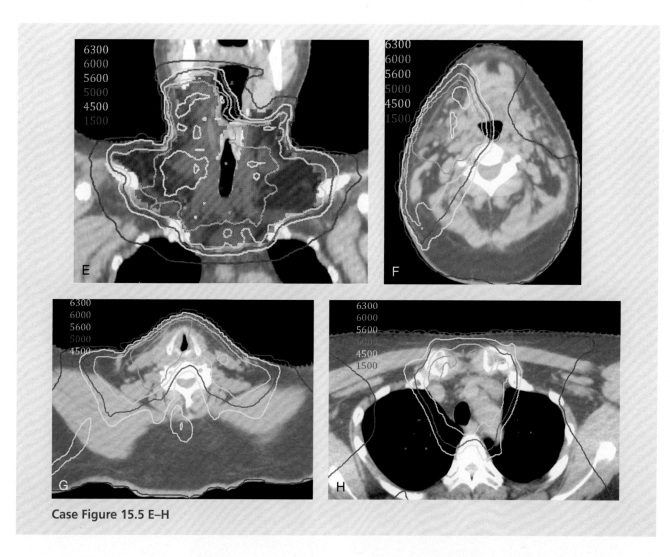

Case Figure 15.5 E–H

Virtual Gross Target Volume

There is no actual gross target volume (GTV) after complete surgical tumor resection. However, it can be useful to formulate a virtual GTV (vGTV) to facilitate target volume definition. The vGTV is the best approximation of the tissues having high likelihood of harboring microscopic tumor reconstructed based on findings of preoperative clinical examination, imaging studies, and surgical–pathologic assessment.

CASE STUDY 15.6

A 76-year-old man presented with hoarseness of voice, dysphagia, and a paretic left true vocal cord. CT neck with contrast revealed a 4-cm ill-defined, mostly isodense mass in the posterior aspect of the left thyroid lobe, with effacement of the esophagus and prevertebral musculature (Fig. 15.6A). Ultrasound-guided fine-needle aspiration biopsy revealed poorly differentiated carcinoma. PET–CT showed this to be an FDG-avid mass (SUV 12.3) without any signs of regional or distant metastases. He underwent total thyroidectomy and left paratracheal lymph node dissection. Due to adherent disease, resection required partial esophageal myectomy and microdissection of the left recurrent laryngeal nerve superiorly to the level of the laryngeal inlet. Final pathology showed a 4.8-cm tumor in the left lobe, poorly differentiated carcinoma, with extrathyroidal extension. All margin resections were negative, including the esophageal muscularis and the left recurrent laryngeal epineurium specimens. There was no tumor present in three left paratracheal lymph nodes resected.

Due to high-risk histology and adherent disease, postoperative radiation therapy was recommended. The left aspect of the glottis, cricoid, laryngeal inlet, upper paratracheal region, and central compartment were included in the CTV_{HD} (60 Gy), the right central compartment in CTV_{ID} (57 Gy), and remainder of the lateral neck at risk (bilateral levels III to IV and left level Vb) and upper mediastinum were included in CTV_{ED} (54 Gy). Treatment was accomplished using volumetric arc-based IMRT, delivered in 30 daily fractions over 6 weeks. Since there was no clinical or pathologic evidence of lymph node involvement, the most superior aspect of the treatment volume was just below the level of the hyoid bone. Figure 15.6B shows CTV_{ED} (54 Gy) in purple and Figure 15.6C the accompanying isodose distributions at that same level. Figure 15.6D shows all three CTVs at the level of the glottis and cricoid and Figure 15.6E the isodose distributions. Likewise, Figure 15.6F,G represents the central aspect of the thyroid resection bed at the level of the surgical scar (note: scar wire with 3-mm bolus over the scar). Figure 15.6H,I is taken from the level of the sternal notch, where the left tracheoesophageal groove (*arrow*) is targeted in the CTV_{HD} and left in the CTV_{ID}. Elective dose was given to the upper mediastinum, inferiorly to level of the aortic arch (Fig. 15.6J,K).

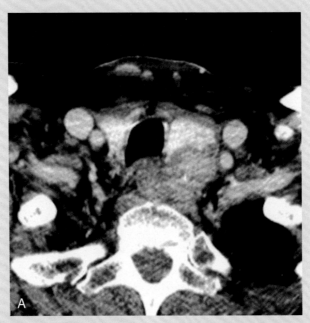

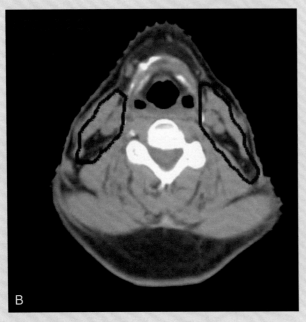

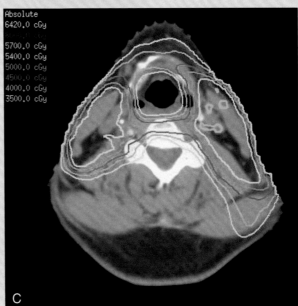

Case Figure 15.6 A–C

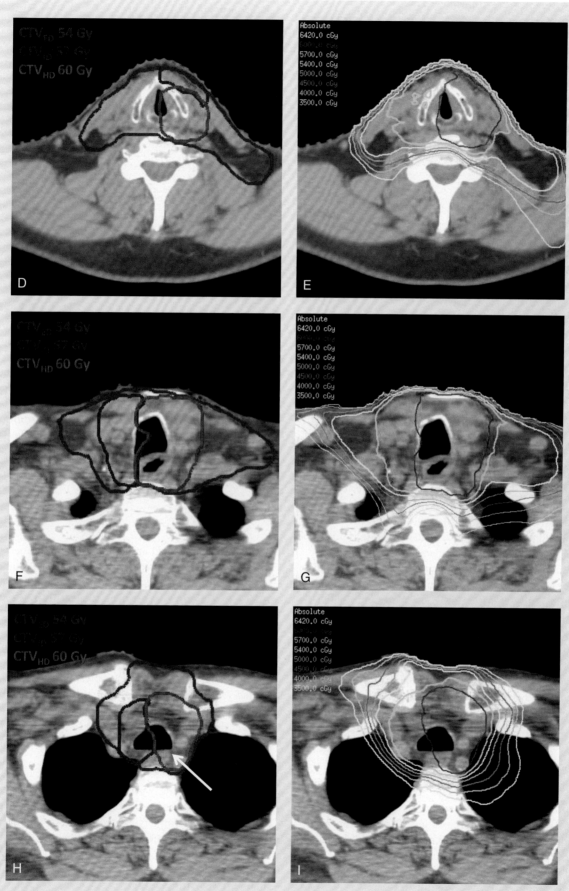

Case Figure 15.6 D–I

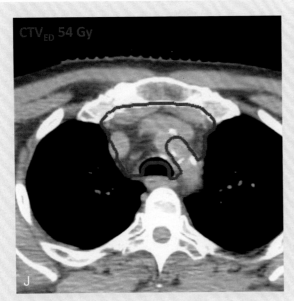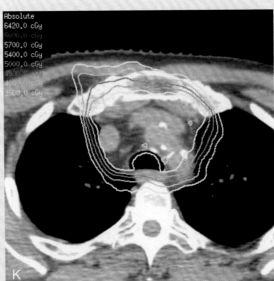

Case Figure 15.6 J,K

Clinical Target Volumes

Three clinical target volumes (CTVs) are generally delineated.

- CTV_{HD} delineates volumes to receive the highest dose. This includes the primary and nodal vGTVs with 1-cm margins. Often, a vGTV cannot be determined due to the absence of preoperative imaging. Contrast CT scans may not be done at many centers for well-differentiated thyroid carcinoma to avoid interference with subsequent potential RAI therapy. It is therefore crucial to be familiar with the anatomy and the routes of thyroid cancer spread, particularly as it pertains to areas near the trachea, esophagus, larynx, and adjacent musculature. CTV_{HD} encompasses the resected tumor and thyroid bed and involved nodal regions, plus the entirety of the central compartment, including tracheal walls and bilateral TE grooves. Adequate coverage of these structures generally necessitates inclusion of much of the cervical esophagus in the target volume, even if not directly involved. Likewise, to ensure coverage of the recurrent laryngeal nerve when directly invaded, sacrificed, or dissected or when upper paratracheal lymph node involvement was present, the entirety of the cricoid and glottis on the side of involvement is often targeted (**Case Study 15.6**). Generally, this volume is often estimated on the basis of surgical and pathologic findings.
- CTV_{ID} delineates volumes to receive an intermediate dose. CTV_{ID} typically encompasses the remaining operative bed or aforementioned structures not included in CTV_{HD}. If the vGTV is very well lateralized, the contralateral structures adjacent to the thyroid bed (such as the superior paratracheal and TE groove) can be in CTV_{ID} rather than CTV_{HD}.

- CTV_{ED} delineates volumes to receive an elective dose for subclinical disease. These include clinically negative and undissected bilateral paratracheal nodes to the level of the top of the aortic arch and level III and IV cervical nodes. If level III nodes harbored disease, CTV_{ED} can include levels II and V on the involved side though in recent years we have stopped treating the uninvolved upper neck with focus on the central compartment.

Dose

With conventional 3-D approach, the initial target volume dose is 44 Gy in 22 fractions. The boost volume dose is 16 Gy in 8 fractions. An additional boost dose of 4 to 6 Gy in 2 to 3 fractions may be given to a relatively small high-risk region.

With IMRT, the doses prescribed to CTV_{HD}, CTV_{ID}, and CTV_{ED} are usually 60, 57, and 54 Gy, respectively, given in 30 fractions. A total dose of 63 to 66 Gy (given in 2.1 to 2.2 Gy per fraction) may be prescribed to a targetable, limited region having an additional high-risk feature (e.g., positive margin, **Case Study 15.7**). If this high-dose target involves the esophagus, therapy may be given in 33 fractions to limit the fraction size to no more than 2 Gy because of risk for esophageal stenosis in this population.

In the treatment of anaplastic thyroid cancers in the postoperative setting various altered fractionation radiation schedules have been used to intensify local therapy, through acceleration, hyperfractionation, or both. Given that concurrent chemotherapy is often incorporated and the treatment volume can be quite large, the potential for significant acute (and late) toxicity must be carefully considered (**Case Study 15.8**).

CASE STUDY 15.7

A 75-year-old man was referred after surgical resection of a 6-cm neck tumor. Histologic examination revealed follicular thyroid carcinoma with extrathyroidal tumor extension. The operative report suggested a close or positive margin at the level of the superior aspect of the trachea. Restaging did not reveal obvious gross disease, so it was elected to treat him with postoperative IMRT.

Four volumes, shown in color wash in Figure 15.7, were delineated. CTV_{HD} (*red*), CTV_{ID} (*blue*), and CTV_{ED} (*yellow*) were prescribed 60, 57, and 54 Gy, respectively. A small volume (*aqua*) thought to be at the highest risk was delineated and prescribed 64 Gy. Treatment was delivered in 30 fractions. CTV_{HD} encompassed the left thyroid bed and left level III nodes. Note that the TE groove is covered due to tumor proximity to this region (Fig. 15.7A). The TE groove is often at risk in patients

with advanced thyroidal disease, whether from primary tumor or paratracheal nodal disease, and should be routinely included in either CTV_{HD} or CTV_{ED} dependent on the clinical situation. A coronal view (Fig. 15.7B) through the larynx also demonstrates the four targets. The dissected uninvolved right neck and right thyroidal bed is covered in CTV_{ID}. An additional margin (1 cm) superior to CTV_{HD} on the left and CTV_{ID} on the right was delineated CTV_{ED}, as is the undissected upper mediastinum. Figure 15.7C,D shows contours in axial slices with isodose lines at the levels of the cricoid and upper mediastinum, respectively. The posterior cervical nodes were also covered in CTV_{ED}. Unfortunately, the patient was subsequently diagnosed with non–small cell carcinoma of the lung and died of complications from distant metastases.

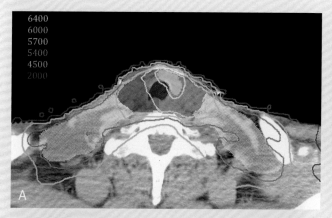

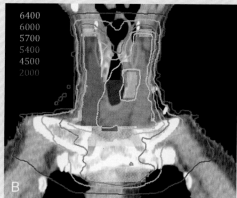

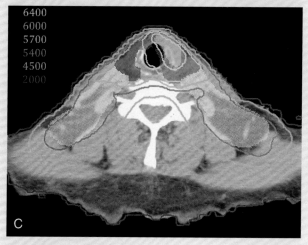

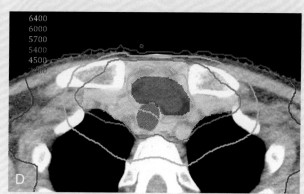

Case Figure 15.7 A–D

CASE STUDY 15.8

A 58-year-old female sought evaluation for a rapidly enlarging, left-sided, lower neck mass and new-onset hoarseness of voice and dysphagia. Ultrasound-guided fine-needle aspiration biopsy was consistent with anaplastic carcinoma. She was then evaluated in our center's anaplastic thyroid cancer fast-track program, where comprehensive staging imaging and multidisciplinary evaluations are completed urgently. CT neck with contrast showed a large heterogeneous left thyroid mass that was displacing central structures with concern for esophageal invasion (Fig. 15.8A). There was no evidence of distant metastases on PET–CT or MRI of the brain. Twelve days after initial diagnosis and 5 days after presenting to our center, she underwent subtotal thyroidectomy, sacrifice and resection of the left recurrent laryngeal nerve, partial esophageal myectomy, and extended left neck dissection. Final pathology showed anaplastic thyroid carcinoma, extraglandular extension, and soft tissue invasion, but surgical margins were negative (R0 resection) and all lymph nodes sampled were negative for tumor.

Postoperative chemoradiation was initiated on postoperative day 14. To facilitate rapid initiation of radiation, initial treatments (the first 6 Gy) were given using conventional techniques while the IMRT plan was being developed. Total dose to the thyroid tumor bed was 66 Gy in 33 fractions, using an accelerated treatment course, giving 6 fractions per week, with two fractions given 1 day per week with a 6-hour interaction interval. Concurrent chemotherapy was carboplatin and paclitaxel.

A nine-field, nonopposing IMRT beam arrangement was used (Fig. 15.8B). As shown in Figure 15.8C,D, the

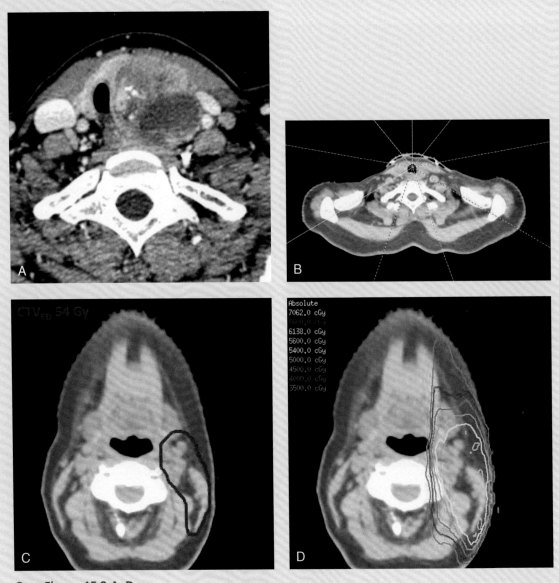

Case Figure 15.8 A–D

ipsilateral (left) upper neck was included in the CTV$_{ED}$. The prelaryngeal soft tissues and left mid neck were included in CTV$_{ID}$ and the contralateral neck in CTV$_{ED}$ (Fig. 15.8E,F). The left aspect of the glottis and cricoid and central compartment were included in the CTV$_{HD}$ (Fig. 15.8G,H). At the level of the thyroid bed (Fig. 15.8I,J) and at the sternal notch (Fig. 15.8K,L), the central compartment was included in the CTV$_{HD}$. Elective dose was given to the upper mediastinum (Fig. 15.8M,N). Representative sagittal (Fig. 15.8O,P) and coronal views (Fig. 15.8Q,R) are shown. Following completion of chemoradiation, she received adjuvant chemotherapy, completing all therapy within 5 months. She remains free of disease, now 20 months after completing radiation therapy. Posttherapy CT neck with contrast shows restoration of normal anatomy (Fig. 15.8S), as compared to initial CT (Fig. 15.8A).

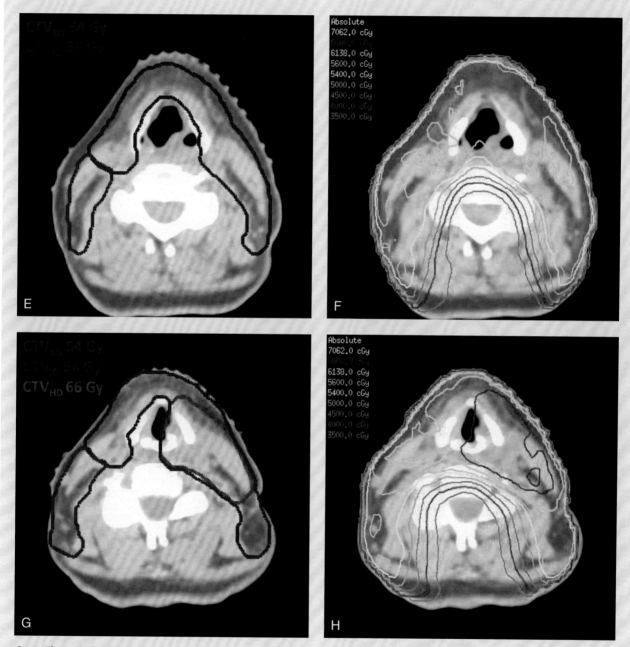

Case Figure 15.8 E–H

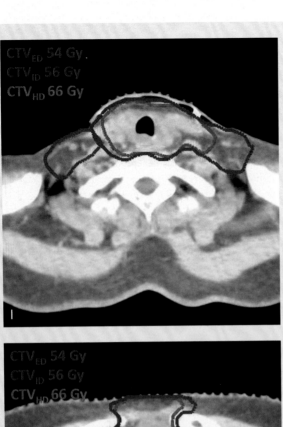

CTV_ED 54 Gy
CTV_ID 56 Gy
CTV_HD 66 Gy

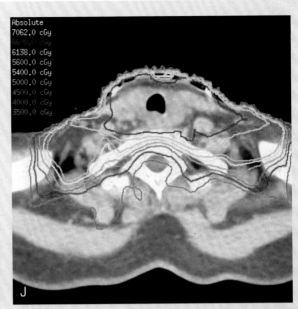

Absolute
7062.0 cGy
6600.0 cGy
6138.0 cGy
5600.0 cGy
5400.0 cGy
5000.0 cGy
4500.0 cGy
4000.0 cGy
3500.0 cGy

I

J

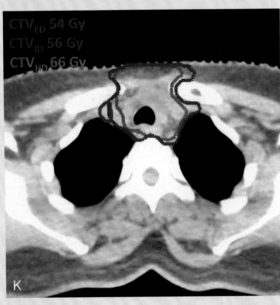

CTV_ED 54 Gy
CTV_ID 56 Gy
CTV_HD 66 Gy

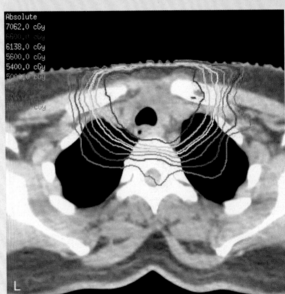

Absolute
7062.0 cGy
6600.0 cGy
6138.0 cGy
5600.0 cGy
5400.0 cGy
5000.0 cGy

K

L

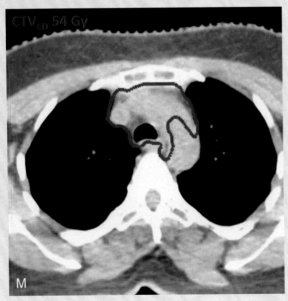

CTV_ED 54 Gy

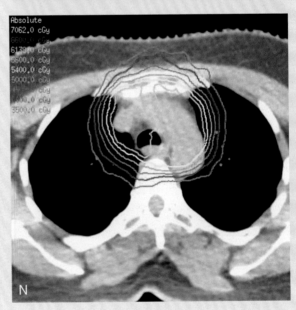

Absolute
7062.0 cGy
6600.0 cGy
6138.0 cGy
5600.0 cGy
5400.0 cGy
5000.0 cGy
cGy
cGy
3500.0 cGy

M

N

Case Figure 15.8 I–N

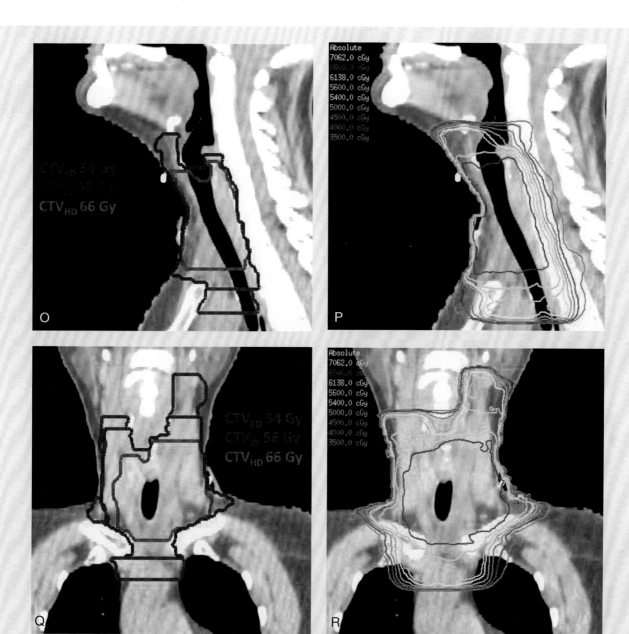

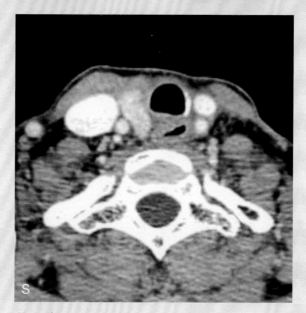

Case Figure 15.8 O–S

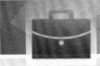

CASE STUDY 15.9

A 65-year-old female was admitted to our hospital with progressive dyspnea on exertion from a rapidly enlarging lower neck mass. CT neck with contrast revealed a large enhancing mass in the right lower neck compressing the trachea and esophagus, which was deemed unresectable (Fig. 15.9A). There was no evidence of distant disease. Core needle biopsy showed anaplastic (undifferentiated) thyroid cancer. There was no stridor or dyspnea at rest. Tracheostomy was not pursued as tumor cut through would be required, and there was perceived short-term benefit with likely problematic symptoms from anticipated tumor progression through the tracheotomy site.

She was admitted for intravenous steroids, airway monitoring, and initiation of palliative chemoradiation.

To facilitate rapid initiation of radiation, initial treatments (the first 6 Gy) were given using conventional techniques and IMRT followed. The gross neck tumor with margin was treated to 66 Gy in 33 fractions, using an accelerated-hyperfractionated treatment course, delivering 1.5 Gy twice daily, with a 6-hour interaction interval. Concurrent chemotherapy was carboplatin and paclitaxel. The GTV at the level of the larynx and associated isodose lines are shown in Figure 15.9B,C. Figure 15.9D,E shows the same at the central aspect of

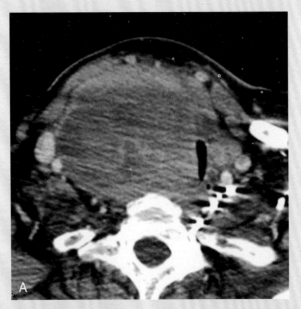

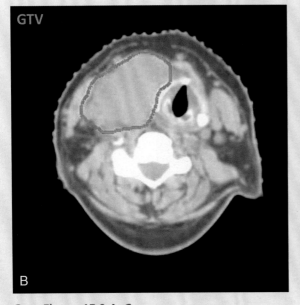

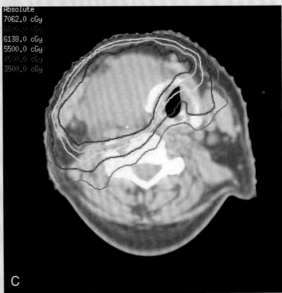

Case Figure 15.9 A–C

the thyroid mass. The tumor extended into the sternal notch (Fig. 15.9F,G) and the upper mediastinum (Fig. 15.9H,I). Figure 15.9J–M depicts the extent of the GTV and isodose lines from sagittal and coronal projections, respectively.

She tolerated treatment well, with improvement in respiratory symptoms. Figure 15.9N shows a representative axial image on a postradiation therapy CT neck with regression of tumor and reduction in tracheal compression. She died from progressive lung and liver metastases 9 months after completion of radiation therapy but lived the remainder of her life free from the morbidity of uncontrolled neck disease and did not require tracheotomy or a feeding tube.

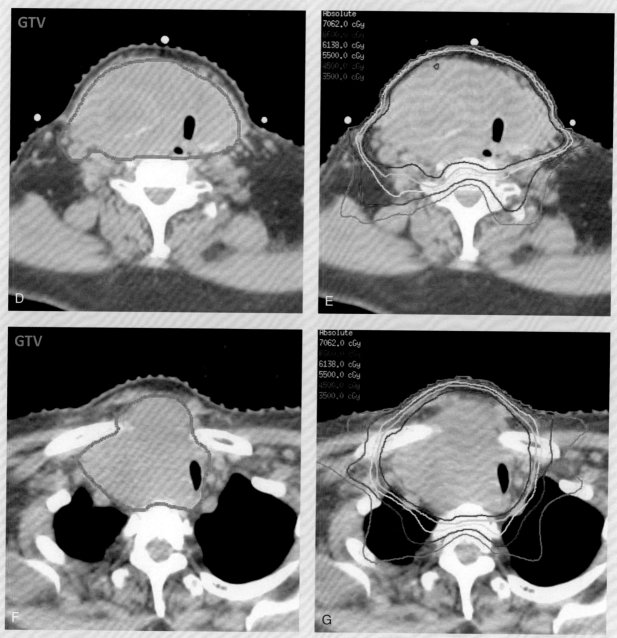

Case Figure 15.9 D–G

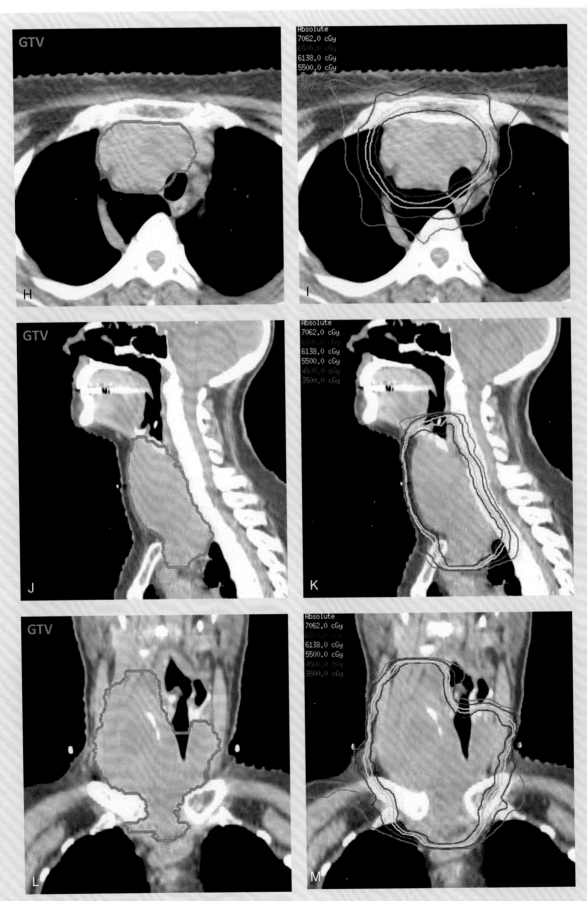

Case Figure 15.9 H–M

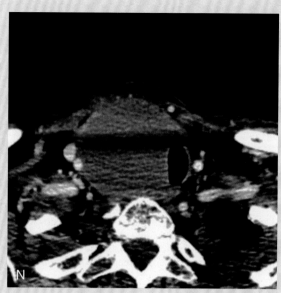

Case Figure 15.9 N

Dose Specification

With conventional or 3-D approaches, treatment is usually given with 6-MV photons for the anterior field and with 18-MV photons for the posterior field. Loading for AP–PA fields is usually 3:2. A CT treatment plan is obtained and adjustment can be made where necessary. The dose is prescribed to an isodose line encompassing the target volume.

Background Data

See Tables 15.1 and 15.2.

Study	Surgery with RAI (%)	Surgery RAI and XRT (%)
TABLE 15.1 Ten-Year Local Recurrence Rates After Therapy for High-Risk Differentiated Thyroid Carcinoma		
Tubiana et al.	21	14
Simpson et al.	18	14
Phlips et al.	21	3
Farahati et al. (includes distant failures)	50	10
Tsang et al. (papillary only)	22	7
Kim et al. (papillary only, 5 yr rates)	37.5	4.8
Keum et al.	89	38
Brierley et al. (patients over 60 who have ETE)*	34.3	13.6

*Extra-thyroidal extension

TABLE 15.2 Outcomes of Conformal Irradiation for Thyroid Cancer: The U.T. M.D. Anderson Experience

Histology	Patient Number (Total/IMRT)	Overall Survival (%)	Disease-Specific Survival (%)	Local–Regional Control (%)
Differentiated carcinoma	131/57	73 (4 yr)	76	79
Medullary carcinoma	34/7	56 (5 yr)	62	87
Anaplastic carcinoma	53/13	19 (1 yr)	19	11

Data from Schwartz DL, Lobo MJ, Ang KK, et al. Postoperative external beam radiotherapy for differentiated thyroid cancer: outcomes and morbidity with conformal treatment. *Int J Radiat Oncol Biol Phys* 2009;74:1083–1091; Schwartz DL, Rana V, Shaw S, et al. Postoperative radiotherapy for advanced medullary thyroid cancer—local disease control in the modern era. *Head Neck* 2008;30:883–888; Bhatia A, Rao A, Ang KK, et al. Anaplastic thyroid cancer: clinical outcomes with conformal therapy. *Head Neck* 2010;32:829–836.

DEFINITIVE RADIATION

General concepts

Definitive Radiation is rarely recommended for well-differentiated cancers. In the unusual situation where tumor is inoperable, the intent of radiation is palliative. The gross disease with appropriate margin is targeted, and the preferred palliative dose-fractionation schedule is chosen. However, in the absence of other disease or life-threatening co-morbidities, higher doses of 60-66 Gy at 2 Gy per fraction to gross disease with margin may be preferred to try to maximize the duration of disease control, though with respect for the adjacent critical structures, as a balance between disease control and potential toxicities needs to be ensured.

For inoperable poorly-differentiated carcinomas, particularly anaplastic carcinoma, in the absence of prohibitive comorbidities and distant disease, the principles of target delineation are similar to the postoperative setting, though GTV does exist. Various altered fractionation radiation schedules have been used to intensify local therapy, through acceleration, hyperfractionation, or both. Given that concurrent chemotherapy is often incorporated and the treatment volume can be quite large, the potential for significant acute (and late) toxicity must be carefully considered **(Case Study 15.9)**. In the event the patient is symptomatic, but has distant disease, or poor performance status, short palliative fractionated radiation may be appropriate.

SUGGESTED READINGS

Benker G, Olbricht T, Reinwein D, et al. Survival rates in patients with differentiated thyroid carcinoma. Influence of postoperative external radiotherapy. *Cancer* 1990;65:1517.

Bhatia A, Rao A, Ang KK, et al. Anaplastic thyroid cancer: clinical outcomes with conformal therapy. *Head Neck* 2010;32:829.

Brierley J, Tsang R, Panzarella T, et al. Prognostic factors and the effect of treatment with radioactive iodine and external beam radiation on patients with differentiated thyroid cancer seen at a single institution over 40 years. *Clin Endocrinol* 2005;63:418.

Brierley J, Tsang R, Simpson WJ, et al. Medullary thyroid cancer: analyses of survival and prognostic factors and the role of radiation therapy in local control. *Thyroid* 1996;6:305.

Cabanillas ME, Dadu R, Hu MI, et al. Thyroid gland malignancies. *Hematol Oncol Clin North Am* 2015;29:1123.

Farahati J, Reiners C, Stuschke M, et al. Differentiated thyroid cancer. Impact of adjuvant external radiotherapy in patients with perithyroidal tumor infiltration (stage T4). *Cancer* 1996;77:172.

Giuliani M and Brierley J. Indications for the use of external beam radiation in thyroid cancer. *Curr Opin Oncol* 2014;26:45.

Kiess AP, Agrawal N, Brierley JD, et al. External-beam radiotherapy for differentiated thyroid cancer locoregional control: a statement of the American Head and Neck Society. *Head Neck* 2016;38:493.

Kwon J, Kim BH, Jung HW, et al. The prognostic impacts of postoperative radiotherapy in the patients with resected anaplastic thyroid carcinoma: a systematic review and meta-analysis. *Eur J Cancer* 2016;59:34.

Nutting CM, Convery DJ, Cosgrove VP, et al. Improvements in target coverage and reduced spinal cord irradiation using intensity-modulated radiotherapy (IMRT) in patients with carcinoma of the thyroid gland. *Radiother Oncol* 2001;60:173.

Salama JK, Golden DW, Yom SS, et al. ACR Appropriateness Criteria® thyroid carcinoma. *Oral Oncol* 2014;50:577.

Schwartz DL, Lobo MJ, Ang KK, et al. Postoperative external beam radiotherapy for differentiated thyroid cancer:

outcomes and morbidity with conformal treatment. *Int J Radiat Oncol Biol Phys* 2009;74:1083.

Schwartz DL, Rana V, Shaw S, et al. Postoperative radiotherapy for advanced medullary thyroid cancer—local disease control in the modern era. *Head Neck* 2008;30:883.

Sia MA, Tsang RW, Panzarella T, et al. Differentiated thyroid cancer with extrathyroidal extension: prognosis and the role of external beam radiotherapy. *J Thyroid Res* 2010;2010:183461.

Smallridge RC, Ain KB, Asa SL, et al. American Thyroid Association guidelines for management of patients with anaplastic thyroid cancer. *Thyroid* 2012;22:1104.

Strong EW. The treatment of thyroid cancer: a summary. In: Najarian JS, Delaney JP, eds. *Advances in cancer surgery.* New York, NY: Stratton, 1976.

Su SY, Milas ZL, Bhatt N, et al. Well-differentiated thyroid cancer with aerodigestive tract invasion: long-term control and functional outcomes. *Head Neck* 2016;38:72.

Tennvall J, Lundell G, Hallquist A, et al. The Swedish Anaplastic Thyroid Cancer Group. Combined doxorubicin, hyperfractionated radiotherapy, and surgery in anaplastic thyroid carcinoma. Report on two protocols. *Cancer* 1994;74:1348.

Tubiana M, Haddad E, Schlumberger M, et al. External radiotherapy in thyroid cancers. *Cancer* 1985;55:2062.

Wilson PC, Millar BM, Brierley JD. The management of advanced thyroid cancer. *Clin Oncol* 2004;16:561.

Wu XL, Hu YH, Li QH, et al. Value of postoperative radiotherapy for thyroid cancer. *Head Neck Surg* 1987; 10:107.

16

Skin

SQUAMOUS CELL CARCINOMA AND BASAL CELL CARCINOMA

Treatment Strategy

Surgery and radiotherapy are equally effective in curing most skin cancers. The choice of treatment modality is determined by several factors, such as functional and cosmetic results, patient age and occupation, treatment time, and cost. Surgery is preferred for most patients, particularly for younger patients who have years of exposure to sunlight ahead of them.

Primary radiotherapy is often indicated for lesions on and around the nose, lower eyelids, and ear, where it can usually attain better functional and cosmetic results than surgery. Extensive lesions of the cheek and oral commissures, which would require full-thickness resection, may also show better results on irradiation.

Postoperative radiotherapy is indicated for positive surgical margins, perineural invasion, and invasion of bone, cartilage, and skeletal muscle.

Rarely, patients have adenopathy at diagnosis. The choice of treatment of the nodal disease is determined by the type of therapy selected for the primary lesion and by the size of the involved node(s). In most situations, surgery is preferred unless there are medical considerations, as these patients are often elderly with comorbidities. For patients who have surgery, adjuvant radiation is recommended if the metastases are to the parotid or if cervical metastases have criteria concerning for an increased risk of recurrence (i.e., ECE, multiple nodes, or nodal size >3 cm).

Primary Radiotherapy

Target Volume

The initial target volume encompasses primary tumor with 1- to 2-cm margins, depending on the size, location, and type of tumor (well-circumscribed vs. ill-defined border). Elective nodal irradiation is not indicated except when the primary is a large, infiltrative squamous cell carcinoma (SCC) or poorly differentiated.

The boost volume encompasses primary tumor with 0.5- to 1-cm margins, depending on the size, location, and type of tumor. The margin size is also dictated by the mode of therapy, as electrons, particularly lower-energy electrons, have wide penumbras and bowing in of the dose necessitating a more generous margin.

Setup and Field Arrangement

The patient is immobilized in a position that gives the best access to irradiate the tumor (preferably the plane of the skin to be treated is parallel to the surface of the treatment couch to avoid the need for gantry rotation).

An appositional field is used in most cases. The borders of the field are chosen to include a 1- to 2-cm margin of normal skin around the tumor (up to 1 cm for lesions <1-cm tumor and 1 to 2 cm for larger tumors). Margins may be smaller when treating areas close to the eye. More generous margins are appropriate for lesions with an ill-defined border.

Radiation treatment is given with orthovoltage x-rays (usually 75 to 125 kilovolt potential [kVp]) or electrons (usually 6 to 9 MeV). The energy of x-rays or electrons is chosen on the basis of the thickness of tumor. The energy of electron beams should be selected so that the distal 90%-isodose line is a few millimeters deeper than the base of the tumor, including surface bolus.

A custom-made lead cutout is used for skin collimation. The cutout should be large enough so that the portal size for an electron beam is at least 4×4 cm.

Skin bolus or a perspex scatter plate is used with electrons to ensure full surface dose.

An internal eye shield is inserted when treating an eyelid lesion with orthovoltage x-rays or with electrons **(Case Study 16.1)**. (*Note:* Eye shields should be individually calibrated with respect to the electron-attenuating properties.)

Dose

Varying fractionation schedules have been recommended for definitive treatment of skin cancers. In general, protracted treatment provides better cosmetic results, but for many patients, particularly elderly with multiple comorbidities for whom multiple fractions can be challenging, shorter schedules are equally effective for tumor eradication. For small tumors (<2 cm), current guidelines for dose fractionation include 64 Gy in 32 fractions, 55 Gy in 20 fractions, 50 Gy in 15 fractions, or 35 Gy in 5 fractions. All schedules are based on once-daily fractions, 5 days per week.

For large tumors close to crucial structures (e.g., eye), maximum tolerance is obtained with a dose of 66 to 70 Gy in 33 to 35 fractions. An alternative if time is a major consideration is 55 Gy in 20 fractions.

Dose Specification

X-rays are prescribed at D_{max}, and electrons are prescribed at the 90% line. This difference in prescription accounts for the relative biologic effectiveness difference between the two beam qualities and the dose coverage differences between the two beams.

Postoperative Radiotherapy

Most frequent indications are lymphatic spread to the parotid gland, upper neck nodes, or both, or perineural extension. Less commonly, postoperative radiation is recommended due to inadequate resection margins **(Case Study 16.2)**.

Target Volume

The initial target volume encompasses the primary tumor bed and ipsilateral parotid and neck nodes, or trigeminal or facial nerve pathways, depending on the indication.

The boost volume encompasses areas of known disease with 1- to 2-cm margins.

Setup and Field Arrangement

For the treatment of parotid and neck nodes or branches of the facial nerve, the technique is similar to that for primary parotid tumors (see Chapter 14). The patient is immobilized in an open neck position. The anterior margin of the parotid portal can be slightly less generous because there is no need to encompass the parotid duct. Treatment is given with an electron beam of appropriate energy (e.g., 12 MeV for parotid and upper neck nodes and 9 MeV for lower neck nodes). However, as the conformality of IMRT and IMPT has continued to improve, these techniques are often replacing electron techniques in the postoperative setting **(Case Study 16.3)**.

For the treatment of perineural extension through the supraorbital, infraorbital, or mandibular branches of the trigeminal nerve, the patient is immobilized in a supine position. The portal margins depend on the tumor extent and particularly the extent of the perineural spread. IMRT, similar to that used for the treatment of sinonasal primary tumors (see Chapter 13), usually provides better coverage for rather convoluted target volumes in such cases while sparing more optic structures and, therefore, has largely replaced conventional technique. IMPT is an attractive alternative, though to date experience is limited.

CASE STUDY 16.1

A 59-year-old man sought medical attention because of a small ulcer at the left lateral dorsum of the nose that gradually increased in size over a 4-year period.

Physical examination showed a ulcerating lesion with raised borders, involving the left lateral dorsum of the nose, the medial aspect of the cheek, and the medial canthus (Fig. 16.1A). The thickest part of the tumor was close to the medial canthus. Biopsy revealed basal cell carcinoma. Computed tomography (CT) scans showed a small soft tissue mass in the medial canthus of the left orbit. The deepest point of this mass was 1.5 cm from the surface. Stage: T2 N0 M0.

The lesion was treated with an appositional left anterior oblique field of 9-MeV electrons. Figure 16.1B–D shows a custom-made eye shield mounted on a contact lens used to protect the cornea and lens (B), a lead mask with extra layers over the contralateral eye for skin collimation (C), and a 1/4-inch scatter plate placed in the beam to eliminate the skin-sparing effect (D). A dose of 60 Gy, prescribed to 90% isodose line, was delivered in 2-Gy fractions, which resulted in local control with good cosmetic and functional outcome (Fig. 16.1E,F).

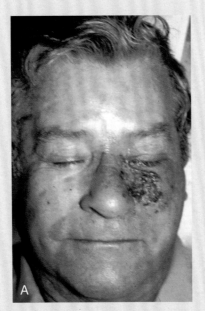

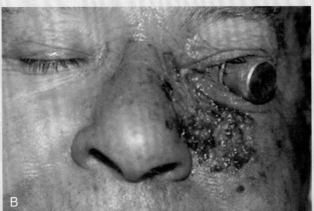

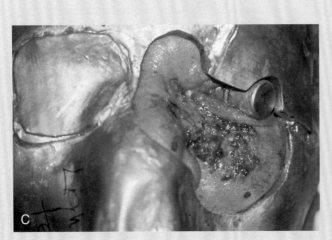

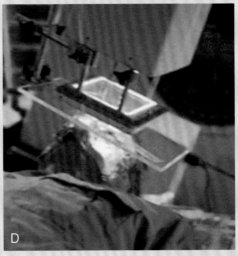

Case Figure 16.1 A–D

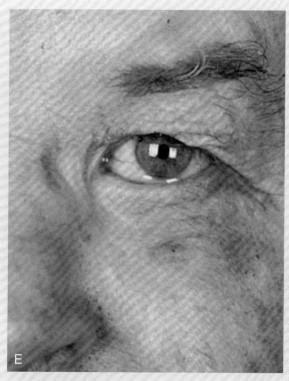
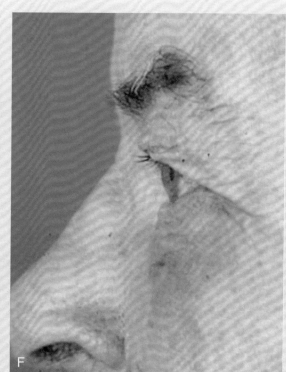

Case Figure 16.1 E,F

CASE STUDY 16.2

A 57-year-old male presented to his local physicians with a lesion of the nasal dorsum. It was excised, and the defect was closed with a rotational flap. Pathology revealed an infiltrative/nodular basal cell carcinoma with diffusely positive margins both at the periphery and deep. It was elected to treat him with postoperative irradiation using a single appositional electron field.

The field was delineated on the patient's face, covering the flap with margin. Figure 16.2A is a photo of the patient as a mold of his face is fabricated. The field borders over the nasal dorsum can be seen. The mold was used to fabricate lead skin collimation, with extra layers of external shielding over the eyes. Figure 16.2B is the patient setup. He is immobilized in a thermoplastic mask, and the lead collimation is applied. In the upper left corner, the bolus that will cover the nose can be seen. Figure 16.2C shows the set up with bolus applied. 60 Gy was prescribed in 30 fractions with dose prescribed to the 90% line, using 12-MeV electrons. Representative isodoses of an axial and a sagittal view are shown in Figure 16.2D,E.

The turquoise coloration is part of the modeling used for the skin collimation.

The patient is doing well 3 years out of therapy.

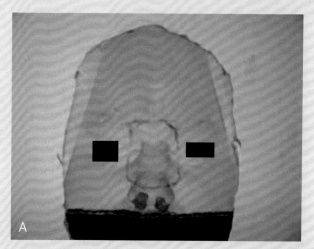

Case Figure 16.2 A

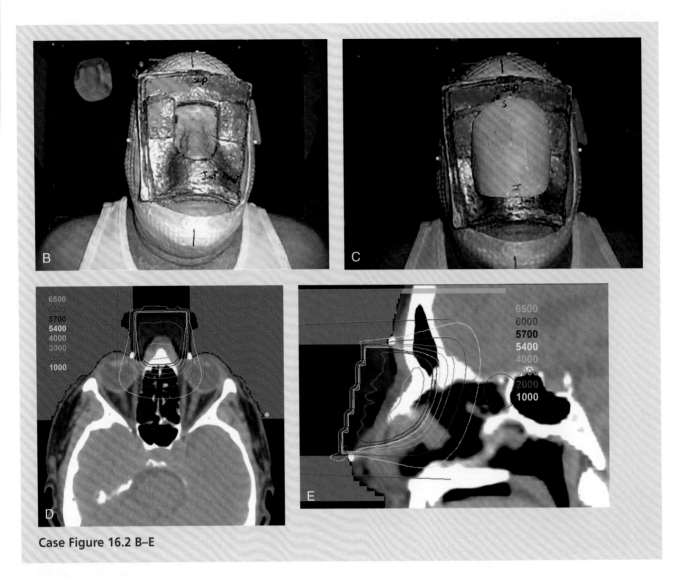

Case Figure 16.2 B–E

CASE STUDY 16.3

A 76-year-old gentleman presented with gradual onset of complete left facial paralysis over previous 14 months. Initial evaluation 8 months ago with MRI of the brain was unremarkable. He was diagnosed with Bell's palsy and treated with steroids without improvement. He then noticed left preauricular mass. He did have a history of multiple basal cell carcinomas of the face and upper chest.

On physical examination facial function overall House-Brackmann grade V/VI on the left with no movement in the left forehead and incomplete left eye closure. There was weakness in the left nasolabial fold and lip depressors, but slight movement was present. Face sensation was intact. There was diffuse fullness of the left parotid bed. There was no skin fixation. The mass was hypomobile.

Otherwise, there was no palpable neck adenopathy. MRI of the face and neck showed a diffuse, enhancing mass of the left superficial parotid (*green arrows* in Fig. 16.3A) but no adenopathy. Fine-needle aspiration of the left parotid mass showed poorly differentiated carcinoma with squamous characteristics.

He underwent multispecialty surgical resection with lateral temporal bone resection, facial nerve decompression, radical parotidectomy, soft tissue resection, left neck dissection (levels 2a/b and 3), and free vastus lateralis muscle flap reconstruction. Operative findings described extensive tumor at the pes anserinus of the facial nerve. Resection required sacrifice of the upper division and main trunk. The lower division was dissected and grafted. There was tumor involving the deep lobe of the parotid. Resection of the adjacent masseter and temporal mandibular joint capsule was required. Final pathology showed multifocal squamous carcinoma in gland and periparotid soft tissue, measuring 3.0 cm; perineural invasion was positive. Carcinoma was abutting the main trunk of the facial nerve, and nerve margin was negative. Periparotid and neck lymph nodes were negative for carcinoma (28 negative nodes).

He was treated with postoperative intensity-modulated proton therapy (IMPT), using active-scanning beam.

He was simulated and treated using a posterior head, neck, and shoulder mold, tongue-deviating stent with bite block, and a full-length custom mask. The parotid tumor bed with margin (CTV$_{HD}$) was treated to 60 Gy (radiobiologic equivalent [RBE]), the operative bed (CTV$_{ID}$) to 56 Gy(RBE), and the remainder of the at-risk neck and nerve tracts (CTV$_{ED}$) to 54 Gy (RBE) all in 30 fractions in a single integrated plan.

The CTVs and IMPT dose distributions are shown in multiple planes in Figure 16.3B–I. Care was taken

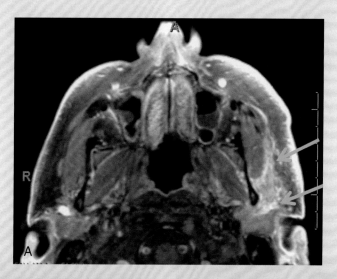

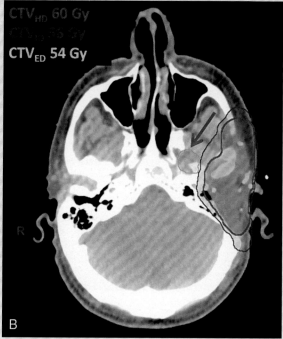

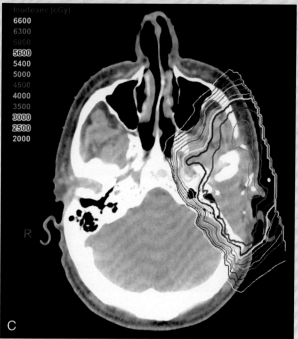

Case Figure 16.3 A–C

to include the temporal bone resection bed, TMJ, and much of the course of the facial nerve in the temporal bone in the target volume. The auriculotemporal branch of the mandibular division of the trigeminal nerve was targeted to foramen ovale as CTV_{ED} (*red arrow* in Fig. 16.3B).

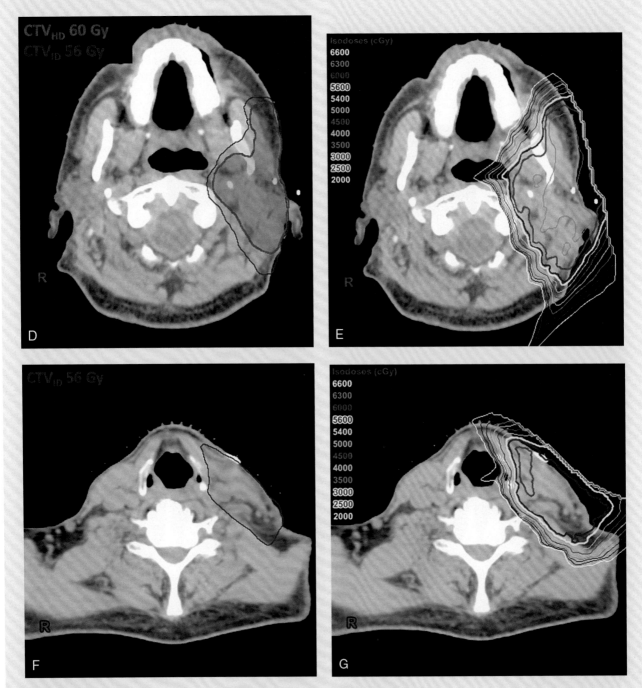

Case Figure 16.3 D–G

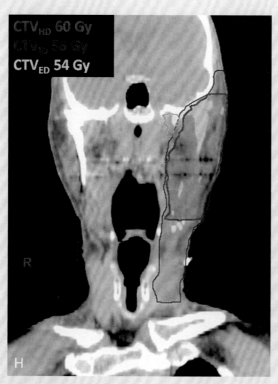
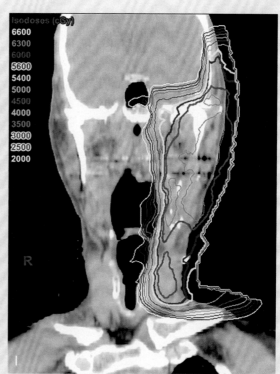

Case Figure 16.3 H,I

Dose

The dose is consistent with other postoperative scenarios. Three targets are typically delineated. CTV_{HD} encompasses the vGTV with a 1- to 2-cm margin, CTV_{ID} encompasses the operative bed outside the CTV_{HD}, and CTV_{ED} encompasses subclinical sites not violated by surgery. CTV_{ED} may include lower neck nodes not operated in patients with node-positive disease, or neural pathways not clinically involved in tumors with perineural extension. For patients whose tumors have minimal (focal) perineural disease, CTV_{ED} will include the adjacent named nerve, and for those with large nerve involvement, CTV_{ED} will include the cavernous sinus and even Meckel's cave.

Doses to CTV_{HD}, CTV_{ID}, and CTV_{ED} are 60, 57, and 54 Gy, respectively, with treatment delivered in 30 fractions. An additional target volume can be delineated to deliver 64 to 66 Gy to a region concerning for high-risk recurrence due to ECE or positive margin. Particularly in cases of perineural invasion, an MRI may detect residual perineural disease, and these "postoperative" cases are often definitive with regard to treatment of the perineural disease **(Case Study 16.4 and Case Study 16.5)**.

Dose Specification: See "General Principles"

Background Data

See Tables 16.1 to 16.3.

MELANOMA

Treatment Strategy

The primary treatment for cutaneous melanoma is complete local excision (which is essential for tissue diagnosis and microstaging) and, for palpable nodes, neck dissection. An exception is large facial lentigo maligna melanoma, which can be treated effectively with primary radiotherapy when wide surgical resection requires an extensive reconstruction or is anticipated to yield poor cosmetic outcome.

Our indications for adjuvant postoperative radiotherapy following therapeutic nodal dissections are as follows:

- Lymph node >3 cm or multiple lymph nodes
- ECE
- Nodal recurrence (in a previously dissected nodal basin) without distant metastases
- Local excision of macroscopic disease only

Sentinel lymph node biopsy with directed lymphadenectomy has replaced routine elective regional radiotherapy following wide local excision of primary lesions ≥1.5 mm thick or Clark's level IV or higher without clinical evidence of lymphadenopathy. Elective nodal irradiation is indicated if the procedure cannot detect the sentinel basin or if the patient's condition precludes a therapeutic dissection.

CASE STUDY 16.4

An 84-year-old male with a history of numerous skin cancers of the face, including a squamous cell cancer surgically removed from the left cheek presented with left cheek numbness. He presented following an orbitotomy that confirmed squamous cell cancer in the floor of the orbit. An MRI performed to evaluate the neuropathy showed evidence of perineural spread with disease in the pterygopalatine fossa and foramen rotundum (Fig. 16.4A) with additional disease in the left middle cranial fossa in the parasellar region (Fig. 16.4B).

He was treated with IMRT. There were three targets: CTV$_{HD}$ (red color wash), which covered GTV with margin, and two elective volumes, CTV$_{ID}$ (blue color wash) and CTV$_{ED}$ (yellow color wash). Treatment was delivered in 30 fractions, with the prescribed doses 66, 60, and 54 Gy, respectively, to the three clinical targets. The distal left optic nerve is color washed in turquoise. Figure 16.4C, D shows two coronal slices demonstrating isodose distributions through the floor of the orbit and more posteriorly through the pterygopalatine fossa and foramen rotundum. Figure 16.4E is a sagittal view, medial to the left orbit, and Figure 16.4F is an axial view. The head is positioned such that anteriorly the superior maxillary sinus is just inferior to the floor of the orbit while posteriorly is the inferior part of the middle cranial fossa just superior to CTV$_{HD}$ that covers the gross disease in the fossa floor.

The patient was last seen 5 years after therapy and was doing well.

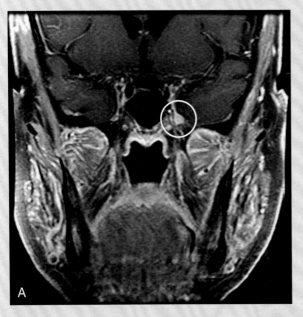

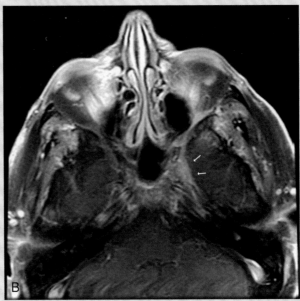

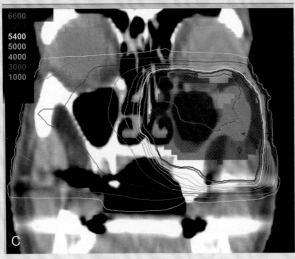

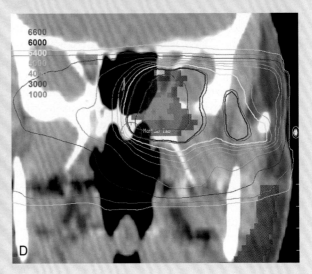

Case Figure 16.4 A–D

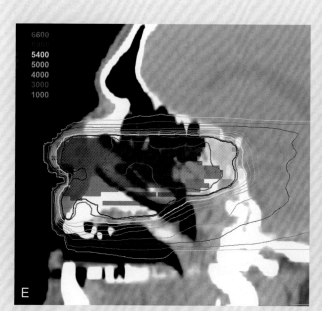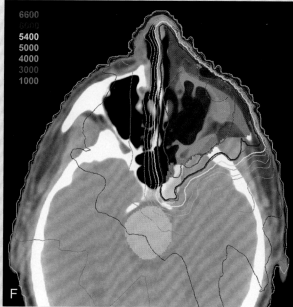

Case Figure 16.4 E,F

CASE STUDY 16.5

An 88-year-old male presented with a history of numerous skin cancers, including seven basal and squamous cell cancers of the right ear treated with multiple limited surgical procedures presented with a basal cell carcinoma of his right external ear canal. He presented following a limited excision. His imaging showed residual disease in the canal and adjacent tissues (Fig. 16.5A). Radiation was recommended.

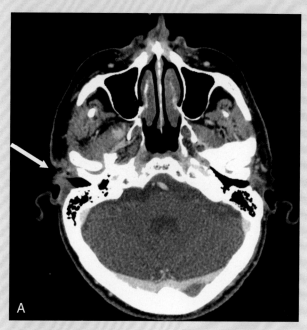

Case Figure 16.5 A

Target volumes included CTV$_{HD}$ (red color wash) encompassing GTV and margin, CTV$_{ID}$ (blue color wash), and CTV$_{ED}$ (yellow color wash), which provided additional margin and parotid coverage. Treatment was delivered in 30 fractions, with doses of 66, 60, and 54 Gy prescribed to the three CTVs. Representative axial slices through the canal (Fig. 16.5B) and TMJ (Fig. 16.5C) and a coronal view through the temporal bone (Fig. 16.5D) with contours of the three CTVs and isodose lines are shown. He remains more than 3 years out from treatment without disease.

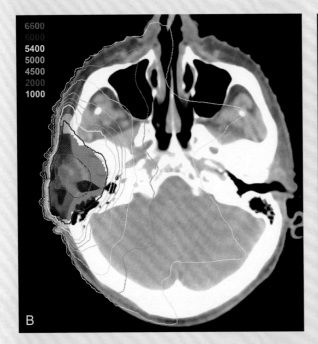

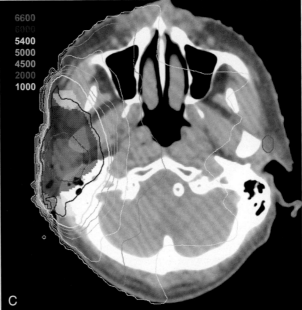

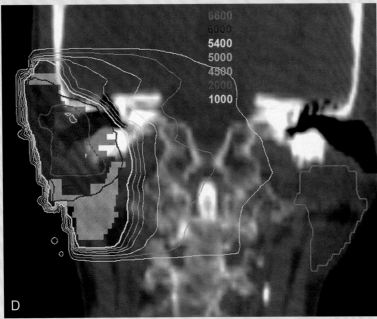

Case Figure 16.5 B–D

TABLE 16.1 Control of Malignant Skin Lesions with Radiation Therapy: Hahnemann University Experience, 1960 to 1980

Diagnosis	No. Treated with Radiotherapy	No. of Treatment Failures	No. of Recurrences Controlled by Reirradiation	No Evidence of Disease 4 yr or Longer (%)
Basal cell carcinoma	444	20	2	426/444 (95.9)
SCC	156	12	—	144/156 (92.3)
Keratoacanthoma	12	0	—	12/12 (100)

Modified from Solan MJ, Brady LW, Binnick SA, et al. Skin cancer. In: Perez CA, Brady LW, eds. *Principles and practice of radiation oncology*, 2nd ed. Philadelphia, PA: JB Lippincott, 1992:479–495.

TABLE 16.2 Clinical Experience with 1,166 Eyelid Tumors Treated by Radiotherapy (1958–1978)[a]

Histologic Finding	Primary Tumors	Recurrent Tumors	Total	5-yr Control	%
Basal cell carcinoma	686	376	1,062	1,009	95.0
SCC	62	42	104	97	93.3
Total	748	418	1,166	1,106	94.8

[a]Most of the primary tumors were controlled and the few failures were salvaged by surgery. Of the 1,166 tumors, 745 (64%) were <2 cm in diameter.
Adapted from Fitzpatrick PJ. Skin cancer of the head—treatment by radiotherapy. *Int J Radiat Oncol Biol Phys* 1984;10:450.

TABLE 16.3 Carcinoma of the Eyelids, Pinna, and Nose Treated with Radiotherapy: Distribution of Patients and Treatment Failure by Lesion Size

Size	No. of Patients	Failures	%
<2 cm	602	42	7
2–5 cm	32	12	37
>5 cm	12	6	50
Total	646	60	9

Modified from Petrovich Z, Kuisk H, Langholz B, et al. Treatment results and patterns of failure in 646 patients with carcinoma of the eyelids, pinna, and nose. *Am J Surg* 1987;154:447.

Postoperative Radiotherapy

Target Volume

For stages II and III, the target volume encompasses the primary tumor bed and ipsilateral draining lymph nodes down to the supraclavicular nodes.

For nodal recurrence, the entire ipsilateral neck is included. The primary tumor bed is also irradiated if excision was carried out <1 year before the nodal recurrence.

Setup and Field Arrangement

Setup and field arrangement vary with the site of the primary lesion. Most patients are treated with electrons of appropriate energies **(Case Study 16.6)**. Patients are usually immobilized in an open neck position. Cutaneous melanoma of frontal, temporal, and preauricular areas, auricle, and cheek are usually treated with two or three fields depending on the distance between the primary and parotid nodes. A field, similar to that of parotid gland tumors, is used to irradiate intraparotid and upper neck nodes with 12-MeV electrons. This field covers most of the tumor beds of lesions arising in these locations. An adjoin-

ing field is added to irradiate the tumor bed with 6- to 9-MeV electrons if the site of the primary tumor is outside the boundary of the parotid field. A matching portal is used to treat the lower neck nodes, as described in the subsequent text.

Cutaneous melanoma of the nose and nasolabial fold is irradiated with the technique described for nasal vestibule, except that lower-energy electrons (<9 MeV) are used for the tumor bed. Field borders encompass nodal areas and the surgical bed with approximately 2-cm margins. Bolus is used to prevent underdosage to the primary tumor bed when 9-MeV electrons or lower-energy electrons are used.

An appositional electron or photon field may be used to treat the mid and lower neck nodes when indicated. The junctions between the fields are moved after the second and fourth radiation fractions to improve dose homogeneity.

Melanoma of some locations, such as lip or suboccipital region, may require irradiation with opposed–lateral photon portal **(Case Study 16.7)**. The use of missing tissue compensator or field-in-field technique is necessary in this setting to avoid hot spots, which can dramatically increase the risk of normal tissue injury by increasing both the fraction size and total dose ("double trouble").

CASE STUDY 16.6

A 51-year-old woman underwent excision of a 2.3-cm skin lesion located in the left cheek (Fig. 16.6). Histologic examination revealed a 6.5-mm thick malignant melanoma. She was referred for further treatment. Physical examination showed a 2-cm excision scar with surrounding erythema and a 1-cm left subdigastric node. Workup for distant metastasis was negative. She then underwent a wide re-excision of the skin of the left cheek along with a left superficial parotidectomy and supraomohyoid neck dissection. Examination of the specimens revealed presence of residual melanoma in the dermis of the cheek and metastatic deposit in three level II and one level III nodes. She received adjuvant radiotherapy to the tumor bed and ipsilateral neck nodes through two abutting appositional fields to a given dose of 30 Gy in 5 fractions (6 Gy per fraction). The left cheek and upper neck nodal basin were irradiated with 12-MeV electrons and the lower neck with 9-MeV electrons. Skin collimation was used around the eye and a 0.5-cm bolus was placed on the cheek. The field junction was moved twice during treatment. She did well until a right parietal brain metastasis was diagnosed 3 years later. There was no evidence of locoregional disease.

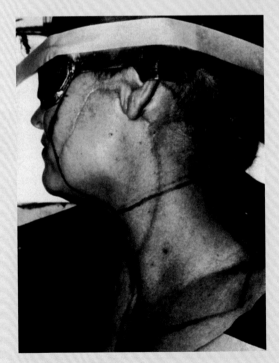

Case Figure 16.6

CASE STUDY 16.7

A 75-year-old man underwent repeated excisions of a lesion in the middle of the lower lip over a period of 1.5 years. Final diagnosis, after review of all slides, was melanoma, and the patient was referred for further therapy. Review of the record of the latest surgery revealed that the excision margin was microscopically positive. It was thought that wide excision would involve removal of most of the lower lip and, therefore, the patient was offered radiotherapy.

On physical examination, there was a scar in the center of the lower lip but no evidence of gross residual disease (Fig. 16.7A). There was no palpable adenopathy. An intraoral stent was used to separate the lips and to displace the tongue posteriorly and cranially (Fig. 16.7B,C).

The lower lip and bilateral upper neck nodes (i.e., submental, submandibular, and subdigastric) were irradiated through left and right parallel–opposed cobalt photon fields. Figure 16.7D shows that with the aid of the stent, the commissures (wired) and the oral tongue could be excluded from the portals. A maximum dose of 30 Gy was delivered in five fractions, twice a week, through the lateral fields. Following this, an additional fraction of 6 Gy was delivered to the tumor bed through an anterior appositional 8-MeV electron beam. A second intraoral stent was constructed; it served to flatten the lower lip and to open the mouth; in addition, lead alloy was inserted in the anterior part of the stent to shield the lower gum (Fig. 16.7E,F).

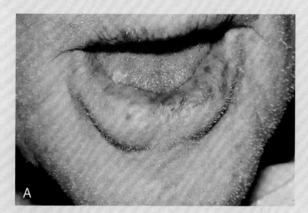

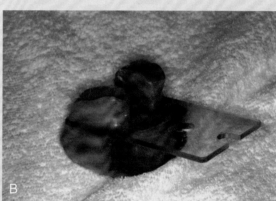

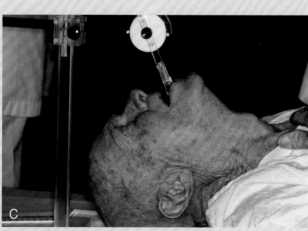

Case Figure 16.7 A–D

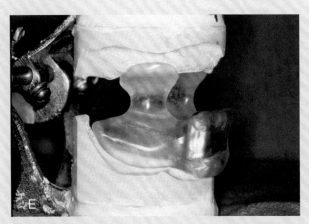

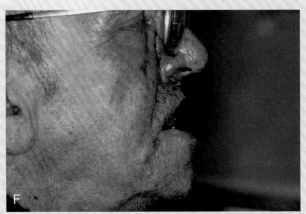

Case Figure 16.7 E,F

Dose

The dose consists of 30 Gy in 5 fractions, 2 fractions per week, for elective irradiation. An additional fraction of 6 Gy may be added to a total dose of 36 Gy in 6 fractions for residual disease **(Case Study 16.8)**. The dose is prescribed to 100% when given with electrons. An alternative dose/fractionation schedule used in a randomized trial is 48 Gy in 20 fractions.

Dose Specification: at D_{max}

The dose to the spinal cord or brachial plexus should not exceed 24 Gy in 4 fractions.

Background Data

See Table 16.4.

MERKEL CELL CARCINOMA

Treatment Strategy

The primary therapy for Merkel cell carcinoma is surgery to establish tissue diagnosis and resect primary tumor and nodal masses. Infrequently, Merkel cell carcinoma can be treated with definitive therapy, as these tumors are very radiosensitive **(Case study 16.9)**.

 CASE STUDY 16.8

A 50-year-old man presented with a melanoma located 2 cm below the right earlobe. It was excised with negative margins. Histologic review showed invasion into the subcutaneous tissue. An additional lesion adjacent to the scar was found and excised as well. This second lesion was a satellite metastasis invading connective tissue. He had no palpable lymphadenopathy. He received adjuvant radiation to the right neck delivered with 12-MeV electrons to a dose of 30 Gy given in 5 fractions. The patient was treated in an open neck position.

Figure 16.8 shows a representative axial isodose through the upper neck.

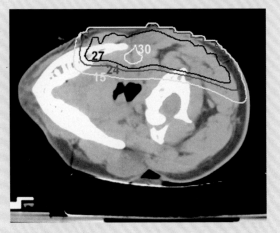

Case Figure 16.8

TABLE 16.4 Pattern of Failure after Elective or Adjuvant Radiotherapy for Cutaneous Melanoma

Status	D	N	D + N	DM	Median Follow-Up	Total
Elective[a]	4	10	5	57	68 mo	157
Adjuvant[b]	5	5	3	81	78 mo	160
Total	9	15	8	138	—	317

[a]Stage I or II cutaneous melanoma treated with wide local excision of the primary followed by elective regional radiation.
[b]Patients with cervical nodal metastases treated with surgery and radiation.
D, dermal recurrence; N, nodal relapse; DM, distant metastasis.
Data from Ballo MT, Bonnen MD, Garden AS, et al. Adjuvant irradiation for cervical lymph node metastases from melanoma. *Cancer* 2003;97:1789–1796; Bonnen MD, Ballo MT, Myers JN, et al. Elective radiotherapy provides regional control for patients with cutaneous melanoma of the head and neck. *Cancer* 2004;100:383–389.

CASE STUDY 16.9

This 63-year-old female presented with a left cheek nodule located approximately 2 cm inferior to the lateral canthus of the eye. A biopsy revealed Merkel cell carcinoma. She was treated with definitive radiation.

Rather than the traditional shrinking field techniques, she was treated with expanding fields. The rationale was that these lesions respond quickly, and as the boost fields are clinically set up, these small boost fields can be set up while the lesion is still visible. The plan was to deliver two sequential boosts to a total of 20 Gy, and then wider field therapy to the tumor and draining lymphatics to 46 Gy.

The initial boost was delivered with orthovoltage therapy. 6 Gy was delivered in 3 fractions using 125-kVp energy with a 4-cm cone. The cone is place on the skin with the tumor nodule in the center (Fig. 16.9A). The boost field was then expanded to treat the tumor with an approximate 2- to 3-mm margin. This was done with 6-MeV electrons and skin collimation. The margin is mainly circular in orientation but is squared off at the inferior eyelid (Fig. 16.9B). In addition to the lead collimation, an internal tungsten eye shield is used. Bolus is applied (Fig. 16.9C), 1 cm thick to ensure the skin receives the full dose, which in this case was 14 Gy in 7 fractions.

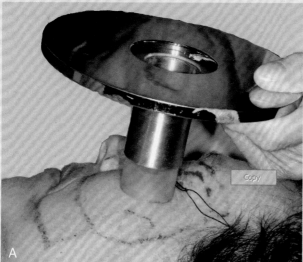
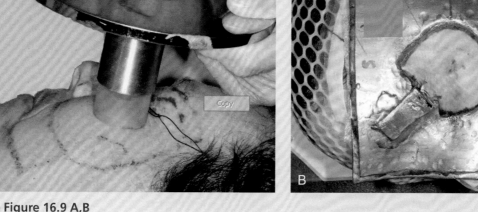

Case Figure 16.9 A,B

The final phase of therapy is delivered with four abutting fields to allow for an approximate 5-cm margin to the lesion and to treat the draining lymphatics (ipsilateral parotid, buccal facial, and cervical nodes). These fields are shown in Figure 16.9D on a rendered image. The purple, yellow, and green are skin renderings of three abutting electron fields. Due to the shape of the face, and to create fields that are approximately perpendicular to the skin to optimize the dosimetry throughout the entire width of the field, the purple field that covers the lesion and periorbital skin has a hinge angle of 160 degrees with the two other fields. While the yellow field covering the superior posterior skin and the green field covering the lymphatics

are oriented in the same plane, they are separated into two fields rather than one due to the skin field only requiring 6-MeV electrons, while the nodal field is treated with 12 MeV electrons. The periorbital skin field is also treated with 6-MeV electrons. The fourth field in red is a 6-MV photon field that treats the lower neck nodes. The superior border is set with a half beam block to minimize divergence. However, due to the dose uncertainty at all the matchlines of all four fields, the junctions between all fields were shifted twice throughout therapy to smooth out these uncertainties, particularly between the electron fields that converged into each other.

The patient remains well 2 years following therapy.

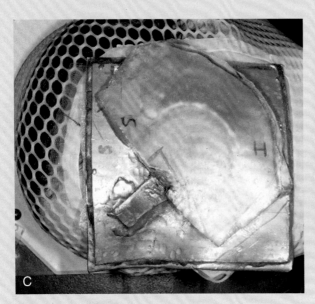
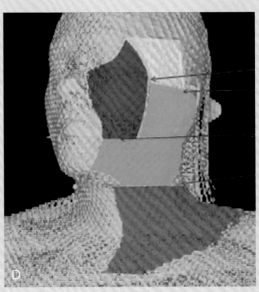

Case Figure 16.9 C,D

Adjuvant postoperative radiotherapy is recommended in most patients because the rate of locoregional relapse after surgery is high.

Postoperative Radiotherapy

Target Volume

The initial target volume encompasses the surgical bed with 4- to 5-cm margins, except when the lesion is situated at or close to crucial structures (e.g., optic apparatus) and the draining lymphatics. For Merkel cell carcinoma of the head and neck region, the whole ipsilateral neck is irradiated.

The boost volume encompasses areas of known disease with 1- to 2-cm margins.

Setup and Field Arrangement

Setup and field arrangement varies with the site of the primary lesion. Most patients are treated with electron beams of appropriate energies, with patients immobilized in an open

neck position, as described for cutaneous melanoma of the head and neck region. However, Merkel cell carcinomas may arise on the scalp, making treatment with electron therapy challenging. IMRT, particularly with VMAT (volumetric arc therapy), can provide the conformality required to treat the skin while minimizing dose to the brain and avoiding dose uncertainty created by matching fields **(Case Study 16.10)**.

Dose

The dose for the initial target volume is 46 Gy in 23 fractions.

The dose for the boost volume is 10 Gy in 5 fractions to the tumor bed, 14 Gy in 7 fractions to positive resection margins, or 20 Gy in 10 fractions to bulky macroscopic disease.

Dose Specification: See "General Principles"

Background Data

See Tables 16.5 and 16.6.

CASE STUDY 16.10

An 80-year-old male presented with a nodule on his left parietal scalp (Fig. 16.10A). Biopsy revealed Merkel cell carcinoma. In addition to the left scalp tumor, his staging revealed a left postauricular node consistent with metastatic spread.

Radiation was the chosen modality of therapy. The treatment was designed to treat the primary tumor with wide margin, and the draining lymphatics including occipital nodes, left parotid and periauricular nodes (including the gross node), and cervical nodes to a subclinical dose of 46 Gy in 23 fractions and boost the two small areas of gross disease to 66 Gy by delivering 20 Gy in 10 fractions to the two sites.

To deliver the 46 Gy to the large volume of scalp and neck, volumetric arc therapy (VMAT) was used. Representative views of the contours of the CTV (*red*), which included the GTV (*green*) and representative isodose lines, are shown in Figure 16.10B–D. Also, 5 mm bolus material is used to cover the target volume and can be seen on the figures. Thermoluminescent dosimetric (TLD) measurements are obtained for dose verification, due to the complexity of this therapy.

The patient is alive 5 years out of therapy. Despite contralateral parotid sparing, he had severe xerostomia, and ultimately required a permanent feeding tube.

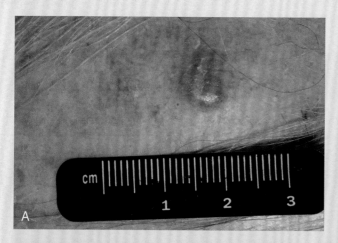

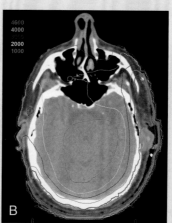

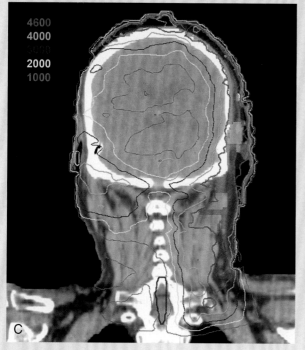

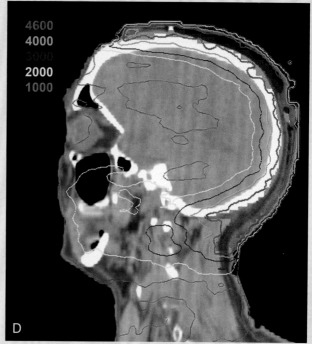

Case Figure 16.10 A–D

TABLE 16.5 Pattern of Failure of Merkel Cell Carcinoma by Treatment Methods

Method	No. of Patients	Local Recurrence	Regional Recurrence	Distant Recurrence	No. Recurrence
Surgery only	34	15 (44%)	29 (85%)	11 (32%)	1 (3%)
Surgery and radiation	26	3 (12%)	7 (27%)	11 (42%)	13 (50%)
Radiation only	6	1 (17%)	4 (44%)	2 (33%)	1 (17%)
P-value (radiation vs. no radiation)		0.01	<0.001	0.59	<0.001

Adapted from Gillenwater AM, Hessel AC, Morrison WH, et al. Merkel cell carcinoma of the head and neck: effect of surgical excision and radiation on recurrence and survival. *Arch Otolaryngol Head Neck Surg* 2001;127:149.

TABLE 16.6 Outcomes of Radiotherapy for Patients with Merkel Cell Carcinoma of the Head and Neck: Results from MD Anderson Cancer Center, 1988–2011

	Patient Number	5-Year Local Control	5-Year Regional Control	5-Year Overall Survival
All patients	106	96%	96%	58%
Node-positive patients	36		97%	
Node-positive patients treated with radiation for gross disease	22		100%	

Patients treated at MD Anderson Cancer Center 1988–2011. Adapted from Bishop AJ, et al. Merkel cell carcinoma of the head and neck: Favorable outcomes with radiotherapy. *Head Neck* 2016;38(Suppl 1):E452–E458.

SUGGESTED READINGS

Abbatucci JS, Boulier N, Laforge T, et al. Radiation therapy of skin carcinomas: results of a hypofractionated irradiation schedule in 675 cases followed more than 2 years. *Radiother Oncol* 1989;14:113.

Ballo MT, Bonnen MD, Garden AS, et al. Adjuvant irradiation for cervical lymph node metastases from melanoma. *Cancer* 2003;97:1789.

Bentzen SM, Overgaard J, Thames HD, et al. Clinical radiobiology of malignant melanoma. *Radiother Oncol* 1989;16:169.

Bishop AJ, Garden AS, Gunn GB, et al. Merkel cell carcinoma of the head and neck: favorable outcomes with radiotherapy. *Head Neck* 2016;38(suppl 1):E452.

Bonnen MD, Ballo MT, Myers JN, et al. Elective radiotherapy provides regional control for patients with cutaneous melanoma of the head and neck. *Cancer* 2004; 100:383.

Creagan ET, Cupps RE, Ivins JC, et al. Adjuvant radiation therapy for regional nodal metastases from malignant melanoma: a randomized, prospective study. *Cancer* 1978;42:2206.

de Wilt JH, Thompson JF, Uren RF, et al. Correlation between preoperative lymphoscintigraphy and metastatic nodal disease sites in 362 patients with cutaneous melanomas of the head and neck. *Ann Surg* 2004;239:544.

Fitzpatrick PJ. Skin cancer of the head—treatment by radiotherapy. *J Otolaryngol* 1984;13:261.

Fitzpatrick PJ. Radiation therapy for tumors of the skin of the head and neck. In: Thawley SE, Panje WR, eds. *Comprehensive management of head and neck tumors.* Philadelphia, PA: WB Saunders, 1987.

Fitzpatrick PJ, Thompson GA, Easterbrook WM, et al. Basal and squamous cell carcinoma of the eyelids and their treatment by radiotherapy. *Int J Radiat Oncol Biol Phys* 1984;10:449.

Guadagnolo BA, Prieto V, Weber R, et al. The role of adjuvant radiotherapy in the local management of desmoplastic melanoma. *Cancer* 2014;120:1361.

Henderson MA, Burmeister BH, Ainslie J, et al. Adjuvant lymph-node field radiotherapy versus observation only in patients with melanoma at high risk of further lymph-node field relapse after lymphadenectomy (ANZMTG 01.02/TROG 02.01): 6-year follow-up of a phase 3, randomised controlled trial. *Lancet Oncol* 2015;16:1049.

Herman MP, Amdur RJ, Werning JW, et al. Elective neck management for squamous cell carcinoma metastatic to the parotid area lymph nodes. *Eur Arch Otorhinolaryngol* 2016;273:3875–3879.

Hliniak A, Maciejewski B, Trott KR. The influence of the number of fractions, overall treatment time and field size on the local control of cancer of the skin. *Br J Radiol* 1983;56:596.

Kearsley JH, Harris TJ, Bourne RG. Radiotherapy for superficial skin cancer at the Queensland Radium Institute: famine in the land of plenty. *Int J Radiat Oncol Biol Phys* 1988;15:995.

Mendenhall WM, Ferlit A, Takes RP, et al. Cutaneous head and neck basal and squamous cell carcinomas with perineural invasion. *Oral Oncol* 2012;48:912.

Morrison WH, Garden AS, Ang KK. Radiation therapy for nonmelanoma skin carcinomas. *Clin Plast Surg* 1997;24:719.

O'Brien CJ, Petersen-Schaefer K, Stevens G, et al. Adjuvant radiotherapy following neck dissection and parotidectomy for metastatic malignant melanoma. *Head Neck* 1997;19:589.

Overgaard J, Hansen PV, Von der Maase H. Some factors of importance in the radiation treatment of malignant melanoma. *Radiother Oncol* 1986;5:183.

Petrovich Z, Kuisk H, Langholz B, et al. Treatment results and patterns of failure in 646 patients with carcinoma of the eyelids, pinna, and nose. *Am J Surg* 1987; 154:447.

Petrovich Z, Parker R, Luxton G, et al. Carcinoma of the lip and selected sites of head and neck skin. A clinical study of 896 patients. *Radiother Oncol* 1987;8:11.

Porceddu SV, Veness MJ, Guminski A. Nonmelanoma cutaneous head and neck cancer and Merkel cell carcinoma: Current concepts, advances and controversies. *J Clin Oncol* 2015;33:3338.

Sause WT, Cooper JS, Rush S, et al. Fraction size in external beam radiation therapy in the treatment of melanoma. *Int J Radiat Oncol Biol Phys* 1991;20:429.

Silva JJ, Tsang RW, Panzarella T, et al. Results of radiotherapy for epithelial skin cancer of the pinna: the Princess Margaret Hospital experience, 1982–1993. *Int J Radiat Oncol Biol Phys* 2000;47:451.

Stevens G, Thompson JF, Firth I, et al. Locally advanced melanoma: results of postoperative hypofractionated radiation therapy. *Cancer* 2000;88:88.

Strom T, Naghavi AO, Messina JL, et al. Improved local and regional control with radiotherapy for Merkel cell carcinoma of the head and neck. *Head Neck* 2017;39: 48–55.

Tapley N. Radiation therapy with the electron beam. *Semin Oncol* 1981;8:49.

Tapley N, Fletcher GH. Applications of the electron beam in the treatment of cancer of the skin and lips. *Radiology* 1973;109:423.

Trott KR, Maciejewski B, Preuss-Bayer G, et al. Dose–response curve and split-dose recovery in human skin cancer. *Radiother Oncol* 1984;2:123.

17

Neck Node Metastasis from Unknown Primary

Key Points

- A thorough search for a primary site is a requisite part of the staging workup and should include an examination under anesthesia, appropriate biopsies of subsites within the pharyngeal axis, and/or tonsillectomy.

- Radiation is recommended in either the frontline or the adjuvant setting to obtain or maintain regional control.

- In the absence of randomized trials, radiation target volumes remain controversial. Many centers recommend comprehensive treatment to bilateral neck lymphatics and putative sources of the primary site, principally the nasopharynx and oropharynx with or without the hypopharynx.

- Early data of IMRT suggest favorable outcomes with regard to disease control and reduced toxicity.

TREATMENT STRATEGY

The diagnosis is usually established by a nodal biopsy or aspiration, which should be followed by an examination under anesthesia, with biopsy of suspicious potential primary sites. Tonsillectomy is usually performed in the absence of suspicious lesions. Historically, after completion of the workup, a neck dissection was performed often followed by postoperative radiation when more than one node is involved, particularly in the presence of extranodal extension. The more common practice today, as many patients present with human papillomavirus (HPV)-associated disease, is to begin with radiation, with concurrent chemotherapy in the presence of large nodal volume or CT evidence of extranodal extension, and perform a neck dissection if the nodal disease does not regress completely. Many centers currently recommend irradiation to the pharyngeal axis and the bilateral neck. Some favor omitting the larynx and hypopharynx, particularly if the disease is HPV associated. Intensity-modulated radiation therapy (IMRT) may allow comprehensive bilateral therapy while providing parotid sparing.

Irradiation to the ipsilateral neck alone is indicated if the histologic findings (e.g., adenocarcinoma) or nodal location (e.g., submental, submandibular, supraclavicular) indicate a low probability of a primary along the pharyngeal axis. It may also be considered when, because of advanced age or poor medical condition, the patient is not expected to tolerate large-volume irradiation to the pharyngeal axis, but residual disease is present or the probability of progression in the neck is high (e.g., presence of extracapsular nodal disease).

Close observation can be considered in patients who had neck dissection, which reveals low risk for recurrence (i.e., a single lymph node <3 cm without extracapsular extension [ECE]).

COMPREHENSIVE RADIOTHERAPY

Target Volume

Initial Target Volume

The initial target volume is composed of oropharynx, nasopharynx, and bilateral neck nodes when the clinical or histologic features suggest primary site origin from the oropharynx or nasopharynx. For example, a nonsmoker with a level II node, particularly with cystic squamous cell carcinoma, nonkeratinizing "nasopharyngeal-like," or undifferentiated carcinoma or carcinoma that is positive by HPV in situ hybridization or p16 immunohistochemical assay would strongly favor an oropharyngeal primary tumor. The presence of involved upper posterior cervical (level V) nodes suggests a nasopharyngeal primary.

In other cases, the initial target volume encompasses nasopharynx, oropharynx, hypopharynx, and bilateral neck nodes **(Case Study 17.1 and Case Study 17.2)**.

The boost or high-dose volume encompasses the involved nodal bed.

Setup and Field Arrangement

The patient is immobilized in a supine position with a thermoplastic mask. Marking of surgical scar facilitates portal design. For 3-D radiotherapy, the initial target volume is irradiated with lateral–opposed photon fields.

- *Superior border:* at midsphenoid sinus or at the bottom of the pituitary fossa to encompass the roof of the nasopharynx
- *Anterior border:* include posterior third of the nasal cavities and the anterior tonsillar pillars; 1-cm falloff for the dissected neck
- *Posterior border:* behind the spinous processes or more posteriorly to encompass the scar
- *Inferior border:* just above the arytenoids or below the cricoid cartilage, depending on whether the hypopharynx is part of the target volume

CASE STUDY 17.1

A 67-year-old man consulted his physician for mild hoarseness. He was found to have leukoplakia on both true vocal cords. Examination of the neck revealed a 2-cm mobile lymph node in the right midjugular region. A fine-needle aspiration from this node showed poorly differentiated squamous cell carcinoma. A computed tomography (CT) scan confirmed the lymphadenopathy in the right jugular chain. An examination under anesthesia showed no abnormalities except for leukoplakia on both true vocal cords. Biopsy specimens were taken from the nasopharynx, tonsils, base of tongue, and both true vocal cords. All results were negative for malignancy. The biopsy specimens of the vocal cords showed only hyperkeratosis. The patient then underwent a right modified radical neck dissection. Histologic examination showed poorly differentiated squamous cell carcinoma in two of the 13 lymph nodes, one located in the midjugular area and the other one at the midposterior cervical chain. There was ECE from the midjugular node (stage: T0 N2b M0). Subsequently, this patient received postoperative radiotherapy.

The entire pharyngeal axis and the upper and mid neck were treated bilaterally with opposed–lateral fields, as shown in Figure 17.1. The lower neck nodes were treated with an anterior appositional field. A total dose of 54 Gy was delivered, and then, the right neck received an additional irradiation dose of 63 Gy with an appositional electron field.

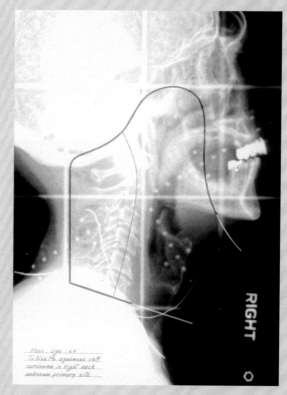

Case Figure 17.1

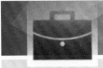

CASE STUDY 17.2

A 50-year-old man presented with bilateral cervical adenopathy (multiple left neck nodes and a 1.5-cm right neck node). He underwent an examination under anesthesia, which did not reveal any primary tumor. Biopsy specimens of both tonsils, the nasopharynx, base of tongue, vallecula, and pyriform sinuses were negative for neoplasm. The patient then underwent bilateral neck dissections. The left neck dissection revealed four of 34 nodes positive for poorly differentiated carcinoma (levels 2 and 3), whereas the right neck dissection was negative for metastases (stage: T0 pN2b M0). He received radiotherapy to both necks and the pharyngeal axis.

Figure 17.2A shows a digitally reconstructed radiograph of the opposed–lateral field. Radiation was delivered with 6-MV photons in 1.8-Gy fractions to a dose of 54 Gy, with an off–spinal cord reduction to 41.4 Gy. A 3-mm tissue equivalent bolus material was placed over the scar. The posterior strips were supplemented with 9-MeV electron beams. Wedges were used to obtain a more homogenous distribution. Isodose distribution of the parallel photon beams at the level of the upper (Fig. 17.2B) and mid necks (Fig. 17.2C) is shown. The low neck was treated with a separate anterior field.

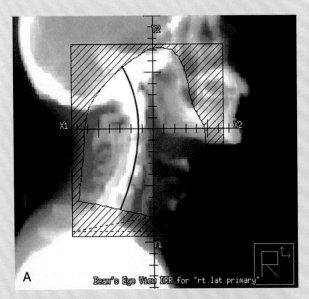

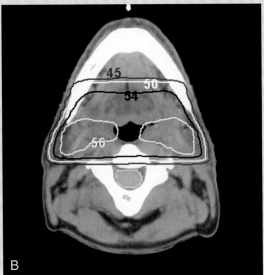

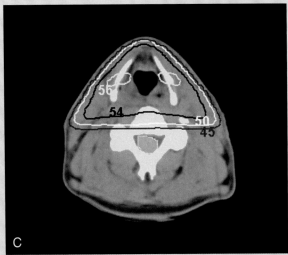

Case Figure 17.2A–C

A matching anterior appositional photon field is used to treat the cervical and supraclavicular nodes below the lateral portals. The boost dose is usually delivered through one or two lateral appositional electron fields. The electron energies are selected based on the depth required to reach the target bed. If the depth is beyond the reach of electrons, glancing photon fields can be used.

Dose

The dose to the initial target volume is 54 Gy in 30 fractions. A boost dose is delivered to the nodal bed at risk. The boost dose is an additional 6 to 10 Gy in 3 to 5 fractions in the postoperative setting. The boost dose can be delivered as a concomitant boost as second daily fractions, with a minimal interval of 6 hours, during the last week of the basic treatment course. In cases of gross nodal disease, a boost dose of 16 Gy in 8 fractions (or in 10 fractions if boost dose is given as second daily fractions) is delivered.

Intensity-Modulated Radiation Therapy Planning

Most patients are now treated with IMRT to spare parotid function **(Case Study 17.3 through Case Study 17.6)**. In the event of gross nodal disease, the nodes with 1-cm margin are outlined as high-dose clinical target volume (CTV$_{HD}$). The neck compartments outside CTV$_{HD}$ with a

CASE STUDY 17.3

A 50-year-old man, with no history of tobacco consumption, presented with an asymptomatic left neck mass. A fine-needle aspiration of this mass revealed squamous cell carcinoma. An examination under anesthesia, with biopsies of the larynx, base of tongue, pharyngeal wall, and nasopharynx, revealed normal-appearing mucosa. CT scan showed two enlarged lymph nodes in level II with additional subcentimeter nodes (stage: T0 N2b M0).

He was treated with IMRT to a dose of 66 Gy to the involved nodes with margin (CTV$_{HD}$—*red*), 60 Gy to the remaining uninvolved ipsilateral upper neck nodes (CTV$_{ID}$—*green*), and 54 Gy to clinically uninvolved contralateral nodes and mucosa of the pharyngeal axis (CTV$_{ED}$—*yellow*) in 30 fractions. The spinal cord dose was limited to <45 Gy.

Figure 17.3 shows CTVs at the levels of the nasopharynx (Fig. 17.3A); superior base of tongue, tonsillar fossae, soft palate, and retropharyngeal nodes anterior to C1 vertebra (Fig. 17.3B); midtongue base, tonsillar fossae, and left level II nodal region (Fig. 17.3C); and inferior base of tongue and bilateral level II nodal level (Fig. 17.3D). Figure 17.3E–G shows axial, sagittal, and coronal dose distributions, respectively.

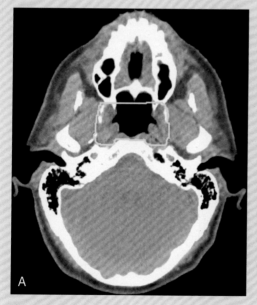
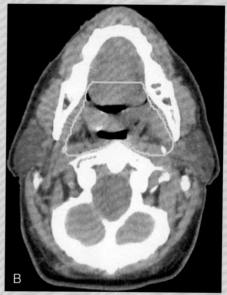

Case Figure 17.3A,B
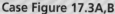

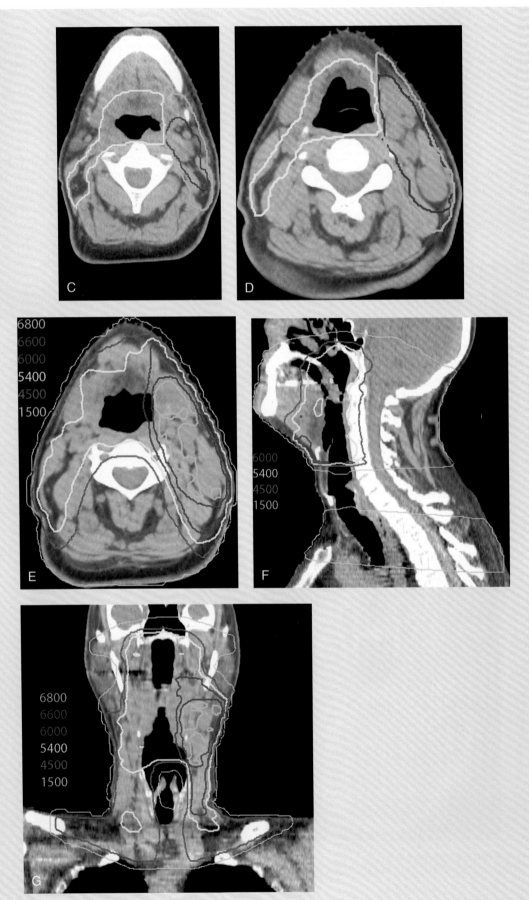

Case Figure 17.3C–G

CASE STUDY 17.4

A 56-year-old man presented with T0 N2b squamous cell carcinoma of the left neck and received IMRT. The involved nodes and margin were outlined as CTV_{HD} (69 Gy), the margins around CTV_{HD} as CTV_{ID} (60 Gy), and the pharyngeal axis (bilateral tonsils, base of tongue, posterior wall), junction of oropharynx and hypopharynx (including vallecula and vestibules of the pyriform sinuses), larynx, and remaining cervical nodes as CTV_{ED} (54 Gy).

Figure 17.4A shows contours delineated on an axial image at nodal level III. The larynx was outlined as a separate CTV_{ED} to allow for the flexibility of planning to minimize hot spots in this structure. Figure 17.4B–D shows isodose distributions at axial sections through the levels of the inferior nasopharynx, the midoropharynx, and the junction of oropharynx and hypopharynx (including vallecula and vestibules of the pyriform sinuses), respectively. The contralateral (*right*) jugular fossa was excluded in the target to allow more sparing of the contralateral parotid gland. CTV_{HD} received 66 Gy with IMRT and then supplemented with 3 Gy in two fractions by appositional 12-MeV electrons (delivered as a second daily fraction). Lower nodal levels III and IV were treated with a matched anterior beam to 50 Gy (with a small midline block to 40 Gy and a full midline block for the remaining 10 Gy). The patient showed complete response and did not undergo neck dissection. He remains without disease for 3½ years and has only grade 1 xerostomia.

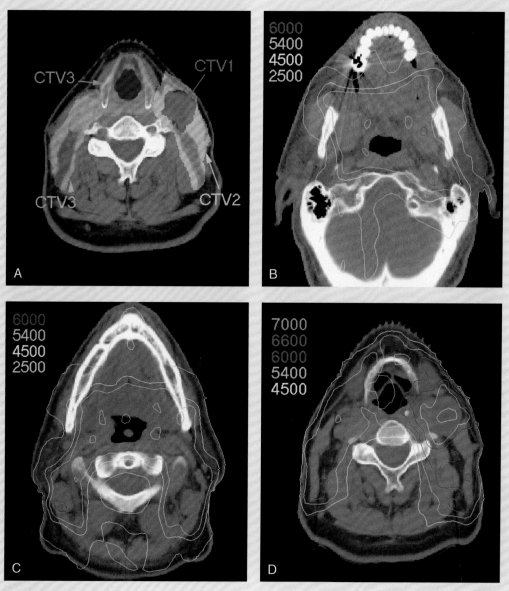

Case Figure 17.4A–D

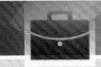

CASE STUDY 17.5

A 66-year-old man, former smoker, presented with right level II adenopathy. He underwent an examination under anesthesia with bilateral tonsillectomies, biopsies of both sides of the nasopharynx and base of tongue as well as the right pyriform sinus, and a right neck dissection. All the results of the mucosal biopsies (including the tonsil specimens) were negative, and the neck dissection revealed squamous cell carcinoma in two level II nodes (largest node measuring 3 cm). He was treated with postoperative IMRT, which was delivered to the entire cervical lymphatics (including level IV and supraclavicular nodes) in 30 fractions.

Contours and isodose distribution are shown on a coronal image (Fig. 17.5). CTV_{HD}, encompassing the right level IIA region with margin, received a dose of 60 Gy (*blue* contour). An additional dose of 4 Gy in 2 fractions was delivered to level II nodal region, with 12-MeV electron beam. The remaining dissected right neck (CTV_{ID}) received a dose of 57 Gy (*maize*). The left neck, pharyngeal axis, and larynx were defined as CTV_{ED} and received a dose of 54 Gy. CTV_{ED} was outlined as three separate structures for flexibility of planning. Notably, portions of the larynx received a slightly lower (within 5%) dose.

He is without disease over 3 years from his treatment. He does have corrected chemical hypothyroidism and minimal xerostomia.

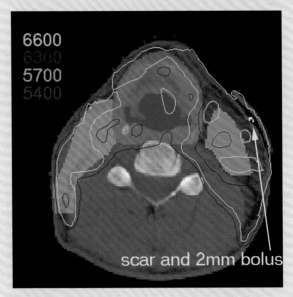

Case Figure 17.5

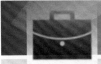

CASE STUDY 17.6

A 45-year-old man presented with a 4-cm left neck mass. It was thought to be a branchial cleft cyst and was excised. Histologic examination, however, revealed squamous cell carcinoma. Complete workup showed no primary lesion, and he was treated with IMRT.

An axial CT image is shown with contours and isodose distribution (Fig. 17.6). CTV_{HD} (*green*), delineated on the basis of original imaging, received a dose of 63 Gy. CTV_{ID} (*purple*) represented margin around the involved nodal bed that encompassed the nodal levels at higher risk. The contour was drawn to just under the skin surface at the surgical scar (*wired*), and bolus was applied for treatment planning. CTV_{ED} included the contralateral neck nodes (*maize*) and putative mucosal sites (*blue*) at the level shown. The doses delivered to CTV_{ID} and CTV_{ED} were 57 and 54 Gy, respectively, in 30 fractions.

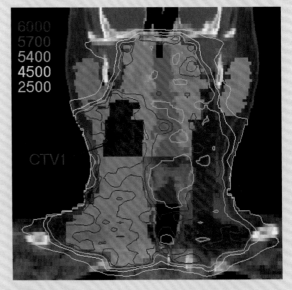

Case Figure 17.6

2-cm margin are delineated as CTV_{ID}. The remaining ipsilateral nodal levels (IB, II, III, IV, and V) on the ipsilateral side, retropharyngeal nodes, and contralateral nodal levels II to IV are contoured as CTV_{ED}. The pharyngeal axis (including the hypopharynx and larynx when indicated) is also delineated as CTV_{ED}.

When treating the pharyngeal axis and bilateral necks, IMRT dosing is typically in 30 fractions, with CTV_{HD}, CTV_{ID}, and CTV_{LD} prescribed 66 Gy, 60 Gy, and 54 Gy, respectively. Bulky adenopathy can be boosted to 70 Gy in 1 or 2 additional fractions with either electron beams or IMRT. Alternatively, CTV_{HD} can be treated to 70 Gy in 33 fractions, with an additional 2 Gy to CTV_{ID} and CTV_{LD}.

In cases where the nodal disease has been surgically excised, the original involved nodal bed with a 1- to 2-cm margin is outlined as CTV_{HD}, the remaining dissected neck is outlined as CTV_{ID}, and CTV_{ED} is similar to the definitive setting.

In the postoperative setting, the prescribed doses are 60 Gy to CTV_{HD} (smaller higher-risk regions may receive 63 to 66 Gy), 57 Gy to CTV_{ID}, and 54 Gy to CTV_{ED}. In the presence of extensive ECE or after only nodal excision, a smaller volume may receive a slightly higher dose **(Case Study 17.5)**. A thin bolus may be used when the nodal disease is close to the skin **(Case Study 17.6)**.

Intensity-modulated proton therapy (IMPT) can also be used to treat patients with carcinoma metastatic to the neck, with a theoretical benefit of reducing the toxicity associated with low and intermediate dose to normal tissues outside the large target volumes **(Case Study 17.7)**.

There are clinical situations when the benefits to comprehensive radiation to both sides of the neck (with only ipsilateral disease), and mucosal irradiation may be minimal in relation to the additional toxicity. In these situations, treatment to the involved neck may be a better alternative for the patient **(Case Study 17.8)**.

Dose Specification

See "General Principles."

Background Data

See Tables 17.1 to 17.3.

CASE STUDY 17.7

A 64-year-old female (never smoker) presented with an otherwise asymptomatic left upper neck lump. CT neck with contrast showed an enhancing, solid left jugulodigastric lymph node measuring 2.3 cm (Fig. 17.7A, *white arrows*). Fine-needle aspiration of this mass revealed squamous carcinoma, positive for p16 and high-risk HPV type 16. Clinical exam and PET/CT showed no additional lesions. She underwent examination under anesthesia, direct laryngoscopy, bilateral tonsillectomy, and directed biopsies of the nasopharynx and base of tongue, which failed to reveal primary site.

She was treated with definitive radiation therapy using a combination of active scanning and passive scatter proton beam. The positive lymph node in the left upper neck was treated to 69.3 Gy (radiobiologic equivalent [RBE]) in 33 fractions. She was initially treated with an IMPT plan using multifield optimization technique. The left upper neck lymph node with margin (CTV_{HD}) was treated to 63 Gy(RBE), the remainder of the left level 2 (CTV_{ID}) to 60 Gy(RBE), and the nasopharynx, oropharynx axis and bilateral neck (CTV_{ED}) to 54 Gy(RBE). This first phase of treatment was accomplished with a single integrated IMPT plan in 30 fractions. The neck volume in CTV_{ED} included left neck levels 1b through 5, right neck levels 2 through 4, and the bilateral lateral retropharyngeal lymph nodes.

Then, the left upper neck lymph node (with margin) was boosted an additional 6.3 Gy(RBE) delivered in 3 fractions using a passive scatter technique, bringing the total dose to the involved lymph node to 69.3. The CTVs and IMPT dose distributions are shown and Figure 17.7B–E. The passive scatter proton boost is shown in Figure 17.7F and a composite plan dose distributions in Figure 17.7G. Figure 17.7F highlights the sharp distal falloff of proton therapy and Figure 17.7E the anterior oral cavity sparing.

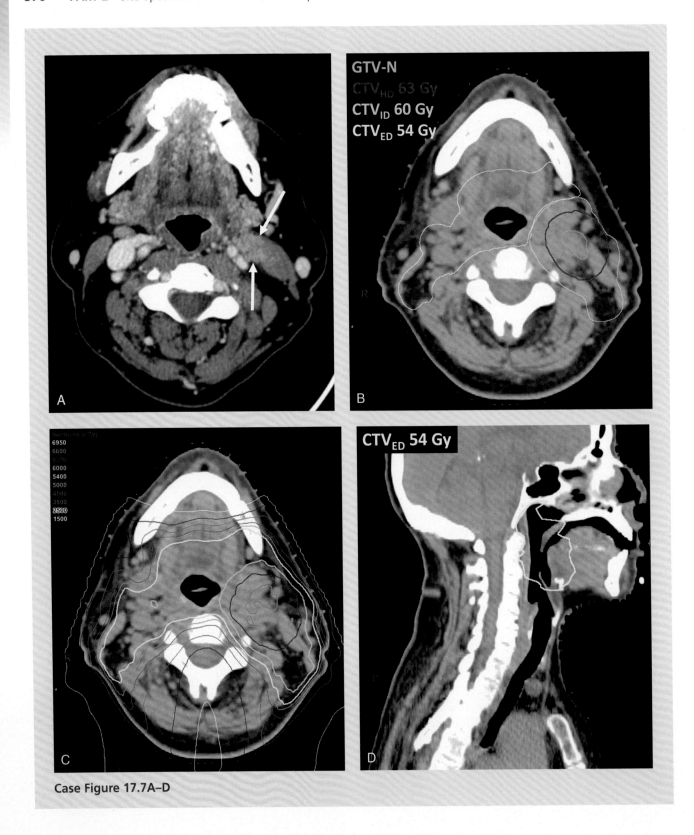

GTV-N
CTV_HD 63 Gy
CTV_ID 60 Gy
CTV_ED 54 Gy

CTV_ED 54 Gy

Case Figure 17.7A–D

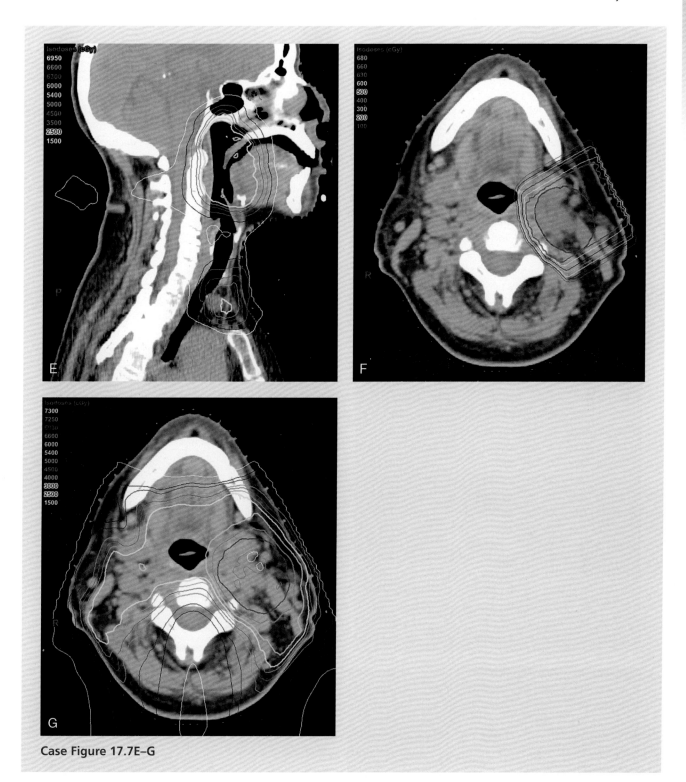

Case Figure 17.7E–G

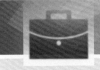

CASE STUDY 17.8

A 66-year-old male with a history of significant cigarette exposure presented with a fixed right neck mass. Fine-needle aspiration confirmed squamous cell cancer, but the tissue specimen was inadequate to determine markers. Clinically, the node palpated to >6 cm, so his staging was T0N3. Imaging did not reveal a primary source and did show that the node was unresectable due to carotid encasement. An examination under anesthesia was performed and his right tonsil felt indurated. However, the biopsy of the tonsil was negative for carcinoma.

It was elected to treat this patient's neck only. However, due to the proximity of the clinically suspicious tonsil to the neck mass, and with PTV expansion of the CTV_{HD} (CTV_{70}), it was believed that much of the tonsil would receive high dose regardless, so it was decided to include the entirety of the tonsil in a subclinical CTV_{66}.

Four CTVs were delineated. Figure 17.8A shows the target delineation on an axial slice through the gross node. CTV_{70} is in *red*, covering the node with margin, CTV_{66} in *magenta* includes the adjacent rim of tonsil, and CTV_{60} in *blue* covers subclinical nodal beds anterior and posterior to CTV_{70}. Figure 17.8B is an axial slice just superior to the nodal disease. CTV_{70} represents the 1-cm expansion above the GTV of the node, CTV_{66} is the adjacent tonsillar bed, and CTV_{60} is the high posterior nodal

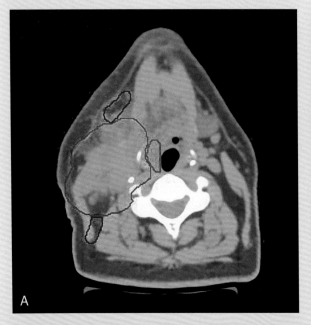

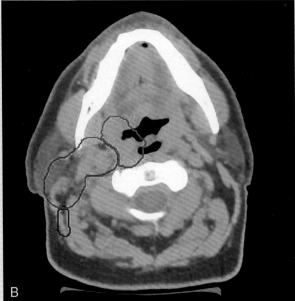

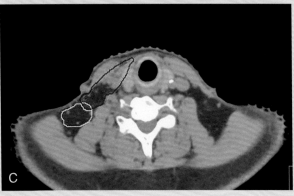

Case Figure 17.8A–C

space. Figure 17.8C is an axial contour through level 4 of the neck demonstrating CTV_{60} covering level 4a within 2 cm of CTV_{70} and CTV_{56} in yellow covering level 5b.

Figure 17.8D shows the isodose distributions on an axial slice just superior to Figure 17.8A with CTVs in color wash. Figure 17.8E is a coronal view without CTVs through the gross node. The patient was treated in 33 fractions with concurrent weekly cisplatin and was without evidence of disease at last follow-up.

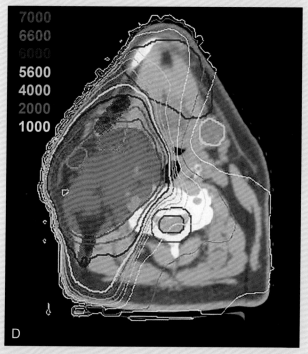

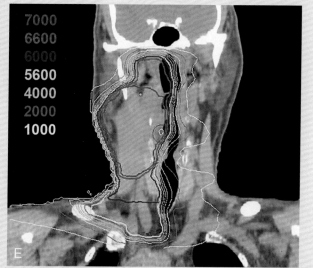

Case Figure 17.8D,E

TABLE 17.1 Therapy Failures by Neck Surgery and Irradiation Technique

Irradiation Site	Incisional Biopsy	Excisional Biopsy	Modified Neck Dissection	Radical Neck Dissection	Total
Neck only	0/2	2/4	1/6	4/8	7/20
Nasopharynx and oropharynx	1/11	0/3	1/6	2/6	4/26
Nasopharynx, oropharynx, and hypopharynx	1/10	0/15	2/12	0/10	3/47
Total	2/23	2/22	4/24	6/24	14/93

Note: The 14 patients who failed therapy are shown by both the type of surgical procedure performed and the irradiation technique used. A greater proportion of patients failed after having received irradiation to the neck only (7/20), as compared to those treated to the naso-oropharynx (4/26) or nasopharynx, oropharynx, and hypopharynx (3/47). No correlation is seen between the incidence of failure and the type of surgery used.
From Carlson LS, Fletcher GH, Oswald MJ. Guidelines for radiotherapeutic techniques for cervical metastases from an unknown primary. *Int J Radiat Oncol Biol Phys* 1986;12:2101–2110, with permission.

TABLE 17.2 Regional Failure and Mucosal Site Occurrence: Literature Review

First Author (Year)	No. of Patients	Neck Treatment	Regional Failure	Radiation Technique	Primary Site Occurrence
Grau (2000)	250	X—224	X—50%	M—224	M—13%
		X + S—26	X + S—38% (5-yr a)	N—26	N—23%
Wallace (2011)	179	X—70	X—73%	M—174	8%
		X + S—109	X + S—82% (5-yr a)	N—5	
Weir (1995)	144	X—144	X—49% (5-yr a)	M—59	M—2%
				N—85	N—7%
Colletier (1998)	136	X + S—136	X + S—9% (c)	M—120	8%
				N—16	
Maulard (1992)	113	X + S—113	X + S—14% (c)	M—113	10%
Ligey (2009)	95	X + S—95 (16 sampled)	A—31% (c)	M—36	M—6%
				N—59	N—12%
Boscolo-Rizzo (2007)	90	X + S—90	A—31% (5-yr a)	M—90	9%
Marcial-Vega (1990)	72	X—41	X—54% (c)	M—53	M—25%
		X + S—31	X + S—58%	N—19	N—16%
Patel (2007)	70	S—19	A—20%	N—60	11%
		X + S—60			

X, radiation alone (following biopsy); X + S, radiation and neck dissection; A, all patients; M, radiation to bilateral necks and mucosal sites; N, radiation to the involved neck only; 5-yr a, 5-year actuarial; c, crude rate.

TABLE 17.3 Results of IMRT for the Treatment of Carcinoma Metastatic to the Neck from Unknown Primary

First Author (Year)	Patient Number	Median Follow-up (Months)	Regional Progression-Free Survival
Klem (2008)	21	24	90% (2-yr)
Madani (2008)	23	17	91% (crude)
Lu (2009)	18	35	89% (2-yr)
Frank (2010)	52	44	94% (5-yr)
Chen (2010)	27	25	92%[a] (2-yr)
Mourad (2014)	68	42	96% (3-yr)

[a]Local–regional control.

SUGGESTED READINGS

Boscolo-Rizzo P, Gava A, Da Mosto MC. Carcinoma metastatic to cervical lymph nodes from an unknown primary tumor: the outcome after combined modality therapy. *Ann Surg Oncol* 2007;14:1575.

Chen AM, Li BQ, Farwell DG, et al. Improved dosimetric and clinical outcomes with intensity-modulated radiotherapy for head-and-neck cancer of unknown primary origin. *Int J Radiat Oncol Biol Phys* 2010;79(3):756–762.

Colletier PJ, Garden AS, Morrison WH, et al. Postoperative radiation for squamous cell carcinoma metastatic to cervical lymph nodes from an unknown primary site: outcomes and patterns of failure. *Head Neck* 1998;20:674–681.

Coster JR, Foote RL, Olsen KD, et al. Cervical node metastasis of squamous cell carcinoma of unknown origin: indications for withholding radiation therapy. *Int J Radiat Oncol Biol Phys* 1992;23:743.

Dixon PR, Au M, Hosni A, et al. Impact of p16 expression, nodal status, and smoking on oncologic outcomes of patients with head and neck unknown primary squamous cell carcinoma. *Head Neck* 2016;38(9):1347–1353.

Frank SJ, Rosenthal DI, Petsuksiri J, et al. Intensity-modulated radiotherapy for cervical node squamous cell carcinoma metastases from unknown head-and-neck primary Site: M. D. Anderson Cancer Center outcomes and patterns of failure. *Int J Radiat Oncol Biol Phys* 2010;78(4):1005–1010.

Friesland S, Lind MG, Lundgren J, et al. Outcome of ipsilateral treatment for patients with metastases to neck nodes of unknown origin. *Acta Oncol* 2001;40:24.

Galloway TJ, Ridge JA. Management of squamous cancer metastatic to cervical lymph nodes with an unknown primary site. *J Clin Oncol* 2015;33:3328

Grau C, Johansen L, Jakobsen J, et al. Cervical lymph node metastases from unknown primary tumours. Results from a national survey by the Danish Society for Head and Neck Oncology. *Radiother Oncol* 2000;55:121.

Klem ML, Mechalakos JG, Wolden SL, et al. Intensity-modulated radiotherapy for head and neck cancer of unknown primary: toxicity and preliminary efficacy. *Int J Radiat Oncol Biol Phys* 2008;70:1100.

Ligey A, Gentil J, Crehange G, et al. Impact of target volumes and radiation technique on loco-regional control and survival for patients with unilateral cervical lymph node metastases from an unknown primary. *Radiother Oncol* 2009;93:483.

Lu H, Yao M, Tan H. Unknown primary head and neck cancer treated with intensity-modulated radiation therapy: to what extent the volume should be irradiated. *Oral Oncol* 2009;45:474.

Madani I, Vakaet L, Bonte K, et al. Intensity-modulated radiotherapy for cervical lymph node metastases from unknown primary cancer. *Int J Radiat Oncol Biol Phys* 2008;71:1158.

Marcial-Vega VA, Cardenes H, Perez CA, et al. Cervical metastases from unknown primaries: radiotherapeutic management and appearance of subsequent primaries. *Int J Radiat Oncol Biol Phys* 1990;19:919.

Maulard C, Housset M, Brunel P, et al. Postoperative radiation therapy for cervical lymph node metastases from an occult squamous cell carcinoma. *Laryngoscope* 1992;102:884.

Mourad WF, Hu KS, Shasha D, et al. Initial experience with oropharynx-targeted radiation therapy for metastatic squamous cell carcinoma of unknown primary of the head and neck. *Anticacer Res* 2014;34:243.

Patel RS, Clark J, Wyten R, et al. Squamous cell carcinoma from an unknown head and neck primary site: a "selective treatment" approach. *Arch Otolaryngol Head Neck Surg* 2007;133:1282.

Strasnick B, Moore DM, Abemayor E, et al. Occult primary tumors. The management of isolated submandibular lymph node metastases. *Arch Otolaryngol Head Neck Surg* 1990;116:173.

Wallace A, Richards GM, Harari PM, et al. Head and neck squamous cell carcinoma from an unknown primary site. *Am J Otolaryngol* 2011;32:286.

Weir L, Keane T, Cummings B, et al. Radiation treatment of cervical lymph node metastases from an unknown primary: an analysis of outcome by treatment volume and other prognostic factors. *Radiother Oncol* 1995;35:206.

18

Treatment of Locoregional Recurrence

Key Points

- Historically, reirradiation for recurrent local or regional disease has been widely discouraged because of concerns of inducing severe complications, including soft tissue and bone necrosis, neurologic deficits, and carotid injury.

- Case series employing modern techniques suggest that reirradiation may be feasible, with durable control, in carefully selected patients. Concern for toxicity remains heightened in this patient population but, in the absence of other curative options, may be considered acceptable after diligent discussion with the patient about expectations and potentially catastrophic complications.

- The use of advanced techniques to minimize dose to previously treated normal tissues is paramount; IMRT, VMAT, proton therapy, SBRT, and brachytherapy may be used to this end.

- In any situation, special attention must be given to minimize dose to critical normal tissues, including the brainstem and spinal cord. If the recurrent disease warrants retreatment of other areas, including the carotid vessels, brachial plexus, or ocular structures, the patient must understand the potential consequences.

- For patients with resectable disease, the recommendation is to proceed with resection and provide adjuvant reirradiation if indicated by significant adverse pathologic features, including positive margins or extensive soft tissue disease.

- For patients with unresectable disease, concurrent chemotherapy is recommended with reirradiation, unless medically contraindicated. Phase II experiences of concurrent chemoreirradiation suggest that this approach is feasible in carefully selected patients and can yield modest long-term control rate; however, complications may be severe.

- In addition to the general indications for radiation, the interval from the first radiation course and the health of the tissues to be reirradiated should be considered in the decision-making process. Reirradiation is strongly discouraged if the interval between the two courses is <6 months.

REIRRADIATION FOR LOCOREGIONAL RECURRENCE

Reirradiation has emerged as a feasible, albeit high risk, treatment for locoregional recurrence of head and neck cancer. Even in the modern era, a proportion of patients treated definitively will have recurrence in the previously irradiated area; the appropriate salvage treatment remains controversial, given concerns for both short- and long-term complications and quality of life. While the focus of this chapter will be on recurrences, similar principles apply to patients who develop second primary tumors in previously irradiated tissues.

Multiple studies suggest that, if possible, surgical salvage should be the first choice for the treatment of a recurrence in a previously irradiated field. However, patient selection is critical to optimal results. Patients with distant metastases, carotid artery encasement, involvement of the prevertebral fascia, or skull base invasion are not typically considered candidates for resection. Furthermore, clinical factors that suggest reduced success with salvage surgery include short disease-free interval, advanced T stage, advanced overall stage, and smoking status. Along with patient selection, treatment by a multidisciplinary team of head and neck cancer experts is important; salvage surgery and reirradiation both require a highly trained group of physicians and ancillary head and neck support personnel to maximize outcomes during treatment in a previously irradiated field and to maximize rehabilitation potential.

If patients are found to be candidates for surgical salvage, the decision about whether to add reirradiation continues to be controversial. Traditional risk factors for postoperative radiation are noted (for instance, perineural invasion, multiple positive lymph nodes), but the decision for reirradiation requires more significant pathologic risk factors for subsequent recurrence (for instance, extensive soft tissue invasion or positive margins) due to the risks for toxicity. If reirradiation is deemed appropriate, it may be delivered using catheter-based brachytherapy, intraoperative radiation, adjuvant external beam radiation (usually IMRT), or stereotactic radiation therapy.

For patients who are not deemed to have surgically resectable recurrences, definitive reirradiation may be used. Careful delineation of the extent of disease, with CT or MRI, is crucial to defining the appropriate target and minimizing dose to previously treated adjacent areas. Furthermore, the prior treatment records must be retrieved, with color isodose plots, to understand the doses previously received; this is important in counseling the patient with regard to potential toxicities (including, but not limited to, brachial plexopathy, necrosis, or carotid damage). The data are mixed in terms of the relevance of disease-free interval with regard to outcomes of salvage reirradiation; however, our recommendation is to only consider offering reirradiation in selected cases in which there has been at least 6 months between the prior course of radiation and the recurrence.

Ultimately, the smaller the volume of recurrent disease, the better the chance of salvage and minimal toxicity. In previously treated areas, the high-dose volume (CTV_{HD}) should include the gross recurrence with a small margin surrounding it (approximately 1 cm). Typically, prophylactic targets (CTV_{ID} and CTV_{ED}) are not treated in the setting of prior radiation, although a small (3 to 5 mm) area of margin around the CTV_{HD} may be delineated. Depending on size and location of adjacent normal tissues, this volume may be best covered using IMRT/VMAT, proton therapy, or SBRT. Data are emerging regarding long-term outcomes and toxicities from the use of proton therapy and SBRT; further follow-up is needed to establish the role of these techniques in reirradiation.

TREATMENT STRATEGY AND PLANNING FOR DEFINITIVE REIRRADIATION

Nasopharyngeal Carcinoma

A large portion of the data on reirradiation has been gained from the treatment of nasopharyngeal carcinoma. Surgical resection is typically not feasible for a local recurrence; isolated neck recurrences may be amenable to surgery. However, with modern techniques, the majority of locoregional nasopharynx cancer recurrences are treated with definitive highly conformal radiation, including IMRT or proton therapy; small volume lesions may be suitable for treatment with SBRT or a combination of external beam radiation and brachytherapy.

The target volume for external beam reirradiation encompasses the clinically and radiologically detectable recurrent disease with an approximately 1 cm margin **(Case Study 18.1 and Case Study 18.2)**. Elective dose levels are not routinely used, but a small area of margin around the high-dose area may be employed. While a composite plan can be generated to understand the total dose delivered over both courses of treatment, the dose and target are typically not adjusted based on the composite plan (other than for critical organ at risk constraints) because the risk of uncontrolled disease is so substantial. The patient should be counseled about potentially significant expected toxicities.

In general, the cumulative external beam dose to the temporal lobes is kept below 105 Gy to minimize the risk of brain necrosis. If the interval between the two courses of radiation is >2 years, the cumulative dose to the spinal cord and brainstem is kept below 65 Gy. More stringent dose constraints are adopted for shorter intervals.

When combined with brachytherapy, the external beam component is delivered first with the aim of flattening the tumor to allow better placement of the intracavitary source and to improve brachytherapy dose distribution. The endocavitary brachytherapy we have used is delivered with an 8- × 3-mm 137-Cesium (^{137}Cs) source afterloaded in a Teflon ball placed into the nasopharynx under general anesthesia. Four sizes of Teflon balls (diameters: 1.5, 2.0, 2.5, and 3.0 cm) are available. The largest that can be inserted snugly is chosen to improve the depth dose distribution. For endocavitary brachytherapy for nasopharyngeal carcinoma, prescribed dose is 40 to 50 Gy (after external beam) delivered at a dose rate of 0.4 to 0.6 Gy per hour.

Other groups have described the use of interstitial therapy with either radioactive gold or iodine seeds for the treatment of recurrent nasopharyngeal cancer. The interstitial therapy is delivered either alone of combined with external beam.

Oropharyngeal Carcinoma

Despite the excellent prognosis of patients with oropharynx cancer, especially in the patients with HPV associated disease, a subset of patients still experience local or regional reirecurrence. Patients should be assessed for surgical resectability. For cases that are not surgically resectable, definitive reirradiation therapy is used often with concurrent chemotherapy **(Case Study 18.3 and Case Study 18.4)**.

CASE STUDY 18.1

A 36-year-old man was treated in Asia with radiation for undifferentiated carcinoma. Treatment records were unavailable. He was found to have recurrent disease on routine follow-up evaluation 4 years later. The restaging workup included a PET–CT scan (Fig. 18.1A), which revealed the recurrent disease confined to the right nasopharynx (stage rT1 N0).

He was reirradiated with IMRT delivered with concurrent cisplatin.

As shown in Figure 18.1B, two targets were defined. CTV_{HD} (66 Gy, *maroon* color wash) encompassed the gross disease in the right nasopharynx with margin and CTV_{ED} (60 Gy, *blue* color wash) encompassed the left nasopharynx. Treatment was delivered in 33 fractions. Figure 18.1B–F shows isodose distributions in axial views, with target volumes delineated, at the level of the tumor epicenter (Fig. 18.1B), inferior (Fig. 18.1C) and superior (Fig. 18.1D) nasopharynx, a sagittal view through midline (Fig. 18.1E), and a coronal view through the nasopharynx (Fig. 18.1F). As the previous records were unavailable, doses to the brainstem and spinal cord were limited to 20 Gy. The patient has no evidence of disease 4 years after reirradiation.

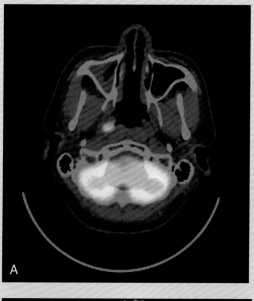
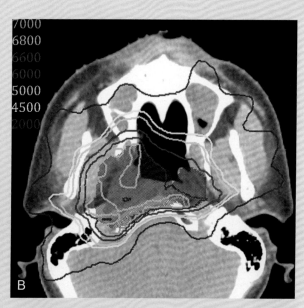
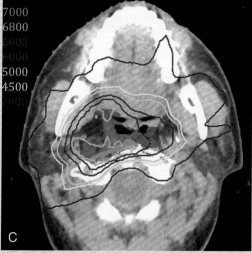
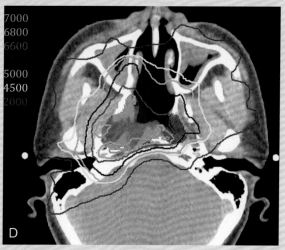

Case Figure 18.1 A–D

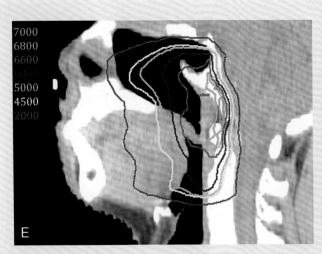

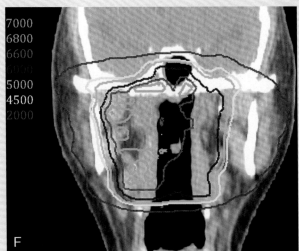

Case Figure 18.1 E,F

CASE STUDY 18.2

A 43-year-old woman was treated for stage T1N1 naso-pharyngeal carcinoma with induction chemotherapy followed by 74 Gy delivered in 69 fractions. Five years later, she presented with facial numbness and was found to have a mass in the left cavernous sinus. Review of her portals revealed that the recurrent tumor was located at the superior edge of the original portals (marginal recurrence) and much of the disease in the cavernous sinus was unirradiated.

She was treated with three cycles of taxane–platin-based induction chemotherapy achieving a partial response. Both the initial and postchemotherapy MRIs were used for planning of reirradiation by fusing them onto the retreatment planning CT scan. Figure 18.2A shows an axial slice on the pretreatment MRI. The gross disease was contoured in two separate volumes. The red contour surrounds the disease in the cavernous sinus, and the aqua contour surrounds the disease in the brainstem (*brown* contour). Figure 18.2B shows the postchemotherapy volume. The

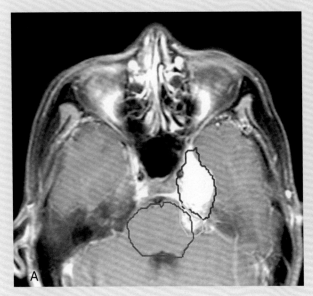

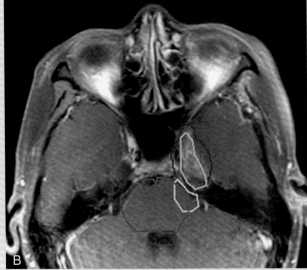

Case Figure 18.2 A,B

red and aqua contours represent pretreatment volumes fused onto this MRI, and the green contour delineates the residual abnormality on the postchemotherapy scan. Figure 18.2C demonstrates the contours fused onto the CT planning scan. Doses were prescribed to these targets without expansion. Daily setup was verified with CT guidance. The residual disease was treated to 64 Gy, the prechemotherapy volume outside the brainstem to 60 Gy, and the prechemotherapy volume abutting the brainstem to 46 Gy.

Treatment was delivered in 32 fractions, with concurrent weekly carboplatin. Figure 18.2D–F shows isodose distributions on an axial (Fig. 18.2D) and on coronal views through the cavernous sinus (Fig. 18.2E) and brainstem (Fig. 18.2F). Noncoplanar beams were used, thus low dose can be appreciated in the superior aspect of the brain. The dose constraints on the brainstem were varied, with more tolerance allowed superiorly outside the initial radiation portal. The patient remains well more than 5 years later.

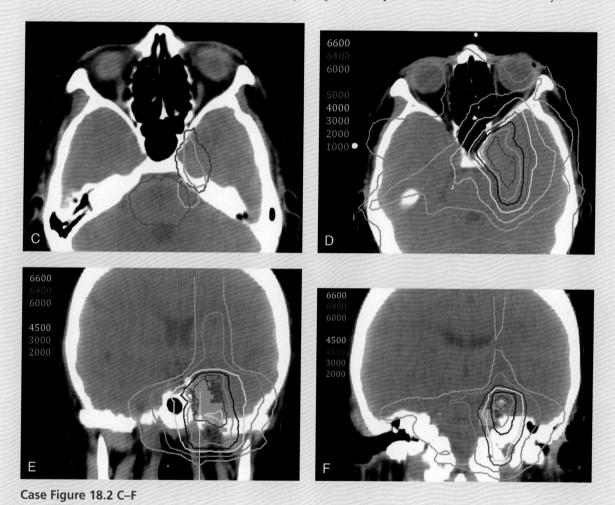

Case Figure 18.2 C–F

CASE STUDY 18.3

A 40-year-old woman was originally treated in 1998 (at age 26) for stage T4 N2c M0 (stage IVa) right tonsil/base of tongue squamous cell carcinoma with induction chemotherapy followed by concomitant boost radiation to a dose of 72 Gy in 42 fractions using conventional radiation fields. In 2012, 14 years after her initial treatment,

she developed progressive dysphagia and odynophagia. Imaging demonstrated two discrete masses in the base of tongue, consistent with recurrence or a second primary (Fig. 18.3A; *arrows* noting two masses). Biopsy confirmed recurrent squamous carcinoma in both nodules. Given the multiple areas of disease, salvage surgery was not advised due to expected toxicity of a total base of tongue resection; she was dispositioned to definitive chemoreirradiation. She was counseled prior to treatment of the risks of soft tissue and bone necrosis, carotid damage leading to stroke or carotid blowout, and dysphagia and aspiration which may require feeding tube dependence or a palliative laryngectomy. She agreed to proceed understanding those risks.

Based on the clinical examination and imaging at the time of the recurrence, reirradiation was planned to encompass both areas of disease in the base of tongue with margin. A mouth-opening, tongue-depressing stent was used to immobilize the tongue and minimize dose

to the adjacent normal structures. Figure 18.3B shows an axial slice on the planning CT delineating the two biopsy-proven nodules (in *green*). The red contour (CTV_{HD}) surrounds the disease with an approximately 1 cm margin in all directions. The blue contour (CTV_{ED}) was used for additional margin of approximately 8 mm. The CTV_{HD} dose was 66 Gy in 33 fractions (2 Gy/fraction) with the blue volume (CTV_{ED}) to 60 Gy (1.8 Gy/fraction). The 3-dimensional IMRT plan is depicted in Figure 18.3C to E. The patient remains with no evidence of disease 3.5 years later. A modified barium swallow reveals moderate oropharyngeal dysphagia with a functional swallow; she does require a feeding tube.

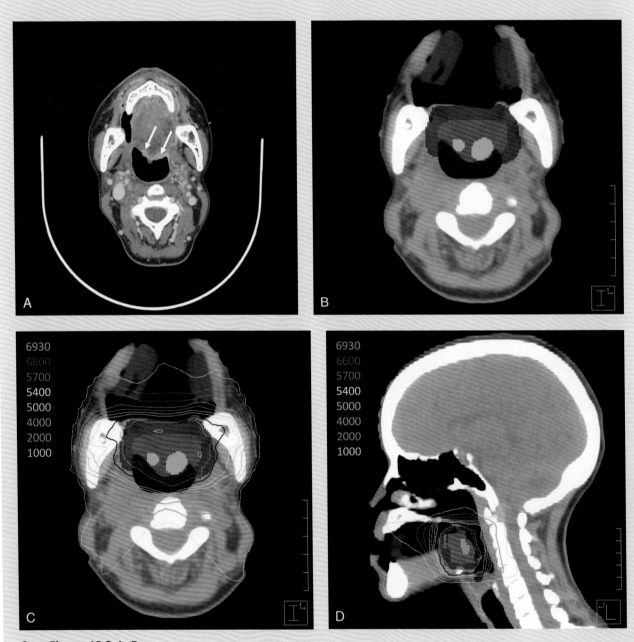

Case Figure 18.3 A–D

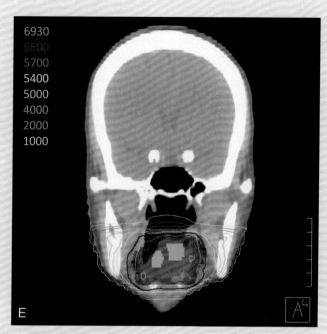

Case Figure 18.3 E

For patients with locoregional recurrence of oropharynx cancer, the target volume encompasses the clinically and radiologically detectable recurrent disease with approximately 1-cm margins. The majority of patients are treated with conformal external beam therapy. The treatment setup is similar to primary radiotherapy as described in individual sites in preceding chapters. Briefly, the GTV is defined based on the clinical information. One or two clinical targets are defined. CTV_{HD} includes the GTV with approximately 1-cm margins. Smaller margins are used, if constrained by proximity to central neural structures (for instance, the brainstem or spinal cord). The general policy is not to systematically administer comprehensive elective irradiation in retreatment setting. Therefore, CTV_{ED} is typically limited or nonexistent.

For definitive external beam reirradiation, a dose of 66 Gy in 33 fractions is prescribed to CTV_{HD}. When applicable, CTV_{ED} generally receives 54 to 60 Gy.

Small volume disease in the tonsil or base of tongue may be suitable for combination of external beam with brachytherapy or, in rare cases, brachytherapy alone. When combined with brachytherapy, the prescribed external beam dose is 20 to 30 Gy in 10 to 15 fractions depending on the thickness of the recurrent lesion and the previous radiation dose.

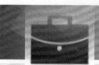

CASE STUDY 18.4

A 78-year-old male underwent surgical resection of a T3 N0 squamous cell carcinoma of the right retromolar trigone. This was followed by postoperative radiation given using a 3-field technique to 50 Gy and an ipsilateral boost to an additional 20 Gy. One year later, he developed a local recurrence and underwent surgical salvage. Disease extended to the palate and pharynx. There was lymphovascular invasion, but the final margins were negative. Therefore, it was elected to observe him. One year later, he presented with odynophagia. Workup revealed multifocal disease in the left base of tongue, and he was thought to be a poor candidate for surgery and was dispositioned to receive reirradiation.

A PET–CT simulation was performed. Sites of disease within the tongue as shown in Figure 18.4A and B (*green arrows*) were outlined as GTV (*aqua* color wash). Due to the lymphvascular space invasion and multifocal nature of the disease, CTV_{HD} (*maroon* color wash) encompassed GTV with a relatively generous margin. The prescription dose to CTV_{HD} was 66 Gy given in 33 fractions with concurrent weekly carboplatin. Figure 18.4C–F illustrates contours and isodoses in axial, sagittal, and coronal views. The spinal cord dose was limited to 20 Gy. The patient remains without disease 2 years later, though he is dependent on a feeding tube for nutritional intake.

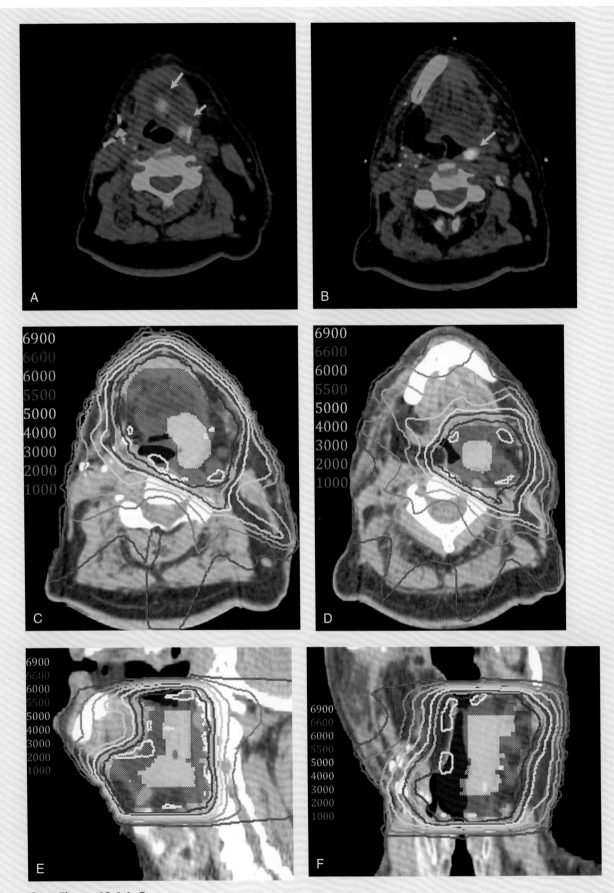

Case Figure 18.4 A–F

Oral Cavity Carcinoma

For the initial presentation of oral cavity carcinomas, the majority of definitive treatment is with surgical resection and reconstruction, followed by adjuvant radiation based on pathologic risk factors. As a result, recurrences are often deep, under reconstructed tissue flaps. In these cases, definitive reirradiation is often preferred since it does not require a complex second surgery in a previously operated and radiated field.

For patients with locoregional recurrence of oral cavity carcinoma, targets and doses are similar to oropharynx cancer. The CTV$_{HD}$ target volume encompasses the clinically and radiologically detectable recurrent disease with approximately 1-cm margins. The majority of patients are treated with IMRT though for small volume disease either brachytherapy or hypofractionated SRT are alternative options. The treatment setup is similar to primary radiotherapy as described in individual sites in preceding chapters. For external beam irradiation alone, a dose of 66 Gy in 33 fractions is prescribed to CTV$_{HD}$. When applicable, CTV$_{ED}$ generally receives 54 to 60 Gy.

Nodal Recurrence

Definitive reirradiation for patients with nodal recurrence is sometimes feasible for patients with small volume unresectable disease **(Case Study 18.5)** and may be preferred for patients with isolated retropharyngeal nodal recurrence **(Case Study 18.6)**. These patients are at high risk for carotid injury, and if considering reirradiation, it is best when the vessel has reasonable tissue coverage.

The options for radiation are varied and include IMRT, proton therapy/IMPT, stereotactic therapy, and brachytherapy. When using IMRT or IMPT, conventional fractionation often with 66 Gy delivered in 33 fractions is favored, delivered to the nodal disease with 0.5- to 1-cm margin (CTV$_{HD}$). Elective targets can be considered if CTV$_{HD}$ is in previously irradiated tissue, but adjacent neck levels are not. Patients with lower neck recurrences are at high risk for brachial plexopathy and should be counseled appropriately.

TREATMENT STRATEGY AND PLANNING FOR POSTOPERATIVE REIRRADIATION

Historically, locoregional recurrences of head and neck cancers were assessed for resectability with an open surgical approach. These procedures were often very morbid due to the necessity to resect adjacent normal tissues and the challenges of perturbed and fibrotic tissue planes as a result of prior radiation therapy. Since 2009, robotic surgery has been approved for use in head and neck cancer; this allows for a minimally invasive surgical approach for selected patients with recurrences. Regardless of the surgical approach, the decision to offer adjuvant reirradiation after salvage surgery should be made based on high risk for subsequent recurrence determined by the surgical findings and pathology.

Recommendation for adjuvant reirradiation after surgical salvage is complex, as its role has not been clearly defined. Factors to consider include the amount of previously irradiated tissue removed by the surgery, the degree of radiation changes in the remaining tissue, and the extent of reconstruction. Patients with extensive surgical resection that removes

CASE STUDY 18.5

A 57-year-old woman was originally treated in 2012 for stage T2 N2b M0 (stage IVa) left tonsil squamous cell carcinoma with induction chemotherapy followed by chemoradiation with cisplatin to a dose of 70 Gy in 33 fractions using IMRT; she had a left neck dissection following treatment for small volume residual disease. She did well for approximately 1 year, at which time he had imaging evidence of a small left neck/supraclavicular recurrence (Fig. 18.5A *arrows* noting recurrent mass); this was biopsy proven to be recurrent disease. Given the location of the disease with respect to the vasculature, salvage surgery was not advised; she was dispositioned to induction chemotherapy followed by definitive chemoreirradiation.

Based on the clinical examination and imaging at the time of the recurrence, reirradiation was planned to

encompass the area of gross disease in the left low neck with a small margin. Given the potential toxicity to adjacent normal tissues, the patient was dispositioned to radiation with passive scattering proton therapy. Figure 18.5B shows an axial slice on the planning CT delineating the target with margin (in *orange* color wash) and the proton beam angles. The CTV$_{HD}$ dose was 66 Gy (radiobiologic equivalent) in 33 fractions. The 3-dimensional proton plan is depicted in Figure 18.5B–D. Proton therapy allowed delivery of definitive dose to the target while significantly minimizing radiation to nontarget structures. The patient remains with no evidence of disease 1 year following reirradiation. She is eating well by mouth and has full use of his left arm without pain or neurologic impairment.

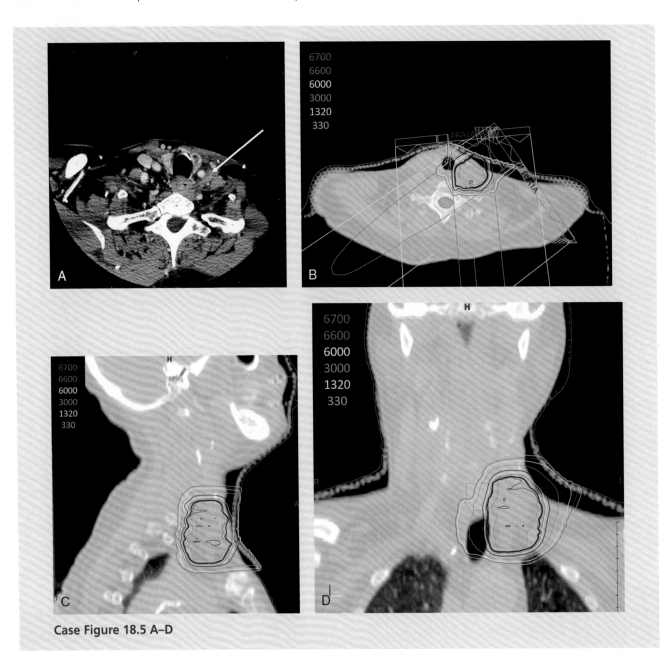

Case Figure 18.5 A–D

CASE STUDY 18.6

A 65-year-old male who was previously treated with postoperative chemoradiation for a T4 N2b M0 (stage IVa) squamous carcinoma of the left retromolar trigone was found to have an isolated left retropharyngeal lymph node recurrence 4 years after his initial treatment. Figure 18.6A shows the area of recurrence (*white arrow*) on PET/CT. CT-guided biopsy confirmed recurrent squamous carcinoma. This area had previously received 60 Gy in 30 fractions via IMRT. He was dispositioned to salvage reirradiation using stereotactic body radiation therapy (SBRT), targeting only the recurrent disease.

He underwent CT simulation and was immobilized using a custom posterior head cradle with a full-length head/neck/shoulder mask with a bite block integrated into the mask (Fig. 18.6B). Volumetric MRI was obtained with the patient immobilized in the treatment position, and the MRI images were registered with the CT planning dataset in order to contour targets and normal structures.

The GTV (Fig. 18.6C) with a 3-mm margin was treated to 45 Gy in 5 fractions, delivered every other day over a 2-week period. Volumetric arc-based IMRT was used (two partial arcs), optimized to minimize dose to the brainstem and spinal cord. Daily cone-beam CT and noncoplanar x-ray verification were used for image guidance. He received concurrent cetuximab. SBRT dose distributions are shown in Figure 18.6D. PET/CT done 3 months after SBRT showed resolution of the disease (Fig. 18.6E). The patient remains free of disease and without significant treatment-related toxicity 8 months after the end of SBRT.

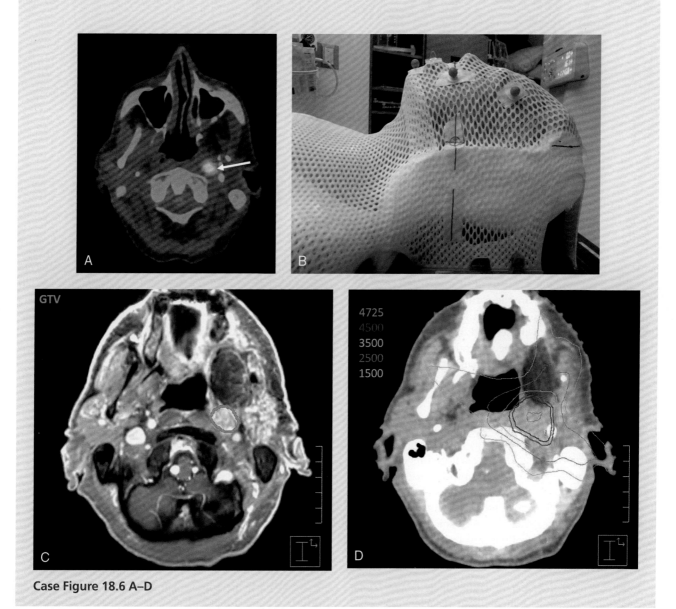

Case Figure 18.6 A–D

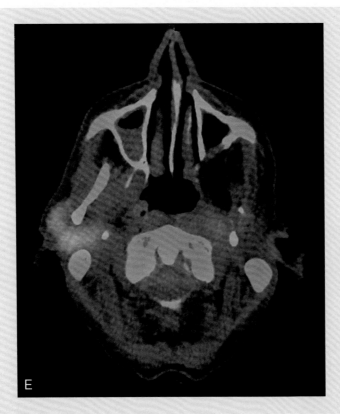

E

Case Figure 18.6 E

substantial amounts of previously irradiated tissues and with free flap reconstructions, especially those that cover the carotid vessels or bones, are the optimal candidates for reirradiation. Only patients considered to be at a significantly high risk for recurrence are selected for adjuvant reirradiation **(Case Study 18.7)**. These indications include positive margins or extensive extranodal extension.

Laryngeal Carcinoma

Patients who were treated with primary radiation therapy to the larynx only for T1–T2 glottic cancers are often candidates for surgical salvage in the event of a recurrence. In selected cases, patients can be treated with voice-preserving procedures, such as transoral laser microsurgery (TLM) or hemilaryngectomy. Reirradiation to the intact larynx has been described in very small series in the literature, but is rarely used, largely due to improved techniques for partial laryngeal surgery, but also due to the high risk of necrosis and aspiration.

Most patients with recurrent larynx cancer require a total laryngectomy. Similarly, patients with recurrent hypopharyngeal cancer who have resectable disease are operated, usually with a total laryngectomy and partial pharyngectomy. Reconstructive surgery is often needed to repair the defect. Consideration for postoperative reirradiation is given if the neopharynx is felt to be at high risk of recurrence. Removal of the larynx facilitates reirradiation, but the nerves

running through the neck and carotid arteries that received prior radiation remain, so there still is the potential for significant toxicity risk.

This risk of toxicity is lessened if the patient had previous radiation to small fields for early larynx cancer. In these cases, postoperative irradiation to the tracheal stoma and/or the neck is recommended when the recurrent lesion extends to the subglottic region or when the neck dissection reveals multiple nodes or extracapsular nodal disease **(Case Study 18.8)**. Since the original fields were confined to the larynx, the volume of tissue reirradiated is small. However, there is not substantive long-term data to truly know if reirradation to small volumes in the neck lead to an increased risk of late events such as stroke or laryngeal and swallowing dysfunction.

Nodal Recurrence

Patients who develop isolated nodal recurrences may be suitable for surgery and either perioperative brachytherapy or intraoperative radiation. We have predominantly used low-dose-rate brachytherapy in conjunction with a neck dissection with the wound closed with a rotational pectoralis major flap **(Case Study 18.9)**. Occasionally, we have used high–dose-rate delivery with the HAM (Harrison–Anderson–Mick) applicator, particularly when the tissues at risk are difficult to access with catheter placement **(Case Study 18.10)**.

Unfortunately, often patients are not referred to radiation oncology until after the neck dissection has been performed.

CASE STUDY 18.7

A 32-year-old woman was diagnosed with left oral tongue cancer. She was treated with partial glossectomy and postoperative IMRT administering 60 Gy in 30 fractions to the primary tumor bed and upper neck. She developed local recurrence 1 year later and underwent resection with negative margins. Three months later, she developed a second recurrence in the left posterior tongue (Fig. 18.7A, *green arrow*) and left level I neck node (Fig. 18.7B, *red arrow*). She was treated with a partial glossectomy, partial mandibulectomy, left neck dissection, and free flap reconstruction. Histologic examination revealed squamous carcinoma in the tongue and soft tissues of left level IA–B regions, but margins were negative. She was treated with postoperative reirradiation with concurrent cisplatin.

As the prior treatment was relatively limited to the left tongue and upper neck, it was felt that elective reirradiation would be beneficial with a relatively low risk for severe complication. Target volumes were designed similar to the routine postoperative situation (see Chapter 7), but the dose constraint for the spinal cord was set at 20 Gy rather than the usual 45 Gy. CTV_{HD} (*red* color wash), CTV_{ID} (*blue* color wash), and CTV_{ED} (*yellow* color wash) were prescribed 60, 57, and 54 Gy, respectively. Figure 18.7C–E shows contours and isodose distributions on axial, sagittal, and coronal views through the tongue. She remains without disease 3 years later.

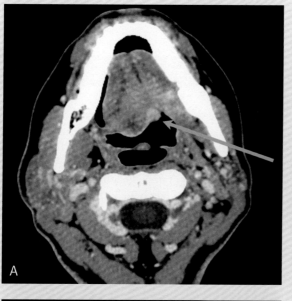

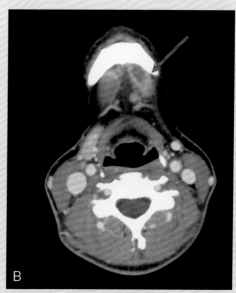

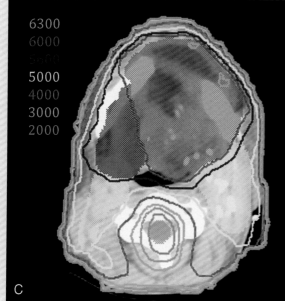

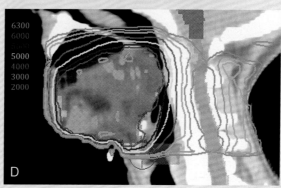

Case Figure 18.7 A–D

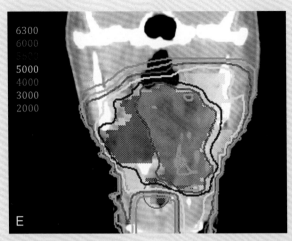

Case Figure 18.7 E

CASE STUDY 18.8

A 70-year-old man was originally treated with definitive radiation to the larynx only using IMRT for a T2 N0 M0 (stage II) glottic squamous carcinoma. He was treated to a dose of 65.25 Gy in 29 fractions at an outside hospital (Fig. 18.8A). Approximately 1 year after treatment ended, he was found to have a local recurrence and underwent salvage laryngectomy and a left neck dissection. He had no adverse features at that time in the primary specimen and no pathologic adenopathy on the left; he was observed. About 6 months after salvage laryngectomy, he developed a right neck mass (Fig. 18.8B). Biopsy confirmed recurrent squamous cell carcinoma. He was dispositioned to surgical resection followed by adjuvant radiation.

The tumor was resected, demonstrating a 5-cm mass diffusely infiltrating the soft tissue. Margins were negative.

Approximately 4 weeks after surgery, the patient was simulated for external beam reirradiation. A plan was created to treat the right neck, including the area of resected disease, to a dose of 60 Gy in 30 fractions using VMAT. The red colorwash is the CTV_{HD} with a dose of 60 Gy; the blue colorwash is CTV_{ID} to 57 Gy. Representative axial, sagittal, and coronal images through the targets are shown in Figure 18.8C–E. The left neck was not treated since the surgical specimen the year before was negative, and he had no evidence of recurrence since that time.

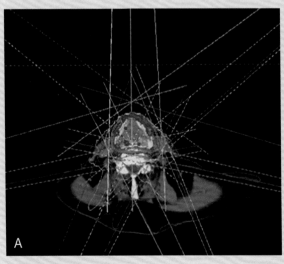

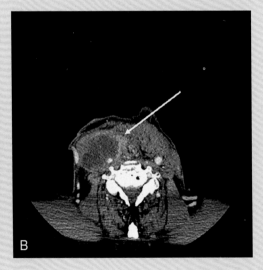

Case Figure 18.8 A,B

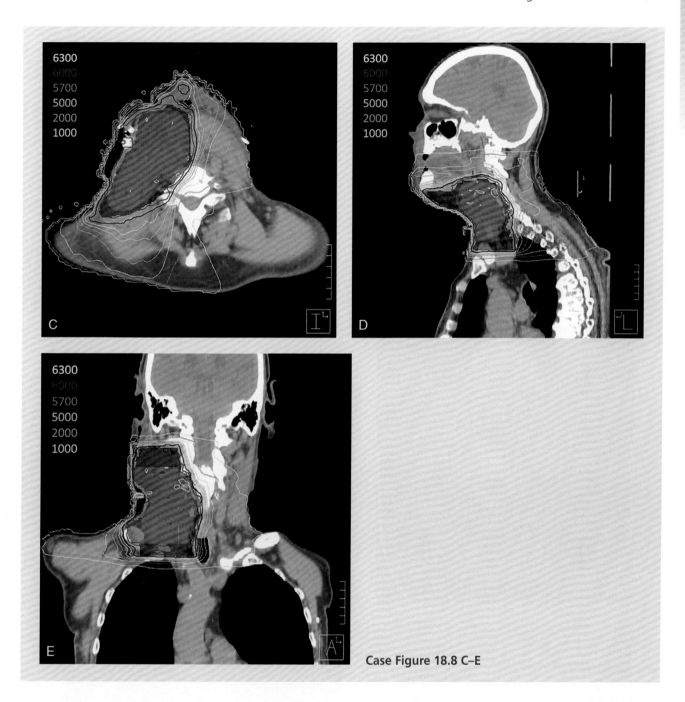

Case Figure 18.8 C–E

In cases where either extensive nodal disease or extracapsular extension is found, external beam reirradiation to the sites of involvement in the neck can be considered.

Technique and Dose

In the modern era, most patients who experience recurrence and require reirradiation are treated with advanced techniques; the most common is IMRT. The treatment setup is similar to primary radiotherapy as described in individual sites in previous chapters. The target encompasses the clinically and radiologically detectable recurrent disease with 1- to 2-cm margins (more generous in the adjuvant setting).

For postoperative reirradiation with IMRT **(Case Study 18.11)**, a virtual GTV (vGTV) is delineated based on the clinical, surgical, and pathologic information. CTV_{HD} includes the vGTV with 1- to 2-cm margins. CTV_{ID} and CTV_{ED} are optional and individualized. In general, elective regions are not reirradiated. When indicated, generally CTV_{ID} can cover CTV_{HD} with an additional 8- to 10-mm margin, and CTV_{ED} encompasses subclinical sites at risk ideally sites that were not previously treated.

The dose for external beam reirradiation in the definitive setting is typically 66 Gy in 33 fractions and following resection typically 60 Gy in 30 fractions. Occasionally, if gross residual disease is highly suspected after surgery, a total dose of 66 Gy is prescribed to a small sub volume

CASE STUDY 18.9

A 53-year-old man was initially treated with external beam radiation therapy for a T2 N2b base of tongue carcinoma. He was found to have a recurrence in the right neck 7 months later. A solitary node (*red arrow*) was seen in the right upper neck (Fig. 18.9A). He underwent a right radical neck dissection and right pectoralis major flap as well as insertion of brachytherapy catheters. Once the lymph node was removed, six afterloading catheters were sutured in place in parallel fashion. Following insertion of the catheters, the wound was covered with the rotational flap and closed. Figure 18.9B,C shows catheters arranged in parallel rows with 1-cm spacing, which were loaded 4 days after surgery

with ^{192}Iridium seeds to deliver 60 Gy at 0.65 Gy per hour to the 5-mm line (Fig. 18.9D). The first catheter had the posterior section significantly <1-cm separation from the second catheter due to proximity to the mastoid. Therefore, a lower activity was loaded in the posterior half of this catheter. Large metal clips were placed during the implant to help localize the bed of the recurrent disease for guiding implants. Histologic examination of surgical specimens showed squamous carcinoma in dense fibroadipose tissue and abutting muscle. The other 21 nodes removed were negative for tumor. The patient remains well 1 year following the implant.

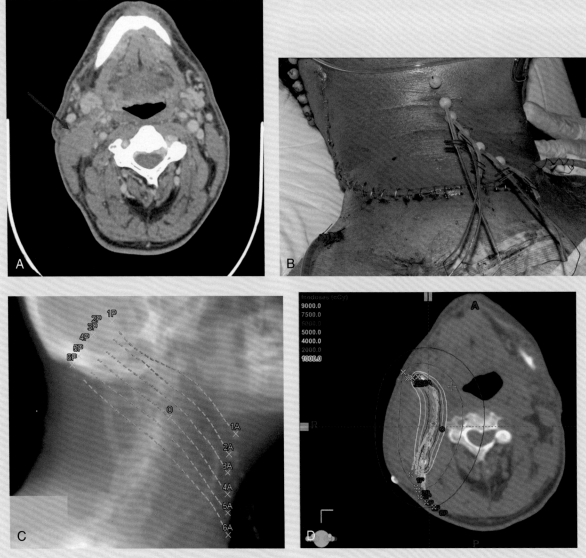

Case Figure 18.9 A–D

CASE STUDY 18.10

A 75-year-old man was originally treated with induction chemotherapy followed by chemoradiation with IMRT for a T3 N2c M0 (stage IVa) right base of tongue carcinoma. His follow-up CT scan at 10 weeks post treatment showed no evidence of disease, with complete resolution of the base of tongue primary and subcentimeter nodal remnants in the treated necks. Two years following the completion of treatment, he was found to have a necrotic lymph node in the left neck (Fig. 18.10A; *arrow* delineates area of recurrence). This was in the low to intermediate-dose volume of the initial treatment (*blue* isodose was 63 Gy and *yellow* was 57 Gy), caudal to the previously identified involved left neck lymph nodes (Fig. 18.10B). The recurrence was biopsy-proved to be squamous carcinoma. He was dispositioned to surgical resection with intraoperative radiation with a HAM applicator, followed by additional external beam reirradiation.

The patient was taken to surgery and underwent a left neck dissection. In Figure 18.10C, the operative bed is noted, with the area of resected disease marked with a circle. While the patient was under anesthesia, a HAM applicator was selected to fully cover this area, with

ample margin. A 9-catheter applicator was chosen, with only the upper eight catheters loaded; the final treatment area was 8 × 8 cm. The applicator was placed over the surgical bed (Fig. 18.10D), and packing was used to displace normal tissue (skin) and to ensure direct contact of the applicator with the tumor bed (Fig. 18.10E). A plan was created to deliver 12.5 Gy to 1 cm (which is 5 mm from the applicator surface). A remote Ir-192 afterloader was used to deliver the treatment while the patient was under anesthesia and with the supervising radiation oncologist and physicist watching from just outside a shielded operating suite.

Approximately 2 weeks after surgery, the patient was simulated for additional external beam radiation, which was started approximately 3 weeks after surgery. A plan was created to treat the area of resection for an additional 46 Gy in 23 fractions using VMAT (Fig. 18.10F–H). The red colorwash is the CTV$_{HD}$ with a dose of 46 Gy; the blue contour is additional margin to 40 Gy. The spinal cord constraint was <10 Gy; the maximum dose to the spinal cord was 7.82 Gy. The patient remains well 8 months following the completion of treatment with no evidence of disease and no significant sequelae.

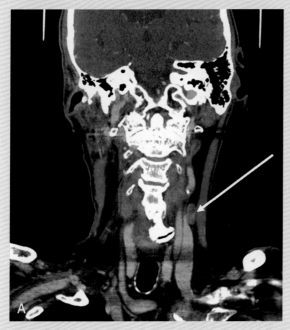
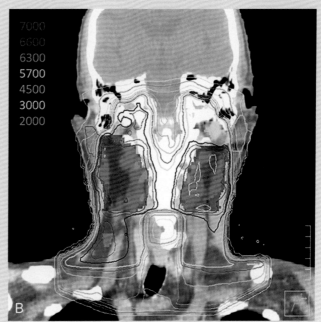

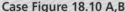

Case Figure 18.10 A,B

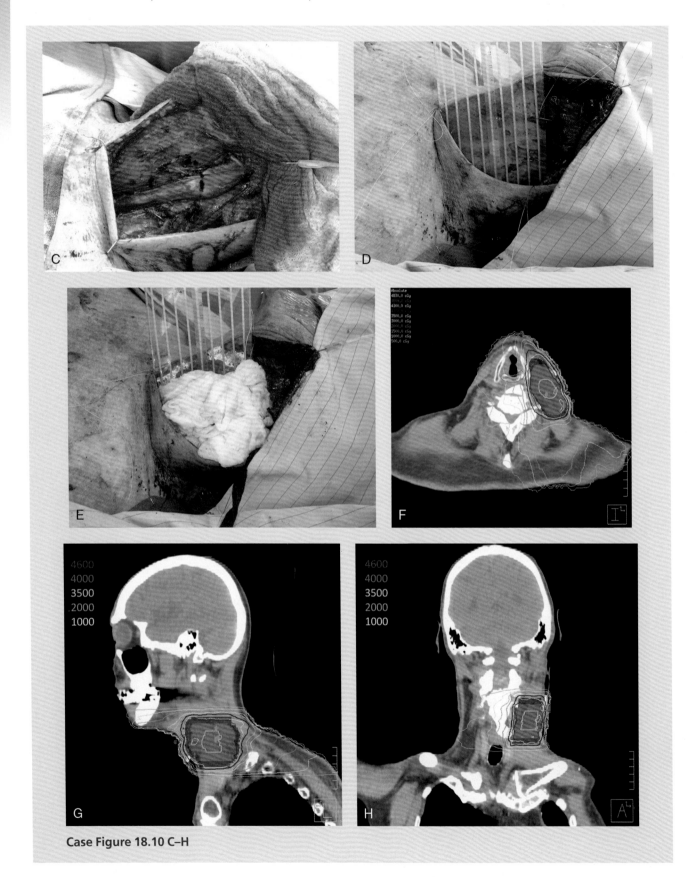

Case Figure 18.10 C–H

(Case Study 18.11). When indicated, generally CTVID can cover CTVHD with an additional 8- to 10-mm margin, and CTVED encompasses subclinical sites at risk ideally sites that were not previously treated. When indicated, the dose to CTV_{ED} is −57 Gy in 30–33 fractions. If the interval between the two courses of radiation is >2 years, the cumulative dose to the spinal cord and brainstem is kept below 65 Gy. More stringent dose constraints are adopted for shorter intervals.

For stoma only irradiation in the setting of postlaryngectomy cases, the typical dose is 50 Gy in 25 fractions delivered with 9- to 12-MeV electrons.

Afterloading catheters used for brachytherapy are generally low-dose-rate Ir-192 prepared in wires or ribbons of seeds. One goal of catheter placement is to achieve a 1-cm separation between individual catheters. The catheters are generally loaded 3 to 5 days after surgical placement. The prescribed dose is usually 60 Gy specified at 5 mm (tissue depth) from the plane of the implant at a dose rate of 0.4 to 0.6 Gy per hour. In recent years we have used pulsed-dose rate Ir-192 afterloading approaches for greater patient/staff safety and convenience.

For cases where individual catheters can not be placed with adequate target coverage, intraoperative high-dose rate Ir-192 with a HAM applicator is a consideration. The dose we have used in this setting is 12.5 Gy in a single fraction specified at 1 cm (5 mm from the applicator surface). Subsequently, external beam is often given to consolidate, with a dose of 46 Gy in 23 fractions prescribed to a CTV_{HD}.

Background Data

See Tables 18.1 and 18.2.

CASE STUDY 18.11

A 56-year-old man was irradiated for nasopharynx cancer using a 3-field conventional technique. The nasopharynx and right neck received 66 Gy. Eight years later, he developed recurrence in the right neck as shown on an axial view on CT scan (Fig. 18.11A, *red arrow*) and coronal view on an MRI (Fig. 18.11B, *red arrow*). He underwent a modified radical neck dissection which revealed nodal disease in level II and III regions. The surgery extended toward the jugular foramen revealing presence of tumor in soft tissue at this site.

Due to the extent of disease and probable residual in the most superior aspect of level II nodal region, it was elected to reirradiate the right neck with IMRT. Four targets were defined. CTV_{HD} (*yellow* color wash), CTV_{ID} (*blue* color wash), and CTV_{ED} (*green–yellow* color wash) were prescribed 60, 56, and 50 Gy, respectively. An additional high-risk target in superior level II and the jugular foramen was also defined (*maroon* color wash) and prescribed 66 Gy. Figure 18.11 also shows contours and isodose distributions on axial views through midlevel II (Fig. 18.11C) and jugular foramen (Fig. 18.11D) and on coronal views through the neck (Fig. 18.11E) and the spinal cord (Fig. 18.11F). The spinal cord dose was limited to 20 Gy. The patient remains without disease 4 years later. He has severe dysphagia, can only eat soft food, and needs a gastrostomy tube to maintain his weight. In addition, he has severe fibrosis of the neck and cannot fully raise his right arm.

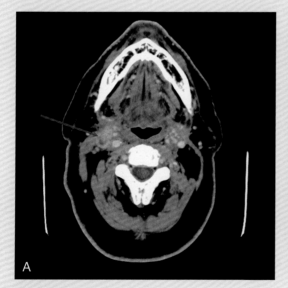
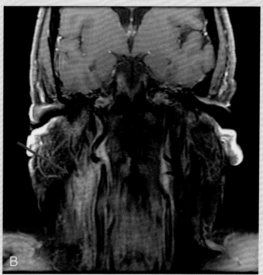

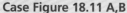
Case Figure 18.11 A,B

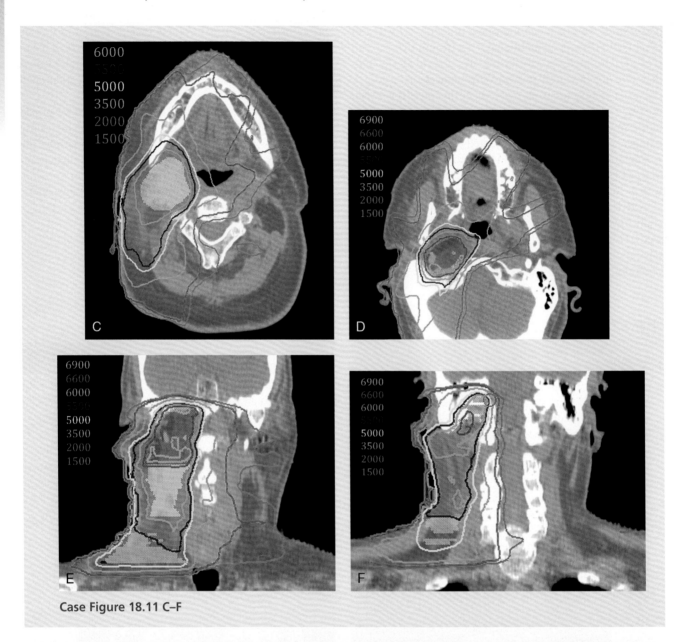

Case Figure 18.11 C–F

TABLE 18.1 Results of Reirradiation of Recurrent Nasopharyngeal Carcinoma (Literature Review)			
Institutions	No. of Patients	Survival (5 Years)	% With Severe Complications
Stanford (Hoppe et al.)	13	Median: 13 mo	Not stated
UCSF (Fu et al.)	42	Overall: 41%	9
Beijing (Yan et al.)	219	Overall: 18%	29
MGH (Wang et al.)	51	T1, T2: 38%; T3, T4: 15%	2
MDACC (Pryzant et al.)	53	Confined to nasopharynx: 32%; larger: 9%	8

From Pryzant RM, et al. Re-treatment of nasopharyngeal carcinoma in 53 patients. *Int J Radiat Oncol Biol Phys* 1992;22:941, with permission.

TABLE 18.2 Results of Reirradiation using Intensity-Modulated Radiotherapy (IMRT)

First Author, Year	Patient Number	Postoperative Radiation (%)	Concurrent Chemotherapy (%)	2-yr Overall Survival	2-yr Local–Regional Control	Grade III+ Toxicity
Biagioli, 2007	41	42%	100%	49%	Not given	5% Fistula 2% Esophagus
Duprez, 2009	84	23%	14%	35%	48%	56% Grade III–V 28% Grade 4
Popovtzer, 2009	66	33%	71%	40%	27%	29% Grade III–V 18% Feeding tube
Sher, 2010	35	49%	100%	48%	67%	43% Grade III–V 49% Esophagus 15% Pulmonary 11% Trismus 6% ORN
Riaz, 2014	257[a]	44%	67%	43%	47%	20% Feeding tube 7% Necrosis 4% Hearing loss 1% Blindness
Curtis, 2016	81[b]	48%	74%	50%	60%	ND
Takiar, 2016	227[c]	43%	62%	51%	59%	35%

[a]78% of patients treated with IMRT.
[b]95% of patients treated with IMRT.
[c]91% treated with definitive intent.
ND, not described.
Adapted from Biagioli MC, et al. Intensity-modulated radiotherapy with concurrent chemotherapy for previously irradiated, recurrent head and neck cancer. *Int J Radiat Oncol Biol Phys* 2007;69:1067–1073; Duprez F, et al. Intensity-modulated radiotherapy for recurrent and second primary head and neck cancer in previously irradiated territory. *Radiother Oncol* 2009;93:563–569; Popovtzer A, et al. The pattern of failure after reirradiation of recurrent squamous cell head and neck cancer: implications for defining the targets. *Int J Radiat Oncol Biol Phys* 2009;74:1342–1347; Sher DJ, et al. Efficacy and toxicity of reirradiation using intensity-modulated radiotherapy for recurrent or second primary head and neck cancer. *Cancer* 2010;116:4761–4768; Riaz N, et al. A nomogram to predict logo-regional control after re-irradiation for head and neck cancer. *Radiother Oncol* 2014;111:382–387; Curtis KK, et al. Outcomes of patients with loco-regionally recurrent or new primary squamous cell carcinomas of the head and neck treated with curative intent reirradiation at Mayo Clinic. *Radiat Oncol* 2016;11:55; Takiar V, et al. Reirradiation of Head and Neck Cancers With Intensity Modulated Radiation Therapy: Outcomes and Analyses. *Int J Radiat Oncol Biol Phys* 2016;95:1117–1131.

SUGGESTED READINGS

Ang KK, Price RE, Stephens LC, et al. The tolerance of primate spinal cord to re-irradiation. *Int J Radiat Oncol Biol Phys* 1993;25:459.

Biagioli MC, et al. Intensity-modulated radiotherapy with concurrent chemotherapy for previously irradiated, recurrent head and neck cancer. *Int J Radiat Oncol Biol Phys* 2007;69:1067.

Delclos L, Moore BE, Sampiere VA. A disposable "afterloadable" nasopharyngeal applicator for radioactive point sources. *Endocuriether Hypertherm Oncol* 1994;10:43.

Duprez F, Madani I, Bonte K, et al. Intensity-modulated radiotherapy for recurrent and second primary head and neck cancer in previously irradiated territory. *Radiother Oncol* 2009;93:563.

Karam I, Poon I, Lee J, et al. Stereotactic body radiotherapy for head and neck cancer: an addition to the armamentarium against head and neck cancer. *Future Oncol* 2015;11:2937.

Kupferman ME, Morrison WH, Santillan AA, et al. The role of interstitial brachytherapy with salvage surgery for the management of recurrent head and neck cancers. *Cancer* 2007;109:2052.

Langer CJ, Harris J, Horwitz EM, et al. Phase II study of low-dose paclitaxel and cisplatin in combination with split-course concomitant twice-daily reirradiation in recurrent squamous cell carcinoma of the head and neck: results of Radiation Therapy Oncology Group Protocol 9911. *J Clin Oncol* 2007;25:4800.

Low JS, Chua ET, Gao F, et al. Stereotactic radiosurgery plus intracavitary irradiation in the salvage of nasopharyngeal carcinoma. *Head Neck* 2006;28:321.

Phan J, Sio T, Nguyen T, et al. Reirradiation of head and neck cancers with proton therapy: outcomes and analyses. *Int J Radiat Oncol Biol Phys* 2016;96:30–41.

Popovtzer A, et al. The pattern of failure after reirradiation of recurrent squamous cell head and neck cancer: implications for defining the targets. *Int J Radiat Oncol Biol Phys* 2009;74:1342.

Pryzant RM, et al. Re-treatment of nasopharyngeal carcinoma in 53 patients. *Int J Radiat Oncol Biol Phys* 1992;22:941.

Riaz N, Hong JC, Sherman EJ, et al. A nomogram to predict logo-regional control after re-irradiation for head and neck cancer. *Radiother Oncol* 2014;111:382.

Romesser RB, Cahlon O, Scher ED, et al. Proton beam reirradiation for recurrent head and neck cancer: multi-institutional report on feasibility and early outcomes. *Int J Radiat Oncol Biol Phys* 2016;95:386.

Salama JK, Vokes EE, Chmura SJ, et al. Long-term outcome of concurrent chemotherapy and reirradiation for recurrent and second primary head-and-neck squamous cell carcinoma. *Int J Radiat Oncol Biol Phys* 2006;64:382.

Scala LM, Hu K, Urken ML, et al. Intraoperative high-dose-rate radiotherapy in the manageet of locoregionally recurrent head and neck cancer. *Head Neck* 2013;35:485.

Spencer SA, Harris J, Wheeler RH, et al. Final report of RTOG 9610, a multi-institutional trial of reirradiation and chemotherapy for unresectable recurrent squamous cell carcinoma of the head and neck. *Head Neck* 2008;30:281.

Takiar V, Garden AS, Ma D, et al. Reirradiation of head and neck cancers with IMRT: outcomes and analyses. *Int J Radiat Oncol Biol Phys* 2016;95:1117–1131.

Teo PML, et al. How successful is high-dose (60 Gy) reirradiation using mainly external beams in salvaging local failures of nasopharyngeal carcinoma? *Int J Radiat Oncol Biol Phys* 1998;40:897.

Vargo JA, Farris RL, Ohr J, et al. A prospective phase 2 trial of reirradiation with stereotactic body radiation therapy plus cetuximab in patients with previously irradiated recurrent squamous cell carcinoma of the head and neck. *Int J Radiat Oncol Biol Phys* 2015;91:480.

Wang CC, McIntyre JT. Re-irradiation of laryngeal carcinoma—techniques and results. *Int J Radiat Oncol Biol Phys* 1993;26:783.

Wu SX, Chua DT, Deng ML, et al. Outcome of fractionated stereotactic radiotherapy for 90 patients with locally persistent and recurrent nasopharyngeal carcinoma. *Int J Radiat Oncol Biol Phys* 2007;69:761.

Index

Note: Page numbers in *italics* denote figures; those followed by a t denote tables.